OXFORD MEDICAL PUBLICATIONS

Autonomic Failure

Autonomic Failure

A Textbook of Clinical Disorders of the Autonomic Nervous System

---

SECOND EDITION

Edited by

SIR ROGER BANNISTER

C.B.E., Hon. LL.D., Hon. D.Sci., M.A.,
M.Sc., D.M.(Oxon), F.R.C.P.
Master, Pembroke College, Oxford;
Consultant Physician, National Hospital for Nervous Diseases, London; Hon. Consultant Neurologist, St. Mary's Hospital, London, Oxford District Health Authority, and Oxford Regional Health Authority

Oxford New York Tokyo
OXFORD UNIVERSITY PRESS

Oxford University Press, Walton Street, Oxford OX2 6DP
Oxford New York Toronto
Delhi Bombay Calcutta Madras Karachi
Petaling Jaya Singapore Hong Kong Tokyo
Nairobi Dar es Salaam Cape Town
Melbourne Auckland
and associated companies in
Berlin Ibadan

Oxford is a trade mark of Oxford University Press

Published in the United States
by Oxford University Press, New York

First published, 1983
Second edition, 1988
Second edition first published in paperback 1989

British Library Cataloguing in Publication Data
Autonomic failure: a textbook of clinical
disorders of the autonomic nervous system.
—2nd ed.—(Oxford medical publications).
1. Nervous system, Autonomic—Diseases
I. Bannister, Sir Roger
616.8′8 RC407
ISBN 0–19–261664–1
ISBN 0–19–261869–5

Library of Congress Cataloging in Publication Data
Autonomic failure.
(Oxford medical publications)
Includes bibliographies and index.
1. Nervous system, Autonomic—Diseases.
I. Bannister, Roger. II. Series. [DNLM:
1. Autonomic Nervous System Diseases. 2. Autonomic
Nervous System—physiopathology. WL 600 A939]
RC407.A95 1988 616.8′8 87–28324
ISBN 0–19–261664–1
ISBN 0–19–261869–5

Printed in Great Britain by
Butler & Tanner Ltd, Frome, Somerset

Preface to the second edition

The second edition aims to provide a comprehensive scientific basis for diagnosis and treatment of the wide range of autonomic disorders which are now being recognized with increasing frequency. It describes these disorders in general diseases such as diabetes and alcoholism as well as in various syndromes of acute, sub-acute, and chronic autonomic failure. Since the first edition there have been many advances in the subject and these have necessitated extensive revision; new chapters have been added on sexual and bladder function, the gut, fainting, cardiac arrhythmias, pain syndromes, sweating disturbances, and porphyria.

In the five years since the first edition many more autonomic investigation units have been set up around the world and this increases the need for methods of testing which can be accepted as comparable internationally. The international approach in this book is helped by the fact that, among the 30 new authors, 14 are from outside Britain, 10 of them from North America. Also a new chapter has been added comparing patients in Britain and in the United States. The standard physiological tests of autonomic function are supplemented in this edition by a wide range of new biochemical, pharmacological, and hormonal tests of autonomic function. These tests are both complex and time-consuming and so the indications for undertaking them need to be clearly described.

Since the last edition there have been rapid advances in the basic science of autonomic transmission, with discovery of many peptides which act as co-transmitters or modulators of transmission. An increasing number of peptides, hormones, and enzymes can now be assayed in man and this has led to the recognition of new causes of disordered autonomic function, such as congenital dopamine-beta-hydroxylase deficiency. Progress in neuropeptide chemistry has been matched by progress in immunocytochemical staining, electron microscopic studies of the ganglia, and fibre counting techniques, all of which give greater precision in pathological diagnosis. Magnetic resonance imaging, positron emission tomography, brainstem evoked potentials, and microneuronography are some of the other promising investigative techniques that are described in this edition.

Better treatment rests on the attempt to bridge the gap between basic neuroscience and clinical medicine, so making diagnosis and treatment increasingly precise. It is hoped that this new edition will continue to provide physicians in different fields, including neurology, diabetology, cardiology, geriatrics, and general medicine, with a rational guide to management.

Oxford
October 1987 R. B.

Acknowledgements

It is a pleasure to acknowledge my gratitude to my clinical colleagues and research associates both at the National Hospital for Nervous Diseases and St. Mary's Hospital, London and, in particular, my colleague Dr Christopher Mathias. I am grateful also to Professor J. F. Mowbray for the interpretation (in Chapter 1) of the significance of the HLA associations in patients with autonomic failure and to Dr R. Frackowiak and Dr D. Brooks for the description of positron emission tomography, illustrated in Fig. 1.3. My thanks are also due to Mrs E. Holly for technical assistance at the National Hospital Autonomic Investigation Unit.

Preface to the first edition

In the past 10 years the clinical syndromes of autonomic failure have been studied by a wide range of new physiological, pharmacological, pathological, and neurochemical techniques, but the information is scattered in papers in many different journals and is not easily available to the clinician. Much is still to be learnt about these syndromes and their management but it is now possible to review these recent advances.

The presenting symptoms of autonomic failure, such as low blood pressure, may overlie unrecognized disturbances of function which are widespread and involve altered control of many different parts of the body including the heart, the kidneys, the pancreas, the bladder, the gut, and the pupils. Symptoms may therefore lead patients to many different specialists who are unfamiliar with these autonomic syndromes. The cardiologist, for example, sees some of the patients with idiopathic orthostatic hypotension and the neurologist, patients with orthostatic hypotension associated with Parkinsonism or multiple system atrophy (Shy-Drager syndrome). The general physician encounters many problems of autonomic failure in association with diseases such as diabetes, alcoholism, or amyloidosis. The geriatrician sees the consequences of failure of body-temperature regulation. The genitourinary surgeon is often presented with a difficult problem of the neurogenic bladder. It would be wrong to think of autonomic failure as a single disease entity but progressive autonomic failure in which pathological lesions are to some degree established provides a model for investigation which can be compared with other diseases in which defective autonomic function is part of a wider picture as in diabetes.

This book aims to provide clinicians in many fields with a guide to useful tests of differing complexity which are now needed to identify autonomic defects of a particular organ in which they have a special interest and should help them to interpret these tests. Interpretation is as important as knowing how to undertake the tests because the autonomic nervous system includes more subtle variations in response than the somatic nervous system and has many compensating mechanisms for impending failure. The practical tests described in the book are set against the more general background of current advances in physiology and pathology of the autonomic nervous system in order to form a basis for rational management in a field which is generally recognized to be exceedingly difficult.

The book also aims to introduce the clinician to new theoretical concepts of the organization of the autonomic nervous system. The old-fashioned notion of a simple duality of a sympathetic-adrenal system causing rather unselective 'fight or flight' responses and a parasympathetic-cholinergic system providing tonic activity, has given way to a new view of a highly selective autonomic nervous system with an integrative action at least as complex as that of the somatic nervous system. New transmitters and modulators abound and receptors, both pre- or postsynaptic, can be blocked, activated, or modified in their numbers and affinities. New general biological principles have emerged with 'up' and 'down' regulation of receptor numbers and affinities and manipulation pharmacologically of pre- and postsynaptic receptors by transmitter depletion or blockade. These fields provide an exciting prospect for future biological as well as medical research. It is appropriate to end with a quotation from my teacher, the late Sir George Pickering, who also concluded a review of autonomic function with the words that it was 'in fact no more than an overture. The main body of the work is to come'.

London R. B.
September 1982

Contents

Contributors

P. Anand, Department of Medicine, Royal Postgraduate Medical School, Hammersmith Hospital, Du Cane Road, London W12 0HS, UK.

Roger Bannister, Autonomic Investigation Department, National Hospital for Nervous Diseases, Queen Square, London WC1, UK.

Terence Bennett, Department of Physiology and Pharmacology, Medical School, Queen's Medical Centre, Clifton Boulevard, Nottingham NG7 2UH, UK.

G. S. Brindley, MRC Neurological Prostheses Unit, Institute of Psychiatry, De Crespigney Park, London SE5, UK.

Sudhansu Chokroverty, Department of Neurology, UMDNJ-Robert Wood Johnson Medical School, New Brunswick, New Jersey; and the Neurology Service, Veterans Administration Medical Center, Lyons, New Jersey, USA.

K. J. Collins, School of Medicine, University College, London; and Department of Geriatric Medicine, St Pancras Hospital, London, UK.

David da Costa, Medical Unit, St Mary's Hospital Medical School, London W2, UK.

I. Bleddyn Davies, Department of Geriatric Medicine, St Tydfil's Hospital, Merthyr Tydfil, Mid-Glamorgan, Wales, UK.

William C. de Groat, Department of Pharmacology and Center for Neuroscience, University of Pittsburgh, Pittsburgh, Pennsylvania 15261, USA.

Michael E. Edmonds, Diabetic Department, King's College Hospital, Denmark Hill, London SE5 9RS, UK.

Marjorie Ellison, National Hospital for Nervous Diseases, Queen Square, London WC1, UK.

David J. Ewing, Department of Medicine, Royal Infirmary, Edinburgh, UK.

Robert D. Fealey, Department of Neurology, Mayo Clinic, Rochester, Minnesota 55905, USA.

Clare J. Fowler, National Hospital for Nervous Diseases, Queen Square, London WC1, UK.

Sheila M. Gardiner, Department of Physiology and Pharmacology, Medical School, Queen's Medical Centre, Clifton Boulevard, Nottingham NG7 2UH, UK.

J. R. Garrett, Department of Oral Pathology, King's College School of Medicine and Dentistry, The Rayne Institute, 123 Coldharbour Lane, London SE5 9NU, UK.

W. R. G. Gibb, National Hospitals for Nervous Diseases, Maida Vale, London W9 1TL, UK.

Abel Gorchein, Department of Clinical Pharmacology, St Mary's Hospital Medical School, London W2, UK.

Roger Hainsworth, Department of Cardiovascular Studies, University of Leeds, Leeds LS2 9JT, UK.

Robert W. Hamill, Department of Neurology, University of Rochester School of Medicine and Dentistry, Rochester, New York, USA.

N. D. Heaton, King's College Hospital, London SE5, UK.

E. R. Howard, King's College Hospital, London SE5, UK.

Ralph H. Johnson, John Radcliffe Hospital, Headington, Oxford OX3 9DU, UK.

John Vann Jones, Cardiology Department, Royal Infirmary, Bristol, UK.

Peter G. E. Kennedy, Department of Neurology and Virology, Glasgow University; and Institute of Neurological Sciences, Southern General Hospital, Glasgow, UK.

Ramesh K. Khurana, Department of Neurology, University of Maryland School of Medicine and University of Maryland Hospital, Baltimore, Maryland, USA.

Roger S. Kirby, Department of Urology, St Bartholomew's Hospital, West Smithfield, London EC1, UK.

Edmund F. La Gamma, Department of Pediatrics, State University of New York at Stonybrook, Stonybrook, New York, USA.

A. J. Lees, National Hospitals for Nervous Diseases, London WC1, UK.

Stafford L. Lightman, Medical Unit, Charing Cross and Westminster Medical School, 17 Page Street, London SW1P 2AP, UK.

Phillip A. Low, Department of Neurology, Mayo Clinic, Rochester, Minnesota 55905, USA.

J. G. McLeod, Department of Medicine, University of Sydney, Sydney, Australia.

Christopher Mathias, Medical Unit, St Mary's Hospital Medical School, London W2, and National Hospital for Nervous Diseases, London WC1, UK.

Margaret R. Matthews, Department of Human Anatomy, Oxford University, Oxford, UK.

John Morgan-Hughes, National Hospital for Nervous Diseases, Queen Square, London WC1, UK.

Peter W. Nathan, National Hospital for Nervous Diseases, Queen Square, London WC1, UK.

David Oppenheimer, Department of Neuropathology, The Radcliffe Infirmary, Oxford, UK.

Ronald Polinsky, Clinical Neuropharmacology Section, Medical Neurology Branch, National Institute of Neurological and Communicative Disorders and Stroke, Bethesda, Maryland 20892, USA.

Donald L. Price, Departments of Pathology, Neurology, and Neuroscience, Neuropathology Laboratory, The Johns Hopkins University School of Medicine, Baltimore, Maryland, USA.

John L. Reid, Department of Materia Medica, Stobhill General Hospital, Glasgow, UK.

P. M. Satchell, Department of Surgery, University of Sydney, Blackburn Building, DO6, Sydney, NSW2006, Australia.

Peter S. Sever, Department of Clinical Pharmacology and Therapeutics, St Mary's Hospital Medical School, London W2, UK.

J. T. Shepherd, Mayo Clinic and Foundation, Rochester, Minnesota 55905, USA.

R. F. J. Shepherd, Mayo Clinic and Foundation, Rochester, Minnesota 55905, USA.

Desmond Sheridan, Department of Cardiology, St Mary's Hospital Medical School, London W2, UK.

Shirley A. Smith, Department of Clinical Pharmacology, United Medical and Dental Schools of Guy's and St Thomas's Hospital, St Thomas's Hospital, London SE1 7EH, UK.

E. G. S. Spokes, Department of Neurology, Leeds General Infirmary, Leeds, UK.

K. Michael Spyer, Department of Physiology, Royal Free Hospital School of Medicine, Rowland Hill Street, London NW3 2PF, UK.

William D. Steers, Departments of Pharmacology and Urology, University of Pittsburgh, Pittsburgh, Pennsylvania 15261, USA.

Phillip Thomas, Department of Cardiology, St Mary's Hospital Medical School, London W2, UK.

B. Gunnar Wallin, Department of Clinical Neurophysiology, University of Göteborg, Sahlgren's Hospital, S 413 45 Göteborg, Sweden.

Peter J. Watkins, Diabetic Department, King's College Hospital, Denmark Hill, London SE5 9RS, UK.

Wouter Wieling, Department of Medicine, Academic Medical Centre, University of Amsterdam, Amsterdam, The Netherlands.

T. D. M. Williams, Medical Unit, Charing Cross and Westminster Medical School, 17 Page Street, London SW1P 2AP, UK.

1. Introduction and classification

Roger Bannister

The autonomic nervous system innervates every visceral organ in the body, creating, as Galen suggested, 'sympathy' between the various parts of the body. It has as complex a neural organization in the brain, spinal cord, and periphery as the somatic nervous system, but remains largely involuntary or automatic. Claude Bernard wrote 'nature thought it provident to remove these important phenomena from the capriciousness of an ignorant will'. Langley, who in 1898 first proposed the term 'autonomic nervous system', based his experiments on the blocking action of nicotine at synapses in ganglia. In 1921 Loewi discovered 'Vagusstoff' which was released by stimulation of the vagus nerve and proved to be acetylcholine. In the same year Cannon discovered that 'sympathin', later shown to be noradrenalin, was produced by stimulation of the sympathetic trunk. The basis was therefore laid for Dale's distinction between cholinergic and adrenergic transmission in the autonomic nervous system.

PERIPHERAL AUTONOMIC FUNCTION

The peripheral autonomic nervous system, an efferent system, is made up of neurons which lie outside the central nervous system and which are concerned with visceral innervation. Both sympathetic and parasympathetic systems have preganglionic neurons in the brain and spinal cord arranged as shown in Fig. 1.1. The afferent limbs of autonomic reflexes may lie in any afferent nerve. The preganglionic sympathetic fibres are myelinated and leave the spinal roots as white rami communicantes and synapse in the ganglia. Unmyelinated postganglionic fibres rejoin the anterior spinal roots by the arrangement shown in Fig. 1.2, although some sympathetic fibres traverse the ganglia and synapse in more peripheral ganglia, following the arrangement of the parasympathetic fibres.

The transmitter at all preganglionic terminals is acetylcholine which is not paralysed by atropine (the nicotinic effect) whereas the action of acetylcholine at the distal end of the cholinergic postganglionic fibres is

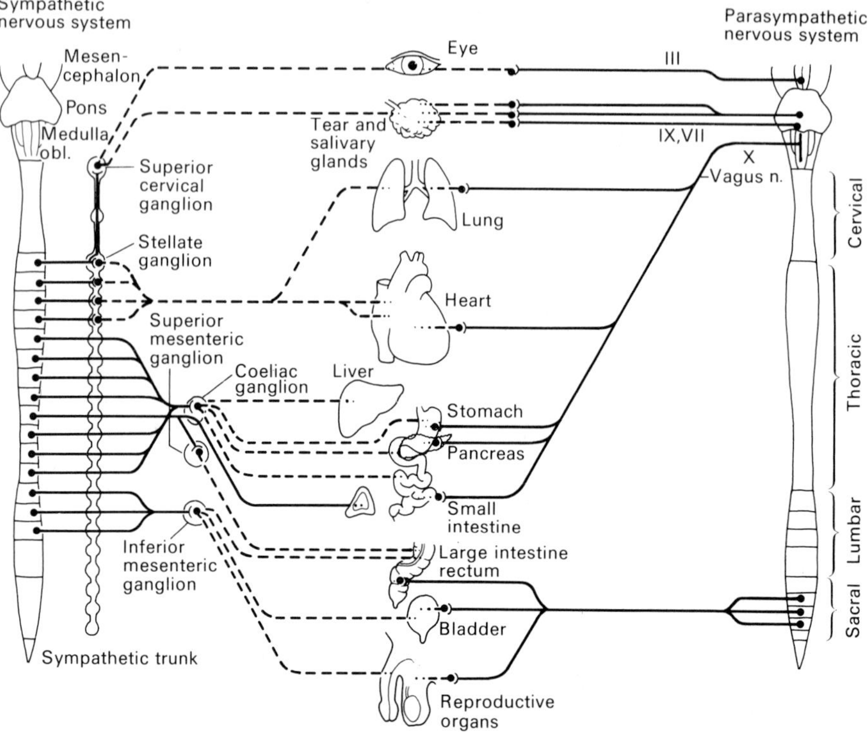

Fig. 1.1. Peripheral autonomic nervous system. The sympathetic innervation of vessels, sweat glands, and piloerector muscles is not shown. Solid lines, preganglionic axons; dashed lines, postganglionic axons. (Taken with permission from Brain (1985).)

paralysed by atropine (the muscarinic effect). Noradrenalin is the principal transmitter for postganglionic sympathetic nerves, the exceptions being sudomotor nerves, which are cholinergic in man, some vasodilator fibres to muscle, and the adrenal medulla which is innervated by preganglionic (cholinergic) fibres and itself secretes both adrenalin and noradrenalin. Noradrenalin is stored in the terminals and is released by nerve activity or by sympathomimetic drugs, which may act partly indirectly on the ganglia or more centrally, e.g. ephedrine and amphetamine, or on the terminals, e.g. phenylephrine or tyramine. The different actions of noradrenalin and adrenalin are caused by relative effects on different receptors. α-receptors mediate vasoconstriction, intestinal relaxation, and dilatation of the pupil (and are blocked by thymoxamine). α-receptors may be either postsynaptic (α_1) or presynaptic (α_2, which when stimulated decrease the release of the transmitter). β-receptors mediate vasodilatation, especially in muscles, increase the rate and force of the heart with a tendency to arrhythmias,

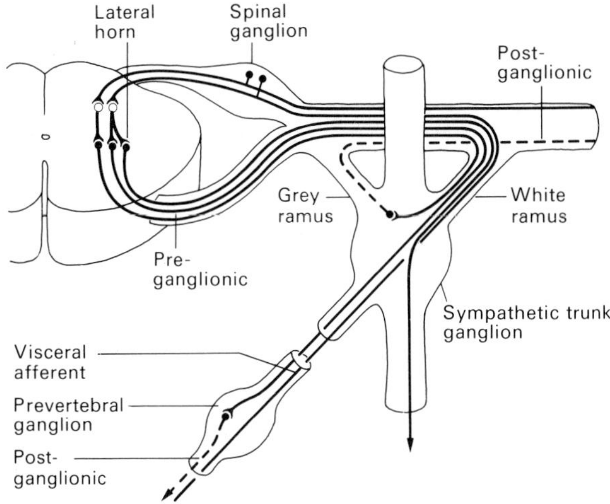

Fig. 1.2. The autonomic spinal reflex arc. (Taken with permission from Brain (1985).)

and cause bronchial relaxation. They are further subdivided into β_1-receptors, mediating the chronotropic cardiac action of isoprenaline, and β_2-receptors which are responsible for most of the peripheral effects of β-adrenergic stimulation (see Chapters 7, 13, and 19). Though descriptions of autonomic sensitivity phenomena were first made more than a century ago, the research was summarized by Cannon and Rosenblueth in 1949 under the title 'The supersensitivity of denervated structures: a law of denervation'. Attention since then has concentrated on the 'up' and 'down' regulation of receptor function depending on the availability of the transmitter.

The cells of the autonomic nervous system tend to act in conjunction and this is achieved mainly by specialized intercellular junctions at the ganglion cells which have been demonstrated by electron microscopy and freeze fracture techniques (see Chapter 29). The autonomic ganglia also contain small intensely fluorescent cells ('SIF' cells) which contain many peptides, thought to act as modulators and transmitters at synaptic sites. Substance P, vasoactive intestinal peptide (VIP), encephalins, and somatostatin have all been identified in autonomic ganglia although their precise role in control of nerve transmission is not yet known (see Chapters 28 and 29).

The previously held distinction between cholinergic and catecholaminergic cells, underlying the dual hypothesis of antagonism in the autonomic nervous system is no longer tenable. Immature ganglion cells in culture contain both acetylcholine and catecholamines (see Chapter 2). Sympathetic ganglia have about 5 per cent of acetylcholine-containing neurons. Within any central pathway there is no simple consistency of a single transmitter and some cells have multiple transmitters; posterior root ganglion cells for example have been found to have as many as 10 neuropeptides and putative transmitters. After birth, sweat glands are switched from adrenergic to cholinergic sympathetic innervation, whereas innervation of some gut structures is switched from sympathetic to cholinergic mechanisms. Presynaptic cholinergic endings may affect noradrenergic sympathetic transmission and noradrenalin may act not only directly as a transmitter but indirectly by modulating the effect of acetylcholine, as has been shown peripherally where small doses of adrenalin and noradrenalin facilitate transmission but in larger doses inhibit it. The complex interactions of central autonomic control require much further study but with advances in biochemical typing of cells and in neuroanatomical and neurophysiological techniques, such complex neuronal effects are now being identified (see Chapter 4).

CENTRAL CONTROL OF THE AUTONOMIC NERVOUS SYSTEM

The hypothalamus can be considered the 'highest' level of integration of autonomic function. It remains under the influence of the cortex and the group of structures known as the 'limbic system' which includes the olfactory areas, the hippocampus and amygdaloid complex, the cingulate cortex, and the septal area. These regions of the brain regulate the hypothalamus and are critical for emotional and affective expression. In phylogenetic development the limbic system represents the older or palaeomammalian cortex as opposed to the neomammalian cortex. Its function is thought to be concerned with levels below cognitive behaviour and inductive and deductive reasoning, though it, nevertheless, is concerned with a feeling of individuality and identity. It analyses the significance of the input of sensation to the organism in relation to the instinctive drives which promote the perpetuation of the individual by satisfying hunger, thirst, and sexual needs.

It is also concerned with maintaining hemeostasis against a changing environment and ensures the perpetuation of the species by sexual and parental drives which can at times override more selfish self-perpetuating drives of the individual. The essence of its function is choice of patterns of behaviour based on sensory information. As it overlaps both with sensory and motor systems it is essential for many aspects of memory and learning. The autonomic nervous system and many metabolic functions are under the control of the limbic system by means of nerve centres, many of which are situated in the hypothalamus, lying ventrally to the thalamus and constituting the floor of the third ventricle. The hypothalamus contains a large number of scattered ganglion cells, which have been differentiated into a number of nuclei (see Appenzeller 1982). The projections of the hypothalamus are not yet completely known and discussion in detail is beyond the scope of this book.

The hypothalamus controls the autonomic nervous system in two ways, by means of the pituitary and hence other endocrine glands (see Chapter 21) and by direct descending nervous pathways (see Chapter 4). Although these descending pathways exist, some regions of the brainstem are to some extent autonomous and function in animals after pontine section of the brainstem. These include cardiac and respiratory function and 'centres' for vomiting and micturition, but under natural circumstances cardiovascular responses never occur in isolation but accompany the processes of exercise, digestion, sexual function, and temperature regulation. The integration of these changes takes place in the hypothalamus. The main course taken by descending sympathetic fibres from the hypothalamus is uncrossed and by way of the lateral tegmentum of the brainstem and lateral medullary formation. Some fibres end directly on the intermediolateral column cells, while others synapse in the reticular formation (see Chapter 4).

DISEASES OF THE AUTONOMIC NERVOUS SYSTEM

The lesions of the nervous system in autonomic failure, with their widespread consequences, are in Claude Bernard's terms 'real experiments by which physicians and physiologists profit'. Some may complain that nature is an imprecise experimentalist, but these lesions can throw much light on the subtle and complex integration of the autonomic nervous system. The syndromes of autonomic failure also offer an example of the system degenerations which are so common in neurology and are yet so baffling. We need to find some common biological basis for this curious selective vulnerability. If we can do this, we shall be closer to finding an effective treatment not only for these particular diseases but possibly also for a wider range of disabling progressive degenerative diseases of the nervous system.

The systematic application of physiological techniques of study to patients with autonomic failure started in the 1960s. Research interest in postural hypotension, the usual presenting symptom of autonomic failure, was stimulated by its occurrence after the weightlessness of space travel (Lamb 1964). Since then there have been striking advances in the investigation and classification of the syndromes of autonomic failure which were until recently both confused and confusing. Peripheral neuropathies with an autonomic component have long been recognized, particularly in diabetes, alcoholism, and amyloid. Sharpey-Schafer and

Taylor (1960) showed that the sympathetic vasoconstrictor pathway to the hands was intact in diabetic autonomic neuropathy and they therefore attributed the absence of circulatory reflexes and the postural hypotension to an afferent lesion. Though an afferent lesion cannot be excluded, their interpretation was probably incorrect because the sympathetic efferent pathway to resistance vessels is often defective in diabetes and the selectivity of lesions on the efferent side is now appreciated.

Much of this book is concerned with the rare chronic or primary neurological disorders in which the autonomic nervous system is selectively involved by both pre- and postganglionic neuronal degeneration (Shy and Drager 1960; Johnson *et al.* 1966; Bannister *et al.* 1967). Some might doubt the worth of such serious attention given to rare diseases but there are many precedents to show that just such studies of rare diseases often lead to the recognition of an entirely new group of disorders of which other examples are then found. It is certain that the detailed study of these diseases, by the extensive range of biochemical, physiological, and histochemical techniques now available, has yielded a rich harvest of knowledge, much of it unexpected, which can now be applied more widely. In one sense we can classify autonomic disorders as changes of receptor function which are one of the major growing points of medicine, especially the development of autoantibodies against receptors (see Chapter 19). The detailed studies of chronic autonomic failure are complemented by the sections of the book which are devoted to diabetes (Chapters 36–38) and alcoholism (Chapter 39), in which sooner or later autonomic disturbances occur. Diabetes is overwhelmingly commoner than other forms of autonomic dysfunction and rapid advances have been made now that the methods of testing, most of which were pioneered in relation to autonomic failure, are being applied to the even more complex disturbances in diabetes and alcoholism.

FIRST SYMPTOMS OF AUTONOMIC FAILURE

Most forms of autonomic failure are insidious in their onset, with mild symptoms which are concealed for years because of autonomic compensatory mechanisms. As Cannon (1929) pointed out, this system can respond to many and varied stresses from the internal and external environment in ways which conceal its dysfunction. When man first took it upon himself millions of years ago to stand on his two legs he posed great strains on the cardiovascular control needed to protect him against the effect of pooling of blood in the lower extremities (Hill 1895). Postural hypotension occurring in emotional syncope raises the intriguing teleological question of whether it has evolutionary significance in avoiding danger by a sudden fall into the horizontal position and the simulation of death. However, true syncope requires an intact autonomic nervous system (see Chapter 9), although persistent postural hypotension is the cardinal feature of autonomic failure. Patients may start with mild symptoms of vague weakness, postural dizziness, or faintness which can very easily be overlooked or result in erroneous referral to a psychiatrist not a neurologist. The crux of the diagnosis is the measurement of blood pressure when standing rather than lying, still often neglected, which can, like the tip of an iceberg, reveal a much more complex underlying autonomic disturbance. The blood-pressure control mechanisms at the lower end of the scale are just as elaborate and fascinating as those which cause the more commonly studied problems of hypertension. Some patients with autonomic failure first have bladder symptoms or impotence, not postural hypotension. A second group of patients may not present with symptoms of autonomic failure at all but with apparent Parkinson's disease. However, there may be subtle features which suggest that the parkinsonism is atypical, with a predominance of rigidity and akinesis over tremor or the presence of mild pyramidal signs. Such parkinsonian patients may develop marked postural hypotension when treated with levodopa. Some may have additional cerebellar or bulbar involvement. These features raise the possibility of more widespread involvement of the central nervous system.

CLASSIFICATION

Accurate diagnosis is essential for proper management of autonomic failure (AF) but in attempting to classify autonomic disease there is a philosophical point to be borne in mind. As in much of medicine, we use a mixed diagnostic classification. We have a list of diseases of largely known pathology such as diabetes and we make a diagnosis of 'secondary' autonomic failure when abnormal tests in life point to a structural disturbance of autonomic reflexes and pathways in patients with these diseases. Other patients, without certainly known pathology in common, share certain autonomic symptoms and, from tests in life and observation of similar patients after death, we choose to use the word 'primary' disease. In such patients tests can hardly be said to prove a disease but this is the only way we can place patients in different categories and hope, by research, to improve their treatment.

Autonomic fibres are damaged secondarily in a variety of medical disorders, most commonly in diabetes and alcoholism, but also in a wide range of acute, subacute, and chronic peripheral neuropathies (see Table 1.1) and this does not provide a problem of classification.

We can now consider the more complex problem of the classification of the group of patients in whom autonomic failure appears to result from a primary or unexplained selective neuronal degeneration. This may occur in association with two quite different degenerations of the

Table 1.1. General classification of autonomic failure

1. Primary

(a) Pure autonomic failure (PAF) formerly called idiopathic orthostatic hypotension (Bradbury and Eggleston 1925)
(b) Autonomic failure (AF) with multiple system atrophy (MSA) which includes striatonigral degeneration (SND) and olivopontocerebellar atrophy (OPCA); AF with MSA first described by Shy and Drager (1960)
(c) Autonomic failure (AF) with Parkinson's disease (PD) (Fichefet *et al.* 1965)

2. Secondary

(a) General medical disorders: diabetes (see Chapters 36–38); amyloid (Rubinstein *et al.* 1978); alcoholism (Chapter 39)
(b) Autoimmune disease: acute and subacute dysautonomia (Chapter 35); Guillain–Barré syndrome (see Chapter 34); mixed connective tissue disease (see Chapter 34); rheumatoid arthritis (Edmonds *et al.* 1979); Eaton–Lambert syndrome (Khurana *et al.* 1983); systematic lupus erythematosus (see Chapter 34)
(c) Carcinomatous autonomic neuropathy (Park *et al.* 1972)
(d) Metabolic diseases: porphyria (see Chapter 40); Fabry's disease; Tangier disease (inherited recessive and lypoprotein deficiency; B_{12}-deficiency (see Chapter 34)
(e) Hereditary sensory neuropathies, dominant or recessive (see Chapter 34)
(f) Infections of the nervous system: syphilis, Chagas' disease (see Chapter 14); HIV infection (Carne and Adler 1986; Craddock *et al.* 1987); botulism (Jenzer *et al.* 1975); herpes zoster (Neville and Sladen 1984)
(g) Central brain lesions: vascular lesions or tumours involving the hypothalamus and midbrain, for example, craniopharyngioma (Thomas *et al.* 1961); multiple sclerosis; Wernicke's encephalopathy; Adie's syndrome
(h) Spinal-cord lesions (Mathias *et al.* 1979; see Chapter 11)
(i) Familial dysautonomia (Dancis and Smith 1966)
(j) Familial hyperbradykininism (Streeten *et al.* 1972)
(k) Renal failure
(l) Dopamine β-hydroxylase deficiency (Robertson *et al.* 1986; Man in't Veld *et al.* 1987)
(m) Other distal transmitter defects (Chapter 31)
(n) Ageing (see Chapter 19)

3. Drugs (see Chapters 10, 34, and 39)

(a) Selective neurotoxic drugs; alcoholism (see Chapter 39) (Low *et al.* 1975); Wernicke's encephalopathy
(b) Tranquillizers; phenothiazines, barbiturates
(c) Antidepressants; tricyclics; monoamine oxidase inhibitors
(d) Vasodilator hypotensive drugs; prazosin, hydralazine
(e) Centrally acting hypotensive drugs; methyldopa, clonidine
(f) Adrenergic neuron blocking drugs; guanethidine, bethanidine, debrisoquine
(g) α-Adrenergic blocking drugs; phenoxybenzamine, labetalol
(h) Ganglion-blocking drugs; hexamethonium, mecamylamine
(i) Angiotensin-converting enzyme inhibitors; captopril

nervous system, Parkinson's disease and multiple system atrophy. Or it may occur in a 'pure' form without any other neurological signs.

Historically, the first reported cases of autonomic failure were described by Bradbury and Eggleston (1925) as 'idiopathic orthostatic hypotension' because of their presenting features. This term is misleading because it stresses only one feature of autonomic failure and ignores the more usually associated neurological disturbances of bladder, sexual function, and sweating, and also because the word 'idiopathic' implies that it is a single disease entity, which is not proven. The term 'pure autonomic failure' (PAF) is preferable for this syndrome though, in America, 'idiopathic orthostatic hypotension' is still sometimes used.

Two cases now recognized as autonomic failure (AF) with multiple system atrophy (MSA) were described by Shy and Drager in 1960 and it is appropriate to quote from their original description. 'The full syndrome comprises the following features; orthostatic hypotension, urinary and rectal incontinence, loss of sweating, iris atrophy, external ocular palsies, rigidity, tremor, loss of associated movements, impotence, the findings of an atonic bladder and loss of rectal sphincter tone, fasciculations, wasting of distal muscles, evidence of a neuropathic lesion in the electromyogram that suggests involvement of the anterior horn cells, and the finding of a neuropathic lesion in the muscle biopsy. The date of onset is usually in the 5th to 7th decade of life.' Though they noted degeneration of the intermediolateral column cells in their pathological report, credit for first specifically linking this with the presenting feature of postural hypotension rests with Johnson *et al.* (1966). At this stage olivopontocerebellar atrophy had not been linked with autonomic failure.

Autonomic failure may also be associated with otherwise apparently typical Parkinson's disease (Vanderhaegan *et al.* 1970). Such cases pathologically have hyaline eosinophilic cytoplasmic neuronal inclusions known as Lewy bodies, also present in Parkinson's disease (see Chapter 26). It is an important fact that Lewy bodies, some of which may contain catecholamine degeneration products, are also found in the brains of patients with pure autonomic failure, without Parkinson's disease, but very rarely in patients with multiple system atrophy. This evidence, discussed below, tends to separate patients with autonomic failure into two groups pathologically.

It must be recognized that at an early stage an accurate prognosis of autonomic failure cannot be given. It may remain as pure autonomic failure for many years, relatively static, or in time it may also come to be associated either with Parkinson's disease or MSA and with care the earliest features of the other condition may be detected clinically. Conversely, the earliest features of autonomic failure may be detected in some patients with Parkinson's disease (PD) or MSA. For example

Miyazaki (1978) has shown that careful study of cases of olivopontocerebellar atrophy with significant postural hypotension shows a high incidence of urinary, pyramidal, and extrapyramidal symptoms and signs, whereas cases without postural hypotension very rarely have these additional features.

There is good evidence (see Chapter 25A) that virtually all patients with primary autonomic failure as opposed to secondary autonomic failure, studied at post-mortem, have severe loss of intermediolateral column cells, the final common pathway cell for the sympathetic nervous system. It is becoming more probable that the pathological process, whether viral, biochemical, or of some other kind, which leads to this loss of intermediolateral column cells differs significantly in pure autonomic failure (and probably in autonomic failure with Parkinson's disease) from that in autonomic failure with multiple system atrophy. In pure autonomic failure, there appears to be an additional loss of ganglionic neurons (see Chapter 29) which are relatively intact in MSA. This suggests the existence of a more distal process in PAF than in MSA. The hypothesis that one of the lesions in pure autonomic failure is more distal accords with the evidence that in general, plasma noradrenalin levels are lower in pure autonomic failure than in autonomic failure with MSA (see Chapters 15, 19, and 31).

When considering the effects of treatment, so that like is compared with like, it is vital to diagnose patients as precisely as possible on the basis of physiological and pharmacological tests and biochemical findings, even though the ultimate criterion of diagnosis is the post-mortem pathological findings. Moreover, it seems probable that there is a number of different types of sympathetic terminal dysfunction in autonomic failure which may be the consequence of pathological processes that differ in degree or kind (Nanda *et al.* 1977; Bannister 1979; Man in't Veld *et al.* 1987) (see Chapter 31). Just as the defects of nicotinic and muscarinic receptors in human disease have proved to be far more complex than was ever expected (Bannister and Hoyes 1981), disturbances of sympathetic receptors will also prove at least as complex (Fraser *et al.* 1981).

AUTONOMIC FAILURE IN HIV INFECTION

Acute and chronic peripheral neuropathy have been described in patients with HIV infection and AIDS (Carne and Adler 1986). Abnormal tests of cardiovascular autonomic function have also been described, implying defective autonomic function (Craddock *et al.* 1987). If confirmed, these may provide an explanation for symptoms such as defective sweating and impotence which occur in AIDS.

NEW TECHNIQUES FOR INVESTIGATION OF CENTRAL AUTONOMIC FUNCTION IN MAN

The detailed information from neurochemical studies at post-mortem (see Chapter 25) is now being extended by positron emission computerized tomography (PET) to living patients. This technique, using injected or inhaled radionucleotides and scanning techniques similar to X-ray computerized tomography, is non-invasive but remains essentially a research investigation because the short-life isotopes have to be prepared by an adjacent cyclotron.

^{18}F-dopa is a positron-emitting tracer analogue of L-dopa. When administered intravenously it is transported across the blood–brain barrier and stored in caudate and putamen synaptosomes as ^{18}F-dopamine. Using positron emission tomography the kinetics of uptake of ^{18}F-dopa in patients with multi-system atrophy (MSA) have been

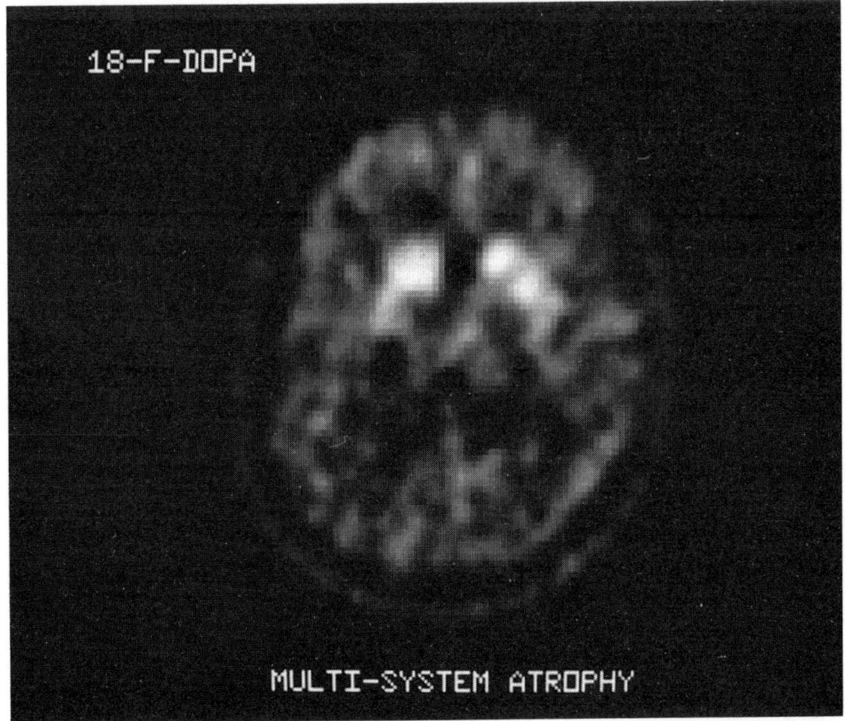

Fig. 1.3. A PET scan of ^{18}F-dopa uptake in a subject with multiple system atrophy. Diminished uptake is seen in the right head of caudate and both putamens. (With permission of Dr R. Frackowiak, Dr D. Brooks, and the Medical Research Council.)

studied. Those MSA patients with clinical evidence of striato-nigral degeneration (SND) showed significantly reduced influx rate constants (K_i) for uptake of ^{18}F-dopa into caudate and putamen. The pattern of normal ^{18}F-dopa is shown in Fig. 1.3. Storage of ^{18}F-dopa was most impaired in the putamen in patients with striato-nigral degeneration, in agreement with published pathological findings. Currently, levels of dopamine re-uptake receptors in the striatum, and noradrenaline re-uptake receptors in the thalamus, are being measured in patients with MSA using ^{11}C-nomifensine and positron emission tomography. Striatal nomifensine binding appears to be diminished in MSA. Ideally study of MSA would require a dopamine D-2-receptor antagonist which has a high affinity for D-2-receptors such as ^{11}C-raclopride

This ligand binds specifically to D-2-receptors and the ratio of activity within the caudate and putamen to a non-specific region of cortex gives a measure of specific D-2-binding and is shown in normal subjects to increase for up to 90 minutes. The changes in tissue activity can also be analysed with reference to plasma tracer activity changes with time. Compartmental analysis allows derivation of factors dependent on receptor numbers and affinities. Repeat measurements in the same subject under conditions of different receptor occupancy (for example following pre-treatment with a pharmacological dose of another 'cold' D-2-blocker such as haloperidol) allows actual measurement of receptor number (B-max) and affinity (Kd) *in vivo* in man (see Chapter 19). The use of raclopride in theory enables Lewy body Parkinson's disease to be distinguished from striato-nigral degeneration.

PREVALENCE OF MULTIPLE SYSTEM ATROPHY AND DIABETIC AUTONOMIC NEUROPATHY

There has been recent evidence of the prevalence of the two commonest causes of involvement of the autonomic nervous system. Lees (see Chapter 33) reports that 15 per cent of patients with presumed Parkinson's disease in life whose brains were examined at the Parkinson's Disease Society's Brain Bank in fact had the pathological changes of striatonigral degeneration which occurs in multiple system atrophy. The prevalence of Parkinson's disease in different studies is between 7 and 19 per 100 000 (Schoenberg 1986) and this suggests that, though not as yet always easy to diagnose in life, multiple system atrophy is in fact far commoner than had hitherto been suspected or indeed than indicated by the relatively few cases so far reported.

The prevalence of autonomic neuropathy in diabetes was estimated by Niel (1987). He and his colleagues conducted a community study using standard non-invasive tests. They found that abnormal cardiovascular reflex tests occurred in 20 per cent of insulin-dependent diabetics and in 15 per cent non-insulin-dependent diabetics. Though this is lower than previous estimates in diabetics attending hospital clinics for obvious reasons, it, nevertheless, represents a large reservoir of patients with autonomic dysfunction in whom, sooner or later, the complications of autonomic disease are likely to arise.

PATHOGENESIS OF PRIMARY AUTONOMIC FAILURE

Some of the difficulties in understanding the pathogenesis of autonomic failure (Bannister 1971, 1979; Bannister and Oppenheimer 1972) have been partially resolved by genetic and HLA studies and by animal experimental work.

Several interrelated questions still need to be answered:

What is the relationship between central, preganglionic, ganglionic, and postganglionic degeneration?

Is the selective vulnerability a result of biochemical factors in common or due to transsynaptic effects or both?

Are these faults solely genetically determined or also the result of some toxic or inflammatory, neonatal, postnatal, or adult influences?

Are these faults defects of maturation or ageing or both?

Genetic studies

In addition to the rare familial cases of AF (Lewis 1964) and olivopontocerebellar atrophy, there are a few cases of AF with a family history of Parkinson's disease (see Chapter 25). The histocompatibility antigen HLA A32 occurs in more than half the cases of AF, irrespective of the group to which they belong, but much less often in PD (Bannister *et al.* 1982). Recently, we examined two siblings with apparent dopamine-beta-hydroxylase deficiency. The siblings both have HLA A32, thereby strengthening the evidence for A32 as a marker associated with autonomic failure. This association has an expected maximum rate of 3 per cent of the population, giving a relative risk of AF of 16, which is almost as high as that of HLA B27 in ankylosing spondylitis and higher than the HLA abnormality in myasthenia gravis or multiple sclerosis.

We have considered several interpretations of the fact that this marker HLA antigen is associated with the presence of autonomic failure. There is a possibility that the disease may be of viral aetiology, and is rare. The HLA association demonstrates, at the very least, a genetic predisposition to the disease, which if of viral origin might be related to susceptibility to infection, or to the damaging effects of the virus. Taking the analogy of viral hepatitis, the presence of virus in the liver may be quite harmless, and in those people incapable of responding there is no liver disease. In the majority who do respond to the virus, acute cellular destruction occurs as a consequence of the patient producing immunity against virus-infected cells. The ability to respond or not is largely genetically determined, and may be HLA-associated. The same may be true of autonomic failure, when the ability of the patient to respond to the virus, presumptively infecting the brain, may cause specific neuronal damage in virus-infected cells. If the genetically determined immune response is not present, the virus may sit unsuspected in the tissue, and the individual remain an asymptomatic carrier. It is possible that the ability of a virus infection to damage may be genetically determined, perhaps by inherited variants of enzymes which are critical for survival of virus-infected cells, when some of the host genome may have been switched off by the virus. This genetic variation may be HLA-linked.

Recent studies of enteroviral infections of tissues, in particular of skeletal and cardiac muscle, suggest that, in the acute initial infection, gross anatomical damage may occur, resulting in permanent changes. The persistent infection which may last for years, does not do this, but only produces defective function of the infected cell. When the infection has gone, the cells are normal, as is their function. We are all aware of the anterior horn-cell destruction produced by one group of enteroviruses, polioviruses, and of the evanescent disease, with complete recovery, that may be seen with acute enteroviral encephalitis, or Guillain–Barré syndrome. The susceptibility of the individual to neuronal damage in the presence of neurotropic viruses may thus be to a great extent dependent on the immune response to infected cells. The ensuing damage will then be very dependent on HLA-linked immune responses to the virus.

Published studies of Parkinson's disease have not shown an HLA association (Leheney *et al.* 1983). Equally it is clear that we found a clear association of AF with A32 and this has been maintained in studies of further patients. Thus the occurrence of AF with PD may imply that PD occurs by another mechanism, but that the appearance of AF is genetically determined, requiring the HLA-linked gene product to do so. At present it is thus most likely that the predisposition to AF, alone or in association with PD, is HLA-linked, although PD itself is not. Certain individuals with autonomic failure, therefore, have clear genetic features in common but, obviously, other factors determine whether autonomic failure occurs, possibly exposure to a neurotropic virus, against a background of altered immunity. Material from the brains of patients inoculated into monkeys has not yet transmitted disease and so a slow virus cannot be incriminated.

Developmental studies (see Chapter 2)

In all kinds of neuronal degenerations affecting several groups of cells we can speculate on the biochemical affinities or synaptic relationships which exist between them. In AF the neuromelanin-containing cells of the brainstem which degenerate are closely associated with catecholamine systems in the brainstem identified in animals (Ungerstedt 1971) and in man (Saper and Petito 1982). They arise from the basal plate of the neural tube, not from the neural crest, and are involved, as well as the cholinergic preganglionic neurons of the brainstem and intermediolateral columns, in AF. The melanin-containing cells, which usually also contain catecholamines, occur in the substantia nigra and in bilateral columns running caudally from near the red nucleus through the locus ceruleus which has complex functions in autonomic control, to the dorsal nucleus of the vagus (where pigmented cells and preganglionic autonomic neurons both occur), and ending in the intermediolateral grey matter of the upper cervical cord. This column follows closely the general visceral efferent column of the brainstem. Cholinergic preganglionic autonomic neurons may degenerate as a result of loss of normal synaptic stimulation from the catecholamine-containing cells in the brainstem or loss of peripheral connections, as is discussed later.

Different pathogenetic factors may play a part in some more peripheral forms of autonomic failure. In early development the primitive autonomic cells migrate from the neural crest to form both melanocytes and the parasympathetic and sympathetic neurons (Burnstock 1981). This occurs under the influence of the protein nerve growth factor (NGF) which is necessary for normal development and maturity of these neurons, but there are probably also other trophic substances which are necessary for normal development of these and other neurons. The autonomic nervous system in the human infant is incomplete at birth and so NGF and other similar factors may, if deficient, have an effect not only on survival of cells, many of which in the normal course of development die, but may also be necessary for the normal function of those that remain. Their presence may determine the length of survival of cells that cannot regenerate, that is the process of ageing. Maternal experiences, viral and drug exposure may all contribute to abnormal development or survival of cells, quite apart from obvious birth defects. Moreover the blood-barrier is never totally competent at the obex region close to the site of many catecholamine cells.

Nerve growth stimulating activity (NGSA) measured by various bioassays in serum, urine, or biopsy material has not yet shown any abnormalities in AF (Mobley *et al.* 1977) but defects of NGSA have been reported in the hereditary sensory neuropathies (type I, dominant and type II, autosomal recessive). The hereditary sensory neuropathies have links with the spinocerebellar degenerations and also, through olivopontocerebellar atrophy (OPCA), therefore, with cases of autonomic failure and MSA. We have studied two patients with AF and MSA with evidence of a sensory neuropathy, in one case also at post-mortem (Bannister and Oppenheimer 1972). It is of interest that NGF is structurally related to insulin and an antiserum to NGF, which causes immunosympathectomy in young animals, might therefore be expected to have structural features in common with autodestructive antibodies to insulin in the diabetic, providing a speculative cause of diabetic autonomic neuropathy as first suggested by Bennett (1984). A nerve growth factor defect may also be present in the autosomal recessive disorder familial dysautonomia, in which there is a reduction in the number of autonomic ganglia (Pearson 1979) (see Chapter 2).

The effects of selective destruction of nuclei such as the locus ceruleus on the descending pathways has not so far been studied. Transection of the spinal cord at C5 in young animals prevents the normal development of both presynaptic terminals and postganglionic neurons but in adult man (see Chapter 19) cord transection causes mild supersensitivity of sympathetic vascular receptors and of α- and β-receptors on platelets and lymphocytes. Transection of the preganglionic cholinergic trunk in young animals prevents the normal sixfold rise of postsynaptic tyrosine hydroxylase (TOH) activity. Destruction of the sympathetic ganglion cells by guanethidine in young animals has retrograde effects and depletes central neurons of noradrenalin as well as affecting the presynaptic choline acetyltransferase (CAT) activity. Sympathetic ganglia require end-organ contact for their normal development, not least for the retrograde axonal transport of NGF. This evidence suggests that transsynaptic regulation by orthograde and retrograde mechanisms, already accepted in visual and auditory systems within the central nervous system, is a general biological phenomenon which also governs the autonomic cholinergic and adrenergic neurons. In turn, their effects influence the first and second order of neurons.

Experimental autonomic neuropathies (see also Chapter 10)

An experimentally induced neuropathy was produced in rabbits by Appenzeller *et al.* (1965) who sensitized animals to antigen extracted from human sympathetic nerves and ganglia. A defect was found in reflex vasomotor function which was attributed to involvement of efferent cholinergic fibres. In a later study they showed a shift to the left of unmyelinated fibres in the paravertebral sympathetic chain in experimental autonomic neuropathy but changes were not specific and also occurred in experimental allergic neuritis (Becker *et al.* 1979). Clearly, further work on animal experimental autonomic neuropathy is needed.

In 1982 Griffiths *et al.* described a disorder in cats presenting with evidence of parasympathetic denervation (dry mucosi, dilated pupils, and gastrointestinal disturbances) but also with some evidence of sympathetic involvement with hypotension. Pathological studies showed loss of neurons in parasympathetic and sympathetic ganglia.

Investigation into the aetiology have so far been unsuccessful. The features resemble no known toxin, no antibodies against viruses have been demonstrated, and, clearly, an immune basis for this disorder remains a possibility.

Relationship between AF and other central neuronal degenerative disorders

There are some pathological associations between AF and other degenerative disorders, at present no more than interesting clues to possible aetiological links. The loss of noradrenergic projections from cells in the locus ceruleus which occurs in AF also occurs in PD, with loss of the striatal projection, and in Alzheimer's disease, with loss of the cholinergic ascending projections from the substance innominata of the reticular formation (Rosser 1981). The locus ceruleus, like the substantia nigra and substantia innominata, has a relatively unspecialized 'isodendritic' pattern suggesting a phylogenetically ancient system of cells. This isodendritic system appears to be tonically active, with less emphasis on spatial and temporal specificity, giving hope that a transmitter replacement therapy in AF may, as in PD, have an important place.

It is now a widely proposed hypothesis that PD results from subclinical environmentally induced damage to the nervous system but that symptoms do not emerge until several decades have elapsed during which normal age-related attrition of nigral neurons occurs. Calne *et al.* (1986), in discussing this, have extended the hypothesis to other chronic neurological diseases such as Alzheimer's disease and motor-neuron disease. Circumstantial evidence would suggest that it is not unreasonable to speculate that autonomic failure might have a similar cause, although epidemiological observations, based on the environment of patients with autonomic failure in early life, have not so far yielded any evidence to support this.

CONCLUSION

The observation that several different chronic neuronal degenerations have features in common accords well with the current view of AF and, apart from increasing our understanding about aetiology, also provides hope that early and effective replacement treatment of neurotransmitters, eventually possibly even by transplant surgery, might delay secondary anterograde or retrograde cell loss. The detailed studies of clinical features, physiology, pathology, pharmacology, and biochemistry described in this book should, in the words of Langley quoted by A. V. Hill (1965), save us from 'unnecessarily protracted discussion of unnecessary hypotheses'. After discussion of possible common pathogenesis we must accept that, in clinical terms, patients with autonomic failure cannot yet all be fitted into recognized groups and each patient has unique features which dictate unique management.

REFERENCES

Appenzeller, O. (1982). *The autonomic nervous system*, 3rd edn. Elsevier/North Holland, Amsterdam.

Appenzeller, O., Arnason, B. G., and Adams, R. D. (1965). Experimental autonomic neuropathy; an immunologically induced disorder of reflex vasomotor function. *J. Neurol. Neurosurg. Psychiat.* **28**, 510–15.

Bannister, R. (1971). Degeneration of the autonomic nervous system. *Lancet* **ii**, 175–9.

Bannister, R. (1979). Chronic autonomic failure with postural hypotension. *Lancet* **ii**, 404–6.

Bannister, R., Ardill, L., and Fentem, P. (1967). Defective autonomic control of blood vessels in idiopathic orthostatic hypotension. *Brain* **90**, 725–46.

Bannister, R., Davies, I. B., Holly, E., Rosenthal, T., and Sever, P. (1979). Defective cardiovascular reflexes and supersensitivity to sympathomimetic drugs in autonomic failure. *Brain* **102**, 163–76.

Bannister, R. and Hoyes, A. D. (1981). Generalized smooth-muscle disease with defective muscarinic receptor function. *Br. med. J.* **282**, 1015–18.

Bannister, R. and Oppenheimer, D. R. (1972). Degenerative diseases of the nervous system associated with autonomic failure. *Brain* **95**, 457–74.

Bannister, R., Sidgwick, A., and Mowbray, J. (1982). Genetic control of progressive autonomic failure: evidence of an association with an HLA antigen. *Lancet* **i**, 1017–18.

Becker, W., Livet, B. G., and Appenzeller, O. (1979). Experimental autonomic neuropathy: ultrastructure and immunohistochemical study of a disorder of reflex vasomotor function. *J. auton. nerv. Syst.* **1**, 53–67.

Bennett, T. (1984). Diabetic autonomic neuropathy and iritis. *Br. med. J.* **289**, 1231.

Bradbury, S. and Eggleston, C. (1925). Postural hypotension: a report of three cases. *Am. Heart J.* **1**, 73–86.

Brain, R., Lord (1985). *Clinical neurology*, 6th edn. (revised by R. Bannister). Oxford University Press, Oxford.

Burnstock, G. (1981). Current approaches to the development of the autonomic nervous system. In *Development of the autonomic nervous system* (ed. K. Elliott and G. Lawrenson), pp. 1–14. Ciba Foundation Symposium, Vol. 83. Pitman Medical, London.

Calne, D. B., Langston, J. W, Martin, W. R., Stoessl, A. J., Ruth, T. J., Adam, M. J., Pate, B. D., and Schulzer, M. (1985). Positron emission tomography after MPTP: observations relating to the cause of Parkinson's disease. *Nature* **317**, 246–8.

Calne, D. B., Eisen, A., McGeer, L., and Spencer, P. (1986). Alzheimer's disease, Parkinson's disease and motoneurone disease: a biotrophic interaction between ageing and environment. *Lancet* **ii**, 1067–70.

Carne, A. C. and Adler, W. M. (1986). Neurological manifestations of human immunodeficiency virus infection. *Br. med. J.* **293**, 462–3.

Cannon, W. B. (1929). Organisation for physiological homeostasis. *Physiol. Rev.* **9**, 399–431.

Cannon, W. B. and Rosenblueth, A. (1949). *The supersensitivity of denervated structures: a law of denervation.* MacMillan, New York.

Craddock, C., Pasvol, G., Bull, R., Protheroe, A., and Hopkin, J. (1987). Cardiorespiratory arrest and autonomic neuropathy in AIDS. *Lancet* **ii**, 16–18.

Dancis, J. and Smith, A. A. (1966). Familial dysautonomia. *New Engl. J. Med.* **274**, 207.

Edmonds, M. E., Jones, T. C., Saunders, W. A., and Sturrock, R. D. (1979). Autonomic neuropathy in rheumatoid arthritis. *Br. med. J.* **ii**, 173–5.

Fichefet, J. P., Sternon, J. E., Franken, L., Demanet, J. C., and Vanderhagen, J. J. (1965). Etude anatomo-clinique d'un cas d'hypotension orthostatique 'idiopathique'. Considerations pathogenique. *Acta cardiol.* **20**, 332–48.

Fraser, C. M., Venter, J. C., and Kaliner, M. (1981). Autonomic abnormalities and auto-antibodies to beta-adrenergic receptors. *New Engl. J. Med.* **305**, 1165–70.

Griffiths, I. R., Nash, A. S., and Sharp, N. J. H. (1982). The Key–Gaskell syndrome. *Vet. Rec.* **111**, 532–3.

Hill, A. V. (1965). *Trails and trials in physiology*, p. 360. Williams and Wilkins, Baltimore.

Hill, L. (1895). The influence of the force of gravity on the circulation. *J. Physiol., London* **18**, 18–53.

Hopkins, A., Neville, B., and Bannister, R. (1974). Autonomic neuropathy of acute onset. *Lancet* **i**, 769–71.

Johnson, R. H., Lambie, D. G., and Spalding, J. M. K. (1984). *Neurocardiology.* Saunders, London.

Johnson, R. H., Lee, G. de J., Oppenheimer, D. R., and Spalding, J. M. K. (1966). Autonomic failure with orthostatic hypotension due to intermediolateral column degeneration. *Quart. J. Med.* **35**, 276–92.

Jenzer, G., Mumenthaler, M., Ludin, H. P., and Robert, E. (1975). Autonomic dysfunction in botulism B: a clinical report. *Neurology* **25**, 150–3.

Khurana, R. K., Koski, C. L., and Mayer, R. F. (1983). Dysautonomia in the Eaton–Lambert syndrome. *Ann. Neurol.* **14**, 123.

Lamb, L. E. (1964). An assessment of the circulatory problem of weightlessness in prolonged space flight. *Aerospace Med.* **35**, 413–19.

Leheney, W. A., Davidson, D. L. W., de Vane, P., House, A. O., and Lenman, A. R. (1983). HLA antigens in Parkinson's disease. *Tissue Antigens* **21**, 260–1.

Lewis, P. (1964). Familial orthostatic hypotension. *Brain* **87**, 719–28.

Low, P. A., Thomas, J. E., and Dyck, P. J. (1975). The sympathetic nervous system in alcoholic neuropathy. *Brain* **98**, 357–64.

Man in't Veld, A. J., Boomsa, H., Moleman, P., and Schalekamp, M. A. D. H. (1987). Congenital dopamine-beta-hydroxylase deficiency. *Lancet* **i**, 183–8.

Mathias, C. J., Christensen, N. J., Frankel, H. L., and Spalding, J. M. K. (1979). Cardiovascular control in recently injured tetraplegics in spinal shock. *Quart. J.*

Med. **48**, 273–87.

Miyazaki, M. (1978). Shy–Drager syndrome—a nosological entity? In *International Symposium on Spinocerebellar Degenerations.* Medical Research Foundation, Tokyo.

Mobley, W. C., Server, A. C., Ishii, D. N., Riopelle, R. J., and Shooter, E. (1977). Nerve growth factor. *N. Engl. J. Med.* **297**, 1211–18.

Nanda, R. N., Boyle, R. C., Gillespie, J. S., Johnson, R. H., and Keogh, H. J. (1977). Idiopathic orthostatic hypotension from failure of noradrenaline release in a patient with vasomotor innervation. *J. Neurol. Neurosurg. Psychiat.* **40**, 11–19.

Neil, H. A. W., Thompson, A. B., John, S., McCarthy, F. T., and Mann, J. L. (1987). Diabetic autonomic neuropathy: its prevalence in a geographically defined population. [Abstract.] *Diabetic Medicine* **4**, 379–80.

Neville, B. G. R. and Sladen, G. E. (1984). Acute autonomic neuropathy following primary herpes simplex infection. *J. Neurol. Neurosurg. Psychiat.* **47**, 648–50.

Oppenheimer, D. R. (1980). Lateral horn cells in progressive autonomic failure. *J. neurol. Sci.* **46**, 393–404.

Park, D. M., Johnson, R. H., Crean, G. P., and Robinson, J. F. (1972). Orthostatic hypotension with recovery after radiotherapy in a patient with bronchial carcinoma. *Br. med. J.* **iii**, 510–11.

Pearson, J. (1979). Familial dysautonomia; a brief review. *J. auton. nerv. Syst.* **1**, 119–26.

Robertson, D., Goldberg, M. R., Onrot, J., Hollister, A. S., Wiley, R., Thompson, J. G., and Robertson, R. M. (1986). Isolated failure of autonomic noradrenergic neurotransmission: evidence for impaired β-hydroxylation of dopamine. *New Engl. J. Med.* **214**, 1494–7.

Rosser, M. N. (1981). Parkinson's disease and Alzheimer's disease as disorders of the isodendritic core. *Br. med. J.* **283**, 1588–90.

Rubinstein, R. E., Yahr, M. D., Mytilineou, C., and Bajaj, K. (1978). Amyloid autonomic neuropathy. *Mt Sinai J. Med.* **45**, 782–9.

Saper, C. B. and Petito, C. F. (1982). Correspondence of melanin-pigmented neurons in human brain with A1–A14 catecholamine cell groups. *Brain* **105**, 87–101.

Schoenberg, B. S. (1986). Descriptive epidemiology of Parkinson's disease; disease distribution and hypothesis formulation. *Adv. Neurol.* **45**, 277–82.

Sharpey-Schafer, E. P. and Taylor, P. J. (1960). Absent circulatory reflexes in diabetic neuritis. *Lancet* **i**, 559–62.

Shy, G. M. and Drager, G. A. (1960). A neurological syndrome associated with orthostatic hypotension. *Arch. Neurol., Chicago* **2**, 511–27.

Streeten, D. H. P., Kerr, L. P., Kerr, C. B., Pior, J. C., and Dalakos, T. G. (1972). Hyperbradykininism: a new orthostatic syndrome. *Lancet* **ii**, 1048–53.

Thomas, J. E., Schirger, A., Love, J. G., and Hoffman, D. L. (1961). Orthostatic hypotension as the presenting sign in craniopharyngioma; case report. *Neurology, Minneapolis* **11**, 418–23.

Ungerstedt, U. (1971). *Acta physiol. scand.* **82** (Suppl. 367), 1–48.

Vanderhaeghan, J. J., Perier, O., and Sternon, J. E. (1970). Pathological findings in idiopathic orthostatic hypotension; its relationship with Parkinson's disease. *Arch. Neurol., Chicago* **22**, 207–14.

Part I

Autonomic integration: scientific aspects of structure and function

2. Autonomic nervous system development

Robert W. Hamill and Edmund F. LaGamma

INTRODUCTION

Since the autonomic nervous system (ANS) has served as a model system to examine developmental mechanisms, a substantial literature on ANS growth and development already exists (for reviews see Black 1978, 1982, 1984; Bunge *et al.* 1978; Burnstock 1981; LeDouarin 1982). This brief review of autonomic development will focus on the embryology and maturation of spinal and peripheral components of the ANS. Specifically, we will address issues relevant to the following areas: developmental stages; regulatory phenomena including genetic encoding, interneuronal influences, environmental influences, and plasticity; clinical issues including normal adaptive autonomic responses and developmental disorders.

A central theme in developmental neurobiology is the interactions between the forces of 'nature' versus 'nurture' (Bunge *et al.* 1978; Black 1982). More specifically, 'nature' refers to the cell's intrinsic potential; i.e. its genetic make-up which provides the potential for a neuron's eventual repertoire of cellular processes and adult characteristics. 'Nurture' refers to extrinsic forces which influence the developmental cascade of neural maturation and serve to shape ontogenetic processes and determine the neuron's adult state. The exact mechanisms of these processes are unknown. Autonomic development has been extensively studied in laboratory animals, especially in chick and rodents. Although several reports characterize areas of human autonomic maturation (Kanerva *et al.* 1974; Pappano 1977), these investigations and others are not as extensive as the animal studies and lack a systematic morphological, neurochemical, and functional approach.

STAGES OF DEVELOPMENT

Embryonic

Embryologically, ANS ontogeny is related to two main processes: basal plate development within the spinal cord and neural crest development, migration, and phenotypic expression. In man neural development begins during the third week when the ectoderm thickens to form the neural plate. Fusion of the neural folds, which form from the elevated lateral edges of the neural plate, results in the formation of the neural tube; neurulation is completed by approximately 26–8 days of gestation (Kissel *et al.* 1981). The walls of the neural tube are composed of neuroepithelial cells which form a pseudostratified epithelium from the lumen to the external limiting membrane. During the process of closing, and shortly thereafter, there is a robust proliferation of neuroepithelial cells. Upon closure these cells become neuroblasts, which form the mantle zone surrounding the neuroepithelial layer. As more neuroblasts accrue, dorsal and ventral thickenings appear and these areas form the alar and basal plates, progenitors of the dorsal and ventral horns. Between these primary accumulations of neuroblasts, a smaller collection of neuroblasts form the intermediolateral horn; the preganglionic neurons of the autonomic nervous system and ventral nerve rootlets are apparent by the fifth week of maturation.

During the fifth week of human intrauterine development the preganglionic fibres (white rami communicans) appear in the midthoracic paravertebral ganglion region and subsequently exist along the entire length of the sympathetic chain (Kanerva *et al.* 1974). The grey rami communicans appear during the sixth week of development and have a more extended developmental phase with completion by the eighth week. Vagal parasympathetic preganglionic fibres are present along the trachea by the fifth week and may be the preferential migratory pathway for vagal and truncal neural crest which apparently are present at the tips of these maturing nerves (Pappano 1977; Kissel *et al.* 1981). Later during the fifth week these vagal nerves reach the pulmonary parenchyma as well as proximal intestinal tract (oesophagus and stomach) and by the end of the sixth week to the beginning of the seventh week the cardiac plexus begins to form (Pappano 1977). The thoracic structures are not substantially innervated until the tenth week when fibres appear in the conduction system of the heart and epithelium of the lung (Kissel *et al.* 1981). Subsequently, as target organ and enteric ganglion development occurs, preganglionic maturation continues in a craniocaudal fashion. Potential mechanisms governing the maturation of preganglionic events are reviewed in the section on 'Regulatory phenomena'.

Neural crest (NC) cells appear early and are first apparent during neurulation. Initially, the NC is located dorsomedially between the neural tube and the overlying ectoderm and is identical along the entire length of the embryo. Before neurulation is complete, crest cells begin to migrate and do so in a rostrocaudal manner along two distinct paths—

dorsolaterally and ventrolaterally. The ventral pathways are quite clearly defined and result in the development of such neuronal populations as autonomic neurons, sensory neurons, paraganglia, and neuroendocrine cells, such as adrenal chromaffin cells. Also, NC cells contribute to chromatophores, non-neuronal (support) cells of the peripheral nervous system. It is apparent that NC cells are the progenitors of a wide variety of neuronal and neuroendocrine populations which are distinct in phenotypic and functional characteristics. The possible mechanisms by which these crest cells arrive at their terminal differentiated adult character have been reviewed (see Weston 1971; Black 1978, 1982; LeDouarin 1982) and it appears that environmental signals exert a major influence on the almost pluripotential nature of crest cells. Table 2.1 summarizes the neural fates and transmitter characteristics of NC.

Normally, cephalic and truncal NC follow quite distinct patterns of migration and eventually populate specific target regions. Studies of chimaeric quail-chick embryos have defined the origin and fate of NC (Le Douarin 1982 for review). During normal ontogeny, mesencephalic NC give rise to the ciliary ganglion and vagal NC (somites 1–7) form the parasympathetic enteric ganglia (Auerbach's and Meissner's plexuses) proximal to the umbilical region. Enteric ganglia distal to this region originate from vagal and lumbosacral NC (crest originating caudal to somite 28). NC from axial regions immediately caudal to the vagal NC (somites 7–28) give rise to the precursors of sympathoblasts of the trunk; adrenomedullary cells originate within this region and are derived largely from the level of somites 18–24. Heterotopic grafts of quail neural primordium into the chick embryo also permitted characterization of the pluripotential nature of NC and the importance of migratory routes and eventual destinations in defining the adult neurochemical character and function of these autonomic precursors.

For instance, mesencephalic and vagal NC transplanted prior to migration to the somitic region, which gives rise to the adrenomedullary cells, eventually formed peripheral sympathetic ganglia and chromaffin cells of the adrenal medulla. Conversely, if NC from the somitic regions which normally form the adrenomedullary cells were grafted to the vagal NC region, they followed a migratory path characteristic of vagal NC and populated the gut—thus forming enteric ganglia. Apparently, the microenvironment both during migration and at target tissue are critical for determining adult phenotypic expression. Thus, somitic mesenchyme, ventral neural tube, and notochord are all important in this regard. These observations in avian systems are supported by studies in mammals which indicate that NC migrating to the gut will express noradrenergic characters (catecholamines and tyrosine hydroxylase) before assuming their final cholinergic state (Cochard *et al.* 1978). As development proceeds, NC form apolar neuroblasts which differentiate

Table 2.1. Neuronal derivatives of neural crest

Primitive cell	*Adult cell/structure*	*Transmitter characteristics (not all inclusive)*
Bipolar neuroblast	**Dorsal root ganglia**	
Multipolar neuroblast	**Sympathetic neurons**	
	Paravertebral ganglia Prevertebral ganglia Terminal ganglia	NA, CCK, Somatostatin, Substance P, ENK, ACH, VIP, 5HT
	Parasympathetic ganglia	
	Major parasympathetic ganglia Ciliary Sphenopalatine Otic Submandibular/sublingual Pelvic ganglia Terminal parasympathetic ganglia (target tissue)	ACH, VIP, SP, CA's–SIF
	Enteric neurons	
	Myenteric plexus (Auerbach's) Submucosal plexus (Meisner's) Enteric ganglia	GABA, ACH, VIP, 5HT, SP, ENK, SRIF, motilin-like peptide, bombesin-like peptide
	Chromaffin cells of adrenal medulla	EPI, NA, ENK, NPY, APUD
	Paraganglia–chromaffin	5HT, DA, A
	Small intensely fluorescent (SIF) cells, ganglia	5HT, DA, A

to bipolar and then multipolar cells. Enteric ganglia maturation in human occurs rostrocaudally; ganglion cells appear in the gut early in the first trimester with Auerbach's plexus visible by 9–10 weeks; Meissner's plexus follows at 13–14 weeks. By 24 weeks ganglion cells have reached the rectum.

The timetable of normal human sympathetic development indicates that by the fifth week migrating NC cells coalesce to form primitive sympathetic chains and during the sixth week the chain extends rostrally into the superior cervical ganglion region and caudally with segmentation (Kanerva *et al.* 1974). Postganglionic fibres are also developing: grey rami appear by the sixth week and fluorescent axons are growing toward targets shortly after the appearance of the catecholamine transmitters at approximately 8–9 weeks (Hervonen 1971).

In the adrenal, fluorescence appears at 9 weeks, adrenalin-like granules with functional release at 16–17 weeks, tyrosine hydroxylase and dopamine-β-hydroxylase at 15 weeks, and phenylethanolamine-*n*-methyltransferase, substance P, and leucine–encephalin at 18–19 weeks (Hervonen 1971; Hervonen and Korkala 1972; Hervonen *et al.* 1981).

Noradrenergic fibres innervate the ductus arteriosus very early and by 8–10 weeks of fetal life catecholaminergic fibres are present within the mesentery and gut wall (Kanerva *et al.* 1974). The heart responds to adrenergic stimuli by 10 weeks, implying adrenergic receptor mechanisms must exist although adrenergic terminals do not appear until after 16 weeks (Partanen and Korkala 1974). Interestingly, the heartbeat is generally not auscultated until 18 weeks of intrauterine life but by 20 weeks clinical judgements can be made regarding changes in fetal heart rate (Walker 1975). The variability and reflex responses from the earlier cholinergic innervation are now counterbalanced by adrenergic influences (Partanen and Korkala 1974; Walker 1975). Some structures such as the iris, pineal, and vas deferens are not substantially innervated until after birth (Kanerva *et al.* 1974).

As the complexity (transmitter characteristics (monoaminergic, cholinergic, peptidergic, purinergic), neural circuitry, and glial satellite cell function) of peripheral autonomic structures becomes more apparent, it is clear that the developmental mechanisms responsible for such diversity are not easily understood. It is also apparent that disease alterations might occur at a number of loci and result in clinical dysfunction (e.g. familial dysautonomia (the Riley–Day syndrome) and Hirschsprung's disease—see below).

Postnatal

The ANS is at various developmental stages at birth. For instance, the rodent is quite immature; there is a 60–100-fold increase in noradrenergic and cholinergic characteristics during the first 2 months of postnatal life and developmental milestones follow a rostrocaudal gradient (Hamill *et al.* 1983; Melvin and Hamill 1986). As discussed below ('Regulatory phenomena'), interruption of mechanisms governing neuronal maturation within the first 2–3 weeks of life will produce life-long developmental deficits in autonomic mechanisms. Postnatal human development is normally gauged by physiological observations (see 'Clinical issues'). Certainly, control over such autonomic functions as blood flow, bowel transit, and bladder emptying depends upon maturation of peripheral neural structures as well as central autonomic control mechanisms. Peripherally, the differentiation of neuroblasts into enteric ganglion cells and mature plexuses is quite delayed; in fact, at birth only approximately one-third of the neuroblasts are differentiated and development continues throughout the first 5 years of life (Kissel *et al.* 1981). Similarly, the development of autonomic ganglia and the innervation of pelvic structures involved in micturition is delayed. Eventually, usually by 2 to 3 years of age, voluntary control over these autonomic functions ensues. Thus, autonomic control occurs in the setting of continued ANS development.

Two clinical areas which have received considerable attention include thermoregulation and cardiovascular control. In brief, although a newborn human infant can initiate vasodilatation and panting in response to hyperthermia and releases catecholamines to vasoconstrict and augment thermogenesis during hypothermia the neonate and infant child adapt poorly to temperature stress. Thus, although functional capabilities are present, they are not fully developed or integrated.

In general, cardiovascular control appears more mature than temperature control. Although incomplete vascular responses to thermal stimuli may be present until about 2 to 3 months of age, cardiovascular responses controlling normal vasomotor tone are present before birth, as early as the end of the second trimester (Gootman and Gootman 1983; LaGamma 1984) and the newborn's cardiovascular response to cold stress is normal, implying intact sympathoadrenal responses and baroreceptor mechanism as well (Gootman and Gootman 1983). Although there are few developmental studies in humans of the neurotransmitter synthesizing or catabolizing enzymes involved in noradrenalin metabolism, studies have examined the transmitters and their metabolites (Dalmaz *et al.* 1979; Saarikoski 1983). All adrenergic compounds are present at birth, but adult levels are not approached until 5 years of age and not reached until adolescence. Laboratory studies in swine and rodent are available which provide a substantial review of the morphological, physiological, and neurochemical development of noradrenergic and baroreceptor systems involved in cardiovascular control (Gootman and Gootman 1983; Slotkin 1984).

REGULATORY PHENOMENA

The factors governing normal autonomic development are not fully known. The following discussion highlights intrinsic and extrinsic mechanisms fully recognizing that all important studies or theoretical aspects relevant to autonomic development cannot be discussed. A schematic diagram illustrating the course of transmitter development is presented in Fig. 2.1.

Intrinsic influences on peripheral autonomic development ('nature')

Genetic encoding

Defining relationships between environmental stimuli and cell responsiveness at the molecular level is central to an understanding of biological adaptation throughout development and to mechanisms of phenotypic expression in maturity (Berridge 1986; Yamamoto 1985; Black *et al.* 1987). Many of these processes require tissue-specific gene control in which factors initiating transcription are critical determinants of physiological function or of choices made during development (Black *et al.* 1987; Yamamoto 1985).

As noted, a central view in regulatory biology envisions many aspects of programmed cellular structure and function originating from processes intrinsic to the cell (nature), and epigenetic factors (i.e. extrinsic factors) which function as critical determinants of cell outcome (nurture). Consequently, during development a dynamic balance must exist between the forces of nature versus nurture. If true, how then do these events transpire; what are the guiding rules? What are the signals and through which intracellular pathways are signals transduced to guide the developing neuron through a myriad of progressively restricted biochemical choices which define cell lineage? Finally, once committed, to what extent may a cell be modified; that is, how 'plastic' or 'mutable' are neurons in maturity?

Answers to these questions are emerging from the convergence of cellular and molecular techniques for characterizing specific molecular signals. Autonomic ganglia/neurons serve as model systems for investigating fundamental mechanisms of developmental neurobiology. In this section, we will review categorical regulatory mechanisms which appear to underlie some of the steps and stages of neuronal growth and development. The reader is referred to original references for details of specific mechanisms where appropriate.

General mechanisms: intra- and intercellular signalling

Communication between cells results from a plethora of biochemical messages including amines, amino acids, peptides, proteins, etc. This

Stage:	Embryo	Fetus		Neonate	Adult
Transmitter mutability:	++++	++++	+++	++	+
Developmental signals	Embryonic	Microenvironment ?NGF		Afferent transsynaptic signals Efferent: target signals Support cell factors NGF Glucocorticoids Gonadal steroids	
Transmitter development	Early expression	Definitive expression	Modulation		Regulation (e.g. inducibility)

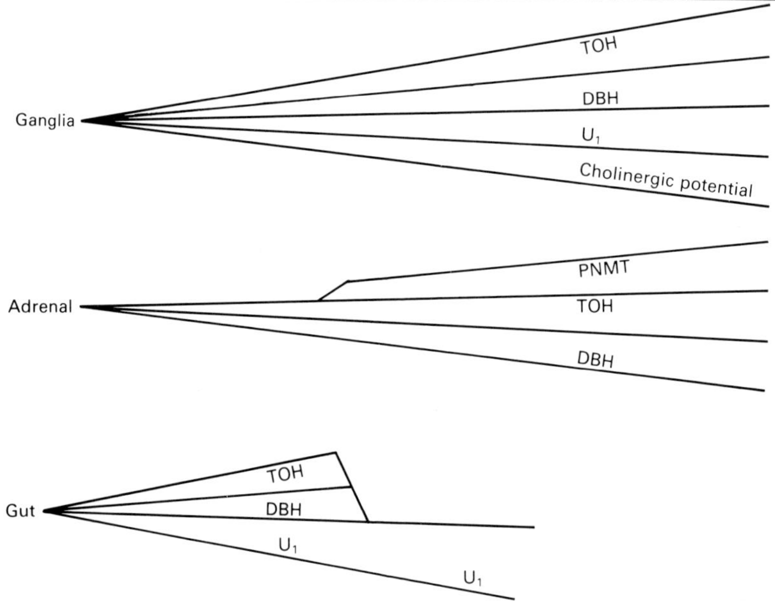

Ganglia

TOH

DBH

U_1

Cholinergic potential

Adrenal

PNMT

TOH

DBH

Gut

TOH

DBH

U_1

U_1

Fig. 2.1. Schematic representation of transmitter development. Developmental age proceeds from left to right in each panel, and vertical alignment among the entries in different panels approximates simultaneous processes or events. Lower segment of schema represents appearance and development of individual transmitter characters for sympathetic ganglia, adrenal chromaffin cells, and the transiently noradrenergic cells of the gut. Phenylethanolamine N-methyltransferase (PNMT) appears during definitive expression in the adrenal and tyrosine hydroxylase (TOH) and dopamine beta-hydroxylase (DBH) disappear in the gut cells, while a high-affinity uptake system for noradrenalin (U_1) persists. NGF denotes nerve growth factor. (Adapted from Black (copyright 1982 by the AAAS).)

method of organized interaction allows only selected cells to respond to specific signals evoked by changes in the cellular environment resulting in integrated responses at the level of the whole animal. The specificity of the signals is imparted largely by cell surface (e.g. acetylcholine, adrenergic, etc.) or intracellular (e.g. glucocorticoids) receptors. However, other mechanisms also exist, for example, the N-CAM (neural cell adhesion molecule) system, glycoprotein cell surface molecules, growth factors (e.g. nerve growth factor (NGF)), cholinergic factors (e.g. ciliary neuronotrophic factors), or myocyte-conditioned medium factors.

Transduction: conversion of extracellular signals to intracellular messages

Neurohormonal messages are detected by cell surface receptors which convert the external biochemical signal into a cellular response (e.g. transmitter release, protein synthesis, etc.). This is often associated with increased transmembrane flux of sodium, potassium, or calcium ions which in turn activates other intracellular transduction systems (Browning *et al.* 1985; Berridge 1986). In contrast, transduction for intracellular receptors differs. For example, activated glucocorticoid receptors cause intracellular responses either directly by activating gene transcription or at epigenetic (i.e. cellular) loci (Yamamoto 1985).

Selective receptor activation is further diversified by intracellular signal-transduction processes providing an additional level of complexity, interaction, and control to expand the cell's functional repetoire. For example, recent research has identified several receptor-linked, signal-transduction mechanisms associated with temporal changes in cell proteins, ion channels, cell function, and proliferation (Berridge 1986; Browning *et al.* 1985; Rozengurt 1986; Nishizuka 1984; Yamamoto 1985). Many of these changes are shown to affect transcriptional events: cell surface receptors linked to membrane-bound G-protein-dependent mechanisms trigger adenylate cyclase-induced increases cAMP production, activating protein kinase A, which phosphorylates numerous cytosolic proteins (Browning *et al.* 1985). This cascade may be involved in transcriptional control as well. Other well-characterized transduction pathways induce calcium-ion mobilization either activating calmodulin or increasing inositol phospholipid turnover and protein kinase-C activity, to phosphorylate proteins (Browning *et al.* 1985; Berridge 1986).

These generalized signal-transduction and second-messenger schemes are central to current thinking in molecular developmental neurobiology, linking biochemical observations with phenotypic expression, neuromodulation, and brain function (Black *et al.* 1987; Berridge 1986). Although limited examples exist for each of these constructs, the important dictum requires transduced extracellular signals to switch on nuclear events in neuronal tissue.

Gene regulation: mechanisms for responding to biochemical messages

Control over the levels of individual messenger RNA (mRNA) species is extremely important in generating the diversity and abundance of proteins encoded by the message. Proteins, in turn, define the phenotype and the function of neuronal cells. Moreover, during development, control over expression of certain genes allows differentiation and clonal cell lines to emerge. Molecular mechanisms governing genomic control resides at several levels. For example, chromatin structure differs in active and inactive genes. Apparently, removal, replacement, or modification of a histone-type DNA-binding protein relaxes the complex chromosomal structure allowing specific regulated-gene subunits the opportunity to be transcriptionally activated by biochemical signals. Additional control is thought to be imparted by other changes in the methylation state of nucleotides in the regulatory region of the gene which may also alter DNA conformation.

Once chromatin geometry is rearranged, current evidence indicates gene activation is predicated on binding of various proteins with site-specific DNA affinity to regulate expression (Dynan and Tjian 1985; Yamamoto 1985). Thus, protein interactions at enhancer, promoter, or repressor sites enhance or repress gene read-out (i.e. transcription) by altering the 'transcriptional efficiency' of the gene. Although key transcriptional regulatory steps are yet to be understood in the context of nervous system development and function, control phenomena are likely to reside at the level of biochemical modification of DNA-binding proteins, in proteins required for splicing RNA transcripts e.g. small nuclear ribonuclearprotein particles, or in mechanisms of message RNA stabilization.

Translation and posttranslational control: extracellular signals result in lasting biochemical responses

Transport of mature mRNA through the nuclear membrane to the cytosol precedes its binding with cytosolic ribosomes for translation. Then the protein product (prohormone) is generated and often biochemically modified (e.g. amidated, glycocylated, etc.) before the mature, active molecule exists. The mature protein (or processed peptide product) can now influence additional effects. Thus, if one of these newly synthesized proteins also serves as a transcriptional control molecule, as is the case with certain oncogenes (Rozengurt 1986), the complexity of interactions that may arise is enormous.

Regulated neuronal communication and gene expression at the molecular level

At present we are still only beginning to identify the multiple stages at which relevant regulatory phenomena occur. However, an emerging area in regulatory molecular neurobiology will focus on identification of regulatory proteins which alter expression of neuronal genes. In more general terms, once regulatory proteins are identified, we can determine when they appear during development. For inducible genes, does the amount of factor increase or is the factor instead modified to increase its affinity for the gene? These questions can only be answered by characterizing appropriate systems, such as the ANS. In this way the role of environmental stimuli on nervous system development or function can be further understood at the cellular and molecular level.

Extrinsic influences on peripheral autonomic development ('nurture')

Environmental signals are known to influence autonomic neuron maturation from the earliest stages of neural crest migration to the development and maintenance of the neuron's adult character. Mature neurons apparently are not immutable since alteration of the environmental milieu during adulthood will alter neuronal characteristics. Our previous discussion has touched on many of these extrinsic/environmental signals. This section will focus on the neuron-humoral issue, in particular hormonal factors, interneuronal influences, and target factors.

Hormonal regulation

Investigations of the hormonal control of peripheral sympathetic neuron development have focused on thyroid hormone, glucocorticoids, and testosterone. Thyroid ablation prevents the normal biochemical development of tyrosine hydroxylase (TOH) activity in the superior cervical ganglion (SCG), and alters SCG catecholamine histofluorescence and noradrenergic terminal development in the submaxillary gland (Black 1978). Similarly, functional adrenal maturation is delayed in the absence of thyroid hormone and prematurely induced in its presence (Slotkin 1984).

Glucocorticoid treatment of neonatal rats appears to influence the appearance of small, intensely fluorescent (SIF) cells in peripheral paravertebral sympathetic ganglia and elevated maternal glucocorticoid hormones may alter phenotypic expression in migrating neural crest cells (Jonakait *et al.* 1980; Black 1982). Glucocorticoids and a normal pituitary–adrenal axis are critical for full development of the adrenalin-synthesizing capacity of adrenal medullary cells, although it is not critical for the initial gene expression of this trait (Bohn *et al.* 1981). In addition, glucocorticoids inhibit neurite outgrowth of adrenal chromaffin cells (Unsicker *et al.* 1980) and influence the transmitter characteristics of SIF cells as well as co-localized catecholamine and opiate peptides (LaGamma and Adler 1987).

Gonadal steroids influence a wide variety of neuronal characteristics throughout life and are thought to act during early critical perinatal periods to permanently organize morphological and biochemical characteristics of neurons associated with sexual function. Subsequently, hormonal influences are activational; i.e. transient changes which only persist as long as the hormonal stimulus is present. Studies in the peripheral sympathetic nervous system indicate that both patterns are operant. Alterations in the hormonal milieu within the first 24 hours of birth and continuing for various times thereafter influence cell number and synaptic input (Wright and Smolen 1983) and neurotransmitter chemistry (Melvin and Hamill 1986) in sympathetic ganglia. Although some of these developmental changes are more prominent in ganglia destined to innervate sex-steroid-dependent targets, many of the abovementioned changes occur in the SCG. The regulatory influence of gonadal steroids persists during adulthood: bilateral castration decreases baseline TOH activity in the hypogastric ganglion and testosterone treatment reverses this effect (Hamill *et al.* 1984).

Interneuronal influences: peripheral regulation of autonomic development

Interneuronal and neuron-target regulatory mechanisms exist during ontogeny and influence not only neuronal characteristics but also neuronal survival. Anterograde transsynaptic influences regulate the development of noradrenergic characteristics of rat sympathetic neurons. Preganglionic neurectomy precludes the development of postsynaptic TOH activity (Black 1978; Smolen *et al.* 1985). In addition, the normal level of noradrenalin fails to accrue with deafferentation of the ganglion (Smolen *et al.* 1985). Similarly, adrenal opiate peptide accumulation fails to occur during development following adrenal denervation (LaGamma and Adler, personal observation).

Conversely, retrograde developmental regulatory influences exist between postsynaptic and presynaptic neural components in ganglia. Ganglionic choline acetyltransferase (CAT) activity, a marker of preganglionic terminal formation within peripheral ganglia, fails to develop following ablation of postsynaptic noradrenergic cells with antinerve growth factor or 6-OH dopamine. In addition, preganglionic cell bodies within the intermediolateral cell column exhibit reduced survival if adrenergic neurons are destroyed in the periphery (Black 1978 for review).

Interneuronal influences: central nervous system regulation of peripheral autonomic development

Sympathetic ontogeny is also influenced by central mechanisms. In rodents, interruption of descending spinal pathways alters the development of preganglionic CAT and postganglionic TOH activities in lumbar sympathetic ganglia (Hamill *et al.* 1983). More recent studies demonstrated that, although ganglion neuron number is not altered in ganglia deprived of central control during development, synapse number within the ganglia is substantially reduced (Lawrence *et al.* 1981). The loss of synapses correlates well with reductions in CAT activity. There appears to be a critical time during development when central lesions alter maturation. Spinal transection at 10 days of age results in complete cessation of adrenergic biochemical maturation and this abnormality persists throughout the first year of life (Hamill *et al.* 1983). Spinal surgery at 30 days of age does not alter the level of CAT or TOH activities.

Target organs regulation

Target organs of peripheral adrenergic neurons also influence the development of the innervating neuron. For instance, removal of the iris or salivary glands prior to any substantial innervation results in a failure in the development of neurotransmitter enzymes in the superior cervical ganglion and a decrease in neuron number within the SCG (Black 1978). In turn, neural crest cells migrating to the embryonic heart contribute to the normal formation of its outlet and influence the intrinsic rate of beating. Removal of these cells prior to migration results in cardiac malformations (Kirby 1987).

The peripheral field of innervation of a neuron may be increased and such studies have demonstrated increased neuronal survival. Studies in the sympathetic system demonstrate that target-organ enlargement increases the survival of peripheral adrenergic neurons (Black 1978 for review). These latter studies are of particular interest. Salivary glands may be enlarged via pharmacological manipulations which either increase acinar cells (isoproterenol treatment) or tubular portions (testosterone treatment) of the glands. Only the latter treatments result in an increase in enzyme activities and cell number. Since the salivary glands are known to contain nerve growth factor (NGF) and since NGF is synthesized in the gland's tubular portions, it is hypothesized that testosterone treatment increases the availability of NGF which is retrogradely transported to the noradrenergic cell bodies in the SCG. Thus, target organs may influence sympathetic development via NGF.

NGF is clearly critical for normal sympathetic development (for a review see Levi-Montalcini and Angeletti 1968). Neonatal treatment with antibodies directed against NGF will result in sympathectomy, and exposure to anti-NGF prenatally, via maternal transfer of antibody or postnatally, via cross-fostering experiments with immunized mothers, precludes the normal morphological and biochemical development of peripheral ganglia (Gorin and Johnson 1979). Thus, NGF plays a critical role both prenatally and postnatally in the growth and development of sympathetic neurons. Furthermore, NGF continues to be important for sympathetic systems during adulthood: treatment of adult mice with anti-NGF decreases catecholamine content in target tissues as well as cell volume of the innervating ganglion and treatment with NGF during adulthood will increase adrenergic characteristics in target organs. In total, NGF exerts regulatory influences on sympathetic systems throughout life.

THE CONCEPT OF PLASTICITY

Traditional teachings concerning neuronal plasticity maintained a restricted view in which neuronal tissue was believed to be committed, unresponsive, or immutable in its ability to adapt to changes in the environment. Recently, the collective work of many investigators has revealed a remarkable degree of synaptic plasticity, transmitter plasticity, receptor plasticity, and, indeed, ongoing neuronal cell division (reviewed Abelson *et al.* 1985). For example, in the SCG and adrenal medulla, molecular mechanisms regulating catecholamine and neuropeptide (e.g. substance P, encephalin, somatostatin, etc.) transmitter expression are subject to transsynaptic regulatory influences (LaGamma *et al.* 1987; Black *et al.* 1987).

CLINICAL ISSUES

Developmental disorders

Two ANS developmental disorders which illustrate ontogenetic aberrations of neural crest cells are familial dysautonomia (Riley–Day syndrome) and Hirschsprung's disease. Familial dysautonomia, an autosomal inherited recessive trait, is essentially confined to Ashkenazic Jews, a pattern suggestive of an altered single mutant allele at one gene locus. Patients experience symptom complexes related to underlying disturbances within autonomic and sensory neurons: cardiovascular instability, swallowing and gastrointestinal transit dysfunction (vomiting crises), tearing and taste bud alterations, and insensitivity to pain and temperature. Since NGF plays a critical role in autonomic development and since animal investigations with anti-NGF (*vide supra*) produce pathological changes similar to those observed in these patients, investigative efforts have centred on whether a defect in NGF exists. Initial studies suggested that the biological activity of β-NGF in serum and fibroblast from these patients is reduced, but more recently, recombinant DNA techniques have been utilized to establish that the structural gene for β-NGF is not defective (Breakefield *et al.* 1984). Whether defects in the processing of NGF or in the NGF receptor exist remains to be explored.

Hirschsprung's disease results from the absence of enteric ganglia from a segment of bowel and presents clinically as intestinal obstruction. Occasionally, intermittent diarrhoea may exist. There is substantial dilatation of the bowel proximal to the aganglionic section and megacolon may result. Hirschsprung's disease occurs in approximately one of every 5000 to 8000 births and 80 per cent of the patients are male. Initial hypotheses suggested that, since the pathology is most frequently localized to the distal bowel, rectum, and rectosigmoid colon—70–80 per cent of cases—a defect in neural crest migration must exist. However, alterations in the differentiation of neuroblasts or a failure of neuroblasts to survive within the bowel because of a defect in the microenvironment are alternative pathophysiological mechanisms.

Functional development

Maturation of integrated sympathoadrenal function has been an area of interest for fetal, neonatal, and perinatal physiologists and clinicians for many years (see reviews by Gootman and Gootman 1983; Phillipe 1983). In the human, catecholamines appear in the adrenal medulla by 8–9 weeks gestation with reflex release by 10 weeks (Hervonen and Korkola 1972). Reflex control of heart rate and integrated distribution of blood flow begins between 10 and 20 weeks gestation and matures considerably thereafter (Pappano 1977; Rudolph *et al.* 1971; Partanen and Korkala 1974). Of interest is the slightly earlier appearance of functional parasympathetic reflex responsiveness (Hervonen 1971; Pappano 1977). For example, well developed baroreflex function exists in nearly all viable preterm neonates (> 24 weeks gestation), but is less sensitive and allows for greater blood-pressure and heart-rate variability (Gootman and Gootman 1983).

At the cellular level, the human fetus will release catecholamines from non-innervated paraganglia to a greater extent than the partially innervated adrenal medulla (Hervonen and Korkala 1972). These responses mature to become qualitatively similar to adult responses by birth where, for example, hypoxia or head-up tilting results in preferential release of noradrenalin over adrenalin. In contrast, insulin, as in the adult, primarily causes release of adrenalin (Phillipe 1983; Slotkin 1984; Lagercrantz 1984).

Finally, although thyroid hormone plays a pivotal role in development of sympathoadrenal function in neonatal rats (Slotkin 1984), in humans this hypothesis has not been adequately tested by experiments of nature or in the laboratory. On the other hand, hypothyroidism profoundly impairs central nervous system maturation resulting in permanent intellectual impairment.

In the broadest sense, the practical issues of neuronal development have achieved a new prominence in perinatal medicine with the survival of increasingly smaller neonates (as early as 24 weeks (400–500 g) gestation). Therefore, the clinical urgency for application of information regarding the neurobiology of neuronal development has become critical. For example, these newborns will undergo a four- to fivefold increase in their birth weight while under the direct care of the clinician in the neonatal intensive care unit, prior to becoming mature enough for discharge from the hospital to parents. Consequently, a failure to comprehend or a lack of appreciation of the ramifications of environmental influences (e.g. drugs, therapy, etc.) on human neonatal development could have disastrous consequences. This is illustrated by the long recognized association of autonomic neuronal dysfunction in infants of drug addicts or in those neonates born to women who abuse ethanol in pregnancy.

Other aspects of sympathoadrenal function are recognized as critical mediators of the successful adaptation to extrauterine life. For example, in the well characterized catecholamine system, catecholamine transmitters serve an important function in temperature regulation, brown fat metabolism, glucose homeostasis, blood pressure, heart rate, and distribution of blood flow regulation as well as in pulmonary surfactant production and release. As stated earlier, the physiological mechanisms evoked by stress-responsiveness at the cellular level utilize the same biochemical signals (i.e. transmitters, hormones, growth factors, cell–cell interactions, etc.) as those necessary during development or for regulated expression and function in maturity. Thus, at many levels, a dynamic interaction is expected among these various factors in the developing human, interactions yet to be defined.

Developmental issues and their relationship to autonomic failure, including the multiple system atrophies

Fundamental to a number of autonomic syndromes is an understanding of why specific cell populations appear uniquely susceptible to disease processes. Relevant questions might include: why do certain chemically defined neuronal populations fail to develop normally; why during adulthood do specific components on the ANS exhibit dysfunction, degenerate, and die; why do specific cell groups appear to exhibit functional decline with age?

Since cellular processes are on a continuum and mechanisms existing during ontogeny probably exist throughout life—from birth through senescence—the aetiologies of various autonomic syndromes may be viewed in terms of developmental mechanisms. It seems reasonable to hypothesize that, throughout life, many of the intrinsic and extrinsic forces described earlier must continue and provide for normal function as well as survival of autonomic neurons. As mentioned, such extrinsic factors as interneuronal mechanisms, hormonal influences, target tissue regulatory influences, and trophic factors are operative throughout life. Accordingly, interruption of these processes may underlie disease expression. The developmental disorders—familial dysautonomia and Hirschsprung's disease—illustrate the potential interrelationships of altered developmental mechanisms and disease. Conceivably, autonomic failure during adulthood may result from interruption of these extrinsic factors. For instance, NGF and insulin are somewhat structurally related and, as mentioned, anti-NGF will result in an immunosympathectomy. Thus, high titres of antibodies to insulin might participate in the autonomic neuropathy in diabetic patients. However, studies to date do not support a clear relationship between autonomic dysfunction and insulin antibody titres. Alternatively, if axoplasmic transport fails in diabetic autonomic neuropathy, an alteration in the availability of NGF from target tissues may occur. It might be of value to measure NGF levels in patients with various autonomic syndromes, but the assay systems are complex and generally either not sensitive or specific enough for us to be sure about the validity of the measures in man. Central and peripheral interneuronal regulatory mechanisms have been examined in pure autononomic failure. Deficits in catecholamine transmitter synthesizing enzymes and morphological abnormalities in catecholaminergic neurons exist peripherally and centrally, whereas cholinergic markers in ganglia appear preserved. These studies suggest that normal regulatory mechanisms are altered in disease states. Disruption of central and peripheral transsynaptic mechanisms results in failed interneuronal communication and trophic interactions, and such alterations might underlie the apparent system degenerations which attend autonomic failure. However, whether these alterations are part of the pathogenesis or secondary to the disease state is not known.

The recent 'explosion' in molecular neuroscience suggests that we may soon begin to examine the effects of altered intrinsic (genetic control) mechanisms in autonomic systems on the pathophysiology and expression of autonomic failure. Certainly in the genetic disorder, the Riley–Day syndrome, the chromosomal and gene locus may eventually be explored utilizing recombinant DNA techniques. Recently, the gene locus of the genetic disease neurofibromatosis (a disorder of neural crest derived Schwann cells) has been located on chromosome 17. Similar studies will eventually permit an understanding of the genetic control of normal as well as abnormal human autonomic growth and development. In addition, studies of the molecular mechanisms influencing neuronal ontogeny and neuroplasticity will provide insights into how neurons respond to disease and possibly permit new understandings of how disease processes alter cell function and how neurons thus fail to function, degenerate, and/or die.

Acknowledgements

Investigations in the authors' laboratories are supported by NINCDS Grant NS22103, University of Rochester/Monroe Community Hospital Research Fund and American Heart Association Grant-in-Aid, and March of Dimes Basil O'Connor Research Award, SUNY Stonybrook.

REFERENCES

Abelson, P. H., Butz, E., and Snyder, S. (Eds.) (1985). *Neuroscience*, pp. 13–132. American Association for the Advancement of Science, Washington, DC.

Berridge, M. (1986). Second messenger dualism in neuromodulation and memory. *Nature* **323**, 294–5.

Black, I. B. (1978). Regulation of autonomic development. *Ann. Rev. Neurosci.* **1**, 183–214.

Black, I. B. (1982). Stages of neutotransmitter development in autonomic neurons. *Science* **215**, 1198–204.

Black, I. B. (1984). *Cellular and molecular biology of neuronal development*, pp. 133–278. Plenum Press, New York.

Black, I. B., Adler, J. E., Dreyfus, C. F., Friedman, W. J., LaGamma, E. F., and Roach, A. H. (1987). Experience, neurotransmitter plasticity and behavior. In *Psychopharmacology: the third generation of progress.* Raven Press, New York. (In press).

Bohn, M. C., Goldstein, M., and Black, I. B. (1981). Role of glucocorticoids in expression of the adrenergic phenotype in rat embryonic adrenal gland. *Devel. Biol.* **82**, 1–10.

Breakefield, X. O., Orloff, G., Castiglione, C., Coussens, L., Axelrod, F. B., and Ullrich, A. (1984). Structural gene for β-nerve growth factor not defective in familial dysautonomia. *Proc. nat. Acad. Sci., USA* **81**, 4213–16.

Browning, M. D., Huganir, R., and Greengard, P. (1985). Protein phosphorylation and neuronal function. *J. Neurochem.* **45**, 11–23.

Bunge, R., Johnson, M., and Ross, C. D. (1978). Nature and nurture in development of the autonomic neuron. *Science* **199**, 1409–16.

Burnstock, G. (1981). Current approaches to the development of the autonomic nervous system. In *Development of the autonomic nervous system* (ed. K. Elliott and G. Lawrenson), pp. 1–14. Ciba Foundation Symposium, Vol. 83. Pitman Medical, London.

Cochard, P., Goldstein, M., and Black, I. B. (1978). Ontogenetic appearance and disappearance of tyrosine hydroxylase and catecholamines in the rat embryo. *Proc. nat. Acad. Sci., USA* **75**, 2986–90.

Dalmaz, Y., Peyrin, L., Sann, L., and Dutruge, J. (1979). Age-related changes in catecholamine metabolites of human urine from birth to adulthood. *J. neural Transmission* **46**, 153–74.

Dynan, W. S. and Tjian, R. (1985). Control of eukaryotic messenger RNA synthesis by sequence-specific DNA binding proteins. *Nature* **316**, 774–7.

Gootman, N. G. and Gootman, P. M. (1983). *Perinatal cardiovascular function.* Marcel Dekker, New York.

Gorin, P. D. and Johnson, E. M. (1979). Experimental auto-immune model of nerve growth factor deprivation: effects on developing peripheral sympathetic and sensory neurons. *Proc. nat. Acad. Sci., USA* **76**, 5382–6.

Hamill, R. W., Cochard, P., and Black, I. B. (1983). Long-term effects of spinal transection on the development and function of sympathetic ganglia. *Brain Res.* **266**, 21–7.

Hamill, R. W., Earley, C. J., and Guernsey, L. A. (1984). Hormonal regulation of adult sympathetic neurons: the effects of castration on tyrosine hydroxylase activity. *Brain Res.* **299**, 331–7.

Hervonen, A. (1971). Development of catecholamine storing cells in human fetal paraganglia and adrenal medulla. *Acta physiol. scand.* **83** (suppl. 368).

Hervonen, A. and Korkala, O. (1972). The effect of hypoxia on catecholamine content of human fetal abdominal paraganglia and adrenal medulla. *Acta obstet. gynecol. scand.* **51**, 17–24.

Hervonen, A., Pickel, W. M., Joh, T. H., Reis, D., Linnoila, I., and Miller, R. J. (1981). Immunohistochemical localization of the catecholamine synthesizing enzymes, substance P and enkephalin in the human fetal sympathetic ganglion. *Cell Tiss. Res.* **213**, 33–42.

Jonakait, G. M., Bohn, M. C., and Black, I. B. (1980). Maternal glucocorticoid hormones influence neurotransmitter phenotypic expression in embryos. *Science* **210**, 551–3.

Kanerva, L., Hervonen, A., and Hervonen, M. (1974). Morphological characteristics of the ontogenesis of the mammalian peripheral adrenergic nervous system with special remarks on the human fetus. *Med. Biol.* **52**, 144–53.

Kirby, M. L. (1987). Cardiac morphogenesis—recent research advances. *Pediat. Res.* **21**(3), 219–24.

Kissel, P., Andre, J. M., and Jacquier, A. (1981). *The neurocristopathies*, pp. 1–15, 165–83, 219–21. Year Book Medical Publishers, Chicago.

LaGamma, E. F. (1984). Endogenous opiates and cardiopulmonary regulation.

Advan. Pediat. **31**, 1–41.

LaGamma, E. F. and Adler, J. E. (1987). Glucocorticoids regulate adrenal opiate peptides. *Mol. Brain Res.* (In press).

LaGamma, E. F., White, J. D., McElvey, J. F., and Black, I. B. (1987). Increased cyclic AMP or calcium ion second messengers reproduce the effects of depolarization on adrenal enkephalin pathways. *Ann. NY Acad. Sci.* (In press).

Lagercrautz, H. (1984). Catecholamine surge at birth in the human infant. In *Catecholamines: basic and peripheral mechanisms* (ed. E. Usdin), pp. 113–20. A. R. Liss, New York.

Lawrence, J. M., Hamill, R. W., Cochard, P., Rasiman, G., and Black, I. B. (1981). Effects of spinal cord transection on synapse numbers and biochemical maturation in rat lumbar sympathetic ganglia. *Brain Res.* **212**, 83–8.

LeDouarin, N. (1982). *The neural crest*, pp. 22–53, 144–97. Cambridge University Press, New York.

Levi-Montalcini, R. and Angeletti, P. U. (1968). Nerve growth factor. *Physiol. Rev.* **48**, 534–69.

Melvin, J. E. and Hamill, R. W. (1986). Gonadal hormone regulation of neurotransmitter synthesizing enzymes in the developing hypogastric ganglion. *Brain Res.* **383**, 38–46.

Nishizuka, Y. (1984). The roles of protein kinase C in cell surface signal transduction and tumor production. *Nature, London* **308**, 693–8.

Pappano, A. J. (1977). Ontogenetic development of autonomic neuroeffector transmission and transmitter reactivity in embryonic and fetal hearts. *Pharmacol. Rev.* **29**, 3–34.

Partanen, S. and Korkala, O. (1974). Catecholamines in human fetal heart. *Experientia* **30**, 798–800.

Phillipe, M. (1983). Fetal catecholamines. *Am. J. Obstet. Gynecol.* **146**, 840–55.

Rozengurt, E. (1986). Early signals in the mitogenic response. *Science* **234**, 161–6.

Rudolph, A. M., Heymann, M. A., Teramo, K. A., Barrett, C. T., and Raiha, N. C. R. (1971). Studies on the circulation of the previable human fetus. *Pediat. Res.* **5**, 452–65.

Saarikoski, S. (1983). Functional development of adrenergic uptake mechanisms in human fetal heart. *Biol. Neonate* **43**, 158–63.

Slotkin, T. A. (1985). Development of the sympathoadrenal axis. Endocrine control of synaptic development in the sympathetic nervous system: the cardiac-sympathetic axis. In *Developmental neurobiology of the autonomic nervous system* (ed. P. M. Gootman), pp. 69–96. Humana Press, New York.

Smolen, A. J., Beaston-Wimmer, P., Wright, L. L., Lindley, T., and Cader, C. (1985). Neurotransmitter synthesis, storage, and turnover in neonatally deafferented sympathetic neurons. *Develop. Brain Res.* **23**, 211–18.

Unsicker, K., Rieffert, B., and Ziegler, W. (1980). Effects of all culture conditions, NGF, dexamethasone, and cAMP, on adrenal chromaffin cells *in vitro*. In *Histochemistry and cell biology of autonomic neurons, SIF cells and paraneurons* (ed. O. Eranko), pp. 51–9. Raven Press, New York.

Walker, D. (1975). Functional development of the autonomic innervation of the human fetal heart. *Biol. Neonate* **25**, 31–43.

Weston, J. A. (1971). Neural crest cell migration and differentiation. In *Cellular aspects of neural growth and differentiation* (ed. D. C. Pease), UCLA Forum Med. Sci. No. 14, pp. 1–22. University of California Press, Los Angeles.

Wright, L. L. and Smolen, A. J. (1983). Neonatal testosterone treatment increases neuron and synapse numbers in male rat superior cervical ganglion. *Develop. Brain Res.* **8**, 145–53.

Yamamoto, K. R. (1985). Steroid receptor regulated transcription of specific genes and gene networks. *Ann. Rev. Genet.* **19**, 209–52.

3. Central and peripheral autonomic control mechanisms

John L. Reid

INTRODUCTION

The autonomic nervous system provides a rapidly responding mechanism to control a wide range of functions. Cardiovascular, respiratory, gastrointestinal, renal, and endocrine and other systems are regulated by either the sympathetic nervous system or the parasympathetic system or both. It is now established that, in the periphery, at the end-organ, responses are determined by chemical transmitters: the catecholamines, noradrenalin at the sympathetic nerve ending, and acetylcholine at the parasympathetic neuron effector junction. In addition, the sympathetic system has a humoral contribution from circulating adrenalin and to a lesser extent noradrenalin from the adrenal medulla.

Over the last 30 years understanding of the actions of these neurotransmitters on their receptors and the development of drugs with specific action on the synthesis and degradation of catecholamines and acetylcholine together with sympathetic agonists (stimulants) or antagonists (blockers) have not only led to important therapeutic developments but these pharmacological studies have themselves permitted a clearer understanding of the mechanisms of autonomic control.

More recently, it has been possible with morphological, pathological, and biochemical developments to investigate the pathways and chemical mediators in the central nervous system which participate in central control of autonomic output. In recent years new concepts, such as existence of transmitters and associated co-release whereby amines and peptides can further modulate each other, have emerged. In this chapter morphological aspects will be briefly discussed together with the evidence from pharmacological studies in man and animals that catecholamines, peptides, and other postulated transmitters in the brain, as in the periphery, participate in autonomic regulation. The emphasis of this review, and indeed of much of the published work on circulatory control, is on baroreceptor reflex influences on autonomic activity.

However, it is likely that the underlying design can be extended to other control systems participating in circulatory regulation.

MORPHOLOGICAL ASPECTS OF AUTONOMIC CONTROL

Peripheral autonomic pathways (Fig. 3.1)

There are two main effector limbs of the autonomic nervous system. Postganglionic parasympathetic fibres from the vagus innervate cardiac, pulmonary, and upper gastrointestinal organs, while pelvic organs are innervated by the sacral parasympathetic outflow.

Sympathetic innervation is derived from the efferent preganglionic fibres whose cell bodies lie in the intermediolateral column of the spinal cord at the level of the thoracic and upper lumbar roots. These nerves synapse in the bilateral chain of sympathetic ganglia with postganglionic sympathetic neurons which innervate widely vascular smooth muscle, heart, kidney, gut, and many other organs. The preganglionic neurons are cholinergic or use acetylcholine as a transmitter while the post-

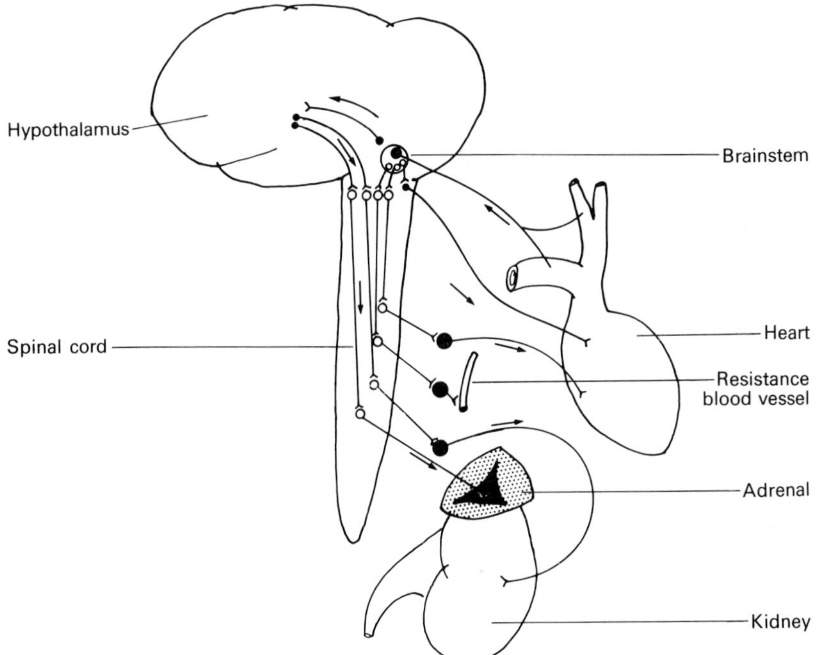

Fig. 3.1. Schematic drawing of the afferent and efferent pathways of the baroreceptor reflex arc.

ganglionic neurons release noradrenalin (noradrenergic). The sympathetic ganglion is not a simple relay station but a site of modulation by short interneurons and a variety of neurotransmitters and receptors.

The adrenal medulla can be considered as a modified sympathetic ganglion. It is cholinergically innervated and releases catecholamine directly into the circulation. The importance of circulating adrenalin in man remains controversial.

Central baroreceptor reflex pathways

The anatomical pathways of the central connections of baroreceptor reflex have been elegantly described (Palkovits 1980) and have assisted in the understanding of the relationships between brainstem nuclei and efferent pathways.

Blood-pressure homeostasis is maintained by a negative-feedback mechanism which is largely under the control of the autonomic nervous system. Changes in blood pressure are detected by baroreceptors in the heart, carotid sinus, aortic arch, and other large vessels. Afferent impulses are transmitted from these structures via the carotid-sinus nerve and the glossopharyngeal and vagus nerves to the brainstem. The carotid-sinus nerve terminates in two areas which play a major role in blood-pressure control: the nuclei of the tractus solitarius (NTS) and the paramedian nucleus.

The major role played by the NTS in blood-pressure control has been clarified by stereotactic destruction by electrolytic lesions. In the rat, when the NTS are ablated bilaterally, baroreflexes are abolished and arterial pressure rises substantially as the result of increased peripheral resistance. Since the fulminating rise in blood pressure could be prevented by administering α-adrenoceptor antagonists, the inference to be drawn is that destruction of the NTS results in an increased sympathetic outflow with α-adrenoceptor-mediated increases in arterial resistance and pressure. Electrical stimulation of the NTS produces the opposite response with a fall in blood pressure. It can reasonably be concluded from these studies that the NTS are intimately involved in blood-pressure control, particularly with respect to integrating information from the baroreceptors.

From the NTS neuronal connections are made both with efferent pathways which are the secondary neurons on the baroreceptor reflex arc and also with ascending neurons which carry information to higher structures in the brain. With respect to the efferent connections, a small lesion in the medial part of the NTS produces diffuse degeneration of fibres in the dorsal vagal nucleus, the nucleus reticularis lateralis, the nucleus reticularis medullae oblongatae, and in the nucleus reticularis gigantocellularis (Palkovits 1980). These various nuclei project directly to the interomediolateral nucleus of the spinal cord and it seems possible that baroreflex information reaches the preganglionic sympathetic cells of the spinal cord by a multisynaptic pathway. The NTS also communicates with the nucleus ambiguus but although baroreceptor neurons might be located in this nucleus definitive evidence has not so far been forthcoming.

The precise neuroanatomical pathways connecting the NTS to higher cardiovascular control centres are still controversial. However, considerable evidence accumulated over many years points to higher brain centres being actively involved in the modulation of the lower cardiovascular reflex control areas.

Hypothalamic and higher centres and autonomic control

The hypothalamus has been implicated as a site of higher cardiovascular control for over half a century. Electrical stimulation of the anterior hypothalamus or of the preoptic area produces bradycardia, a fall in blood pressure, and an inhibition of the baroreceptor reflexes. Conversely, bilateral destruction of these areas decreases the baroreflex response to afferent stimulation (Hilton and Spyer 1971). Beyond the hypothalamus there is little doubt that the highest brain centres can influence blood-pressure control. For example, mental arithmetic has been shown to elevate blood pressure while various relaxation techniques such as biofeedback and transcendental meditation have been shown to lower blood pressure.

The anterior and posterior hypothalamus both modify efferent autonomic outflow as discussed above, in experiments in which the areas were stimulated electrically, destroyed, or activated pharmacologically. However, although similar experiments undoubtedly implicate limbic, cortical pontine, and mesencephalic modulation, gross studies, whether by lesions or stimulation, at present cannot characterize the precise mechanisms by which these higher centres influence circulatory control. It is, however, of some clinical relevance that sympathetic activity can be activated directly from higher centres even when baroreceptor function is disturbed or destroyed. Mental arithmetic and physical exercise will increase blood pressure in patients in whom afferent baroreceptor reflex mechanisms are absent (Johnson *et al.* 1971).

PHARMACOLOGICAL ASPECTS OF AUTONOMIC CONTROL

Catecholamines

There is compelling evidence to implicate a role of catecholamines in the control of blood pressure both in the periphery and in the brain. The recent description of a patient with orthostatic hypotension and an apparent isolated deficiency or absence of dopamine-β-hydroxylase in brain and the periphery emphasizes the role of noradrenalin in blood-pressure control (Man in t'Veld *et al.* 1987). The relatively normal behavioural and sexual development of this patient does however cast doubt on the role of noradrenalin in other functions.

The areas in the brain which appear to be involved in blood-pressure control contain many catecholaminergic cell bodies or terminals. Higher concentrations of catecholamines have been reported in the NTS and dorsal vagal nucleus than in other nuclei of the medulla oblongata (Saavedra *et al.* 1979). The nucleus reticularis lateralis in the medulla oblongata also contains both noradrenergic (Dahlstrom and Fuxe 1964) and adrenergic neurons (Hokfelt *et al.* 1974).

In the spinal cord high concentrations of catecholamine-containing nerve fibres have been located in the intermediolateral horn of the thoracic and lumbar cord which synapses with sympathetic preganglionic neurons.

In the periphery, postganglionic sympathetic fibres are noradrenergic and have been observed in the majority of vascular beds with particularly dense innervation being found in the small arterioles which play an important role in determining peripheral resistance.

Controversy has existed as to whether descending bulbospinal catecholaminergic tracts play a role in the baroreflex arc and, if they do, whether this role is excitatory or inhibitory. Although there is dispute about precise mechanisms there is good evidence that central noradrenergic neurons play a role in central autonomic control.

Although noradrenergic neurons were the first to be identified and implicated in central cardiovascular control, there is now persuasive evidence that adrenalin-containing neurons are also involved. Adrenalin-containing neurons have been identified in the medulla oblongata, particularly in association with NTS. These adrenalin-containing fibres have been found to project to other brainstem areas and to the hypothalamus (Hokfelt *et al.* 1974). The findings of high activity of phenylethanolamine N-methyltransferase (PNMT) (Saavedra *et al.* 1979) and high adrenalin concentrations in hypothalamic nuclei and brainstem supports a significant role for adrenalin as do pharmacological studies. When adrenalin is injected into the anterior hypothalamus of the rat, it not only produces a fall in blood pressure and heart rate, but it is about 10 times more effective in this regard than noradrenalin (Struyker-Boudier and Beker 1975).

In the periphery, postganglionic sympathetic fibres are noradrenergic while the adrenal medulla releases both noradrenalin and adrenalin which exert circulating humoral actions.

In the periphery and in the brain the effects of noradrenalin and adrenalin are a result of activation of α- or β-receptors. Both receptor types have been identified in brain and more recently radioligand studies have demonstrated the presence of both α_1- and α_2-receptor types in preparations of neuronal membranes (Miach *et al.* 1978). As will be discussed in detail later, in the brain α_2-receptors are of particular importance in autonomic control.

Neuropeptide Y (NPY) is a 36 amino-acid peptide which has been identified in sympathetic nerve endings in the periphery and in the adrenal medulla (Allen *et al.* 1983). It is also found in brain and is co-localized with adrenalin and noradrenalin in most if not all brainstem catecholaminergic neurons (Hokfelt *et al.* 1983). NPY has long-lasting peripheral pressor actions and can also facilitate response to other neurogenic and humoral pressor stimuli (Lundberg *et al.* 1982). Injection of NPY into some brainstem areas results in hypotension and bradycardia. NPY may be an important modulator of catecholamine effects on the circulation both in the brain and the periphery.

Peptides

There has been considerable interest in recent years in the role of peptides in central autonomic regulation. This has been reviewed in detail elsewhere (Kreiger 1983; Reid and Rubin 1987).

Just as the recognition of the peripheral role of catecholamines preceded recognition of their central nervous role, so, with the octapeptide angiotensin II, its peripheral vasoconstrictor and autonomic modulator role was recognized first and only recently has its central role been identified.

In the periphery angiotensin II increases noradrenalin release, blocks re-uptake, and stimulates adrenal adrenalin release. In the central nervous system angiotensin II has been shown to have a variety of actions. It increases blood pressure, heart rate, and cardiac output via the area postrema of the brainstem and stimulates thirst and sympathetic outflow by actions at hypothalamic and other forebrain sites (Fitzsimmons 1980). In addition to the central effort of peripheral angiotensin II it has been proposed that an endogenous brain angiotensin II can be formed in the brain by the actions of the brain isorenin system. All the components of the renin–angiotensin system have been described in brain tissue (Ganong 1984; Ganten *et al.* 1984). Immunofluorescence studies have demonstrated angiotensin II in specific nerve terminals and a neuromodulatory role has been proposed in the brain. When angiotensin II is injected directly into forebrain areas, sympathetic activity is increased resulting in rises in blood pressure. Although central angiotensin II has been proposed to be involved in control of sympathetic activity, the precise mechanism and interrelationships with catecholamines and other putative transmitters remain to be determined.

Several other peptides may be involved in central blood-pressure control. The NTS has been shown to contain endogenous opioids, substance P, somatostatin, and neurotensin-immunoreactive nerve terminals. Evidence is accumulating that endogenous opioids are involved in blood-pressure control. Not only are they and their receptors localized in the NTS, but injection of β-endorphins into the cisterna magna of dogs produces a fall in both heart rate and blood pressure. Stable encephalin analogues and opiates modify the blood pressure of spontaneously hypertensive rats (Schaz *et al.* 1980). Centrally-administered encephalins attenuate baroreceptor-reflex function in rabbits (Petty and Reid 1981) and this effect is prevented by naloxone. Preliminary studies in man are also consistent with a central action of encephalins on autonomic control. It is not clear whether opioids interact with catecholamines in the brain but there is evidence that the two systems influence each other. Further studies are indicated with opioid drugs with different agonist and antagonist effects on opioid receptor subtypes and on interrelations at a brainstem and hypothalamic level with catecholamines.

Substance P, an undecapeptide which has been proposed as a possible sensory transmitter at afferent sensory terminals in the dorsal horn of the spinal cord may also be involved in the transduction of afferent baroreceptor impulses. While there is evidence of a neuromodulator role for substance P at the brainstem level (Petty and Reid 1981), alternative agents such as glycine must be considered as the primary baroreceptor afferent transmitter.

Other neurotransmitters

Over the past 25 years an increasing number of amines, amino acids, and peptides have been identified in the brain and put forward as putative neurotransmitters (Kreiger 1983; Reid and Rubin 1987). Developments in histochemistry and analytical methods have supported many of these claims and in several cases a role in central autonomic regulation proposed. Acetylcholine and gamma aminobutyric acid (GABA) have all been reported to modify blood pressure and heart rate by central nervous mechanisms. Serotonin may modulate efferent sympathetic activity in several ways including via descending bulbospinal neurons in the spinal cord. Thus an increasing number of chemical mediators in the nervous system have been implicated in autonomic regulation. In view of the complex interaction at many levels it is perhaps not surprising that the precise role, location, and interrelationships of these transmitters are unclear at present.

CLINICAL PHARMACOLOGICAL ASPECTS OF AUTONOMIC CONTROL

The assessment of central and peripheral effects in man

The importance of the integrity of the sympathetic nervous system to circulatory regulation can be explored in man using drugs with well-characterized actions. Blockade of ganglionic transmission with pentolinium or of postganglionic neuronal transmission with guanethidine or bethanidine leads to a failure of orthostatic regulation and response to exercise, but has little effect on supine resting blood pressure and heart rate. If the drugs used do not enter the central nervous system, their peripheral actions will account for the haemodynamic consequences. More recently using selective and polar β-antagonists of α- and β-adrenoceptors, the role of these receptors can be explored. It is more difficult to assess directly in man the central contribution to autonomic control. It is not practical (or ethical) to administer drugs directly into the brain or cerebrospinal fluid. When given orally or intravenously, the observed effects are usually a result of peripheral and central actions. It has been possible to derive indirect evidence for central mechanisms by examining the actions of drugs, which in animals have well-characterized actions, in patients with known selective neurological lesions and comparing the responses to those in normal intact man (Reid *et al.* 1977). It is also possible to compare the effects of lipid-soluble drugs which readily enter the brain with polar compounds which have a low penetration of the blood–brain barrier, at least after acute or short-term dosing. The anticholinergic drug, atropine, and its polar analogue, methylatropine, have been used to assess central and peripheral cholinergic mechanisms of parasympathetic control. The similarity of the effects of polar β-adrenoceptor blockers like atenolol with lipophilic agents such as propranolol has been taken as circumstantial evidence against a significant central contribution to the antihypertensive action of β-blockers (Reid *et al.* 1977). β-adrenoceptors are present in brain and animal experiments indicate that blockade of central β-receptors can lower blood pressure. However, in man β-blockers do not lower sympathetic activity as measured by plasma noradrenalin and their haemodynamic effects in man can probably be accounted for by peripheral β-receptor blockade. Thus central α- and not β-receptors appear to be the principal vehicle of expression of catecholamine effect.

Central α-adrenoceptors and autonomic regulation in normal man

In the late-1960s several groups demonstrated that drugs with α-adrenoceptor stimulant or agonist properties could lower blood pressure in animals by a direct action on lowered blood pressure after injection into the cerebrospinal fluid (Kobinger and Walland 1967). Methyldopa was also suggested to act centrally after metabolism to α-methylnoradrenalin (Henning 1969). Some, but not all, α-blockers could antagonize the fall in blood pressure after clonidine (Schmitt *et al.* 1973).

As clonidine and α-methylnoradrenalin have a higher affinity for the presynaptic α-receptors which modulate transmitter release (Langer 1977) than classical postsynaptic α-receptors, a subclassification has been proposed. The central effects of clonidine appear to depend on activation of receptors similar to but not identical with presynaptic receptors. However, as there is now evidence for the location of this receptor type in many tissues including platelet membranes and as the anatomical location in brain is not established, it is preferable to use the term α_1 to refer to classical α-receptors and α_2 for those with properties resembling presynaptic receptors (Berthelsen and Pettinger 1977).

Clonidine and other α_2-receptor agonists lower blood pressure in normal man (Reid 1981). Qualitatively, the effects of clonidine are similar in normotensive and hypertensive subjects. Methyldopa also causes modest falls in blood pressure in normal subjects as do other α_2-agonists. The fall in blood pressure is associated with a fall in plasma noradrenalin consistent with a central inhibition of sympathetic tone. Clonidine and analogues cause sedation probably also mediated by α_2-receptor activation (Reid 1981). However, the hypotensive and sympathoinhibitory effects of centrally acting antihypertensive drugs are not simply a secondary consequence of a sedative action. Benzodiazepine-induced sedation does not lead to a similar magnitude of fall in blood pressure or fall in catecholamines as does clonidine (Hossman *et al.* 1980). However, the best evidence for a central hypotensive action of clonidine in man comes from the studies of patients with neurological disease. In addition, the results of these studies can provide valuable information on the location and extent of central catecholaminergic involvement via α_2-receptors in autonomic regulation.

Patients with traumatic transection of the spinal cord at a high cervical level are not only tetraplegic but also have anatomically severed connections between the brain and the spinal efferent sympathetic outflow. However, vagal reflexes are present and sympathetic efferent outflow at a spinal level is intact. Careful study of such patients has extended understanding of circulatory control in man and the role of renin release. In a group of tetraplegic subjects, clonidine did not lower blood pressure, although heart rate fell and central sedative side-effects were similar to those in normal subjects (Reid *et al.* 1977). Thus, in the absence of descending bulbospinal pathways, clonidine did not lower blood pressure. The results are consistent with animal experiments indicating that an important site of action of clonidine is in the brainstem. These studies in tetraplegics, however, also revealed an additional peripheral action manifest as a reduction in the spinal-reflex induced rise in pressure and plasma noradrenalin during bladder distension (Reid *et al.* 1980). This peripheral action is consistent with an effect on peripheral presynaptic receptors at least when sympathetic activity is increased.

Administration of clonidine to patients with autonomic neuropathy reveals differences in responses depending on the likely site of the lesion. A 67-year-old man with severe symptomatic postural hypotension, very low resting plasma noradrenalin which did not change on tilting, and greatly increased pressor sensitivity to noradrenalin had no evidence of focal or generalized neurological disease. Clonidine (300 mg) had no significant effect on blood pressure or on plasma or urinary catecholamine excretion (Reid *et al.* 1980), although he experienced the same degree of sedation as normal subjects. It appeared that this man had a primary efferent autonomic neuropathy and that, in the absence of intact efferent connections, neither the depressor nor sympathoinhibitory actions of clonidine could be observed.

In contrast, in a patient with clinical features of tabes dorsalis and orthostatic hypotension, clonidine (300 mg) had a profound hypotensive effect. This patient had a blocked response to Valsalva's manoeuvre but a relatively normal response to cold stress and mental stress and plasma noradrenalin at the lower end of the normal range. In view of these features and the associated tabes, it was proposed that the lesion in this instance was predominantly of one of the baroreceptor afferents and that he had an afferent autonomic neuropathy. The persistence of a hypotensive action of clonidine in this patient suggested that the central α_2-receptors causing hypotension were not dependent on the integrity of baroreceptor afferent fibres (Reid *et al.* 1977).

CONCLUSIONS

Monoamines and peptides are involved both peripherally and in the central nervous system in autonomic regulation and the control of blood pressure. The demonstration of coexistence of several transmitters in the same neuron and the implications of cotransmitters, particularly NPY with adrenalin and noradrenalin, remain to be further evaluated. A range of studies strongly suggest that the catecholamines noradrenalin and adrenalin are important central neurotransmitters expressing their effect on circulatory control mainly via α_2-adrenoceptors. Clinical experiments with selective agonists and antagonists which enter the brain have supported such a role of central α_2-receptors in man. Administration of these drugs to patients with defined neurological disease or localized lesions of the brain or spinal cord indicate that in man as in animals α_2-adrenoceptors in the brainstem are an important factor in autonomic control. Recent observations suggest that several peptides, in particular NPY, encephalins, substance P, and angiotensin II in addition to monoamine and amino acid transmitters, have an important role in circulatory control in the brainstem and hypothalamus. Future experiments in man will confirm and clarify the role of these peptides in the regulation of central sympathetic and parasympathetic tone.

REFERENCES

Allen, J. M., Adrian, T. E., Polak, J. M., and Bloom, S. R. (1983). Neuropeptide Y (NPY) in the adrenal gland. *J. auton. nerv. Syst.* **9**, 559–63.

Berthelsen, S. and Pettinger, W. A. (1977). A functional basis for classification of alpha-adrenergic receptors. *Life Sci.* **21**, 595–606.

Dahlstrom, A. and Fuxe, K. (1964). Evidence for the existence of monoamine neurones in the central nervous system. I. Demonstration of monoamines in the cell bodies of brain stem neurones. *Acta physiol. scand.* **62** (Suppl. 232) 1–55.

Fitzsimmons, J. T. (1980). Angiotensin and other peptides in the control of water and sodium intake. *Proc. R. Soc.* **B210**, 165–80.

Ganong, W. F. (1984). The brain renin–angiotensin system. *Ann. Rev. Physiol.* **46**, 17–31.

Ganten, D., Lang, R. E., Lehmann, E., and Unger, T. (1984). Brain angiotensin: on the way to becoming a well studied neuropeptide system. *Biochem. Pharmacol.* **33**, 3523–8.

Henning, M. (1969). Interactions of dopa decarboxylase inhibition with the effect of alpha methyldopa on blood pressure and tissue monoamines of rats. *Acta pharmacol. tox.* **27**, 135–48.

Hilton, S. M. and Spyer, K. M. (1971). Participation of the anterior hypothalamus in the baroreceptor reflex. *J. Physiol., London* **218**, 279–93.

Hokfelt, T., Fuxe, K., Goldstein, M., and Johansson, O. (1974). Immunological evidence for the existence of adrenaline neuron in the rat brain. *Brain Res.* **66**, 235–51.

Hokfelt, T., Lundberg, J. M., Tatemoto, K., Mutt, V., Terenius, L., Polak, J., Bloom, S., Asake, C., Elde, R., and Goldstein, M. (1983). Neuropeptide Y (NPY) and FMR amide neuropeptide-like immunoreactivities in catecholamine neurons in rat medulla oblongata. *Acta physiol. scand.* **117**, 315–18.

Hossmann, V., Maling, T. J. B., Hamilton, C. A., Reid, J. L., and Dollery, C. T. (1980). Sedative and cardiovascular effects of clonidine and nitrazepam. *Clin. Pharmacol. Ther.* **28**, 167–76.

Johnson, R. H., McLellan, D. L., and Love, D. R. (1971). Orthostatic hypotension and the Holmes–Adie syndrome: a study of two patients with afferent baroreceptor block. *J. Neurol. Neurosurg.* **34**, 562–70.

Kobinger, W. and Walland, A. (1967). Investigation into the mechanism of hypotensive effect of 2, (2, 6-dichlorophenylamino)-2-imidazoline HCl. *Eur. J. Pharmacol.* **2**, 155–62.

Kreiger, D. T. (1983). Brain peptides: what, where and why? *Science* **222**, 975–84.

Langer, S. Z. (1977). Presynaptic receptors and their role in the regulation of transmitter release. *Br. J. Pharmacol.* **60**, 481–98.

Lundberg, J. M., Terenius, L., Hokfelt, T., Martling, C. R., Tatemoto, K., Mutt, V., Polak, J., Bloom, S., and Goldstein, M. (1982). Neuropeptide Y like immunoreactivity in peripheral noradrenergic neurons and effects of NPY on sympathetic function. *Acta physiol. scand.* **116**, 477–80.

Man in t'Veld, A. J., Boomsma, F., Moleman, P., and Schalekamp, M. A. D. H. (1987). Congenital dopamine beta hydroxylase deficiency: a novel orthostatic syndrome. *Lancet* **i**, 183–8.

Miach, P. J., Dausse, J. P., and Meyer, P. (1978). Direct biochemical demonstration of two types of alpha-adrenoceptor in rat brain. *Nature, London* **274**, 492.

Palkovits, M. (1980). The anatomy of central cardiovascular neurones. In *Central adrenaline neurons* (ed. K. Fuxe, M. Goldstein, T. Hokfelt, and B. Hokfelt), pp. 3–17. Pergamon Press, Oxford.

Petty, M. A. and Reid, J. L. (1981). Opiate analogs, substance P, and baroreceptor reflexes in the rabbit. *Hypertension* **3** (Suppl. 1), 142–7.

Reid, J. L. (1981). The clinical pharmacology of Clonidine and related central antihypertensive agents. *Br. J. clin. Pharmacol.* **12**, 295–302.

Reid, J. L., Mathias, C. J., Jones, D. H., and Wing, L. M. H. (1980). The contribution of central and peripheral adrenoceptors to the action of clonidine and alpha methyldopa in man. In *Central adrenaline neurons: basic aspects and their role in cardiovascular functions*, Wennergren Symposium 33 (ed. K. Fuxe, M. Goldstein, B. Hokfelt, and T. Hokfelt). Pergamon Press, Oxford.

Reid, J. L. and Rubin, P. C. (1987). Peptides and central neural regulation of the circulation. *Physiol. Rev.* **67**, 725–49.

Reid, J. L., Tangri, K. K., and Wing, L. M. H. (1977). The central hypotensive action of clonidine and propranolol in animals and man. In *Hypertension and brain mechanism* (ed. W. de Jong, A. P. Provoost, and A. P. Shapiro), Progress in Brain Research Vol. 47, pp. 369–84. North-Holland, Amsterdam.

Saavedra, N. M., del Carmine, R., Awai, J., and Alexander, N. (1979). Catecholamines in discrete areas of the rat brain in the different forms of genetic and experimental hypertension. In *Radioimmunoassay of drugs and hormones in cardiovascular medicine* (ed. M. Albertini, M. da Prada, and B. A. Peskar), pp. 199–215, North-Holland, Amsterdam.

Schaz, K., Stock, G., Simon, W., Schlor, K. H., Unger, T., Rockhold, R., and Ganten, D. (1980). Enkephalin effects on blood pressure, heart rate, and baroreceptor reflex. *Hypertension* **2**, 395–407.

Schmitt, H., Schmitt, H., and Fenard, S. (1973). Action of alpha-adrenergic blocking drugs on the sympathetic centres and their interactions with the central sympatho-inhibitory effect of clonidine. *Arzneimittel-Forsch.* **23**, 40–5.

Struyker-Boudier, H. A. J. and Beker, A. (1975). Adrenaline-induced cardiovascular changes after intrahypothalamic administration to rats. *Eur. J. Pharmacol.* **31**, 153–5.

4. Central nervous system control of the cardiovascular system

K. Michael Spyer

INTRODUCTION

During the last 20 years considerable changes have occurred in our appreciation of the role of the central nervous system in the control of the cardiovascular system as a consequence of the application of contemporary neuroanatomical and neurophysiological approaches. Formerly, this control had been thought to be exercised via a restricted 'vasomotor centre' located in the medulla oblongata (Alexander 1946) whose major function was the maintenance of arterial blood pressure. This concept held that a pool of medullary neurons determined the level of ongoing sympathetic activity through an integration of peripheral afferent inputs and descending inputs from 'higher centres' thus determining both peripheral vascular resistance and cardiac output (Alexander 1946). This model required some small modification to include the vagal component of cardiac control (see Spyer 1981 for discussion).

The location of this centre has been delineated using electrical stimulation via microelectrodes but must be viewed as an abstraction since stimulating within this same region was seen to lead to changes in general autonomic function and also in motor activity, respiration, the sleep–wakefulness cycle, etc. (see Spyer 1984 for discussion). However, the detailed cerebral transection and lesion experiments of the past century cannot be so easily dismissed and it is clear that neural elements at the bulbar level may indeed play an important role in generating vasomotor tone and mediating the cardiovascular components of behavioural responses (see later). To that extent this review will seek to identify the central substrate of cardiovascular control by, first, assessing the physiological and anatomical basis of the central organization of reflex circulatory control using the baroreceptor reflex as the main experimental model (Spyer 1981). It will then concentrate on how, and by what means, the hypothalamus and amygdala exert their influences on circulation as an integral part of behavioural activity. Finally, an attempt will be made to understand the interactions of reflex control and central drive.

THE CENTRAL ORGANIZATION OF THE BARORECEPTOR REFLEX

It is well documented that several groups of peripheral receptors contribute to the reflex control of the circulation with the role and characteristics of the baroreceptor reflex being outlined in most detail (Spyer 1981).

The primary site of interaction within the central nervous system (CNS) of most afferents with an influence on the cardiovascular system (CVS) is the nucleus of the tractus solitarius (NTS) (Spyer 1981, 1982, 1984; Jordan and Spyer 1986 for detailed reviews). Neurophysiological studies have shown that specific areas of the NTS receive an innervation from the arterial baroreceptors (Jordan and Spyer 1986) and that these same regions of the nucleus receive a variable innervation from other vagal afferents and the arterial chemoreceptors. In particular, the dorsolateral and dorsomedial regions of the NTS at levels rostral to the obex have been shown using an antidromic mapping technique to receive input from both myelinated and unmyelinated carotid-sinus baroreceptor afferents (Donoghue *et al.* 1984) and the aortic baroreceptors also send a marked input to this region (Donoghue *et al.* 1982*a*). Since the NTS receives such a patterned input from afferents arising from receptors which reflexly affect both the cardiovascular and respiratory systems (Fig. 4.1) and also receives input from many regions of the CNS, it is a potential site of integration (see Jordan and Spyer 1986 for discussion). Accordingly, interest has been aroused in elucidating the synaptic processes underlying transmission of baroreceptor inputs. The importance of these considerations resides in the fact that, while sinoaortic denervation leads to a lability in arterial pressure, destruction of the NTS leads acutely to fulminating hypertension with concomitant pulmonary oedema and chronically to maintained hypertension (see Spyer 1981 for discussion).

The majority of these neurophysiological studies have involved extracellular recordings of unit activity while stimulating electrically a number of potential afferent inputs or activating receptors with natural stimuli. An extensive survey indicated a marked convergence of input on neurons located in the vicinity of the NTS from the glossopharyngeal, carotid-sinus, aortic-depressor, and superior laryngeal nerves, although few were actually localized to the NTS (Biscoe and Sampson 1970). A limited convergence of carotid-sinus, aortic-depressor, and vagus nerve inputs specifically within the NTS has been reported. Ciriello and

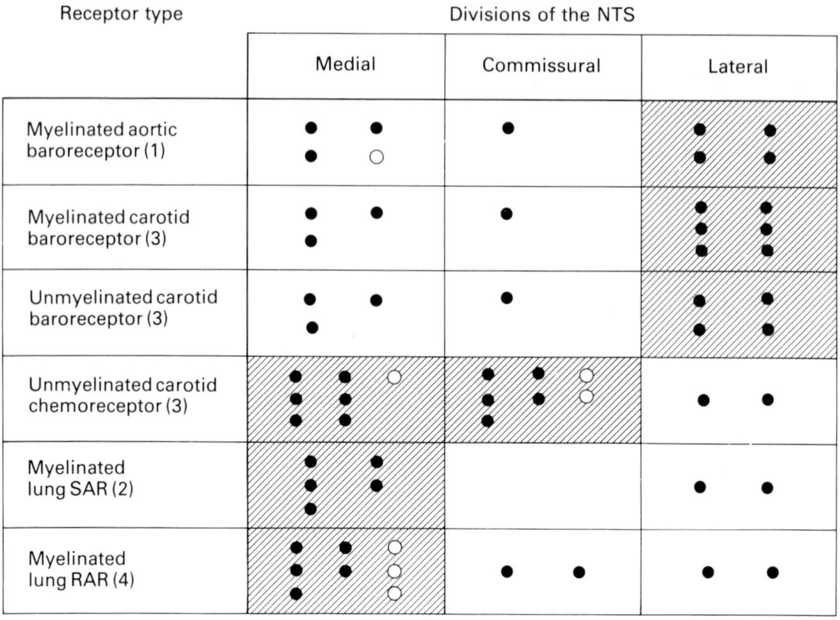

Receptor type	Divisions of the NTS: Medial	Commissural	Lateral
Myelinated aortic baroreceptor (1)	● ● ● ○	●	● ● ● ●
Myelinated carotid baroreceptor (3)	● ● ●	●	● ● ● ● ● ●
Unmyelinated carotid baroreceptor (3)	● ● ●	●	● ● ● ●
Unmyelinated carotid chemoreceptor (3)	● ● ● ● ● ● ○	● ● ● ● ● ○ ○	● ●
Myelinated lung SAR (2)	● ● ● ● ●		● ●
Myelinated lung RAR (4)	● ● ● ● ● ● ○ ○ ○	● ●	● ●

Fig. 4.1. Terminations within the cat NTS of cardiovascular and pulmonary afferents. A summary of the relative density of ipsilateral (●) and contralateral (○) regions of termination based on antidromic mapping studies. (1) Donoghue *et al.* (1982*a*); (2) Donoghue *et al.* (1982*b*); (3) Donoghue *et al.* (1984); (4) Kubin and Davies (1985). Shading represents the major projection for each afferent. SAR—slowly adapting vagal lung stretch afferent; RAR—rapidly adapting lung stretch afferent. (Reproduced with permission from Jordan and Spyer (1986).)

Calaresu (1981) have shown a significant convergence of carotid-sinus and aortic-depressor nerve inputs on neurons in the medial and lateral NTS and the interstitial nucleus. In an intracellular study, Donoghue *et al.* (1985) provided clear evidence for this form of convergence with regard to excitatory inputs but also observed inhibitory inputs of a more exclusive nature. In a more detailed intracellular study, short-latency excitatory postsynaptic potentials have been observed in NTS neurons, primarily in lateral divisions of the nucleus, evoked from carotid-sinus, aortic-depressor, and vagus nerves in neurons which were also excited by inflation of a balloon-tipped catheter within the ipsilateral carotid sinus (Mifflin *et al.* 1986*a,b*). The detailed synaptic organization of the NTS remains to be resolved; this will require a combined physiological and neuroanatomical approach.

Regarding the efferent outflow from the NTS there is considerable literature describing projections to the ventrolateral medulla; the nucleus ambiguus (NA), nucleus parabrachialis, and other midbrain regions; the spinal cord; hypothalamus; and amygdala resulting from neuroanatomical tracing studies (Loewy and Burton 1978 amongst others). The significance of many of these connections to cardiovascular control had been a matter of speculation until some very recent studies in several laboratories. The connections between NTS and NA, that have been demonstrated in several species, are responsible for the baroreceptor control of heart rate as the NA contains the cell bodies of the vagal cardioinhibitory neurons (McAllen and Spyer 1976, 1978*a,b*). In respect of the control of sympathetic outflow, there is now evidence to suggest several pathways by which the activity of sympathetic preganglionic neurons may be controlled. One of the exciting developments has been the realization that cell groups in the rostral ventrolateral medulla which may contain either adrenalin, the C1 group (Ross *et al.* 1984), or substance P (Helke *et al.* 1982) are likely to be a major source for the generation of sympathetic activity. This area in both cat (Barman and Gebber 1985) and rat (Brown and Guyunet 1985; Sun and Guyunet 1985) contains bulbospinal neurons with the appropriate slow conduction velocities (4 m/s) to account for the long central delay of the baroreceptor-sympathetic reflex. In an elegant study, Barman and Gebber (1985) demonstrated, using an antidromic mapping approach, that these descending fibres innervate the intermediolateral cell column (IML) of the thoracic spinal cord at several levels. They also showed that these neurons have a firing pattern closely correlated to the level of arterial pressure and are specifically inhibited by baroreceptor stimulation (Fig. 4.2). Their ongoing discharge has a close, and appropriate, temporal relationship with sympathetic efferent discharge. From the study of Sun and Guyenet (1985) it is likely that the baroreceptor-evoked inhibition of these neurons is mediated by gamma aminobutyric acid (GABA) and not glycine. The existence of a direct connection from the NTS to the vicinity of the C1, has been shown by Ross *et al.* (1985) who suggest that this involves a synapse on local GABA-containing interneurons. These observations, however, raise other questions. First, is this pathway from the ventrolateral medulla the sole pathway for baroreceptor control of sympathetic activity? The evidence for spinally mediated inhibition has been reviewed elsewhere (Spyer 1981). Figure 4.3 illustrates the many descending pathways that have been shown anatomically to converge on to the IML and recent neurophysiological studies have emphasized the importance of raphe-spinal pathways (Morrison and Gebber 1982; and see later). The likely role of spinal inhibition is enhanced by the fact that the catecholamines have been shown to be generally inhibitory in their actions on sympathetic preganglionic neurons, making the direct excitatory role of C1 neurons difficult to rationalize. There is, however, evidence that substance P has an excitatory action when applied iontophoretically on to sympathetic preganglionic neurons (Gilbey *et al.* 1983) and the IML contains a large

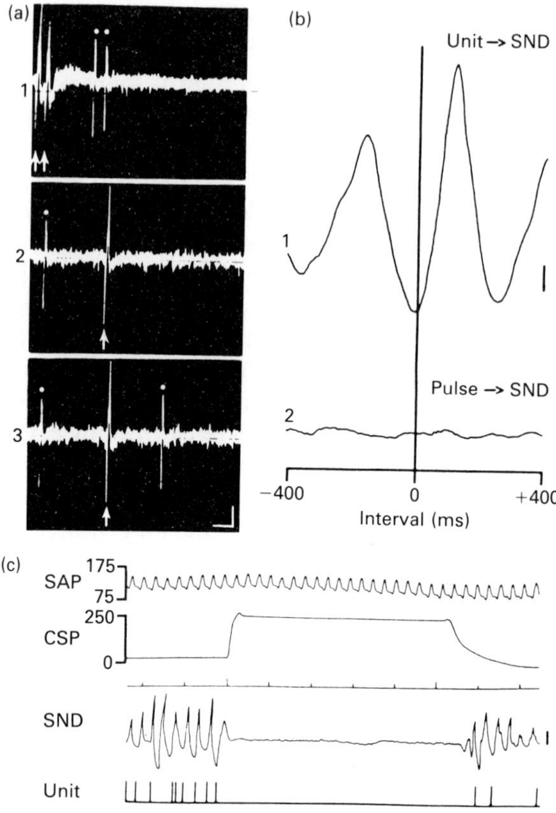

Fig. 4.2. Discharge characteristics of a ventrolateral medullospinal sympathoexcitatory neuron in a baroreceptor-innervated cat. (a) antidromic responses initiated by stimulation in grey matter of second thoracic spinal segment. Four superimposed traces appear in each panel. Dots mark spontaneous and stimulus-induced action potentials; arrows mark spinal stimuli. Panel 1, estimation of axonal refractory period with paired stimuli. Panels 2 and 3, time-controlled collision test for antidromic activation. Stimulus current was 1.5 × threshold. Horizontal calibration is 10 ms; vertical calibration is 50 μV. (b) normalized midsignal spike-triggered (panel 1) and 'dummy' (panel 2) averages of inferior cardiac sympathetic nerve discharge (SND), each based on 700 trials. Bin width is 0.8 s and vertical calibration is 30 μV. (c) baroreceptor reflex response. Traces show (top to bottom): systemic arterial pressure (SAP; mm Hg), carotid sinus pressure (CSP; mm Hg), time base (1 s/division), SND, and standardized pulses derived from action potentials of the neuron. Vertical calibration is 100 μV. (Reproduced with permission from Barman and Gebber (1985).)

number of substance-P binding sites (Takano *et al.* 1984). Current studies using an *in vitro* slice preparation of the thoracic spinal cord of the cat are beginning to resolve the complexities of the pharmacology of the synaptic regulation of sympathetic activity (Nishi *et al.* 1987). The

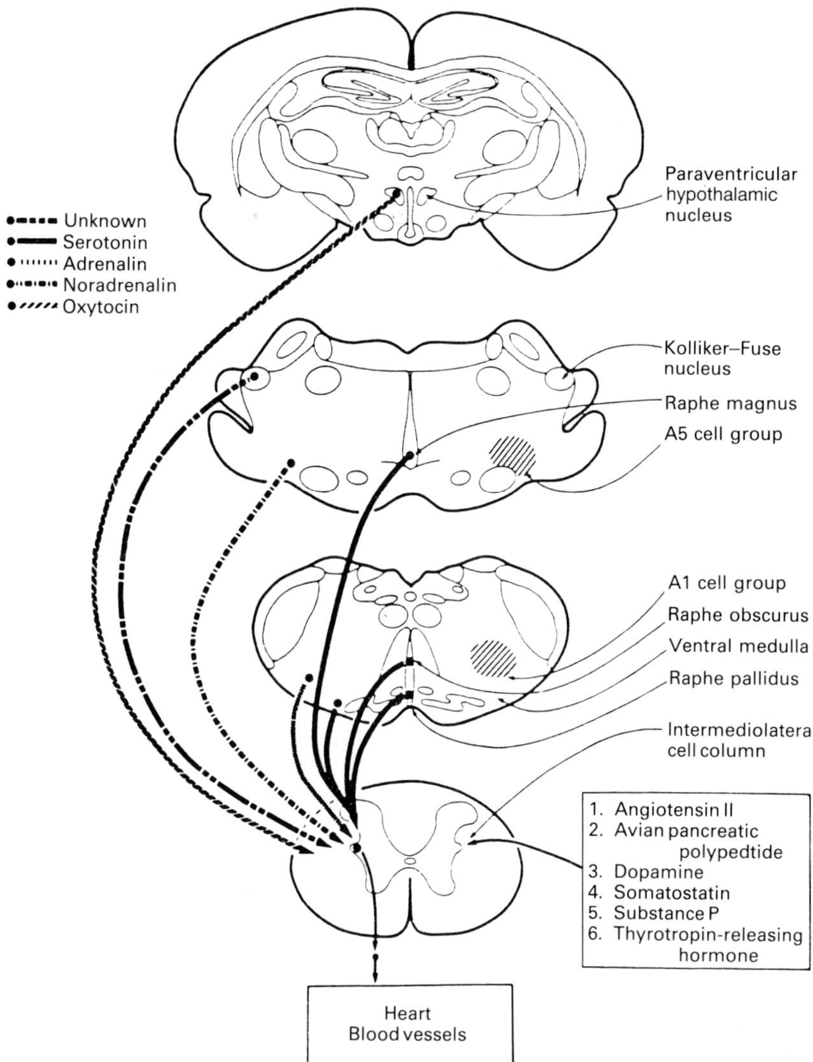

Fig. 4.3. Summary of the inputs to the intermediolateral cell column. The serotonergic inputs arise from the raphe pallidus, raphe obscurus, raphe magnus, and ventral medulla. The adrenalin input appears to arise from the region of the A1 cell group. The noradrenalin input arises from the A5 cell group. Other inputs come from the Kolliker–Fuse nucleus and paraventricular hypothalamic nucleus. The latter appears to be an oxytocin fibre system. Other neuropeptides are known to be present in the intermediolateral cell column but their site of origin is unknown. (Reproduced with permission from Loewy and Neil (1981).)

outcome of these investigations will have particular significance for the understanding of bulbospinal mechanisms mediating cardiovascular control.

The connection from the NTS to the ventrolateral medulla may also be more complicated than indicated so far since neurons in the lateral tegmental field, which are not bulbospinal, show similar properties in other respects to ventrolateral medullary neurons (Gebber and Barman 1985). Their discharge has a temporal relationship to sympathetic discharge which suggests that they may be antecedent to the C1 neurons, i.e. provide their excitatory input and so generate their ongoing cardiac rhythmicity. However, as proposed by Spyer (1981), there appears to be a marked lateralization of the baroreceptor reflex pathway within the medulla; the close association of the NA (and its action in cardiac control) with the ventrolateral medulla and its control of sympathetic efferent activity emphasizes this.

In addition to this evidence of a major sympathoexcitatory role for a bulbospinal pathway, there is also considerable evidence that additional excitatory and inhibitory pathways may arise from the raphe nuclei (Gilbey *et al.* 1981; Morrison and Gebber 1984, 1985). Morrison and Gebber (1984) describe raphe-spinal neurons with properties to be expected of those mediating excitation and inhibition. For the latter group there is now precise electrophysiological evidence that these neurons innervate the IML at thoracic levels and are excited by baroreceptor inputs (Morrison and Gebber 1985). Those raphe-spinal neurons with properties indicating a sympathoexcitatory role have not been shown to directly innervate the IML (Morrison and Gebber 1984). A proportion of raphe-spinal neurons with fine myelinated axons are known to contain 5-hydroxytryptamine (5HT). The microiontophoretic application of 5HT on to sympathetic preganglionic neurons produces excitation with few exceptions (Coote *et al.* 1981), while 5HT antagonists applied directly to the spinal cord, or intravenously, block raphe-induced inhibition of sympathetic preganglionic neurons (Gilbey *et al.* 1981). This would suggest that the raphe-spinal evoked inhibition is mediated via an inhibitory interneuron within the IML (see Gilbey *et al.* 1981) and such an interneuron role may explain the apparent discrepancy between catecholamine-containing descending pathways evoking excitation, while the catecholamines applied iontophoretically evoke inhibition (see Ross *et al.* 1983; Coote *et al.* 1981; Guyenet 1984; Spyer 1981 for discussion). The appropriate receptors for catecholamines are certainly located within the IML (Dashwood *et al.* 1985). It has a particularly dense concentration of α_2-adrenoceptors. As yet nothing is known of spinal integrative processes in the regulation of sympathetic preganglionic neuron activity, although the study of Dembowsky *et al.* (1985) using intracellular recordings from preganglionic neurons in the cat probably heralds the era where these controversies will be resolved as indicated in the elegant study of Nishi *et al.* (1987).

The connections of the baroreceptor reflex described so far have concentrated on the involvement of the medulla in its integration (Fig. 4.4). In addition, there is evidence of important suprabulbar components to the baroreceptor reflex involving midbrain and hypothalamus (see Spyer 1981 for discussion), which may imply that the other descending pathways known to innervate the IML (see Fig. 4.3) are involved in mediating the reflex control of sympathetic discharge. Whatever the resolution of this particular question, it is certain that both baroreceptor, and general, regulation of sympathetic preganglionic neuron activity involves the interplay of both descending excitatory and inhibitory inputs at the level of the IML. This becomes even more evident with the demonstration of a powerful respiratory patterning of sympathetic preganglionic neuron activity that is generated through classical respiratory pathways (Gilbey *et al.* 1986; Millhorn 1986).

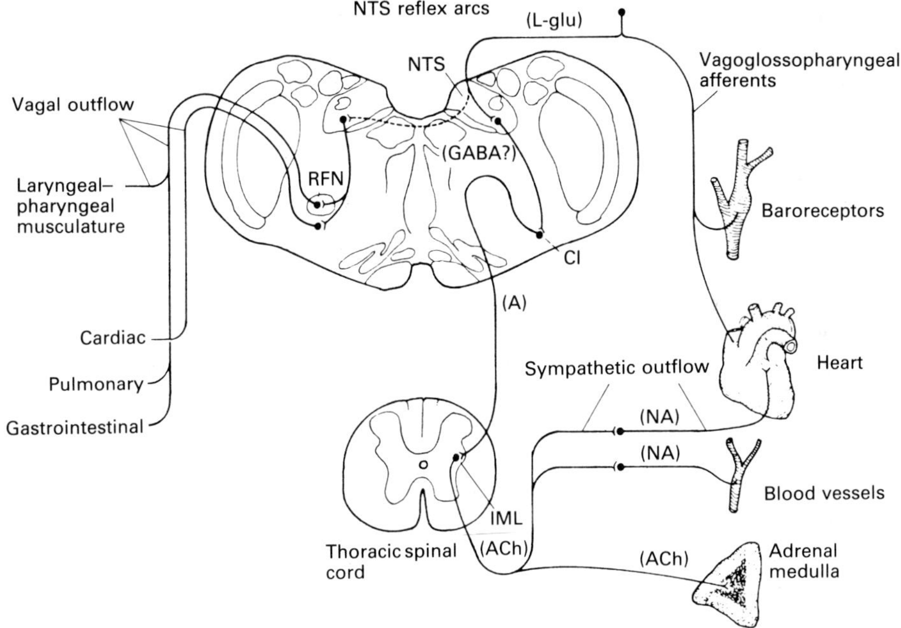

Fig. 4.4. Summary of the proposed substrates for baroreceptor and other visceral reflexes. Afferent projections in the vagal and glossopharyngeal nerves terminate in the NTS. The NTS projects (right side of the figure) to the C1 region, which in turn projects to the intermediolateral cell column (IML) of the spinal cord, controlling the sympathetic outflow. The NTS also projects (left side of the figure) to the vagal complex controlling the parasympathetic outflow. RFN, retrofascial nucleus; ACh, acetylcholine. (Reproduced with permission from Ross *et al.* (1985).)

SUPRAMEDULLARY CONTROL OF THE CARDIOVASCULAR SYSTEM

The cardiovascular system plays a pivotal role in homeostasis largely by adjusting the blood supply to various vascular beds in proportion to the level of activity in the particular organ. Basically, the nervous system achieves this by maintaining arterial pressure and regulating cardiac output in the face of different behavioural demands through the interplay of reflex inputs (see above) and central drives. To achieve the latter characteristic of cardiovascular responses, the autonomic outflows are patterned and these patterns are highly specific for the different repertoire of responses, although components may overlap in varying behavioural activities. From studies in man and experimental observations in a range of vertebrates much has been learned of the cardiovascular responses that accompany sleep, exercise (including diving), and emotional responses; yet it is only with respect to affective behaviour that we have a detailed description of the central nervous structures involved in mediating these changes. The investigations on the defence reaction in the cat by Hilton and his colleagues (see Hilton 1966) and on the 'playing-dead' or freezing response of the rabbit (Applegate *et al.* 1983) have shed considerable light on the role of the amygdala and hypothalamus in organizing these responses. These two distinct animal models of behaviour may have considerable significance in developing an understanding of the human adaptations to environmental and emotional stress.

The defence reaction

In terms of the organization of affective behaviour, the hypothalamus has long been recognized as having an essential role. Hilton (1966) emphasized the role of the perifornical region of the hypothalamus which could be activated either directly by electrical stimulation through microelectrodes or via the activation of central or peripheral afferent inputs. Similar studies have since been undertaken in a number of species (see Spyer 1984 for references). From these studies the cardiovascular pattern of response accompanying the defence reaction has been shown to involve a rise in heart rate and aortic blood flow (and hence cardiac output), a widespread vasoconstriction but a characteristic withdrawal of vasoconstrictor tone to the vasculature of skeletal muscle, and, in the cat, an activation of sympathetic cholinergic vasodilator fibres in this bed (Hilton 1966; Janig 1985) (Fig. 4.5). In all species the vasodilatation in skeletal muscle is also enhanced by an increased outpouring of catecholamines from the adrenal medulla (see Hilton 1966). Cutaneous, renal, and mesenteric blood flow is diminished and arterial pressure and pulse pressure rise dramatically (Timms 1981).

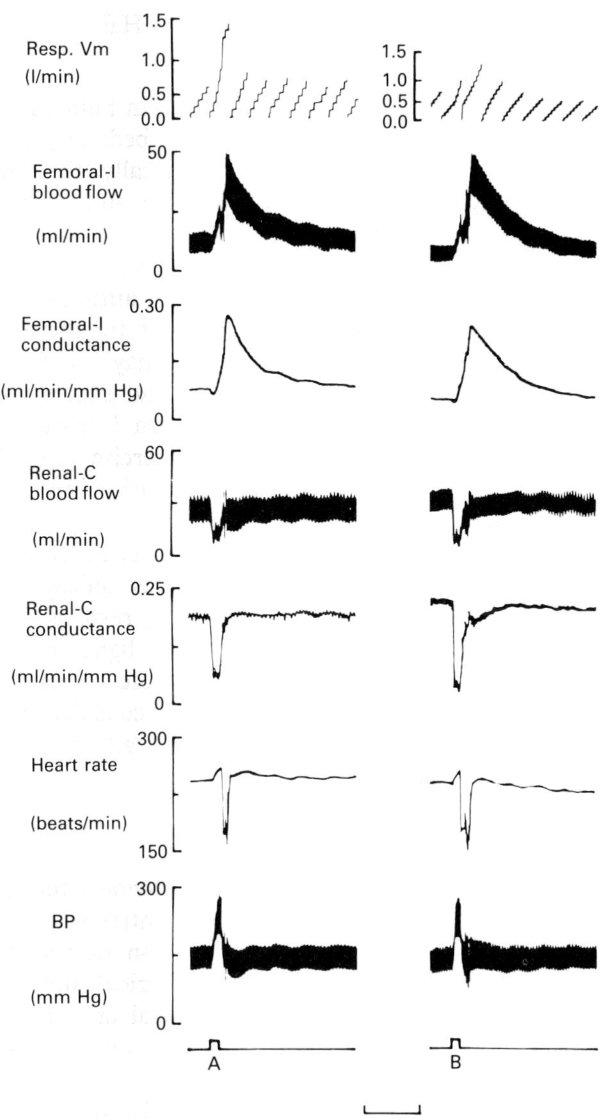

Fig. 4.5. Cat, Althesin. Comparison of the responses to stimulation in the ventral amygdalofugal pathway and in the hypothalamic defence area. Records, from above down, of respiratory minute volume (Resp. Vm), blood flow, and conductance from: femoral artery ipsilateral (I) and renal artery contralateral (C) to the sites of stimulation, heart-rate, and arterial blood pressure (BP). Stimulus markers indicate: (A) stimulation in the ventral amygdalofugal pathway for 10 s at 100 μA; (B) stimulation in the hypothalamic defence area for 8 s at 75 μA. (Reproduced with permission from Timms (1981).)

Further, under appropriate experimental conditions, a similar pattern of response can be elicited on electrical stimulation of the central nucleus of the amygdala in the cat (Timms 1981) and there is good evidence that at least a part of the forebrain control of behaviour is mediated by the amygdala which is 'afferent' to the hypothalamus (Timms 1981).

Recent studies have questioned the importance of the hypothalamus in the integration of the response (Smith *et al.* 1982). In the baboon, Smith *et al.* (1980) describe how lesions in the perifornical region abolish the cardiovascular component but spare the behavioural component of conditioned aversive responses. Equally, it has proved difficult to elicit defence responses on chemical activation of neurons in this region when applying excitant amino acids thought to activate preferentially cell bodies rather than affecting axons of passage (Smith *et al.* 1982). Accordingly, the focus of attention has moved to the amygdala (see above), and the midbrain periaqueductal grey, from where both electrical (Abrahams *et al.* 1960; Coote *et al.* 1973) and chemical (Yardley and Hilton 1986) stimulation are effective in eliciting the characteristic response.

'Playing dead' response

While stimulation in the perifornical region of the rabbit's hypothalamus may evoke similar cardiovascular responses to those seen in other species (Azevedo *et al.* 1983), affective behaviour in this species is usually associated with a bradycardia and hypotension and a suppression of motor activity—freezing or playing dead (see Applegate *et al.* 1983). This is accompanied by rapid shallow breathing. This is the characteristic response that can also be evoked from the central nucleus of the amygdala (CEN) in both anaesthetized (Kapp *et al.* 1982) and conscious preparations (Applegate *et al.* 1983; Pascoe and Kapp 1984).

EFFERENT PATHWAYS FOR AFFECTIVE BEHAVIOUR

In considering the organization of the patterning of cardiovascular activity in relation to behaviour it is necessary to review the neuroanatomical pathways that mediate autonomic outflow (see Fig. 4.6). It is probably easiest to begin with the connection of the CEN which is known to provide both an afferent input to the hypothalamus (Timms 1981 for review) and descending connections beyond. The CEN directly innervates the midbrain, Kolliker–Fuse nucleus, the NTS, dorsal vagal nucleus, and NA with the heaviest innervation being to the dorsomedial NTS in the rabbit (Schwaber *et al.* 1982). Reciprocal connections

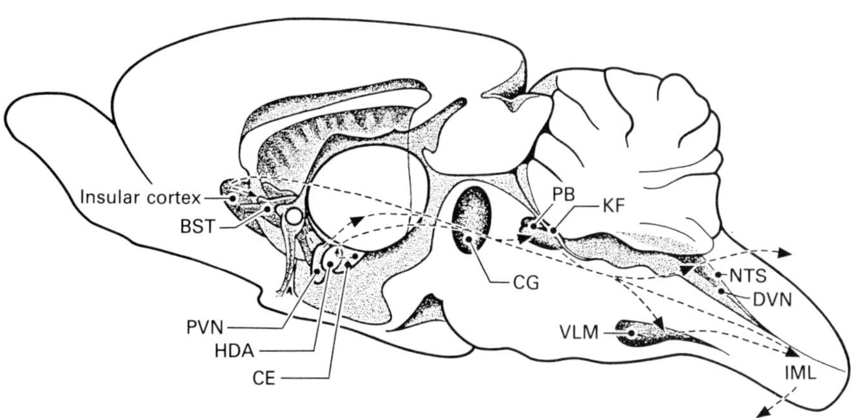

Fig. 4.6. Diagrammatic representation of the descending pathways in the rat that are responsible for the cardiovascular component of affective behaviour. For simplicity, the dorsal vagal nucleus (DVN) is used for the source of cardioinhibitory output although the nucleus ambiguus is in many species the source of this output. BST, bed nucleus of the stria terminalis; CE, central nucleus of amygdala; CG, central gram; DVN, dorsal vagal nucleus; HDA, hypothalamic defence area; IML, intermediolateral cell column of thoracic spinal cord; KF, Kolliker–Fuse nucleus; NTS, nucleus tractus solitarius; PB, parabrachial nucleus; PVN, paraventricular nucleus; VLM, ventrolateral medulla (see text for additional information).

between the NTS and CEN have been demonstrated (Hopkins and Holstege 1978). The descending connections of the hypothalamic defence areas have been mapped electrophysiologically and include the periaqueductal grey (see above) and a dorsal strip running through the pons and medulla (Coote *et al.* 1973) but also a separate pathway pursuing a ventral course (Hilton 1966, 1980). This latter pathway appears to involve a synapse close to the ventral surface of the medulla, probably amongst a population of bulbospinal neurons (McAllen *et al.* 1982; Guyenet 1984) which may be equivalent to those that have been implicated as generating vasomotor 'tone' and which are in part involved in mediating baroreceptor control of sympathetic activity as described above.

There also may be several connections with the pathways indicated in Fig. 4.3 as innervating the IML, including those descending from the paraventricular nucleus containing neurophysins and oxytocin. This is not an exhaustive list of potential connections involved in mediating these responses. Other pathways have been demonstrated with neuroanatomical tracing techniques to descend from several areas of the hypothalamus to the spinal cord (Kuypers 1981) although a direct role for these in cardiovascular control remains to be discerned. However, the potential to influence the activity of the sympathetic outflow through anatomically defined pathways is now firmly established. Further, there is ample evidence of influences on the dorsal vagal nucleus and NA—both direct and indirect—resulting from activation of disencephalic structures organizing affective behaviour (Schwaber *et al.* 1982; Cox *et al.* 1986; among others). The third mechanism by which a control of the cardiovascular system may be exerted is through a modulation of cardiovascular reflexes at the level of the NTS.

REFLEX MODIFICATION

One of the striking features of the defence reaction elicited on electrical stimulation of the hypothalamus and amygdala in the cat is the concomitant rise in arterial pressure and heart rate (Hilton 1966). This suggested a central suppression of the baroreceptor reflex (Hilton 1963; Coote *et al.* 1973). In part, this may be a consequence of the increase in respiratory activity that is evoked which effectively exerts a profound inhibition of cardiac vagal efferent motoneurons to block the cardiac component of the reflex (Spyer 1982; for detailed discussion, 1984). In contrast, in the rabbit, the bradycardia and hypotension resulting from CEN stimulation appear to involve a modulation of the baroreceptor reflex (Cox *et al.* 1986). The most obvious site for the interactions resulting in these modifications of the reflex has been suggested to be the NTS. In the cat, McAllen and Spyer (1976) provided evidence that stimulation within the hypothalamus can inhibit the activity of neurons in the vicinity of the NTS which receive excitatory inputs from the sinus nerve and arterial baroreceptors. The specificity of this mechanism has been the subject of an extensive experimental review undertaken in both cat and rabbit (Cox *et al.* 1986; Mifflin *et al.* 1986*a*) involving both intra- and extracellular recordings from neurons located within the NTS.

Taking the study in the rabbit first, stimulating within the CEN at sites evoking the characteristic bradycardia and hypotension excited NTS neurons receiving an excitatory input from the aortic depressor nerve (Cox *et al.* 1986). These convergent excitatory responses (Fig. 4.7) were consistent with the neuroanatomical demonstration that amygdalofugal pathways provide a relatively dense innervation of the dorsomedial NTS, in a region which also receives an overlapping aortic depressor nerve input (Higgins and Schwaber 1983). A similar pattern of excitatory convergence was also seen in respect to vagal neurons in the dorsal vagal nucleus, in the case of those considered to be cardioinhibitory and also those without cardiac function (Cox *et al.* 1986). It is probable that the major influence of the CEN on cardioinhibitory neurons is mediated, however, via the NTS since its innervation of the dorsal vagal nucleus is sparse and restricted to regions of the dorsal vagal nucleus which do not contain cardioinhibitory neurons (Schwaber *et al.* 1982; Jordan *et al.*

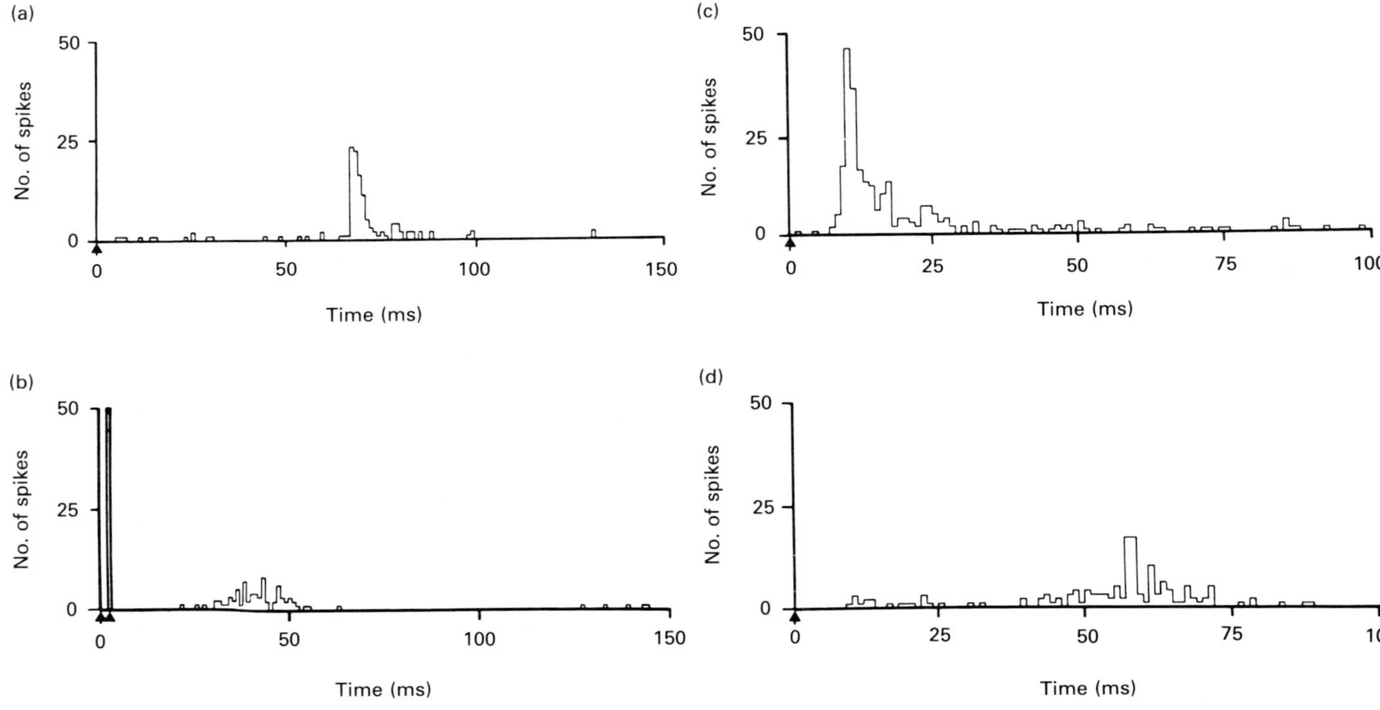

Fig. 4.7. Post-stimulus time histogram of spike activity recorded in two NTS neurons (a and b; c and d). On the left and right, respectively, are the responses of the two neurons to stimulation of the aortic nerve (a and c) and central nucleus (b and d) at ▲. Each histogram consists of 100 sweeps, 1 ms bins; 150 bins in (a) and (b), 100 bins in (c) and (d). Stimuli to the aortic nerve were single 0.1-ms pulses given at 1 Hz, 7 V in (a) and 15 V in (c). Stimuli to the central nucleus were given at 1 Hz, two pulses, 0.2 ms at 100 μA in (b) and one pulse, 0.1 ms at 150 μA in (d). (Reproduced with permission from Cox *et al.* (1986).)

1982). This suggests that, in part, the cardiovascular responses evoked from the CEN are mediated through accessing, and modulating, the baroreceptors reflex at a synapse, or synapses, early in the central pathway.

In contrast to this facilitatory innervation, observations in the cat confirm the inhibitory influence of diencephalic stimulation on NTS neurons that had been indicated in earlier studies. Neurons within the NTS receiving short-latency inputs from the sinus, aortic, and vagal nerves were inhibited on stimulation within the hypothalamic defence area, and the amygdalofugal pathway as it passes over the optic tract into the hypothalamus (Mifflin *et al.* 1986*a*; Spyer *et al.* 1987). From intracellular recordings it was shown that an inhibitory postsynaptic potential was evoked in these neurons with an onset latency of around 10 ms and that, with temporal and spatial summation, this could last for 150–220 ms (Fig. 4.8). It effectively suppressed the excitatory influences evoked from sinus, aortic, and vagal nerves and, more specifically, this occurred in every neuron shown to receive a specific baroreceptor input on inflation of a balloon-tipped catheter in the ipsilateral carotid sinus. Stimulating at sites in the hypothalamus which did not evoke a block of the baroreceptor reflex, although exerting significant cardiovascular effects, was ineffective in suppressing the action of excitatory inputs from the sinus nerves and arterial baroreceptors in the vast majority of

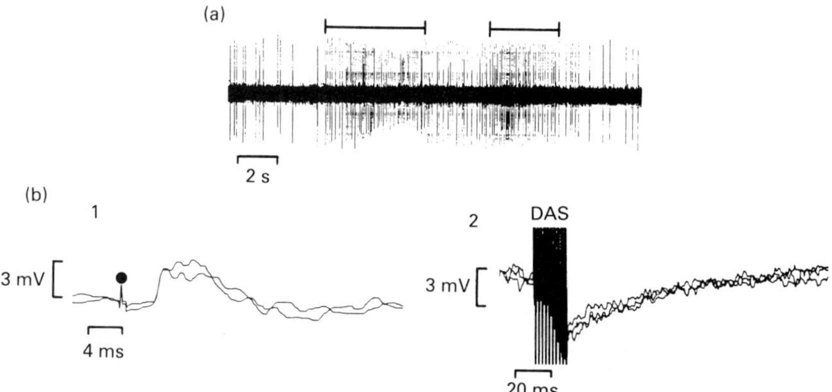

Fig. 4.8. Response of unit with carotid sinus baroreceptor input to defence area stimulation (DAS). (a) Extracellularly recorded increase in action potential discharge evoked by stimulation of the carotid sinus baroreceptors. The inflations of the intrasinus balloon are indicated by the bars above the neurogram unit recording. (b) Intracellularly recorded responses of the same unit to: (1) electrical stimulation of the carotid sinus nerve (stimulus artefact indicated by filled circle): two sweeps superimposed; (2) electrical stimulation of the hypothalamic defence area. The hypothalamus was stimulated for 20 ms, 500 Hz, 1-ms pulses of 120 μA during the period indicated by the DAS. Three sweeps superimposed. (Reproduced by permission from Spyer *et al.* (1987).)

cases. In addition, a significant number of neurons were identified in the NTS which were inhibited by the activation of the arterial baroreceptors but, conversely, excited on stimulation within the hypothalamic 'defence area'. One could speculate that these represent interneurons mediating the inhibition of the former population. These data provide an insight into the neural substrate through which the effectiveness of the baroreceptor reflex may be modified in relation to emotion.

In other studies, the influence of such hypothalamic stimulation on the activity of medullary respiratory neurons has indicated powerful inhibitory actions on expiratory neurons, and the alteration of the balance of both inhibitory and excitatory influences on inspiratory neurons. It is well documented that hypothalamic stimulation in the cat inhibits vagal cardioinhibitory neurons and evidence in favour of a relatively direct inhibition of these has been obtained (Spyer 1984). It is clear that part of this vagal inhibition may also result from disfacilitation through the action of diencephalic descending inputs acting at the level of the NTS. The nature and sites of action of diencephalic outputs on the sympathetic outflow remain to be elucidated.

CARDIORESPIRATORY INTERACTIONS

There is a body of evidence in the literature indicating an extensive interaction between reflexes in the moment-by-moment regulation of the cardiovascular and respiratory systems (see Daly 1985). Indeed, the influences exerted by these inputs cannot be explained by a simple algebraic summation of their individual effects but involve a complex, and as yet unresolved, set of interactions at a synaptic level, or levels, within the central nervous system. The non-linearities of both postganglionic sympathetic and vagal actions on their appropriate effectors may provide an additional contribution to this situation. As yet, relatively little is known of the nature of the central processes underlying these interactions, although some recent studies reviewed above and others from a number of different laboratories are beginning to shed some light on the basic mechanisms of integration. Notwithstanding this deficit, it has emerged from numerous studies that respiration can markedly modify the performance of both cardiovascular and respiratory reflexes; these studies are now providing some important clues in the unravelling of the action of the central nervous system in cardiovascular regulation.

The fundamental observations that led to the current interest in this field can be attributed to Anrep and his colleagues (Anrep *et al.* 1936*a*, *b*) who demonstrated that sinus arrhythmia was the consequence of a respiratory control of the vagal outflow to heart. Anrep *et al.* (1936*a*, *b*) identified that two factors were responsible for this—one due to the central generation of respiratory activity, the second as a consequence of reflexes evoked during respiratory movements.

Electrophysiological studies in the cat have now identified the nature of the central mechanism and have shown it to be specifically related to inspiratory activity (Gilbey *et al.* 1984). In this study vagal cardiomotor neurons of the NA were shown to be actively hyperpolarized during inspiration by a wave of Cl^- dependent inhibitory postsynaptic potentials (Fig. 4.9). This resulted in a fall of membrane input resistance of sufficient magnitude to effectively shunt the excitatory influences of the arterial baroreceptors. Hence, any influence which increases inspiratory drive will lead by this process both to a suppression of vagal efferent discharge and a reduced sensitivity of these neurons to excitatory input, and, thus, will result in tachycardia. There is also a profound influence of central respiratory activity on the discharge of sympathetic efferents. This patterning of their discharge is certainly more complicated than the

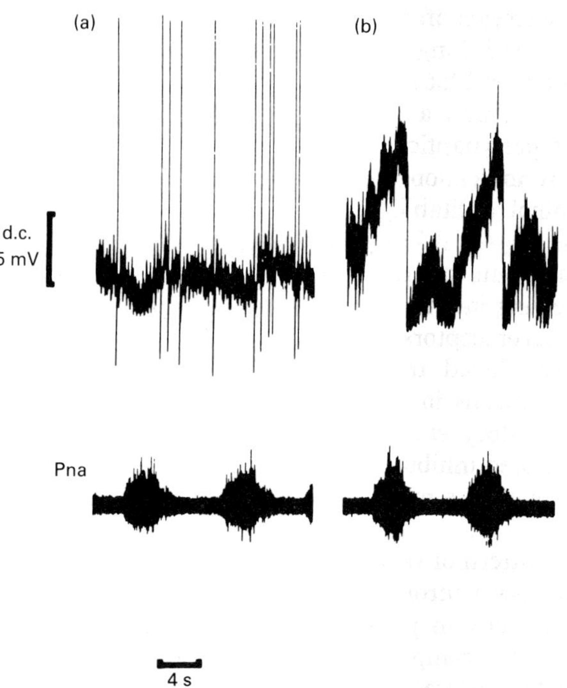

Fig. 4.9. Intracellular recording from a cardiovascular motoneuron showing changes in membrane potential in relation to phrenic nerve activity (a). Passage of negative hyperpolarizing current (1 nA for 3 min) resulted in reversal of the hyperpolarizing waves. Record (b) was taken after current injection ended. In each panel traces from above: high-gain d.c. recording of membrane potential and phrenic nerve activity (Pna). (Reproduced with permission from Gilbey *et al.* (1986).)

homogeneous influence on cardiomotor neurons since individual sympathetic pre- and postganglionic neurons exhibit distinctly different patterns of discharge with respect to respiration (Janig 1985; Gilbey *et al.* 1986). In this respect there is now evidence that the inspiratory component of sympathetic discharge is mediated by the activity of medullary inspiratory neurons (Millhorn 1986).

The suppressive action of lung inflation inputs on reflexly evoked bradycardias is well characterized (Daly 1985) but the central site of action of slowly adapting vagal lung stretch afferents has yet to be discerned. From a study investigating the influence of this input on baroreceptor-evoked vagal discharge, Potter (1981) suggested that lung inflation was effective in inhibiting vagal activity only when vagal tone was high and only then when discharge was evoked by baroreceptor stimulation, the input failing to affect ongoing activity. Conversely, inspiratory activity was effective in suppressing both components of vagal activity.

Recent electrophysiological studies have failed to reveal the site of action of lung stretch afferents. In these the premise was that, since both baroreceptors and lung stretch afferents terminate within the NTS (Jordan and Spyer 1986), this might be the site of interaction since this nucleus also contains a major population of inspiratory neurons. No evidence of a presynaptic interaction of these afferents was revealed nor was there any indication of an influence of central respiratory activity on the terminal excitability of baroreceptors afferents (Richter *et al.* 1986). Subsequently, it has proved impossible to reveal any influence of lung stretch inputs on the activity, or membrane potential, of NTS neurons receiving inputs, excitatory or inhibitory, from the sinus nerves and arterial baroreceptors within the NTS (Mifflin *et al.* 1986*b*). Since we had previously failed to observe changes in membrane potential in cardiomotor neurons in relation to lung inflation (McAllen and Spyer 1976, 1978*a*; Gilbey *et al.* 1984), their activity being dominated by the inspiratory-related inhibition described above, it appears that any action of lung stretch inputs must be mediated at sites between the NTS and NA.

The firing pattern of vagal cardiomotor neurons resembles closely that of postinspiratory neurons of the medulla described by Richter (1982) which show activity in phase with the discharge of phrenic nerve that continues after the ramp inspiratory discharge. This is known as Stage 1 expiration, which precedes activity in expiratory motoneurons. As with postinspiratory neurons, cardiomotor neurons are particularly sensitive to inputs from irritant receptors in the airways and may be excited on electrical stimulation of the superior laryngeal nerve (Lopes and Palmer 1976). Such stimulation evokes a prolonged respiratory pause with continuing activity in the phrenic nerve and a vagal bradycardia. This may provide at least one potential source for the hazardous consequence of periods of apnoea; should such an event occur, cardiomotor neurons will be in a heightened state of excitability so that any other concomitant input, such as an input from the arterial chemoreceptors, could then evoke a potentially fatal bradycardia (see Daly 1985). This might form at least one facet in the aetiology of the sudden infant death syndrome.

Aside from providing, at least a plausible, explanation for this syndrome, the apparently tight coupling of cardiac control to respiratory activity that this neural mechanism ensures has major physiological consequences. It provides an immediate mechanism to match cardiac output to respiratory minute volume in such diverse situations as exercise and breath-hold diving. The underlying neural processes so far considered thus provide a framework on which to base further studies into the central nervous control of the circulation.

CONCLUSIONS

In endeavouring to provide a contemporary analysis of the central nervous control of the cardiovascular system, this review has been restricted to an assessment of the organization and control of the baroreceptor reflex since this appears the most appropriate physiological model for which a body of data exists. The neuroanatomical pathways mediating the reflex have been reviewed and the underlying synaptic mechanisms described. It is clear that the central nervous system exerts its control of the circulation in relationship to behaviour in part through a modification of the performance of reflexes that are responsible for homeostatic regulation. This is partially organized by controlling transmission at stages early in the reflex pathway and secondarily by actions at the level of the autonomic preganglionic neurons. In addition, the demonstration of powerful synaptic coupling of respiratory activity to autonomic preganglionic neurons ensures that any evoked changes in respiration elicit appropriate, and immediate, responses in the cardiovascular system.

These observations indicate that the central nervous system exerts its control over autonomic function, and specifically the cardiovascular system, in a manner analogous to the way in which motor activities are controlled. In particular, the modification of reflex action which can be exerted by rostral brainstem and cortical areas may provide an indication of potential mechanisms whereby stress and emotion can cause profound changes in the cardiovascular system. Whether the acute, and clearly reversible, changes of the type reviewed above may be converted on repetition to prolonged and irreversible alterations remain to be investigated.

Acknowledgements

The financial support of the Medical Research Council and British Heart Foundation is gratefully acknowledged.

REFERENCES

Abrahams, V. C., Hilton, S. M., and Zbrozyna, A. (1960). Active muscle vasodilatation produced by stimulation of the brain stem: its significance in the defence reaction. *J. Physiol.* **154**, 491–513.

Alexander, R. S. (1946). Tonic and reflex functions of medullary sympathetic cardiovascular centres. *J. Neurophysiol.* **9**, 205–17.

Anrep, G. V., Pascual, W., and Rössler, R. (1936*a*). Respiratory variations of heart rate. I. The reflex mechanism of the respiratory arrhythmia. *Proc. R. Soc., London* **B119**, 191–217.

Anrep, G. V., Pascual, W., and Rössler, R. (1936*b*). Respiratory variations of heart rate. II. The central mechanism of respiratory arrhythmia and the inter-relationships between central and reflex mechanisms. *Proc. R. Soc., London* **B119**, 218–30.

Applegate, C. D., Kapp, B. S., Underwood, M. D., and McNall, C. L. (1983). Autonomic and somatomotor effects of amygdala central nucleus stimulation in awake rabbits. *Physiol. Behav.* **31**, 353–60.

Azevedo, A. D., Hilton, S. M., and Timms, R. J. (1983). The defence reaction elicited by midbrain and hypothalamic stimulation in the rabbit. *J. Physiol.* **301**, 56–7.

Barman, S. M. and Gebber, G. L. (1985). Axonal projection patterns of ventrolateral medullospinal sympathoexcitatory neurons. *J. Neurophysiol.* **53**, 1551–66.

Biscoe, T. J. and Sampson, S. R. (1970). Responses of cells in the brain stem of the cat to stimulation of the sinus, glosso-pharyngeal aortic and superior laryngeal nerves. *J. Physiol.* **209**, 359–73.

Brown, D. L. and Guyunet, P. G. (1985). Electrophysiological study of cardiovascular neurons in the rostral ventrolateral medulla in rats. *Circulation Res.* **56**, 359–69.

Ciriello, J. and Calaresu, F. R. (1981). Projections from buffer nerves to the nucleus of the solitary tract: an anatomical and electrophysiological study in the cat. *J. autonom. nerv. Syst.* **3**, 299–310.

Coote, J. H., Hilton, S. M., and Zbrozyna, A. W. (1973). The ponto-medullary area integrating the defence reaction in the cat and its influence on muscle blood flow. *J. Physiol.* **229**, 257–74.

Coote, J. H., Macleod, V. H., Fleetwood-Walker, S., and Gilbey, M. P. (1981). The response of individual sympathetic preganglionic neurons to microelectrophoretically applied endogenous monoamines. *Brain Res.* **213**, 135–45.

Cox, G. E., Jordan, D., Moruzzi, P., Schwaber, J. S., Spyer, K. M., and Turner, S. A. (1986). Amygdaloid influences on brainstem neurones in the rabbit. *J. Physiol.* **381**, 135–48.

Daly, M. de Burgh (1985). Interactions between respiration and circulation. In *Handbook of physiology—the respiratory system II*, Chapter 16, pp. 529–94. American Physiological Society, Bethesda, Maryland.

Dashwood, M. R., Gilbey, M. P., and Spyer, K. M. (1985). The localization of adrenoceptors and opiate receptors in regions of the cat central nervous system involved in cardiovascular control. *Neuroscience* **15**, 537–51.

Dembowsky, K., Czachurski, J., and Seller, H. (1985). Morphology of sympathetic preganglionic neurons in the thoracic spinal cord of the cat: An intracellular horseradish peroxidase study. *J. comp. Neurol.* **238**, 453–65.

Donoghue, S., Felder, R. B., Gilbey, M. P., Jordan, D., and Spyer, K. M. (1985). Post-synaptic activity evoked in the nucleus tractus solitarius by carotid sinus and aortic nerve afferents in the cat. *J. Physiol.* **360**, 261–73.

Donoghue, S., Felder, R. B., Jordan, D., and Spyer, K. M. (1984). The central projections of carotid baroreceptors and chemoreceptors in the cat: a neurophysiological study. *J. Physiol.* **347**, 397–410.

Donoghue, S., Garcia, M., Jordan, D., and Spyer, K. M. (1982*a*). Identification and brain-stem projections of aortic baroreceptor afferent neurones in nodose ganglia of cats and rabbits. *J. Physiol.* **322**, 337–52.

Donoghue, S., Garcia, M., Jordan, D., and Spyer, K. M. (1982*b*). The brain-stem projections of pulmonary stretch afferent neurones in cats and rabbits. *J. Physiol.* **322**, 353–63.

Gebber, G. L. and Barman, S. M. (1985). Lateral tegmental field neurons of cat medulla: a potential source of basal sympathetic nerve discharge. *J. Neurophysiol.* **54**, 1498–512.

Gilbey, M. P., Coote, J. H., Macleod, V. H., and Peterson, D. F. (1981). Inhibition of sympathetic nerve activity by stimulating in the raphe nuclei and the role of 5-hydroxytryptamine in this effect. *Brain Res.* **226**, 131–42.

Gilbey, M. P., Jordan, D., Richter, D. W., and Spyer, K. M. (1984). Synaptic mechanisms involved in the inspiratory modulation of vagal cardio-inhibitory neurones in the cat. *J. Physiol.* **356**, 65–78.

Gilbey, M. P., McKenna, K. E., and Schramm, L. P. (1983). Effects of substance P on sympathetic preganglionic neurones. *Neurosci. Lett.* **41**, 157–9.

Gilbey, M. P., Numao, Y., and Spyer, K. M. (1986). Discharge patterns of cervical sympathetic preganglionic neurones related to central respiratory drive in the rat. *J. Physiol.* **378**, 253–65.

Guyenet, P. G. (1984). Baroreceptor-mediated inhibition of A5 noradrenergic neurons. *Brain Res.* **303**, 31–40.

Helke, C. J., Neil, J. J., Massari, V. J., and Loewy, A. D. (1982). Substance P neurons project from the ventral medulla to the intermediolateral cell column in the rat. *Brain Res.* **243**, 147–52.

Higgins, G. A. and Schwaber, J. S. (1983). Somatostatinergic projections from the central nucleus of the amygdala ot the vagal nuclei. *Peptides* **4**, 657–62.

Hilton, S. M. (1963). Inhibition of baroreceptor reflexes on hypothalamic stimulation. *J. Physiol.* **165**, 56–7.

Hilton, S. M. (1966). Hypothalamic regulation of the cardiovascular system. *Br. med. Bull.* **22**, 243–8.

Hilton, S. M. (1980). Central nervous origin of vasomotor tone. In *Cardiovascular physiology, heart, peripheral circulation and methodology. Advances in Physiological Sciences*, Vol. 8, pp. 1–11. Pergamon, Oxford.

Hopkins, D. A. and Holstege, G. (1978). Amygdaloid projections to the mesencephalon, pons and medulla oblongata in the cat. *Exp. Brain Res.* **32**, 529–47.

Janig, W. (1985). Organization of the lumbar sympathetic outflow to skeletal muscle and skin of the cat hindlimb and tail. *Rev. Physiol., Biochem., Pharmacol.* **102**, 119–213.

Jordan, D., Khalid, M. E. M., Schneiderman, N., and Spyer, K. M. (1982). The location and properties of preganglionic vagal cardiomotor neurones in the rabbit. *Pflüger's Arch.* **395**, 244–50.

Jordan, D. and Spyer, K. M. (1986). Brainstem integration of cardiovascular and pulmonary afferent activity. In *Progress in brain research*, Vol. 67 (ed. F. Cervero and J. F. B. Morrison), pp. 295–314. Elsevier Science Publishers, Amsterdam.

Kapp, B. S., Gallagher, M., Underwood, M. D., McNall, C. C., and Whitehorn, D. (1982). Cardiovascular responses elicited by electrical stimulation of the amygdala central nucleus in the rabbit. *Brain Res.* **234**, 251–62.

Kubin, L. and Davies, R. O. (1985). In *Neurogenesis of central respiratory rhythm* (ed. A. L. Bianchi and M. Denavit-Saubie), pp. 262–5. MTP Press Ltd, Lancaster.

Kuypers, H. G. J. M. (1981). Anatomy of descending pathways. In *Handbook of Physiology, The Nervous System. Motor Control*, Section 1, Vol. 11, Pt. 1, Chapter 13, pp. 597–666. American Physiology Society, Bethesda, Maryland.

Loewy, A. D. and Burton, H. (1978). Nuclei of the solitary tract; efferent projection to the lower brainstem and spinal cord of the cat. *J. comp. Neurol.* **181**, 421–50.

Loewy, A. D. and Neil, J. J. (1981). The role of descending monoaminergic systems in central control of blood pressure. *Fed. Proc.* **40**, 2278–85.

Lopes, O. U. and Palmer, J. F. (1976). Proposed respiratory 'gating' mechanism for cardiac slowing. *Nature* **264**, 454–6.

McAllen, R. M., Neil, J. J., and Loewy, A. D. (1982). Effects of kainic acid applied to the ventral surface of the medulla oblongata on vasomotor tone, the baroreceptor reflex and hypothalamic autonomic responses. *Brain Res.* **238**, 65–70.

McAllen, R. M. and Spyer, K. M. (1976). The location of cardiac vagal preganglionic motoneurones in the medulla of the cat. *J. Physiol.* **258**, 187–204.

McAllen, R. M. and Spyer, K. M. (1978*a*). Two types of vagal preganglionic motoneurones projecting to the heart and lungs. *J. Physiol.* **282**, 353–64.

McAllen, R. M. and Spyer, K. M. (1978*b*). The baroreceptor input to cardiac vagal motoneurones. *J. Physiol.* **282**, 365–74.

Mifflin, S. W., Spyer, K. M., and Withington-Wray, D. J. (1986*a*). Hypothalamic inhibition of baroreceptor inputs in the nucleus of the tractus solitarius of the cat. *J. Physiol.* **373**, 58P.

Mifflin, S. W., Spyer, K. M., and Withington-Wray, D. J. (1986*b*). Lack of respiratory modulation of baroreceptor inputs in the nucleus of the tractus solitarius of the cat. *J. Physiol.* **376**, 33P.

Millhorn, D. E. (1986). Neural respiratory and circulatory interaction during chemoreceptor stimulation and cooling of ventral medulla in cats. *J. Physiol.* **370**, 217–31.

Morrison, S. F. and Gebber, G. L. (1982). Classification of raphe neurons with cardiac-related activity. *Am. J. Physiol.* **243**, R49–R59.

Morrison, S. F. and Gebber, G. L. (1984). Raphe neurons with sypathetic-related activity: baroreceptor responses and spinal connections. *Am. J. Physiol.* **246**, R338–R348.

Morrison, S. F. and Gebber, G. L. (1985). Axonal branching patterns and funicular trajectories of raphe spinal sympathoinhibitory neurons. *J. Neurophysiol.* **53**, 759–72.

Nishi, S., Yoshimura, M., and Polosa, C. (1987). Synaptic potentials and putative transmitter actions in sympathetic preganglionic neurons. In *Organisation of the autonomic nervous system: central and peripheral mechanisms* (ed. J. Ciriello, F. R. Calaresu, and C. Polosa), pp. 15–26. Alan R. Liss, New York.

Pascoe, J. P. and Kapp, B. S. (1984). Electrophysiological characteristics of amygdaloid central nucleus neurons during Pavlovian fear conditioning in the rabbit. *Behav. brain res.* **16**, 117–33.

Potter, E. K. (1981). Inspiratory inhibition of vagal responses to baroreceptor and chemoreceptor stimuli in the dog. *J. Physiol.* **316**, 177–90.

Richter, D. W. (1982). Generation and maintenance of the respiratory rhythm. *J. exp. Biol.* **100**, 93–107.

Richter, D. W., Jordan, D., Ballantyne, D., Meesmann, M., and Spyer, K. M. (1986). Presynaptic depolarization in myelinated vagal afferent fibres terminating in the nucleus of the tractus solitarius in the cat. *Pflüger's Arch.* **406**, 12–19.

Ross, C. A., Ruggiero, D. A., Joh, T. H., Park, D. H., and Reis, D. J. (1983). Adrenaline synthesizing neurons in the rostral ventrolateral medulla: a possible role in tonic vasomotor control. *Brain Res.* **273**, 356–61.

Ross, C. A., Ruggiero, D. A., Joh, T. H., Park, D. H., and Reis, D. J. (1984). Rostral ventrolateral medulla: selective projections to the thoracic autonomic cell column from the region containing C1 adrenaline neurons. *J. comp. Neurol.* **228**, 168–85.

Ross, C. A., Ruggiero, D. A., and Reis, D. J. (1985). Projections from the nucleus tractus solitarii to the rostral ventrolateral medulla. *J. comp. Neurol.* **242**, 511–34.

Schwaber, J. S., Kapp, B. S., Higgins, G. A., and Rapp, P. R. (1982). Amygdaloid and basal forebrain direct connections with the nucleus of the solitary tract and the dorsal motor nucleus. *J. Neurosci.* **2**(10), 1424–38.

Smith, O. A., Astley, C. A., De Vito, J. L., Stein, J. M., and Walsh, K. E. (1980). Functional analysis of hypothalamic control of cardiovascular responses accompanying emotional behaviour. *Fed. Proc.* **39**, 2487–94.

Smith, O. A., De Vito, J. L., and Astley, C. A. (1982). The hypothalamus in emotional behaviour and associated cardiovascular correlates. In *Changing concepts of the nervous system* (ed. Morrison and Struck), pp. 569–84. Academic Press, New York.

Spyer, K. M. (1981). Neural organisation and control of the baroreceptor reflex. *Rev. Physiol., Biochem., Pharmacol.* **88**, 23–124.

Spyer, K. M. (1982). Central nervous integration of cardiovascular control. *J. exp. Biol.* **100**, 109–28.

Spyer, K. M. (1984). Central control of the cardiovascular system. In *Recent advances in physiology, Vol. 10* (ed. P. F. Baker), pp. 163–200. Churchill Livingstone, Edinburgh.

Spyer, K. M., Mifflin, S. W., and Withington-Wray, D. J. (1987). Diencephalic control of the baroreceptor reflex at the level of the nucleus of the tractus solitarius. In *Organisation of the autonomic nervous system: central and peripheral mechanisms* (ed. F. R. Calaresu, J. Ciriello, and C. Polosa), pp. 307–14. Alan R. Liss, New York.

Sun, M.-K. and Guyunet, P. G. (1985). GABA-mediated baroreceptor inhibition of reticulospinal neurons. *Am. J. Physiol.* **249**, R672–R680.

Takano, Y., Martin, J. E., Leeman, S. E., and Loewy, A. D. (1984). Substance P immunoreactivity released from rat spinal cord after kainic acid excitation of the ventral medulla oblongata: a correlation with increases in blood pressure. *Brain Res.* **291**, 168–72.

Timms, R. J. (1981). A study of the amygdaloid defence reaction showing the value of althesin anaesthesia in studies of the functions of the fore-brain in cats. *Pflüger's Arch.* **391**, 49–56.

Yardley, C. P. and Hilton, S. M. (1986). The hypothalamic and brainstem areas from which the cardiovascular and behavioural components of the defence reaction are elicited in the rat. *J. autonom. nerv. Syst.* **15**, 227–44.

5. Control of blood pressure and the circulation in man

R. F. J. Shepherd and J. T. Shepherd

INTRODUCTION

The mechanisms which regulate the arterial blood pressure are complex indeed, involving peripheral sensors, centres in the nervous system, autonomic nerves, and humoral and local factors.

Continuous measurements over a 24-hour period, during which normal activities are pursued, have shown that, in healthy individuals, arterial blood pressure varies widely as a consequence of continuous adjustments in autonomic outflow. These adjustments originate directly from centres in the brain and also from the reflexogenic zones in the systemic circulation. They provide the body with the perfusion pressure appropriate to meet, in conjunction with the local regulation of the resistance blood vessels, the changing metabolic requirements of the organs and tissues of the body in response to the many stresses to which the cardiovascular system is subjected.

CIRCADIAN PATTERN

Systolic and diastolic pressures move in the same direction over the 24-hour cycle, so that there is little change in pulse pressure. The arterial baroreflexes exert a buffering influence on the magnitude of the day and night variations in blood pressure. They act to reduce the size of the centrally induced blood-pressure oscillations. They induce short-lived changes in heart rate opposite in direction to the changes in blood pressure, thus increasing heart-rate variability. Hence, when the arterial baroreceptors are functioning normally, there occur smaller blood-pressure and larger heart-rate oscillations; if the arterial baroreceptors are ineffective, there are larger blood-pressure and smaller heart-rate oscillations (Mancia and Zanchetti 1986).

Blood-pressure variability increases with ageing. In patients with essential hypertension the arterial pressure variability increases progressively with increasing levels of blood pressure (Mancia and Zanchetti 1986).

Patients with autonomic failure who exhibit postural hypotension retain a circadian variation in pressure; however, this is the inverse of the normal pattern, with the highest pressures being at night and the lowest in the morning. This is consistent with the fact that postural dizziness is most common in the morning. They also have a reduction in heart-rate variability (Mann *et al.* 1983).

Studies in animals and man have demonstrated that normal blood-pressure control depends on the proper functioning of the sympathetic nervous system to the systemic vessels. While the autonomic nerves to the heart have important roles in regulating heart rate, arteriovenous (AV) conduction, and cardiac contractility, both humans and animals have no problem in blood-pressure regulation in the absence of the autonomic nerves to the heart. Some increase in heart rate occurs during exercise due to an intrinsic mechanism and the denervated heart is supersensitive to circulating noradrenalin.

SYMPATHETIC ACTIVITY

Changes in sympathetic outflow are governed by arterial baroreceptors and chemoreceptors, cardiopulmonary mechanoreceptors, and receptors in skeletal muscles activated by muscular contraction. Changes in sympathetic outflow also occur from primary changes in the activity of brain centres, including the 'central command' originating in the cerebral cortex during exercise and in the hypothalamic centres with emotional stress. It is not surprising, in view of the complexity of these peripheral sensors and of the brain centres that control the cardiovascular system, that the sympathetic outflow is not uniformly altered to meet the various stresses to which the body is subjected. Rather, the sympathetic nerve discharge occurs in a highly differentiated pattern, Thus, in response to reflex or central stimuli, the efferent sympathetic activity varies between the different organs and tissues, and, in the same organ or tissue, can vary between resistance and capacitance vessels. In some instances, it may increase in some organs and decrease in others (Shepherd 1982). Multiunit recordings of efferent sympathetic activity in human limb nerves, using tungsten microelectrodes, have shown that, in skin fascicles, the resting activity consists of irregular bursts of impulses, unrelated to the arterial blood pressure. In muscle fascicles the activity occurs in pulse-synchronous bursts which correlate with variations in diastolic but not systolic blood pressure; the changes in activity are greater when the blood pressure is decreasing than when it is increasing. Thus acute decreases in arterial blood pressure are buffered more efficiently than acute increases, and variations in sympathetic outflow to skeletal muscle vessels are determined mainly by fluctuations in diastolic blood pressure (Wallin 1986).

Plasma levels of noradrenalin are frequently used as an index of sympathetic activity. Such levels are governed by the balance between release of noradrenalin from sympathetic nerve endings, re-uptake into the endings, and catabolism of the amine. Also, the plasma level of noradrenalin gives no indication of the relative changes in sympathetic outflow to the different components of the circulation. The skeletal muscles contribute about one-fifth of the plasma noradrenalin level, whereas the splanchnic bed contributes little since the liver clears catecholamines from the blood (Keller *et al.* 1984; Shepherd and Mancia 1986).

ADRENOCEPTORS

The noradrenalin released from the sympathetic nerves activates α- and β-adrenoceptors in the circulatory system. β-adrenoceptors are present on the sinus and atrioventricular nodes, the conducting system and muscle cells of the heart, and the large coronary arteries. When activated, they cause an increase in heart rate, a shortening of the refractory period, enhancement of ventricular contractility, and dilatation of the coronary arteries. They are also present on the sympathetic adrenergic nerve endings and, if activated, increase the output of noradrenalin. In the kidney they are present on the juxtaglomerular cells where they are involved in the control of renin release (Fig. 5.1).

The β-adrenoceptors have been divided into two subtypes, β_1 and β_2. If adrenalin and noradrenalin are equipotent in activating them, the receptors are considered to be of the β_1 subtype, and if they have a greater affinity for adrenalin than for noradrenalin they are classified as β_2. The majority of the receptors innervated by the sympathetic nerves are of the β_1 subtype, including those affecting heart rate and cardiac contractility and the release of renin from the juxtaglomerular cells. The receptors in the muscle resistance vessels, which are not innervated, are classified as β_2.

The function of the β-adrenoceptors is to adjust the circulation to help meet the stresses imposed by gravitational forces, by muscular exercise, and by emotional stress. Thus, after pharmacological blockade of the β-adrenoceptors, it is only when the cardiovascular system is severely taxed that deficiencies in its performance are apparent (Shepherd 1985*a*).

The α-adrenoceptors are present on the resistance and capacitance vessels of the systemic circulation (Fig. 5.1). These postsynaptic receptors are classified as α_1 and α_2. In general α_1-adrenoceptors

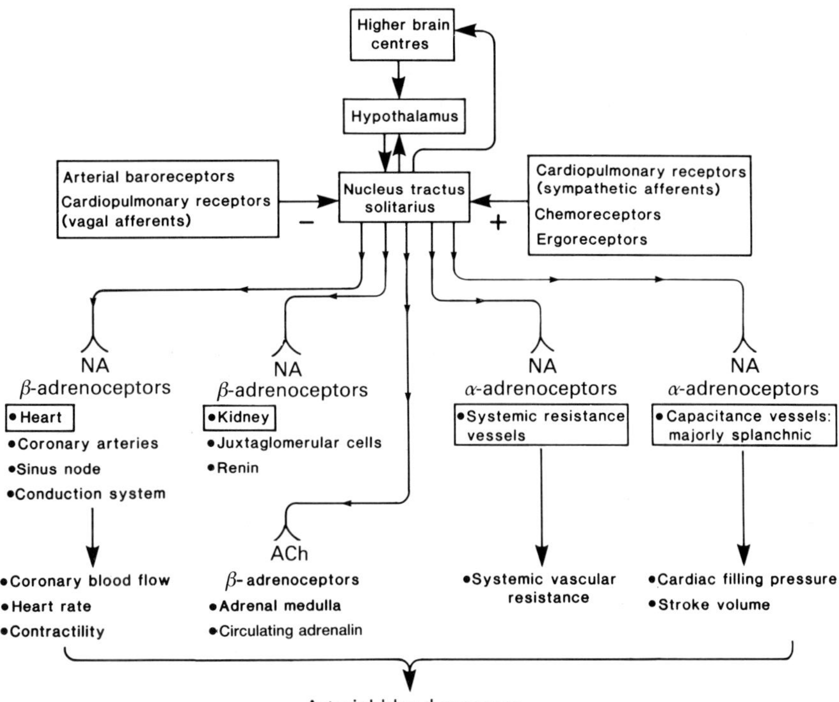

Fig. 5.1. Reflex control of the cardiovascular system. The arterial baroreceptors and the cardiopulmonary receptors with vagal afferents tonically inhibit (−) the vasomotor centres. The cardiopulmonary receptors with sympathetic afferents, the arterial chemoreceptors, and ergoreceptors in the skeletal muscles (when activated by their contraction) stimulate (+) the centres. All these afferent signals are integrated in the central nervous system. As a consequence the sympathetic outflow is modified selectively to adjust appropriately the performance of the cardiovascular system. The noradrenalin (NA) released at the sympathetic terminals acts on β-adrenoceptors in the heart and the coronary vessels and on the juxtaglomerular cells of the kidney to regulate the release of renin. As a consequence the heart rate and cardiac contractility are augmented, and the main coronary arteries are relaxed. This relaxation is enhanced by a flow-induced release of an endothelium-derived relaxing factor (Rubanyi *et al.* 1986). The sympathetic outflow to the adrenal medulla regulates adrenalin release. The circulating adrenalin also activates the β-adrenoceptors. The noradrenalin released also activates α-adrenoceptors to cause constriction of the resistance vessels and a decrease in the capacitance of the splanchnic vascular bed. As a consequence the systemic vascular resistance and the cardiac filling pressure (and hence the stroke volume and cardiac output) are adjusted to maintain the arterial blood pressure at the appropriate level for the proper perfusion of the organs and tissues of the body.

predominate in arterial smooth muscle. In the capacitance vessels, including the human saphenous vein, both types mediate vasoconstriction in response to neuronally released and circulating noradrenalin (Elsner *et al.* 1986; Steen *et al.* 1986).

The activity of the sympathetic nerves is not the only determinant of the amount of noradrenalin released. Studies on isolated vessels have shown that noradrenalin released from the sympathetic nerve endings can activate α-adrenoceptors of the α_2 subtype on prejunctional neuronal cell membranes, thus providing a mechanism for negative feedback on the further release of noradrenalin. As mentioned previously, the β_2-adrenoceptors on these endings, when activated by adrenalin, enhance the exocytotic release of noradrenalin.

OTHER RECEPTORS

Other receptors at this site include muscarinic receptors for acetylcholine, which, when activated in isolated blood vessels, reduce the output of noradrenalin during sympathetic nerve stimulation. Adenosine, histamine, and 5-hydroxytryptamine can also reduce the output of noradrenalin by activating prejunctional P_1-purinergic receptors, H_2-histaminergic receptors, and S_1-serotonergic receptors, respectively. Angiotensin II augments the constrictor response to sympathetic nerve stimulation in part by acting on prejunctional receptors to facilitate the release of noradrenalin (Fig. 5.2). The importance of the regulation of noradrenalin release via any of these prejunctional receptors in intact animals and man remains to be determined (Shepherd and Vanhoutte 1981).

The output of noradrenalin can also be modified by local metabolic changes at the neuroeffector junction (Fig. 5.2). During muscular exercise, metabolites in the active muscles, in addition to their direct relaxing action on the vascular smooth muscles of the resistance vessels, can simultaneously depress the output of noradrenalin from these nerves (Shepherd and Vanhoutte 1981).

CARDIOVASCULAR REFLEXES

The cardiovascular reflexes initiated from the peripheral sensors can be divided into those which inhibit and those which excite the vasomotor centres in the brain (Fig. 5.1).

The carotid and aortic baroreflexes

A commonly used approach to study the carotid baroreflex in man is to apply negative and positive pressures to the neck to cause increases and

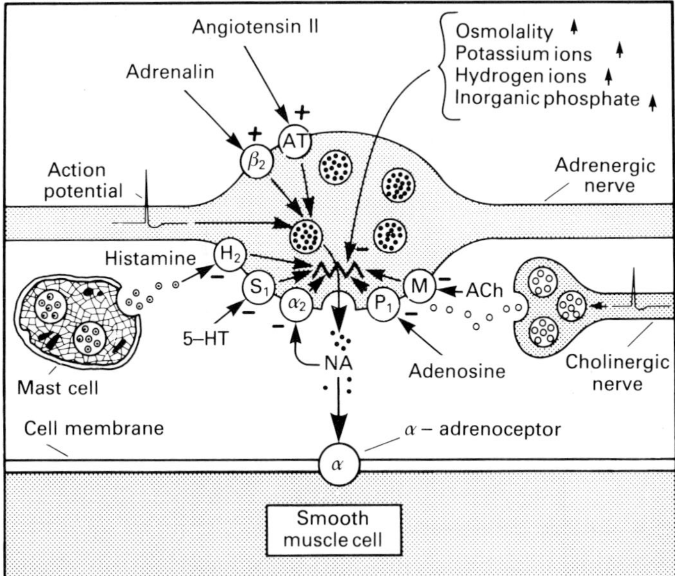

Fig. 5.2. Modulation of the neurotransmitter noradrenalin release at the sympathetic neuroeffector junction by prejunctional receptors and by local metabolic changes. Vasoactive substances can activate receptors on the sympathetic nerve endings to reduce (−) or increase (+) the output of noradrenalin when the sympathetic nerves are active. NA, noradrenalin; 5-HT, 5-hydroxytryptamine; ACh, acetylcholine; M, muscarinic; P_1, purinergic; H_2, histaminergic; S, serotonergic; α_1, α_1-adrenoceptor; AT, angiotensin receptor; β_2, β_2-adrenoceptor. The postjunctional α-adrenoceptors belong to either the α_1 or α_2-subtypes, the prejunctional ones to the α_2-subtype. An increased osmolarity in the interstitial fluid, or increased concentration of metabolic products including potassium, hydrogen, and/or inorganic phosphate ions can reduce the amount of neurotransmitter released during activation of the adrenergic nerves.

decreases, respectively, in carotid-sinus transmural pressure. This alters the degree of activation of the carotid-sinus baroreceptors. The main limitation of the method is that the alterations of systemic arterial blood pressure induced by changes in the activity of the carotid-sinus baroreceptors affect in an opposite manner the aortic baroreceptors and possibly also receptors in the left ventricle.

Other approaches to studying the role of the combined influence of carotid and aortic baroreceptors in the control of heart rate involve using drugs to alter arterial blood pressure and then examining the resultant changes in heart rate. Usually, phenylephrine is used to raise the pressure and amyl nitrite, nitroglycerin, or nitroprusside are used to lower it. The same changes in pressure are sensed by the carotid and aortic baroreceptors, but no information, of course, can be obtained by this approach on the relationship between baroreceptor activity and arterial blood pressure. Heart rate is only one component of the many complex events which determine the latter.

The primary role of the arterial baroreflexes is the rapid adjustment of arterial blood pressure around the existing mean pressure. This is accomplished by changes in heart rate, stroke volume, cardiac contractility, total systemic vascular resistance, and venous capacitance in response to changes in the activity of these stretch receptors in the carotid sinus and ascending aorta.

Carotid baroreflexes

The heart rate decreases and increases rapidly in response to increases and decreases, respectively, in the activity of the carotid baroreceptors. This is due to the variations in vagal activity to the sinus node. The speed of the response permits the rate to be regulated on a beat-to-beat basis. An increase in sympathetic outflow to the sinus node, which is slower in onset, contributes to the cardioacceleration during a sustained decrease in carotid-sinus pressure. The change in heart rate also depends on the period during the respiratory cycle in which the signal to the baroreceptors is changed; it is less in early- and mid-inspiration and greatest in early expiration. This is explained by modulation of the vagal cardioinhibitory neurons by a central respiratory oscillator (Mancia and Mark 1983).

The arterial pressure decreases when the carotid baroreceptors are activated by the application of negative pressure to the neck and increased when they are deactivated by positive pressure. In normal subjects the set-point on the curve relating the stimulus to the baroreceptors to the changes in arterial blood pressure is closer to the saturation limit. This makes the reflex more effective in buffering a reduction than an increase in pressure (Mancia and Mark 1983).

The changes in arterial blood pressure with activation or deactivation of the carotid baroreceptors result from the balance of changes in cardiac output and in total systemic vascular resistance. However, the buffering action of the carotid sinus baroreceptors is not impaired by combined β-adrenergic and parasympathetic blockade (Mancia and Mark 1983). This implies that adjustments in cardiac output are not essential and that the moment-to-moment control of blood pressure by the arterial baroreceptors depends primarily on changes in total systemic vascular resistance through sympathetically mediated adjustments in vasoconstrictor tone. While these receptors can exert considerable transient control of the resistance vessels in the skeletal muscles suitable for rapid and short-lasting adjustments in blood pressure, they seem to have little sustained influence on these vessels during static changes in arterial blood pressure (Lindblad *et al.* 1982; Mancia and Mark 1983; Wallin 1986). These receptors also govern the splanchnic vascular resistance (Mancia and Mark 1983). No data is available in man on changes in renal blood flow or in splanchnic capacitance. Animal studies have shown the importance of both the arterial and cardiopulmonary receptors in regulating the renal resistance vessels and in causing rapid changes in the capacity of the splanchnic venous system to regulate the filling pressure of the heart (Shepherd 1986). Both skin-resistance vessels and veins are usually unresponsive to alteration in the activity of the arterial and cardiopulmonary mechanoreceptors, unless there is a marked decrease in their activity (Shepherd and Mancia 1986).

During rhythmic (dynamic) and isometric (static) exercise the carotid baroreceptors are adjusted quickly to a higher level. This permits the arterial pressure to increase to help meet the metabolic demands of the active muscles. The gain of the reflex is unchanged so that it operates normally around the higher set point. This adjustment presumably is mediated centrally (Shepherd and Mancia 1986).

Studies in dogs have demonstrated that the arterial baroreceptors regulate the overall systemic vascular resistance during and after exercise, while the heart rate and cardiac output are controlled by other mechanisms. If, in dogs with chronic aortic denervation, the influence of the carotid baroreceptors is acutely removed, there is a greater decrease in arterial blood pressure at the onset of exercise and as the severity of the exercise is increased the blood pressure rises progressively and remains elevated for some time after the exercise ceases (Fig. 5.3). The cardiac-output and heart-rate changes are similar with and without the carotid sinuses operative. It seems that the function of the carotid sinus is to oppose the hypotension that develops at the onset of exercise and to limit the elevation in pressure that develops with increasing work load.

Aortic baroreflexes

Due to the obvious limitations in man of causing a selective activation of a particular set of mechanoreceptors, and especially those on the ascending aorta, the importance of the aortic baroreceptors in the control of arterial blood pressure in man is not known. Some studies have indicated that the aortic baroreceptors are more important than the carotid in the control of heart rate (Ferguson *et al.* 1985).

Cardiopulmonary reflexes

In addition to its key mechanical function, the heart also serves as a sensory and an endocrine organ. Concerning its sensory function, studies in animals have demonstrated that the heart and lungs contain numerous mechanoreceptors whose afferent fibres, both myelinated and unmyelinated, course in the vagal nerves to the brainstem (Fig. 5.4). Large unencapsulated endings, confined mainly to the atria and the

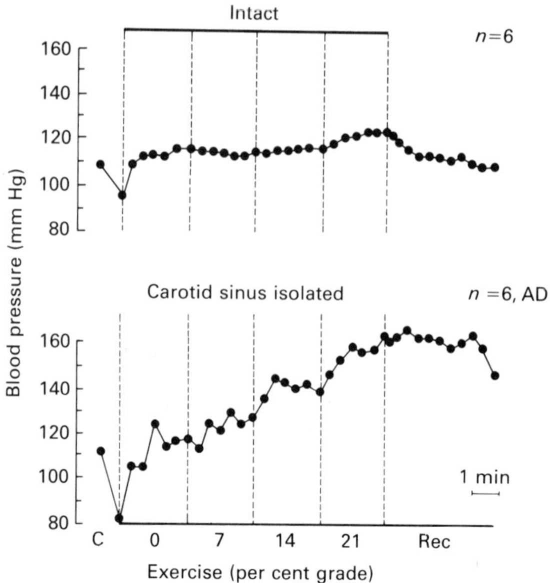

Fig. 5.3. Mean arterial pressure during continuous graded exercise in dogs with aortic-arch denervation before (top) and after (bottom) vascular isolation and pressurization of carotid sinuses. AD, aortic denervation; C, control; Rec, recovery. (Data from Walgenbach and Donald (1983).)

vein–atrial junctions are subserved by fast-conducting myelinated vagal afferents; one group signals atrial contraction and the other atrial filling. Their different discharge patterns seem to be related to their location rather than to any basic difference in their characteristics. When their activity is increased they cause an increase in heart rate by activating selectively sympathetic fibres to the sinus node. The activity to the myocardium is not increased while that to the kidney is inhibited. This illustrates the reflex selectivity that can occur in the sympathetic outflow (Linden and Kappagoda 1982). These receptors are also involved in the release of vasopressin and hence in the regulation of water reabsorption in renal tubules (Bennett *et al.* 1983).

Like the arterial baroreceptors, the cardiopulmonary receptors with unmyelinated vagal afferents act continuously to inhibit the vasomotor centre. Receptors in the atria, ventricles, and lungs each contribute to this tonic inhibition. In anaesthetized and atropinized dogs, with the arterial baroreceptors denervated and the vagi sectioned below the diaphragm, interruption of the afferent vagal traffic from the heart and lungs results in an increase in arterial blood pressure, increased mesenteric, muscle, and renal vascular resistance, decreased splanchnic

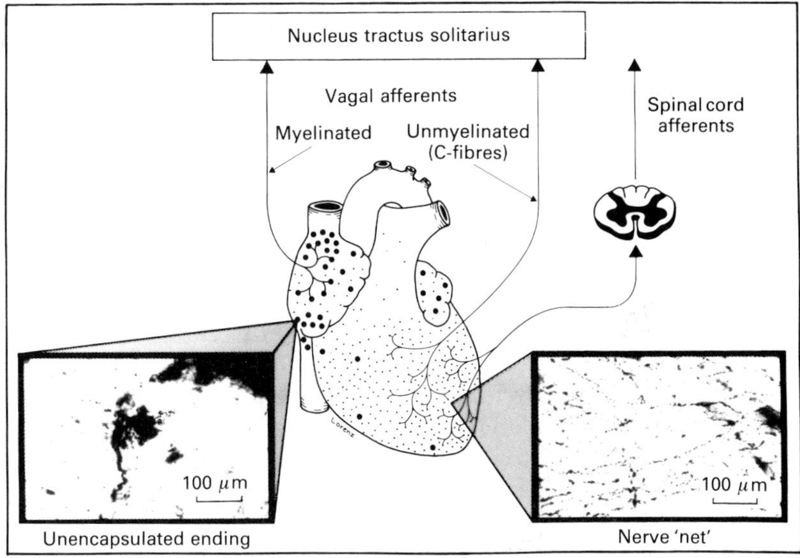

Fig. 5.4. Mechanoreceptors in the heart and their afferent fibres. The unencapsulated endings subserved by myelinated vagal afferent nerves are localized to the vein–atrial junctions: the nerve 'nets' subserved by unmyelinated vagal afferents and those by spinal cord afferent nerves (sympathetic afferents, myelinated and unmyelinated) are present in all the chambers of the heart. (Taken with permission from Shepherd (1985*b*).)

capacitance, and tachycardia. These changes are due to an increase in sympathetic outflow (Shepherd 1982).

When humans change from the supine to the upright position, there is a gravitational shift of blood from the cardiopulmonary region of the dependent parts. This results in a decrease in the activity of the cardiopulmonary and arterial mechanoreceptors. There follow an increase in heart rate, a decrease in stroke volume, a reflex constriction of muscle, splanchnic, and renal resistance vessels, and an increase in plasma renin activity and in plasma noradrenalin. The mechanisms involved in the fluctuations in heart rate and arterial blood pressure in the first 20–30 seconds of tilting upright (passive change in posture) and standing (active change in posture) are complex. In the latter case, the contraction of the postural muscles contributes to the cardiovascular changes (see Chapter 15).

The application of lower-body negative pressure has been used to study reflexes from the heart and lungs in man. By pulling blood from the central circulation to the periphery this reduces the cardiac filling pressure and hence the stimulus to mechanoreceptors in the low-pressure side of the central circulation. When small negative pressures are used, the central venous pressure can be reduced without a change in mean arterial pressure or pulse pressure or in arterial dP/dt. Thus, it is assumed that the activity of the arterial baroreceptors is unchanged (Mark and Mancia 1983).

These studies indicate that in man these low-pressure receptors have an important action in reflexly controlling the calibre of the resistance vessels in the forearm muscles. Since the muscle of the human body constitutes about 45 per cent of the body mass, if this reflex involved the majority of these muscles, it would have a key role in regulating systemic vascular resistance and hence arterial blood pressure, particularly in response to gravitational shifts of blood. However, simultaneous studies of the resistance vessels of the calf indicate that these vessels do not constrict as much as those in the forearm until enough blood is pooled in the lower part of the body to deactivate both the low- and high-pressure mechanoreceptors (Essandoh *et al.* 1986). In the calf this constriction can be reinforced by a local sympathetic axon reflex. Both in skin and muscle, this can be triggered by venous congestion. The receptors appear to be in small veins in skin, muscle, and subcutaneous adipose tissue and the effector site in the arterioles supplying these tissues. This axon reflex is an important adjunct to the postural reflexes mediated through the central nervous system so that, on assuming the upright position, the resultant increase in hydrostatic pressure in the veins of the lower limbs causes a local constriction of the resistance vessels (Henriksen 1986). A myogenic response of the smooth muscle of the resistance vessels to the increased transmural pressure also contributes.

The relative importance of the cardiopulmonary receptors and of the arterial baroreceptors in the control of renin release in man is not established. However, the evidence suggests that the cardiopulmonary receptors play an important role in the secretion of renin on changing from supine to the upright position (Grassi *et al.* 1985). The increased levels of angiotensin II would reinforce the sympathetic constriction of the systemic vessels by a direct effect on the vascular smooth muscle, its central actions, and the facilitation of noradrenalin release by its effects on the prejunctional sympathetic nerves.

Vasopressin (antidiuretic hormone (ADH)) is synthesized in the supraoptic and paraventricular nuclei in the hypothalamus. The neurosecretory granules pass along the supraoptic hypophyseal tract to the neurohypothesis. It is released by increases in plasma osmolarity which are detected by osmoreceptors in the hypothalamus. It is also released in response to decreases in blood volume; in dogs this release is governed by cardiopulmonary receptors with vagal afferents, and primarily by large unencapsulated endings at the vein–atrial junctions. These endings, which detect changes in atrial transmural pressure are subserved by fast-conducting, myelinated vagal afferents (Linden and Kappagoda 1982). The role of the cardiopulmonary receptors versus the arterial baroreceptors in regulating the release of this hormone in man is still uncertain. The plasma vasopressin levels are increased in the upright position; in patients with orthostatic hypotension, tilting upright evoked a greater decrease in arterial blood pressure in those subjects with a subnormal increase in plasma vasopressin. However, if the sympathetic nervous system and the renin–angiotensin system are activated normally by standing, these serve to maintain the arterial pressure in the absence of any increase in circulating vasopressin levels. In studies in which lower-body negative pressure (40 mm Hg for 10 min) was applied to normal subjects, the decrease in mean arterial blood pressure was no greater before and after administration of an angiotensin-converting enzyme inhibitor, indicating again that when the renin–angiotensin system is inhibited, the sympathetic nervous system and vasopressin can compensate (Bennett and Gardiner 1985).

Studies in dogs have shown that vasopressin acts on the endothelium of the cerebral arteries to cause release of a factor which relaxes the underlying smooth muscle. Since the response is prevented by indomethacin, this indicates that the vasodilator substance is a cyclo-oxygenase derivative. In the coronary arteries vasopressin causes relaxation both by an endothelium-dependent mechanism and by a direct relaxing action on the smooth muscle. In the systemic circulation, it causes constriction which is due to a direct action on the smooth muscle and is not affected by removal of the endothelium (Katusic *et al.* 1987). Since the major cerebral arteries make a significant contribution to cerebral vascular resistance, these various actions serve to preserve blood flow to the brain and the myocardium while maintaining arterial blood pressure by constriction of systemic resistance vessels. This is of particular importance during hypotensive haemorrhage.

Animals studies have demonstrated that some of the cardiopulmonary and aortic mechanoreceptors have afferent fibres which travel in the sympathetic nerves to the spinal cord. One group with myelinated afferents has a spontaneous discharge at normal intracardiac pressures. Another group with unmyelinated afferents discharges irregularly with no apparent relation to cardiac events. Stimulation of the spinal input of these sympathetic afferents causes cardiovascular reflexes that are mainly excitatory although inhibition can also occur. However, it remains to be demonstrated that cardiovascular reflex responses can be induced by natural stimulation of sympathetic mechanoreceptors (Bishop *et al.* 1983).

The cardiocytes of mammalian atria contain secretory granules that synthesize and, in response to an increase in atrial transmural pressure, release a series of related peptides (cardiac hormones) with diuretic, natriuretic, and vasoactive properties. These are referred to as atriopeptins and are released in response to atrial distension. Together with vasopressin, they have the key role in the regulation of the plasma volume. When injected into healthy humans atriopeptins cause, in addition to diuresis and natriuresis, an inhibition of vasopressin and renin release and result in the synthesis of aldosterone and a reduction of systemic atrial blood pressure (Burnett *et al.* 1984; Goetz 1986).

Ergoreflexes

A strong static contraction of the skeletal muscles, or rapid powerful rhythmic contractions, cause a marked increase in arterial blood pressure, the so-called blood pressure-raising reflex. This increase helps to oppose the reduction in blood flow to the muscles resulting from the mechanical compression. The evidence indicates that this rise is due to products of muscle metabolism activating chemosensitive endings in the muscles; while the metabolic products have not been identified, it is tempting to suggest that these are the same metabolites which cause the local vasodilatation. The afferent fibres involved are the small myelinated (Group III) and unmyelinated (Group IV) (Mitchell and Schmidt 1983). The pressor response, which is caused by increased sympathetic outflow to the circulation, is proportional to the degree of ischaemia in the exercising muscles and to the mass of the ischaemic muscle.

In addition to the reflex from the active muscles, there is a 'central command' from the cerebral cortex to the cardiovascular and respiratory centres in the brainstem (Mitchell and Schmidt 1983). It seems that central command has a key role in increasing the heart rate with isometric or strong dynamic exercise, while the stimulation of the chemosensitive muscle afferents increases the sympathetic outflow (Mark *et al.* 1986). The increase in arterial blood pressure is due both to an increase in cardiac output and in systemic vascular resistance. In healthy subjects the increased output usually makes the major contribution, whereas, if the output cannot increase normally, the same increase in pressure for the same isometric exercise is attained by a greater increase in resistance. Thus the prime purpose of the reflex seems to be to increase the flow to the contracting muscles and it calls on any combination of cardiac output and peripheral resistance to achieve this goal. For unknown reasons, the arterial and the cardiopulmonary mechanoreceptors are rendered unable to prevent the marked pressure increase. The arterial baroreceptors, however, retain their ability to modulate the pressure around the increased level (Shepherd and Mancia 1986). The reflex response to stimulation of somatic afferents (by isometric exercise of one arm) is augmented when the input of the cardiopulmonary afferents is reduced by lower-body negative pressure (Bishop *et al.* 1983).

The afferent projections of the various peripheral sensors that provide information to the brain centres on the functioning of the cardiovascular system terminate in the nucleus tractus solitarius (NTS) or closely associated structures. The potential neurotransmitters that have been identified in the NTS include acetylcholine, noradrenalin, oxytocin, vasopressin, and serotonin. It is suggested, however, that glutamate and substance P may have a primary neurotransmitter role in the baro-receptor reflex. In cats the paramedian reticular nucleus, via connections from the fastigial nucleus of the cerebellum, has an important role in the increase in sympathetic outflow that serves to maintain the arterial blood pressure when the upright position is assumed (Brody 1986).

There are numerous connections between the NTS and other centres in the brain and spinal cord, and many potential neurotransmitters have been identified (see Chapter 4).

In view of the complexity of the autonomic control of the circulation, it is not surprising that lesions at many sites can interfere with its proper function. Abnormalities of the peripheral sensors and their afferent pathways, in the brain centres, in the spinal cord, in the efferent nerves, or in the adrenoceptors, could cause disturbances in arterial blood-pressure regulation. Chronic autonomic dysfunction can be caused by multiple lesions, from those in brain centres (multiple system atrophy) to a deficit in the sympathetic nerves with impaired response of the blood vessels (pure autononomic failure). In addition to the fall in arterial blood pressure on standing, which is a classic manifestation of autonomic dysfunction, hypotension can occur following a meal in patients with pure autonomic failure (Mathias *et al.* 1986) and in response to mild supine leg exercise. The postcibal and the post-exercise hypotension can be explained by the dilatation in the splanchnic bed and active muscles, respectively, which is not counteracted by reflex constriction in other systemic vascular beds. Patients with multiple system atrophy have a defective pressure–volume mediated vasopressin release and a normal osmotically mediated release. This indicates that the site of damage is in the afferent pathways from the cardiovascular mechanoreceptors (Bannister *et al.* 1983). In patients with multiple-system atrophy and autonomic failure (Shy–Drager syndrome) spinal reflexes are absent because of intermediolateral column degeneration. Plasma noradrenalin levels are decreased and there are excessive pressor responses to an intravenous infusion of noradrenalin (Bannister *et al.* 1980). Also, there are increased numbers of β-adrenoceptors as measured by [H^3] dihydroalprenolol ((H^3) DHA) binding to β-receptors on lymphocytes. If these receptors on the lymphocytes reflect the status of cardiac β-adrenoceptors, increased numbers of the latter may contribute to the denervation sensitivity to isoprenaline in multiple system atrophy with sympathetic degeneration (Bannister *et al.* 1981).

In sympathotonic orthostatic hypotension, the patients have normal levels of noradrenalin and low mean arterial pressure when reclining. They also have reduced sensitivity to infused noradrenalin. On standing they have marked tachycardia and the plasma noradrenalin levels sometimes increase excessively. It is suggested that this disorder is caused by an impaired response of the effector organ (Polinsky *et al.* 1981). Abnormalities of adrenergic physiology also occur in parkinsonism and diabetes. Some of the patients with relatively severe diabetes have hypoadrenergic postural hypotension due to adrenergic neuropathy and hence have a lessened increase in plasma noradrenalin on standing. Some, however, have hyperadrenergic postural hypotension and it is suggested that this might be due to vascular resistance to endogenous noradrenalin (Cryer *et al.* 1978).

REFERENCES

Bannister, R., Boylston, A. W., Davies, I. B., Mathias, C. J., Sever, P. S., and Sudera, D. (1981). Beta-receptor numbers and thermodynamics in denervation supersensitivity. *J. Physiol., London* **319**, 369–77.

Bannister, R., Davies, B., Holly, E., Lethbridge, K., Mathias, C., Sever, P., and Sudera, D. (1980). Different alpha-receptor properties and baroreflex loss in alpha-adrenergic denervation in man. *J. Physiol., London* **308**, 44–45P.

Bannister, R., Lightman, S. L., and Williams, T. D. M. (1983). Vasopressin secretion in chronic autonomic failure: normal response to an osmotic stimulus. *J. Physiol., London* **346**, 109P.

Bennett, K. L., Linden, R. J., and Mary, P. A. S. G. (1983). The effect of stimulation of atrial receptors on the plasma concentration of vasopressin. *Quart. J. exp. Physiol.* **68**, 579–89.

Bennett, T. and Gardiner, S. M. (1985). Involvement of vasopressin in cardiovascular regulation. *Cardiovasc. Res.* **19**, 57–68.

Bishop, V. S., Malliani, A., and Thorén, P. (1983). Cardiac mechanoreceptors. In Handbook of Physiology, Sec 2. *The cardiovascular system* (ed. J. T. Shepherd and F. M. Abboud), Vol. III, Part 2, pp. 497–556. Published for the American Physiological Society by Williams and Wilkins, Washington, DC.

Brody, M. J. (1986). Central nervous system mechanisms of arterial pressure regulation. *Fed. Proc.* **45**, 2700–6.

Burnett, J. C., Granger, J. P., and Opgenorth, T. J. (1984). Effects of synthetic atrial natriuretic factor on renal function and renin release. *Am. J. Physiol.* **247**, F863–F866.

Cryer, P. E., Silverberg, A. B., Santiago, J. V., and Shah, S. H. (1978). Plasma catecholamines in diabetes; the syndromes of hypoadrenergic and hyperadrenergic postural hypotension. *Am. J. Med.* **64**, 407–16.

Elsner, D., Stewart, D. J., Sommer, O., Holz, J., and Bassenge, E. (1986). Postsynaptic α_1- and α_2-adrenergic receptors in adrenergic control of capacitance vessel tone *in vivo. Hypertension* **8**, 1003–14.

Essandoh, L. K., Houston, D. S., Vanhoutte, P. M., and Shepherd, J. T. (1986). Differential effects of lower body negative pressure on forearm and calf blood flow. *J. appl. Physiol.* **61**(3), 994–8.

Ferguson, D. W., Kempf, J. S., and Mark, A. L. (1985). The importance of aortic baroreflexes in the heart rate response to dynamic increase in arterial pressure in normal man. *J. Am. Coll. Cardiol.* **5**, 415 (Abstract).

Goetz, K. L. (1986). Atrial receptors, natriuretic peptides and the kidney. Current understanding. *Mayo Clinic Proc.* **61**, 600–3.

Grassi, G., Gavazzi, C., Ramirez, A., Sabadini, E., Turulo, L., and Mancia, G. (1985). Role of cardiopulmonary receptors in reflex control of renin release in man. *J. Hypertens.* (Suppl. 3), 263–5.

Henriksen, O. (1986). Circulatory studies: local sympathetic venoarteriolar axon 'reflex'. In *The sympathoadrenal system* (ed. N. J. Christensen, O. Henriksen, and N. A. Lassen), pp. 67–80. Alfred Benzon Symposium, No. 23. Munksgaard, Copenhagen,

Katusic, Z. S., Shepherd, J. T., and Vanhoutte, P. M. (1987). Endothelium-dependent contraction to stretch in canine basilar arteries. *Am. J. Physiol.* (In press).

Keller, U., Gerber, P. G., Buhler, F. R., and Stauffacher, W. (1984). Role of the splanchnic bed in extracting circulating adrenaline and noradrenaline in normal subjects and in patients with cirrhosis of the liver. *Clin. Sci.* **67**, 45–9.

Lindblad, L. E., Wallin, B. G., and Bevegård, S. (1982). Transient vasodilatation in forearm on stimulation of carotid baroreceptors in man. *J. auton. nerv. Syst.* **5**, 373–9.

Linden, R. J. and Kappagoda, C. T. (1982). *Atrial receptors.* Mongraphs of the Physiological Soc., No. 39. Cambridge University Press, Cambridge.

Mancia, G. and Zanchetti, A. (1986). Blood pressure variability. Handbook of Hypertension, Vol. 7. *Pathophysiology of hypertension—cardiovascular aspects* (ed. A. Zanchetti and R. C. Tarazi), pp. 125–52. Elsevier Science Publications, Amsterdam.

Mancia, G. and Mark, A. L. (1983). Arterial baroreflexes in humans. In Handbook of Physiology, Sect. 2. *The cardiovascular system* (ed. J. T. Shepherd and F. M. Abboud), Vol. III, Part 2, pp. 775–93. Published for the American Physiological Society by Williams and Wilkins, Washington, DC.

Mann, S., Altman, D. G., Raftery, E. B., and Bannister, R. (1983). Circadian variation of blood pressure in autonomic failure. *Circulation* **68**, 477–83.

Mark, A. L., Victor, R. G., Nerhed, C., Seals, D. R., and Wallin, B. G. (1986). Mechanisms of sympathetic nerve responses to static and rhythmic exercise: new insight from direct intraneural recordings in humans. In *The sympathoadrenal system* (ed. N. J. Christensen, O. Henriksen, and N. A. Lassen), pp. 221–33. Alfred Benzon Symposium, No. 23. Munksgaard, Copenhagen.

Mathias, C. J., da Costa, D. F., Fosbraey, P., Bannister, R., and Christensen, N. J. (1986). Post-cibal hypotension in autonomic failure. *The sympathoadrenal system* (ed. N. J. Christensen, O. Henriksen, and N. A. Lassen), pp. 402–13. Alfred Benzon Symposium, No. 23. Munksgaard, Copenhagen.

Mitchell, J. H. and Schmidt, R. F. (1983). Cardiovascular control by afferent fibers from skeletal muscle receptors. In Handbook of Physiology, Sect. 2. *The cardiovascular system* (ed. J. T. Shepherd and F. M. Abboud), Vol. III, Part 2, pp. 623–

58. Published for the American Physiological Society by Williams and Wilkins, Washington, DC.

Polinsky, R. J., Kopin, I. J., Ebert, M. H., and Weise, V. (1981). Pharmacological distinction of different orthostatic hypotension syndromes. *Neurology* **31**, 1–7.

Rubanyi, G. M., Carlos-Romero, J., and Vanhoutte, P. M. (1986). Flow induced release of endothelium derived relaxing factor. *Am. J. Physiol.* **250**, H1145.

Shepherd, J. T. (1982). Reflex control of arterial blood pressure. *Cardiovasc. Res.* **16**, 357–83.

Shepherd, J. T. (1985*a*). Circulatory response to beta-adrenergic blockade at rest and during exercise. *Am. J. Cardiol.* **55**, 87D–94D.

Shepherd, J. T. (1985*b*). The heart as a sensory organ. *J. Am. Coll. Cardiol.* **5**, 83b.

Shepherd, J. T. (1986). Role of venoconstriction for circulatory adjustments to orthostatic stress. In *The sympathoadrenal system* (ed. N. J. Christensen, O. Henriksen, and N. A. Lassen), pp. 103–15. Alfred Benzon Symposium, No. 23. Munksgaard, Copenhagen.

Shepherd, J. T. and Mancia, G. (1986). Reflex control of the human cardiovascular system. *Rev. Physiol. Biochem. Pharmacol.* **105**, 1–99.

Shepherd, J. T. and Vanhoutte, P. M. (1981). Local modulation of adrenergic neurotransmission. *Circulation* **64**, 655–66.

Steen, S., Castenfors, J., Sjöberg, T., Skarby, T., Andersson, K-E., and Norgren, L. (1986). Effects of alpha-adrenoceptor subtype-selective antagonists on the human saphenous veins *in vivo*. *Acta physiol. scand.* **126**, 15–19.

Walgenbach, S. C. and Donald, D. E. (1983). Inhibition by carotid baroreflex of exercise-induced increases in arterial pressure. *Circ. Res.* **52**, 253.

Wallin, B. G. (1986). Functional organization of sympathetic outflow in man. In *The sympathoadrenal system* (ed. N. J. Christensen, O. Henriksen, and N. A. Lassen), pp. 52–66. Alfred Benzon Symposium, No. 23. Munksgaard, Copenhagen.

6. Pathophysiology of autonomic dysregulation in heart failure

Phillip Thomas and D. J. Sheridan

INTRODUCTION

Definitions and historical background

Heart failure is a well established condition in medical practice; since Thomas Withering's observations, published in 1785, that preparations from foxgloves slowed the heart rate and improved urinary output in cardiac dropsy, our understanding of the syndrome of congestive heart failure has continued to improve.

The term heart failure appears at first sight self-explanatory, but as with so many other well established terms in medicine, the complete answer to the question 'What is heart failure?' is far from clear and an acceptable definition encompassing all aspects of the syndrome has not so far been agreed. Braunwald (1981) defined heart failure as 'the pathophysiological state in which an abnormality of cardiac function is responsible for failure of the heart to pump blood at a rate commensurate with the requirements of the metabolising tissues'. However, even this apparently straightforward definition has been challenged. What are the tissue requirements and the body needs? If oxygen is the requirement, why is the consumption of this vital element not reduced in heart failure? Despite these questions, Braunwald's definition does incorporate all the clinical situations termed heart failure.

Early workers approached the investigation of heart failure by attempting to explain the symptoms and signs as a direct result of pump dysfunction. They were limited by their lack of understanding of normal myocardial mechanics and the details of circulatory control. In 1832, James Hope proposed his backward-failure hypothesis suggesting that, if a particular cardiac chamber failed to pump adequately, pressure would increase in the components of the circulation proximal to it. In 1913, MacKenzie challenged this view, advancing his forward-failure hypothesis, stating that the clinical manifestations of heart failure were related to an inadequate cardiac output to other organs and that the impaired renal blood flow in particular led to the congestive state. Since the output from the right and left heart must be balanced, MacKenzie concluded that the heart failed 'as a whole'. It now appears that both hypotheses apply to most situations of heart failure. Following the work of Frank (1895) and Starling (1918), one of the most important cardiac compensatory mechanisms in pump dysfunction was elucidated, namely that an increase in cardiac filling pressure, or preload, maintains pump performance. It has since been recognized that increased afterload, manifested as an increase in systolic wall stress, produces myocardial hypertrophy as a second compensation in impaired pump function. The relationship between preload, afterload, and contractility for the normal and failing heart can be illustrated by pressure–volume loops (Fig. 6.1). Finally, since the worth of Wiggers and Katz in 1950 and Sarnoff in 1960, the important contribution of the stimulation of the sympathetic nervous system to compensation for inadequate pump performance has been realized.

Although investigation of the abnormal myocardial mechanics in heart failure has greatly improved our understanding of the heart's performance and although molecular biology is improving our knowledge of

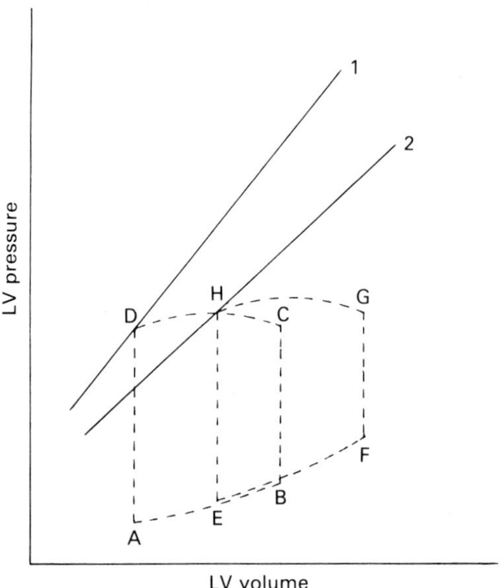

Fig. 6.1. Left ventricular (LV) pressure–volume loops for the normal (ABCD) and failing (EFGH) heart. Curves 1 and 2 represent the end-systolic pressure–volume relationship, an index of contractility, for the normal and failing heart, respectively. AB is the diastolic filling curve; BC is the isovolumic contraction period; CD is the ejection phase; and DA is the isovolumic relaxation period. In heart failure the preload is higher, represented by point F, in order to maintain stroke volume in the presence of reduced contractility, curve 2, and higher afterload, point G.

the subcellular events occurring during myocardial contraction, since the early-1960s a new focus of investigational interest has opened up. From regarding the heart as the centre of attention in heart failure, many investigators have attempted to move towards a clearer understanding of the role of the neurohumoral systems controlling the haemodynamic responses in this syndrome, with great implications for the management and eventually, one hopes, the prognosis of the condition.

The neurohumoral systems active in heart failure

Heart failure is a dynamic process: its effects vary with the duration and severity of the condition. Riegger and Liebau (1982) studied the time course of neurohumoral changes in the development and regression of congestive heart failure in dogs. They observed that plasma levels of noradrenalin, adrenalin, renin, angiotensin II, and aldosterone increased during the development of heart failure and, simultaneously, that cardiac output fell and pulmonary wedge pressure (an indirect haemodynamic measure of left heart filling pressure and therefore of preload) rose. In addition, plasma osmolality fell while plasma arginine–vasopressin increased significantly. During regression of the failure state, mean body weight decreased as excess fluid was excreted. Plasma catecholamine and hormone levels returned to baseline values and normal plasma osmolality was reachieved. They demonstrated the increased activity of the renin–angiotensin system in heart failure and its probable contribution to maintenance of tissue perfusion pressure. This increased activity has been confirmed in man, although the relative contribution of the renin–angiotensin system to maintenance of systemic perfusion pressure in congestive heart failure is very variable and is likely to depend on the duration, severity, and form of treatment of the condition.

Renin is released from the endothelium of the terminal part of the afferent renal arterioles. It is released in response to three types of stimuli: (1) an increase in renal sympathetic nerve activity producing β-adrenoceptor stimulation of the juxtaglomerular cells; (2) a reduction in wall tension in the afferent arterioles; and (3) a reduction in sodium concentration sensed by the macula densa cells of the distal tubule. All three potential stimuli are present in congestive heart failure.

Renin is also present in other vascular walls and may provide local modulating effects on vascular tone, although the importance of this aspect in heart failure is unclear. Circulating renin acts on an α_2-globulin, angiotensinogen, originating in the liver to form the decapeptide angiotensin I which is then transformed to the octapeptide angiotensin II by the converting enzyme present in the capillary endothelium. This enzyme, also known as kininase II, degrades the vasodilator substance, bradykinin. Angiotensin II has many actions, the best known of which is its ability to accelerate the production and release of aldosterone from the zona glomerulosa of the adrenal cortex, so resulting in increased sodium and, hence, water reabsorption by the kidney. In addition, angiotensin II interacts extensively with the autonomic nervous system (Fig. 6.2). It increases sympathetic output by its action on the area postrema and increases adrenal catecholamine release. It potentiates ganglionic transmission and increases available noradrenalin through its action on presynaptic angiotensin receptors at the nerve terminal, accelerating the synthesis and release of noradrenalin and inhibiting uptake$_1$. Angiotensin II is also a powerful vasoconstrictor of vascular smooth muscle and acts as a stimulus to arginine–vasopressin release.

Arginine–vasopressin, the antidiuretic hormone, is elevated in the plasma in congestive heart failure in animal models and in man (Cohn *et*

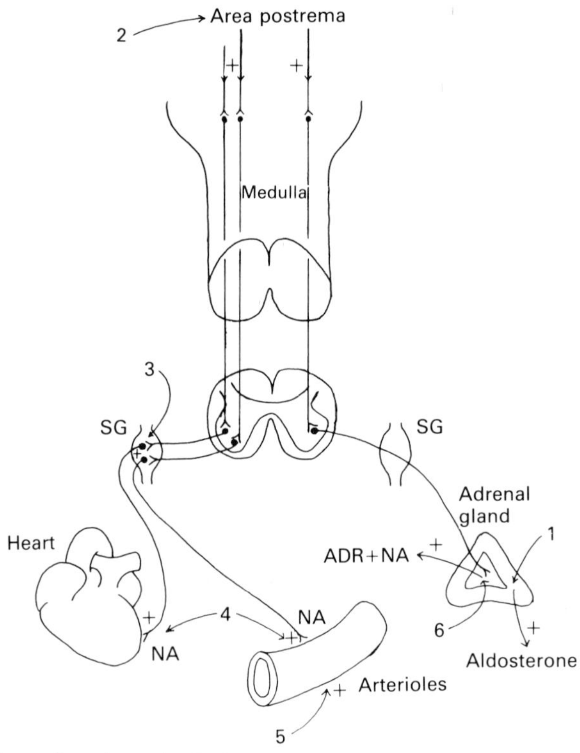

Fig. 6.2. Actions of angiotensin II. 1. Increased production and release of aldosterone from the adrenal medulla. 2. Increased central sympathetic output by an action on the area postrema. 3. Potentiation of ganglionic transmission. 4. Increased available noradrenalin at the synapses. 5. Direct vasoconstrictor action on the arterioles. 6. Increased adrenal catecholamine release. ADR, adrenalin; NA, noradrenalin; SG, sympathetic ganglion.

al. 1981) but its role in the pathophysiology of heart failure is so far unclear. It is released from the posterior pituitary gland in response to osmotic stimuli and angiotensin II as well as other non-specific stimuli such as anxiety and discomfort. Arginine–vasopressin, in addition to its action on the collecting ducts, potentiates the vasoconstrictor effects of noradrenalin and angiotensin II.

Recently, atrial natriuretic peptides have aroused interest. The peptides are secreted by the atrial wall in response to stretch and there is some evidence that an intact nerve supply is required (Knapp *et al.* 1986). Their role in volume control, both under normal circumstances and in pathophysiological states such as heart failure, remains to be elucidated. Infusions of atrial natriuretic factor produce a diuresis and natriuresis, relax vascular smooth muscle, and decrease renin release. Initial reports suggest elevated levels in heart failure in man and reduced atrial levels have been documented in at least one animal model of failure (Chimoskey *et al.* 1984). It is possible that this system in some way participates in the compensation for the volume-overloaded state.

From the above it is clear that the three neurohumoral systems active in congestive heart failure are closely interrelated, although it would appear that the stimuli for their respective activation is different. The purpose of this chapter is to review our present understanding of the role of autonomic dysfunction in congestive heart failure and its interaction with other humoral systems. Potential areas for future research with particular reference to points for therapeutic intervention will be highlighted.

THE HEART AND CENTRAL CIRCULATION

Autonomic contribution to heart failure

In congestive heart failure receptors responsible for the modulation of autonomic nervous system activities fail to differentiate between circulatory and cardiac causes of impaired tissue perfusion. Thus, the sympathetic nervous system responses which, in association with the activation of humoral systems, apparently evolved to compensate for a low blood volume, result in similar compensatory effects in heart failure. The negative feedback becomes a positive feedback and a dangerous cycle evolves. The systemic arteriolar vasoconstriction increases afterload and thus produces compensatory myocardial hypertrophy in response to the increased systolic wall stress; this in turn increases myocardial oxygen demand, often where oxygen supply is in any case diminished. The high afterload eventually further impairs cardiac performance, adding to the stimulus to maintain increased sympathetic nervous-system activity. Renal vasoconstriction impairs urinary output in a situation where fluid excretion should be encouraged. Systemic venoconstriction reduces venous capacitance, thus increasing cardiac filling pressure which will further increase tissue congestion and produce myocardial dilatation and eventually hypertrophy in response to the increased end-diastolic wall stress. Enhanced cardiac stimulation increases myocardial oxygen demand still further with little incremental gain in chronotropy or inotropy since the intrinsic cardiac disease is usually too severe. The overall effect is to add to the deterioration of the condition: opposing many of the actions of the dysregulated autonomic nervous system in heart failure is imperative if the patient is to improve.

Autonomic afferent limb dysfunction

The stimulus (or stimuli) which precipitates activation of the sympathetic nervous system in heart failure is not clearly defined, although it is likely that circulatory receptors such as baroreceptors, mechanoreceptors, and perhaps chemoreceptors and osmoreceptors are the points where the stimulus (or stimuli) is perceived (Fig. 6.3). The decrease in

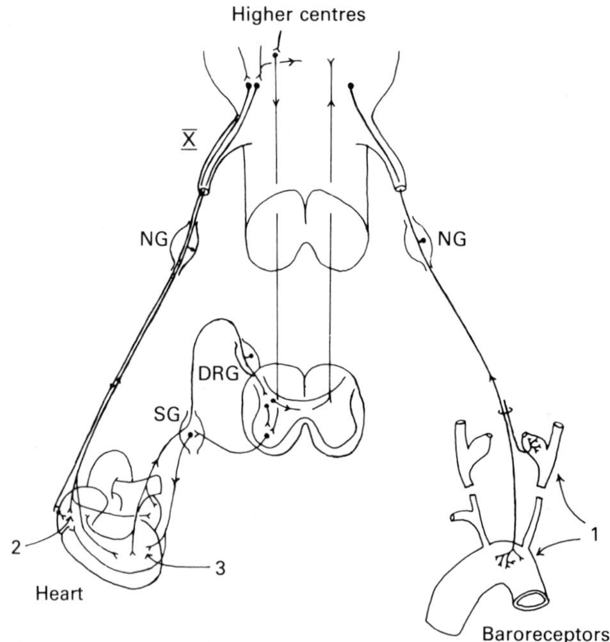

Fig. 6.3. Probable areas of autonomic afferent limb dysfunction in heart failure. 1. Alteration of carotid-sinus and/or aortic-arch baroreceptor sensitivity and reduction in vagal afferent activity. 2. Alteration of left atrial stretch receptor sensitivity and reduction in vagal afferent activity. 3. Alteration of the balance between vagal afferent and sympathetic afferent activity (may be partly central). DRG, dorsal root ganglion; NG, nodose ganglion; SG, sympathetic ganglion; X, vagus nerve.

impulse traffic in the unmyelinated vagal afferent fibres from the baroreceptors results in a reduction of the continuous inhibition of the nucleus tractus solitarius in the medulla allowing accentuation of central sympathetic outflow and inhibition of vagal activity. Several studies report that the baroreflex mechanisms are less responsive in congestive heart failure—responses to the Valsalva manoeuvre, upright tilt, vasodilator substances, and the cold pressor test are all depressed and the degree of attenuation appears to be related to the severity of the condition.

Abraham (1967) suggested an anatomical abnormality—degeneration of neuronal end-plates—to account for the dysfunction of the baroreceptors of the aortic arch and carotid sinuses, while others (Goldstein *et al.* 1975) postulated central defects and/or defects at effector sites to explain the receptor dysfunction. It has been proposed that the electrolyte changes associated with heart failure may affect arterial wall compliance and hence baroreceptor function—sodium retention can increase vascular wall water content and alter afferent transmembrane electrophysiological function. Hyponatraemia, often a feature of congestive heart failure, could also contribute to the dysfunction since a low plasma sodium concentration has been shown to impair carotid sinus baroreceptor sensitivity (Cunns and Brown 1978).

Niebauer and Zucher (1985) suggested that sympathetic efferent activity may affect baroreceptor function in volume-overloaded heart failure and, to support this, rich innervation of the carotid sinus with sympathetic fibres has been described (Abraham 1969). Since sympathetic nervous system activity is increased in heart failure, alteration of baroreceptor characteristics could occur as a result of the prolonged influence of this system's activity. In addition, angiotensin II or arginine–vasopressin may influence baroreceptor function, although this seems less likely.

A reduction in baroreflex sensitivity as described above, may partly explain this persistent sympathetic outflow. However, other abnormalities in the afferent limbs of reflexes concerned with circulatory control have been described. Under normal conditions an increase in left atrial volume stimulates left atrial stretch receptors, resulting in increased activity of myelinated and unmyelinated fibre afferents which inhibits the release of arginine–vasopressin from the pituitary gland and decreases renal sympathetic nerve activity; thus, by two mechanisms, increasing water excretion by the kidney and so maintaining plasma osmolality. Zucher *et al.* (1979) demonstrated a defect in the sensitivity of left atrial stretch receptors in congestive heart failure and proposed that this may be a result of chronic left atrial dilatation which alters the stress/strain relationship of atrial type-B nerve endings impairing their ability to sense changes in atrial diastolic size.

Pagani *et al.* (1982) proposed an alternative explanation for the increased sympathetic discharge. They demonstrated an increase in heart rate following volume loading in unanaesthetized cats with chronic spinal section at C8. In this model, two reflex cardiovascular loops are involved, vasovagal and sympathosympathetic. In their experiments the vagal reflex was blocked with atropine and the observed tachycardia was attributed to the sympathosympathetic reflex. The response was abolished by interruption of the afferent limb by sectioning the dorsal roots from T1 to T6 and performing a spinal section at T6/T7. Sympathetic afferent activity has been reported to decrease cardiac vagal efferent activity and reduce baroreflex sensitivity. Malliani and Pagani propose that, in congestive heart failure, some central modulating influence determines the 'gain' of vagal and sympathetic afferent limbs which interact in a complex manner. The precise mechanisms responsible for afferent reflex limb dysfunction in heart failure remain to be elucidated but these observations have directed a line of enquiry into an important aspect of autonomic reflex dysfunction in congestive heart failure.

Sympathetic efferent limb dysfunction

Catecholamine turnover

In heart failure circulating plasma noradrenalin and adrenalin are increased at rest and there is markedly elevated urinary 24-hour noradrenalin excretion. Although the relative contribution of the sympathetic nervous system to circulatory support in congestive heart failure is unclear, the deleterious effect of removing this support, as during β-blockade, has long been known. Paradoxically, however, in some circumstances β-blockade may be beneficial, for example in dilated cardiomyopathy (Waagstein *et al.* 1983), presumably by reducing heart rate and improving diastolic filling time. It may also allow 'up-regulation' of myocardial β-adrenoceptors promoting improved responsiveness to circulating catecholamines (see below). The increase in plasma noradrenalin concentration correlates well with the degree of left ventricular impairment (Thomas and Marks 1978).

The origin of the elevated plasma noradrenalin is probably neuronal, although a small proportion originates in the adrenal medulla. In normal subjects only about 2 per cent of cardiac neuronal noradrenalin enters the circulation. The rest is removed by re-uptake into neuronal endings or by diffusion into the coronary circulation and only a small proportion is taken up by extraneuronal tissues. The increased circulating level of neurotransmitter is likely to reflect the high sympathetic nervous system activity present in congestive heart failure; however, a defect in neuronal uptake of noradrenalin is probably also involved.

Neuronal biosynthesis of noradrenalin appears to be defective in some models of heart failure; for example, Poole *et al.* (1967) demonstrated a reduction in activity of the rate-limiting enzyme tyrosine hydroxylase, responsible for the production of 3,4-dihydroxyphenylalanine (dopa), in dogs with heart failure.

Myocardial catecholamine stores

The presence of low myocardial noradrenalin stores in heart failure has long been recognized. It has long been known that reduction in total myocardial noradrenalin content was not simply a dilutional process associated with an increased muscle mass of one chamber but also occurred in the chambers uninvolved in the hypertrophic process. Impaired uptake of exogenous noradrenalin into depleted myocardial nerve terminals in dogs and guinea pigs with heart failure has been described (Spann *et al.* 1965) suggesting there is either a reduction in the total number of neurons supplying the myocardium or a decrease in intraneuronal catecholamine binding sites in this condition. The low myocardial noradrenalin content is likely to be a consequence rather than a cause of the poor contractile state in heart failure since Spann *et al.* (1966) demonstrated similar contraction of cat papillary muscle from normals and from those with noradrenalin depletion produced by chronic cardiac denervation or reserpine pretreatment. Overall reduction in myocardial noradrenalin stores is likely to reflect increased sympathetic nervous system activity: the nerve terminals appear to be unable to maintain turnover in the presence of a greatly increased sympathetic nerve impulse traffic and apparent defects in catecholamine uptake, biosynthesis, or both.

Changes in the adrenoceptors

As heart failure progresses, the myocardium loses an important source of inotropic support; gradually the intrinsic noradrenalin stores are decreased and the heart becomes more and more dependent on circulating catecholamines as its means of maintaining, if not improving, the degree of contractility. Even this source, however, is not without its disadvantages. In 1978 Thomas and Marks described a reduction in the cyclic AMP response to isoprenaline in isolated lymphocytes in patients with heart failure and in 1981 Colucci and co-workers demonstrated a reduction in β-adrenoceptor surface density of lymphocytes from heart failure patients. They termed this a 'down-regulation' of the adrenoceptors in response to the high circulating catecholamine pool. Since then with the onset of the heart transplantation programme and its huge potential for research in this field, Bristow and his co-workers (1982) have demonstrated that there is a significant β-adrenoceptor down-regulation in the myocardium of patients with heart failure. In contrast to myocardial noradrenalin content, β-adrenoceptor down-regulation appears to be 'chamber-specific' and is likely to be related to the severity of the condition.

Although the β_1-adrenoceptor has, until recently, been considered as the exclusive subtype associated with myocardial function, it now seems likely that in man chronotropic effects are mediated by the β_2-adrenoceptor and that this subpopulation of β-adrenoceptors also has a role in inotropic responses. From recent work it is also likely that down-regulation is 'adrenoceptor subtype-specific' (Bristow *et al.* 1986)—selective β_1-adrenoceptor down-regulation appears to be present in human failing myocardium. Noradrenalin has a tenfold greater affinity for β_1-adrenoceptors than for β_2-adrenoceptors and this may partly explain the selective down-regulation of this β-adrenoceptor subtype in heart failure in man. Since there is a higher proportion of β_2-adrenoceptors in the myocardium of heart failure patients, this could provide a useful basis for inotropic intervention in the future and warrants further investigation.

The role of myocardial α-adrenoceptors in heart failure has not been clearly elucidated. Postsynaptic α_1-adrenoceptors are present in the myocardium of many species including man. They mediate a positive inotropic response without any significant chronotropic effect. α-adrenoceptor numbers have been reported to be increased (Karliner *et al.* 1980) or remain unchanged (Chang *et al.* 1982) in animal models of heart failure. Platelet α_2-adrenoceptor number has been reported to be decreased in patients with severe heart failure (Weiss *et al.* 1983) and the decrease correlates well with the increased circulating noradrenalin levels. If the decrease in α_2-adrenoceptors is mainly of the presynaptic type, this would contribute to the elevation of plasma noradrenalin by impairing re-uptake into the neuronal endings and could be an important mechanism to explain the observed elevation of circulating catecholamines.

Other receptors such as H_2-receptors and dopamine receptors appear to be unchanged in heart failure and could provide an alternative mechanism for inotropic support.

Parasympathetic efferent-limb dysfunction

Abnormal parasympathetic nervous-system activity has been observed in a wide variety of heart disease, but documentation and understanding of the pathophysiology has not been as extensive as for the sympathetic nervous system. The major disturbance reported is an alteration in the heart rate response to various stimuli. A decrease in baroreceptor-mediated responses to increased systemic pressure has been observed in dogs (Higgins *et al.* 1972*a*) and in man impaired increments in heart rate have been observed following glyceryl trinitrate and on standing. It seems likely that the chronotropic abnormality reflects an impaired ability to increase adrenergic activity and to withdraw parasympathetic activity. Higgins *et al.* (1972*a*) demonstrated that the sinoatrial node in dogs with heart failure reacts normally to vagal stimulation suggesting that a baroreceptor or central abnormality is more likely than an efferent or end-organ defect. In the cardiomyopathic Syrian hamster a decrease in activity of choline acetyltransferase in the cardiac vagal nerve terminals has been reported but the acetylcholine content of failing hearts is normal. Where there is an impaired ability to increase stroke volume in response to standing and exercise as in heart failure, the contribution of an increased heart rate would be invaluable. Parasympathetic nervous system dysfunction may be a contributory mechanism for deterioration in heart failure and deserves further attention.

Central dysfunction

It seems unlikely that in the presence of so many peripheral autonomic nervous-system derangements the central regulating process should remain completely intact. A central cause for autonomic dysregulation in heart failure is appealing, yet little, if any, direct evidence has accumulated to incriminate it. Defects of the hypothalamic osmoregulatory centre have been proposed to explain the elevated levels of antidiuretic hormone in heart failure. In addition, many of the neurohumoral components active in heart failure have themselves central influences, for example, angiotensin II, which may explain some of the observed changes.

THE PERIPHERAL CIRCULATION

The circulation at rest

An important hallmark of heart failure is peripheral vasoconstriction. At rest in mild heart failure it may be minimal or absent but on exercise, inappropriate vasoconstriction always develops. In mild cases it may be selective, affecting splanchnic and renal beds but in severe cases it becomes more widespread involving cutaneous and muscle vascular beds, significantly increasing peripheral resistance, and further impairing cardiac performance. The sympathetic nervous system and the renin–angiotensin system are primarily responsible for this inappropriate vasoconstriction. In addition, arginine–vasopressin may have a role. In heart failure the compliance of the vasculature is also decreased probably related to increased vascular wall sodium concentration and extrinsic compression by tissue oedema. Stimulation of the renin–angiotensin system by the increased renal sympathetic nerve activity and by renal efferent arteriolar vasoconstriction further potentiates sympathetic nerve activity and a positive feedback circuit results.

Arteriolar vasoconstriction is the major determinant of cardiac afterload while systemic venoconstriction and fluid retention are the main determinants of left ventricular preload. The splanchnic veins, in particular, play the dominant role in modulation of venous capacitance, the cutaneous veins being essentially involved in thermoregulation. In congestive heart failure most studies of venous tone in man have been restricted to the limb vessels and showed increased tone at rest. The increased venous tone may partly explain the attenuation of normal haemodynamic responses to tilt. In severe heart failure peripheral venous pooling is absent and stimulation of mechano- and baroreceptors in response to a decreased cardiac output does not occur on standing. There is therefore, little increase in heart rate and vascular tone remains relatively fixed.

Plasma noradrenalin and adrenalin are both elevated at rest in heart failure. Peripherally, noradrenalin appears to act predominantly on α-adrenoceptors increasing arteriolar resistance and reducing venous capacitance, while adrenalin causes vasodilatation especially in skeletal and splanchnic vascular beds via its action on β-adrenoceptors.

Relatively little is known about vascular adrenoceptor function in heart failure and results of studies to assess the catecholamine content of vascular tissue in heart failure also conflict.

Responses to exercise

During exercise an increased proportion of the cardiac output enters the muscle vascular bed to meet the increased requirements of the tissues. The source of the increased muscle blood flow is the increased cardiac output, often up to fivefold in normal subjects. Vasoconstriction in other vascular beds (i.e. cutaneous, splanchnic, and renal) allows some diversion of blood to the muscle beds concerned in addition to maintaining flow to cerebral and coronary beds. Although coronary blood flow is increased on exercise, often up to fivefold, cerebral flow changes little.

In heart failure, the muscle vascular beds receive proportionally less blood flow than under normal circumstances which effect is partly related to the decreased compliance of the vasculature and partly due to an appreciably lower cardiac output for a particular level of exercise. Greater reductions in flow occur to renal, splanchnic, and cutaneous circulations due to inappropriately elevated adrenergic and renin–angiotensin system activity. Cutaneous vasoconstriction is prominent in severe heart failure at rest and throughout exercise impairing thermoregulation and producing slight hyperthermia. Vasoconstriction on exercise may be such that ischaemic damage occurs to the viscera.

Higgins *et al.* (1972*b*) demonstrated the important contribution of the autonomic nervous system to vasoconstrictor responses in dogs with heart failure induced by tricuspid regurgitation and pulmonary artery constriction. Following denervation of one kidney, they observed that blood flow to the contralateral kidney was more reduced on exercise than that to the denervated kidney, indicating the importance of renal sympathetic-nerve activity in mediating this response.

The intense peripheral vasoconstriction helps to maintain pressure in the central circulation despite an inappropriate cardiac output for the degree of exercise but with the risk that this excessive vasoconstriction may impair function of the failing heart still further. Although cerebral blood flow usually remains unaltered, coronary flow rarely increases to the extent found in normals. The systemic arterial pressure in heart failure is often unchanged during exercise (unlike in normal subjects whose pressure increases) and may even decrease with resulting syncope (Higgins *et al.* 1972*b*). Left ventricular filling pressure is also inappropriately elevated on exercise and the risk of developing pulmonary oedema during activity is therefore greater.

THERAPEUTIC INTERVENTIONS

New methods in the management of heart failure are gaining wider acceptance. From the concept that the patient with heart failure is 'waterlogged' requiring large doses of diuretics, treatment has moved, based on pathophysiological data, to a more rational approach using smaller quantities of diuretics but introducing vasodilators earlier in the treatment. Vasodilators may act like diuretics achieving a reduction in filling pressure by venodilatation or they may decrease systemic vasoconstriction and, thus, left ventricular afterload improving cardiac performance. Balanced vasodilators achieving both objectives would theoretically be the most beneficial. The introduction of the converting enzyme inhibitors, in particular, has been a major advance in this respect and these, in addition to decreasing plasma angiotensin II levels, decrease bradykinin degradation, decrease plasma catecholamine levels, and alter encephalin degradation. Interventions which directly antagonize the sympathetic nervous system in heart failure are at present experimental, although their use in heart failure is logical in view of the intricate involvement of the sympathetic nervous system in the pathophysiology of the condition. Possible areas of intervention include central, ganglionic, and effector sites.

Centrally-acting α-agonists may reduce sympathetic outflow. Preliminary acute studies in heart failure have shown some improvement following clonidine (Hermilier *et al.* 1983). Bromocriptine, a presynaptic dopa agonist, has been shown to reduce plasma noradrenalin by 50 per cent with some haemodynamic improvement (Francis *et al.* 1983). Some benzodiazepines may also be of future benefit by reducing catecholamine levels through central activation of gamma aminobutyric acid (GABA) (Stratton and Halter 1985) and morphine probably produces many of its peripheral effects through its central action. Treatment aimed at impairing ganglionic transmission has many adverse effects and its efficacy in congestive heart failure has not been pursued.

In addition to the converting enzyme inhibitors, other vasodilators act specifically at effector sites to reduce peripheral catecholamine effects. The non-selective α-adrenoceptor antagonist phentolamine increases venous capacitance in the forearm in patients with congestive heart failure (Villani *et al.* 1974) while the selective α_1-antagonist prazosin has beneficial effects at least in the short term (Elkayam *et al.* 1979). Therapy aimed at activating presynaptic receptors to increase noradrenalin uptake may also be beneficial, and peripheral β_2-adrenoceptor stimulation should reduce afterload and improve myocardial performance.

CONCLUSION

Research over the past two decades into the pathophysiological processes active in congestive heart failure has raised important questions about the role of the various autonomic and humoral mechanisms involved. A unified hypothesis to explain all the neurohumoral changes in heart failure has not, as yet, been provided. Investigation in different species, at different stages of heart failure, and during different therapeutic interventions has produced a complex picture. There seems little doubt that further investigation of these important aspects of heart failure will contribute significantly to unravelling the intricacies of this most tantalizing of syndromes—superficially simple yet deeply complex.

REFERENCES

Abraham, D. (1967). The structure of baroreceptors in pathological conditions in man. In *Baroreceptors and hypertension* (ed. P. Kezdi), p. 273. Pergamon Press, Oxford.

Abraham, A. (1969). *Microscopic innervation of the heart and blood vessels in vertebrates, including man.* Pergamon Press, Oxford.

Braunwald, E. (1981). Heart failure: pathophysiology and treatment. *Am. Heart J.* **102**, 486–90.

Bristow, M. R., Ginsberg, R., Minobe, W., Cubicciotti, R. S., Sageman, W. S., Lurie, K., Billingham, M. E., Harrison, D. C., and Stinson, E. B. (1982). Reduced catecholamine sensitivity and beta adrenergic receptor density in failing human hearts. *New Engl. J. Med.* **307**, 205–11.

Bristow, M. R., Ginsberg, R., Umans, V., Fowler, M., Minobe, W., Rasmussen, R., Zera, P., Menlove, R., Shah, P., Jamieson, S., and Stinson, E. B. (1986). Beta 1 and beta 2 adrenergic receptor subpopulations in non-failing and failing human ventricular myocardium: coupling of both receptor subtypes to muscle contraction and selective beta 1 receptor down regulation in heart failure. *Circulation Res.* **59**, 297–309.

Chang, H. Y., Klein, R. M., and Kunos, G. (1982). Selective desensitisation of cardiac beta receptors by prolonged *in vivo* infusion of catecholamines in rats. *J. Pharmacol. exp. Ther.* **221**, 784–9.

Chimoskey, J. E., Spielman, W. S., Brant, M. A., and Hiederman, S. R. (1984). Cardiac atria of BIO 14.6 hamsters are deficient in natriuretic factor. *Science* **223**, 820–2.

Cohn, J. N., Levine, T. B., Francis, G. S., and Goldsmith, S. (1981). Neurohumoral control mechanisms in congestive heart failure. *Am. Heart J.* **102**, 509–14.

Colucci, W. S., Alexander, R. W., Williams, G. H., Orud, R. A., Holerman, B. L., Konstan, M. A., Wynne, J., Muj, G. J., and Braunwald, E. (1981). Reduced lymphocyte beta-adrenergic receptor density in patients with heart failure and tolerance to the beta-adrenergic agonist pirbuterol. *New Engl. J. Med.* **305**, 185–90.

Cunns, D. L. and Brown, A. M. (1978). Sodium sensivity of baroreceptors. Reflex effects of blood pressure and fluid volume in the cat. *Circulation Res.* **42**, 714–20.

Elkayam, U., Lejemtel, T. H., and Mathur, M. (1979). Marked daily attenuation of oral prazosin therapy in chronic congestive heart failure. *Am. J. Cardiol.* **44**, 540–5.

Francis, G. S., Parks, R., and Cohn, J. N. (1983). The effects of bromocriptine in patients with heart failure. *Am. Heart J.* **106**, 100–6.

Goldstein, R. E., Beiser, G. D., Stampfer, N., and Epstein, S.E. (1975). Impairment of autonomically mediated heart rate control in patients with cardiac dysfunction. *Circulation Res.* **36**, 571–8.

Hermilier, J. B., Magorien, R. D., Leithe, M. E., Unverferth, D. V., and Leier, C. V. (1983). Clonidine in congestive heart failure. *Am. J. Cardiol.* **51**, 791–5.

Higgins, C. B., Vatner, F. F., Ekberg, D. L., and Braunwald, E. (1972*a*). Alteration in the baroreceptor reflex in conscious dogs with heart failure. *J. clin. Invest.* **51**, 715–24.

Higgins, C. B., Vatner, F. F., Franklin, D., and Braunwald, E. (1972*b*). Effects of experimentally produced heart failure on the peripheral vascular response to severe exercise in conscious dogs. *Circulation Res.* **31**, 186–94.

Karliner, J. S., Barnes, P., Brown, M., and Dollery, C. (1980). Chronic heart failure in the guinea pig increases cardiac alpha and beta adrenoceptors. *Eur. J. Pharmacol.* **67**, 115–18.

Knapp, M. F., Hicks, M. N., Linden, R. G., and Mary, D. A. S. G. (1986). Evidence against atrial natriuretic peptide as a natriuretic hormone during atrial distension. *J. Endocrinol.* **109**, R5–R8.

Niebauer, M. and Zucher, I. H. (1985). Static and dynamic responses of carotid sinus baroreceptors in dogs with chronic volume overload. *J. Physiol.* **369**, 295–310.

Pagani, M., Fizzinelli, P., Bergamaschi, M., and Malliani, A. (1982). A positive feedback sympathetic pressor reflex during stretch of the thoracic aorta in conscious dogs. *Circulation Res.* **50**, 125–32.

Poole, P. E., Covell, G. W., Levitt, M., Gibb, J., and Braunwald, E. (1967). Reduction of cardiac tyrosine hydroxylase activity in experimental congestive heart failure. Its role in depletion of cardiac norepinephrine stores. *Circulation Res.* **20**, 349–53.

Riegger, A. J. G. and Liebau, G. (1982). The renin–angiotensin–aldosterone system, antidiuretic hormone and sympathetic nerve activity in an experimental model of congestive heart failure in the dog. *Clin. Sci.* **62**, 645–9.

Spann, J. F., Chidsey, C. A., Poole, P. E., and Braunwald, E. (1965). Mechanism of norepinephrine depletion in experimental heart failure produced by aortic constriction in the guinea pig. *Circulation Res.* **17**, 312–21.

Spann, J. F., Sonnenblick, E. H., Cooper, T., Chidsey, C. A., Wilman, V. L., and Braunwald, E. (1966). Cardiac norepinephrine stores and the contractile state of heart muscle. *Circulation Res.* **19**, 317–25.

Stratton, J. R. and Halter, J. B. (1985). Inhibition of epinephrine and norepinephrine released by a benzodiazepine in man. *J. Am. Coll. Cardiol.* **5**, 47 (Abstract).

Thomas, J. A. and Marks, B. H. (1978). Plasma norepinephrine in congestive heart failure. *Am. J. Cardiol.* **41**, 233–43.

Villani, F., Petter, C., Jequier, E., and Schelling, J. C. (1974). Effect of phentolamine on peripheral venous distensibility in congestive heart failure. *Eur. J. clin. Pharmacol.* **7**, 11–16.

Waagstein, F., Hjalmarson, A., Swedeberg, K., and Wallentin, I. (1983). Beta-blockers in dilated cardiomyopathies: they work. *Eur. Heart J.* **4P**, 173–8.

Weiss, R. J., Tobes, M., Wertz, C. E., and Smith, C. B. (1983). Platelet alpha$_2$ adrenoceptors in chronic congestive heart failure. *Am. J. Cardiol.* **52**, 101–5.

Zucker, I. H., Earle, A. M., and Gilmore, J. P. (1979). Changes in the sensitivity of left atrial receptors following reversal of heart failure. *Am. J. Physiol.* **237**, H555.

7. Autonomic regulation of heart rhythm

D. J. Sheridan

INTRODUCTION

Regulation of the rate and rhythm of cardiac contraction is a major function of the autonomic nervous system. By regulating heart rate at rest and during exercise, it is an important determinant of cardiac reserve. It facilitates the rapid cardiac response to the needs of the body associated with variations in the level of physical and mental activity, by providing rapid communication between the heart and the midbrain. The performance and efficiency of the body in health is therefore dependent upon normal autonomic function. Abnormal autonomic activity can lead to serious problems in regulation of heart rate and blood pressure during alterations in posture and physical activity, causing weakness and even syncope. The management of such cases presents a considerable challenge to clinicians, both from the diagnostic and therapeutic points of view. This requires an understanding of the electrophysiological regulation of the heart rhythm and how the autonomic system interacts with it in health and disease.

In addition to arrhythmias which may result from the effect of abnormal autonomic influences on the normal heart, there is increasing evidence that autonomic factors may contribute to the genesis of arrhythmias in abnormal cardiac states, particularly during acute myocardial ischaemia. Sudden cardiac death is nearly always due to ventricular fibrillation and accounts for about 70 000 deaths annually in the UK. Coronary heart disease is virtually always present in such cases and, although acute myocardial ischaemia is the major precipitating factor, there is convincing evidence that transient disturbances in autonomic regulation of myocardial function, particularly in ischaemic zones, may contribute significantly to the genesis of the arrhythmias responsible. In this chapter, the mechanisms by which sinus rhythm is regulated will be discussed and mechanisms by which autonomic dysfunction may produce arrhythmias in normal and diseased hearts will be reviewed.

SINUS RHYTHM

The sinus node is richly innervated with sympathetic and parasympathetic fibres and, through them, the autonomic nervous system exerts its control of heart rate. Central regulation of autonomic outflow takes place in the brainstem where information is received from peripheral receptors. This is relayed to other parts of the brain from where, in turn, signals are also received, integrated, and ultimately used to adjust the level of autonomic outflow to various parts of the circulation to allow appropriate adaptation to different stresses.

Input to the central regulating structures is received from systemic and pulmonary baroreceptors, chemoreceptors, and sensors of respiratory inflation, via the ninth and tenth cranial nerves. Additional information is received from the heart and aorta via spinal afferents as well as from peripheral and central thermoreceptors. Most afferents terminate in the nucleus tractus salutarius (NTS), where information from peripheral receptors and higher centres is integrated. From there information is relayed to the vasomotor centre and vagal nucleus to regulate sympathetic and parasympathetic outflow.

Vagal preganglionic efferents arise from the nucleus ambiguus and dorsal nucleus of the vagus and leave the medulla via the vagus nerve. They pass through the neck in the carotid sheath and after entering the chest, course in apposition to the caudal sympathetic ganglia, close to the stellate ganglia. From there postganglionic sympathetic and preganglionic parasympathetic fibres course together in a plexus of mixed nerves. The preganglionic sympathetic fibres which eventually relay through this plexus have their origin in the vasomotor centre, from which several nuclei, most notably the paramedian reticular nucleus, radiate to the intermediolateral column of the spinal cord. Cardiac preganglionic sympathetic fibres arise from neurons in the intermediolateral columns of the upper eight thoracic segments of the spinal cord. They emerge in the rami communicantes of the upper six thoracic segments and in some animals in the ventral roots of the fifth to eighth cervical segments. Virtually all cardiac sympathetic fibres pass through the stellate ganglia and from there in the ventral or dorsal ansa subclavia to join the vagal sympathetic trunk forming the plexus of mixed nerves referred to above (Fig. 7.1). While the autonomic nerves which innervate the sinus node are those which regulate the heart rate during sinus rhythm, autonomic influences on the atrioventricular (AV) node and ventricular myocardium can also be important factors in the development of arrhythmias.

Innervation of the heart

As described above, autonomic nerves course to the heart as a plexus of

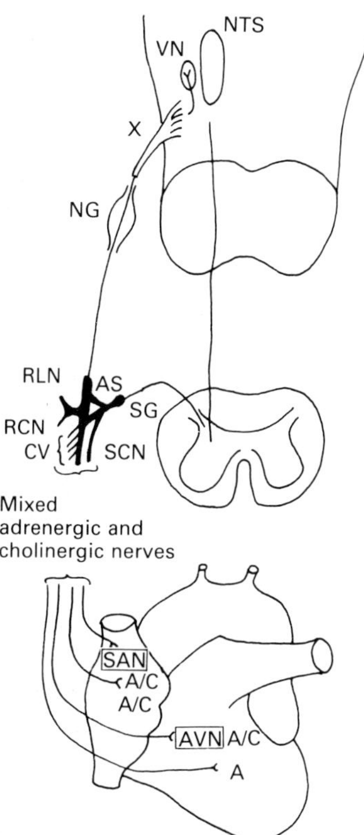

Fig. 7.1. Efferent pathways of autonomic innervation of the heart. Preganglionic sympathetic fibres emerge from the spinal cord via the rami communicantes and through the stellate ganglion (SG). Some postganglionic fibres continue in the stellate cardiac nerve (SCN), but most course in the ansa subclavia (AS). Parasympathetic fibres arise in the vagal nucleus (VN) and emerge from the brainstem in the vagus nerve (X). After passing through the carotid sheath, they join with the ansa subclavia to form the vagosympathetic trunk and continue to the heart as a plexus of mixed nerves innervating the sinoatrial node (SAN) and the atrioventricular (AVN) node (adrenergic and cholenergic) and ventricles (mainly adrenergic).

NTS, Nucleus tractus salutarius; VN, vagal nucleus; X, vagus nerve; NG, nodose ganglion; RLN, recurrent laryngeal nerve; RCN, recurrent cardiac nerve; CV, cardiovagal nerves; AS, ansa subclavia; SG, stellate ganglion; SAN, sinoatrial node; A/C, adrenergic and cholinergic; AVN, atrioventricular node; A, adrenergic.

mixed sympathetic and parasympathetic nerves. The anatomy of these nerves varies considerably within species and on the two sides. From the cardiac plexus, sympathetic and parasympathetic fibres pass to the heart to supply the sinus node, AV node, atria, ventricles, and coronary arteries. Sympathetic efferents are distributed to the sinus node, atria, AV node, ventricles, and coronary arteries. Parasympathetic efferents pass preferentially to the sinus node, AV node, and to a lesser extent to the atria (Fig. 7.1).

Regulation of sinus rhythm

Early studies suggested that right-sided autonomic nerves regulated sinus-node function while left-sided nerves regulated AV-node function. Electrical stimulation of either left or right stellate ganglia produces a positive chronotropic effect; however, right-sided stimulation produces a greater response (Meek and Eyster 1914). In a recent study of the dog, in which electrophysiological mapping of the cardiac activation sequence was carried out, stimulation of autonomic nerves on both sides produced changes in heart rate (Schuessler *et al.* 1986). In this study, tachycardia was most frequently produced by stimulation of left-sided nerves. Thus, node, and to a lesser extent in the AV node. When the latter occurred, it was most frequently produced by stimulation of lef-sided nerves. Thus, while right-sided sympathetic fibres have a greater effect on sinus-node function, left-sided nerves also exert a considerable influence. In general the magnitude of chronotropic responses follows a similar pattern. Stimulation of individual sympathetic and parasympathetic nerves on the right produces greater positive and negative chronotropic responses than stimulation of left-sided nerves, suggesting greater control by the former on sinus-node function.

Mechanisms of changes in sinus-node discharge rate

Activation of postganglionic sympathetic and parasympathetic fibres causes a local release of noradrenalin and acetylcholine, respectively. The time course of release and removal of transmitter differs considerably between the two systems. Electrical stimulation of cardiac sympathetic nerves produces an increase in heart rate, which reaches a steady state after about 30 seconds and takes a similar period to return to normal on cessation of stimulation (Warner and Cox 1962). The removal of released noradrenalin is achieved by re-uptake into sympathetic nerve terminals, by local tissue metabolism, and by wash-out into the coronary circulation. Electrical stimulation of parasympathetic nerves produces a reduction in heart rate which reaches a steady state within a few seconds and the effect wears off on cessation of stimulation over a similar period, reflecting rapid hydrolysis of acetylcholine. The response to electrical stimulation of both systems is frequency-dependent, the maximal response with sympathetic nerves being approximately 20 Hz and with parasympathetic nerves approximately 10 Hz.

In addition to changing the rate of sinus-node discharge, autonomic stimulation produces a shift in the focus within the sinus node from which activation spreads. Detailed mapping of electrical activation of the sinus node has shown that sympathetic stimulation causes a cranial shift in the pacemaker focus within the sinus node in association with the usual positive of chronotropic response (Geesbreght and Randall 1971). Parasympathetic stimulation produces a caudal shift in association with its negative chronotropic effect (Scheussler *et al.* 1986). A differential distribution of receptors on cells within the sinus node, resulting in greater sensitivity in some cells, is likely to account for this shift in impulse origin. Thus, several studies have shown that infusion of isoprenaline, a β-adrenoceptor agonist, which would be expected to be uniformly distributed, also produces a cranial shift in the impulse origin.

The electrophysiological basis by which sympathetic and parasympathetic activity regulate sinus-node discharge rate are only understood in part. The property of spontaneous diastolic depolarization characterizes all cells with pacemaker activity (Fig. 7.2). This means that the transmembrane potential changes in a positive direction during diastole (membrane potential remains unchanged in non-pacemaker cells). Diastolic depolarization eventually allows the transmembrane potential to reach the threshold potential and thereby initiates an action potential. The electrophysiological properties which determine the rate of discharge are: (1) the rate of diastolic depolarization; (2) the threshold potential; and (3) the maximum diastolic potential. Cholinergic stimulation of sinoatrial cells has been studied experimentally by vagal-nerve stimulation and by application of acetylcholine. Such experiments show

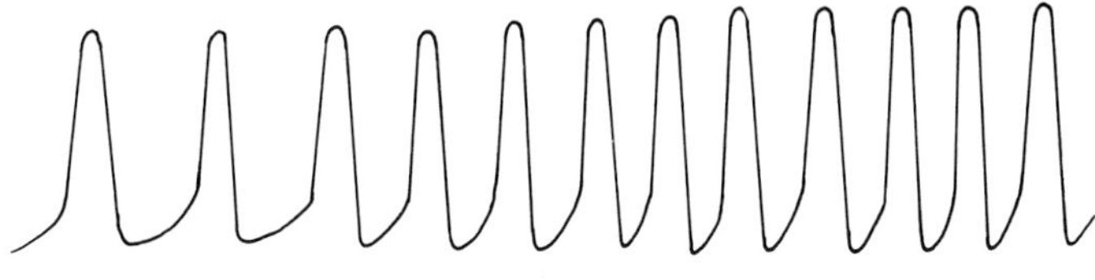

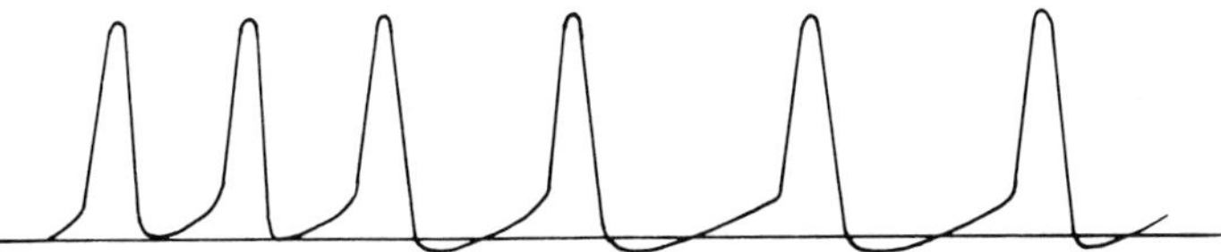

Fig. 7.2. Effects of sympathetic (upper trace) and parasympathetic (lower trace) stimulation on sinoatrial electrophysiology. Sympathetic stimulation accelerates heart rate by increasing the rate of diastolic depolarization. In contrast, parasympathetic stimulation has no effect on diastolic depolarization but slows discharge rate by causing diastolic hyperpolarization.

that parasympathetic-mediated negative chronotropism is achieved by diastolic hyperpolarization (Fig. 7.2) (Hutter and Trautwein 1956). This results from increased membrane permeability for potassium ions, the ionic current responsible for repolarization. The resulting hyperpolarization prolongs the interval between successive action potentials by increasing the difference between the maximum diastolic potential and threshold potential (Fig. 7.2).

The acceleration in firing rate associated with β-adrenoceptor stimulation is produced by an increased rate of diastolic depolarization (Fig. 7.2). Other effects are also observed, however, i.e. increased action potential amplitude and decreased action potential duration. These changes indicate that the ionic currents responsible are more complex than is the case for a cholinergic stimulation. The slow inward current, which in sinoatrial cells is carried by sodium ions, is enhanced, thereby increasing action potential amplitude. The outward current responsible for repolarization is activated earlier accounting for the reduction in action potential duration and slight diastolic hyperpolarization which often occurs.

The chain of events regulating heart rate is complex. Information is gathered from all parts of the cardiovascular system and higher cerebral centres integrated in the brainstem. Sympathetic and parasympathetic outflow are then adjusted accordingly to alter the distribution of autonomic activity within the sinus node to alter permeability of sinus-node cells to sodium and potassium ions, which in turn results in a change in their discharge rate. Under normal circumstances the acceleration in heart rate which occurs in association with exercise, for example, is achieved initially by a reduction in parasympathetic tone followed by an increase in sympathetic-nerve activity.

Variation in sinus rhythm

Children and young adults usually show a variation in heart rate and if this exceeds 0.12 seconds between the longest and shortest cycles, it is called sinus arrhythmia. It is a normal finding which tends to disappear with advancing years. It reflects variations in vagal tone during each respiratory cycle mediated through Bainbridge's reflex. The attenuation of sinus arrhythmia which occurs with increasing age is associated with a general attenuation of heart-rate variability. Thus, the heart-rate response to the Valsalva manoeuvre and deep breathing declines with age in normal subjects. This almost certainly reflects other changes which take place in the autonomic nervous system with age. Thus, for example, with increasing years there is evidence to suggest a gradual increase in plasma noradrenalin concentrations (Ewing *et al.* 1978) and altered adrenoceptor function (Box and Cox 1964) due to reduced responsiveness to adrenergic stimulation (Rowe and Troen 1980).

Measurement of heart-rate responses to a variety of standardized stimuli has become an important method for assessment of autonomic function. These tests consist of measuring reflex changes in heart rate in response to stimuli designed to alter activation of afferent inputs involved in autonomic regulation of the cardiovascular system. The Valsalva manoeuvre, deep breathing, passive changes in posture, compression and decompression of the carotid sinus, and injection of pharmacological pressure agents are used to stimulate different sensors and the evoked autonomic reflex is assessed by measurement of heart-rate change. These tests are discussed in more detail in Chapter 8. It has now been recognized that age-related changes in autonomic function may modify the results of such tests and a range of values for normal subjects of various ages has been derived (O'Brien *et al.* 1986) which should significantly improve their value.

Sinus tachycardia is most frequently a physiological response to a need for increased cardiac output during exercise or emotional stress. It is an integral part of the 'flight-or-flight' reaction mediated by increased sympathetic and reduced parasympathetic activity. Physiological sinus tachycardia may reach 190–200 beats/min during maximal exercise in young athletes, but for most healthy adults maximum rates of 160–170 beats/min are usual. Sinus tachycardia is also an important sign of increased sympathetic activity in association with conditions such as shock, myocardial infarction, infections, and heart failure. Tachycardia has the potential short-term benefit of offsetting harmful effects of certain conditions, i.e. it may increase cardiac output in heart failure. Given that it represents a response to increased physiological demand, it is perhaps not surprising that it is inappropriate and may be deleterious in certain other conditions. In acute myocardial infarction, for example, the increased cardiac work and inappropriate hypertension may increase oxygen demand and extend the necrotic process. Even in heart failure, chronically increased sympathetic stimulation may have wide-ranging disadvantages which are discussed in Chapter 6. Sinus tachycardia may be a clinical feature of autonomic neuropathy; however, a more usual feature is reduced variability in heart rate particularly in diabetic autonomic neuropathy. This can be readily demonstrated by plotting R–R intervals from 24-hour ECG recordings.

Sinus bradycardia (heart rate <60 beats/min) is common in healthy adults, particularly in those who are physically fit, and represents a normal reaction to vagal stimulation. It may also occur in conditions associated with increased vagal stimulation such as in raised intracranial pressure, or vomiting. Increased vagal stimulation is also frequently seen following acute myocardial infarction and is particularly likely to occur following inferior infarctions; it may be sufficient to cause second- or third-degree heart block. This explains why heart block is almost always transient following acute myocardial infarction and why atropine is often dramatically effective in restoring normal sinus rhythm. The most important clinical aspect of sinus bradycardia is that it may indicate the presence of sinus-node disease (sick sinus syndrome, brady-tachy syndrome). The occurrence of bradycardia in association with syncope or a history of palpitations should always lead to suspicion of this syndrome, in which intermittent bradycardia and tachycardia may cause syncope. Bradycardia may occur only occasionally, but may be intense with episodes of sinus arrest. Such episodes are particularly likely to occur at the termination of a tachycardia before sinus rhythm becomes re-established. There is no good evidence that autonomic dysregulation is a primary cause of this condition; however, drug-induced changes in autonomic function such as increased vagal stimulation with digoxin or reduced β-adrenergic stimulation with β-blockade may precipitate a serious deterioration or even sudden death in such patients.

The atrioventricular (AV) node is also richly innervated with sympathetic and parasympathetic fibres. In normal hearts the AV node provides the only bridge of electrical continuity between the atria and ventricles. As a result of its peculiarly slow conduction velocity (2–3 mm/s) it accounts for virtually all of the delay inherent in the P–R interval. Sympathetic and parasympathetic stimulation advance or retard conduction velocity within the AV node, and thereby serve the function of adjusting ventricular filling as the heart rate is increased and decreased, respectively. Under normal circumstances, autonomic stimulation of the AV node plays no significant role in sinus-node rhythm, although, as mentioned previously, intense vagal tone may cause AV block. In contrast, AV node function has in important role in the clinical effects of atrial fibrillation. In this condition, the AV node is bombarded with atrial impulses in excess of 350 impulses/min and, if all were conducted to the ventricles, a state identical to ventricular fibrillation would follow. The normal slow-conducting properties of the AV node prevents this but the precise rate of ventricular activation will depend on the level of autonomic stimulation of the AV node. Thus, with increased sympathetic activity, as is likely to occur following the abrupt onset of atrial firbillation, the ventricular rate may be so rapid that filling is impaired. Treatment is aimed at slowing the ventricular rate by reducing AV-node conduction with digoxin which acts directly on the AV node and indirectly by increasing vagal tone. The addition of β-blockade is useful in refractory cases as it also reduces AV-node conduction indirectly by reducing sympathetic tone.

Atrioventricular node function may play a crucial role in certain other arrhythmias which require antegrade (atrioventricular) or retrograde (ventriculoatrial) conduction. For example, in supraventricular tachycardia associated with an accessory pathway as in the Wolff–Parkinson–

White syndrome, a circular propagation of activity (re-entrant circuit) occurs. This usually takes the form of antegrade AV conduction with retrograde conduction by the accessory pathway. The occurrence and maintenance of such re-entrant arrhythmias is crucially dependent on conduction properties in all parts of the circuit, so that autonomic stimulation of the AV node is important. It is significant, for example, that drug-induced termination of such arrhythmias is most frequently achieved by slowing AV conduction using drugs such as verapamil. Changes in AV-node function, due to vagal or increased sympathetic tone such as occurs during normal activity, may therefore be important for the initiation and propagation of such arrhythmias. This explains why β-adrenoceptor blockade may be useful in preventing paroxysms of tachycardia in such patients.

During sinus rhythm, conduction through the AV node is exclusively in the antegrade direction. Many re-entry tachycardias which require retrograde ventriculoatrial conduction achieve this through the AV node. Examples of such arrhythmias are AV-nodal re-entry, antidromic supraventricular tachycardia in the Wolff–Parkinson–White syndrome, and pacemaker-mediated tachycardias. Studies based on pharmacological autonomic blockade (Hamilton Dougherty *et al.* 1986) indicate that ventriculoatrial conduction through the AV node is modulated by sympathetic and parasympathetic activity in a balanced fashion, as in the case of atrioventricular conduction. It follows that autonomic influences may also suppress or facilitate arrhythmias dependent on such abnormal propagation.

AUTONOMIC INFLUENCES ON ARRHYTHMIAS ASSOCIATED WITH MYOCARDIAL ISCHAEMIA

Sudden cardiac death is almost always due to ventricular fibrillation. Although myocardial ischaemia is its most common cause, the precise mechanisms are not well understood. Coronary atheroma is almost always severe in such cases, but complete occlusion is often absent and experimental studies indicate that both transient ischaemia and subsequent reperfusion may cause ventricular fibrillation (Sheridan *et al.* 1980). Considerable evidence has accumulated in recent decades linking disturbances in autonomic function with ventricular arrhythmias during myocardial ischaemia. The anxiety of patients in the early stages of myocardial infarction is intense and the sweating and tachycardia usually present suggest enhanced sympathetic activity. The finding of elevated levels of plasma and urinary catecholamines in patients following a myocardial infarction (Strang *et al.* 1974) supports this. In addition, rapid release of noradrenalin has been demonstrated in hearts following experimental ischaemia and reperfusion (Wollenberger and

Shahab 1965; Gauduel *et al.* 1979). The changing patterns of myocardial blood flow during ischaemia and reperfusion complicate the assessment of noradrenalin release and re-uptake; however, it is generally accepted that adrenergic stimulation is an important contributing factor in the genesis of arrhythmias during myocardial ischaemia and reperfusion. Since catecholamine release occurs in isolated perfused hearts (Wollenberger and Shahab 1965), it is likely that local factors related to the ischaemic process are responsible for producing this effect. This is supported by the finding that catecholamine release is greater in ischaemic than non-ischaemic regions of the heart following coronary ligation (Mathes and Gudbjarnason 1971).

Many studies have been undertaken to assess the importance of adrenergic stimulation in the arrhythmogenesis of myocardial ischaemia and reperfusion.

Denervation studies

Denervation studies have been carried out by surgical denervation and by depletion of noradrenalin content of nerve endings by treatment with 6-hydroxydopamine or reserpine. Surgical denervation of the heart significantly reduces the incidence of ventricular fibrillation following coronary ligation; however, this is only effective if carried out long enough prior to coronary ligation to permit catecholamine depletion to occur (Ebert *et al.* 1970). Myocardial catecholamine depletion also protects isolated buffer-perfused hearts from arrhythmias during ischaemia and reperfusion (Culling *et al.* 1984), suggesting that local release of catecholamines within the ischaemic territory is critically important. Thus, pre-treatment with 6-hydroxydopamine almost completely abolished ventricular tachycardia and fibrillation during acute myocardial ischaemia and reperfusion (Culling *et al.* 1984). Depletion of myocardial catecholamines using reserpine is also effective against arrhythmias during reperfusion but is much less so against arrhythmias during ischaemia. The basis for this apparent discrepancy is not clear, but it may reflect incomplete depletion of catecholamines coupled with adrenoceptor hypersensitivity. Studies using 6-hydroxydopamine suggest that myocardial noradrenalin content must be reduced to about 5 per cent of control values in order to prevent ventricular fibrillation during ischaemia and reperfusion (Culling *et al.* 1984). That catecholamines contribute to the general adverse effects of ischaemia is indicated by studies in which release of myocardial enzymes was used as a marker of myocardial damage (Gauduel *et al.* 1979). These studies showed that enzyme release was reduced by depletion of myocardial catecholamines. In addition, a temporal correlation has been demonstrated in the pig between the onset of arrhythmias and increased coronary arteriovenous noradrenalin differences.

Pharmacological blockade

A substantial number of studies have been undertaken to examine the effect of β-adrenoceptor blockade on arrhythmias during experimental myocardial ischaemia (for review see Fitzgerald 1982). Most studies have demonstrated some anti-arrhythmic effect; however, the degree of protection varies considerably. Thus, in some experiments a marked reduction in the incidence of ventricular fibrillation and improved survival have been observed, while in others a reduction in the number of ectopic beats has occurred without altering the incidence of ventricular fibrillation (Sheridan *et al.* 1980). Establishment of chronic β-blockade prior to coronary ligation may be more effective, suggesting that additional factors may be involved. Chronic β-blockade in man reduces overall mortality in patients following myocardial infarction and this includes a reduction in sudden cardiac death. The latter finding suggests that the protective effect is mediated in part by reducing the incidence of life-threatening arrhythmias.

Interest in the possibility that α-adrenoceptor blockade might prevent arrhythmias during ischaemia and reperfusion arose from studies in which phentolamine was found to prevent arrhythmias induced by a variety of techniques including intravenous administration of noradrenalin, nicotine, aconitine, or inhalation of chloroform (for review see Sheridan 1982). In addition, uncontrolled studies in man suggest that phentolamine may also prevent ventricular arrhythmias following myocardial infarction (Gould *et al.* 1975). Detailed studies in the cat and dog have demonstrated a significant anti-arrhythmic effect during coronary ligation and during subsequent reperfusion (Sheridan *et al.* 1980; Stewart *et al.* 1980) in response to acute administration of phentolamine. A drawback to the use of phentolamine is its blockade of α_1- and α_2-adrenoceptor subtypes and the fact that it has direct effects on myocardial electrophysiology (Rosen *et al.* 1971); however, a number of other more selective blocking agents have been shown to afford protection (Fig. 7.3). Thus, acute administration of prazosin (Sheridan *et al.* 1980) or indoramin (Penny *et al.* 1985) have been shown to be protective in the cat and guinea pig, respectively. The anti-arrhythmic effect of these agents has been suggested to result from either increased myocardial blood flow (due to blockade of α-adrenoceptor mediated coronary vasoconstriction) or direct myocardial electrophysiological actions. Available evidence however, suggests that this is unlikely; myocardial blood flow measured using radiolabelled microspheres was not altered in ischaemic myocardium pre-treated with phentolamine and reversal of the peripheral haemodynamic effects of phentolamine does not alter its anti-arrhythmic action (Sheridan *et al.* 1980). Direct electrophysiological actions of phentolamine have been documented in studies using isolated superfused Purkinje fibres (Rosen *et al.* 1971). The

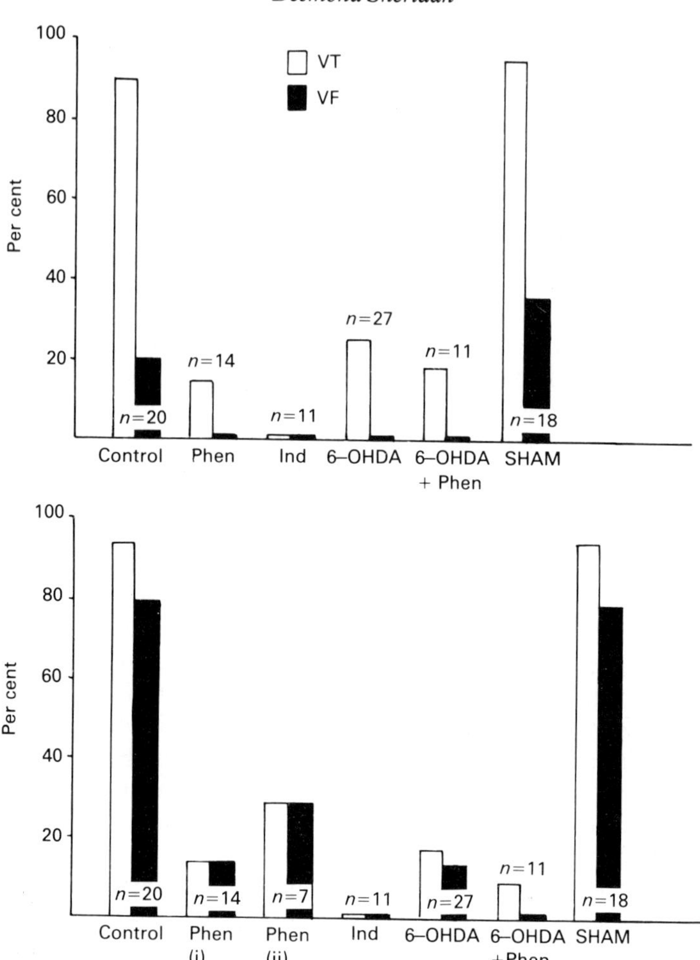

Fig. 7.3. Incidence of ventricular tachycardia (VT) and ventricular fibrillation (VF) during 30 minutes of ischaemia (upper panel) and reperfusion (lower panel) in Langendorf-perfused guinea pig hearts. α-adrenoceptor blockade with phentolamine or indoramin or myocardial catecholamine depletion significantly reduced both arrhythmias during ischaemia and reperfusion. Phentolamine was equally effective during reperfusion when added prior to the onset of ischaemia (i) or just prior to the onset of reperfusion (ii). Phen, phentolamine; Ind, indoramine; 6-OHDA, pre-treatment with 6 hydroxydopamine to deplete myocardial catecholamines.

concentrations of phentolamine required to prevent arrhythmias during experimental myocardial ischaemia are significantly lower than those used to demonstrate direct electrophysiological actions, suggesting that this is unlikely to be the relevant mode of action. In addition, electrophysiological studies in hearts depleted of endogenous catecholamines (Penny *et al.* 1985) indicate that its electrophysiological effects during ischaemia and reperfusion are dependent on the presence of endogenous catecholamines. A more likely explanation is that myocardial α-adrenoceptor stimulation is an important contributing factor in the production of arrhythmias during ischaemia and that the anti-arrhythmic action of α-blockade is due to its action on the myocardium.

Adrenergic stimulation

There is considerable circumstantial evidence that sympathetic activity is increased during experimental ischaemia and in patients with myocardial infarction (see above). More direct evidence is provided by the finding that efferent sympathetic neural activity is increased within 5 minutes following coronary ligation in the cat (Gillis 1971). Electrical stimulation of the left stellate ganglion or higher sympathetic centres in the dog can cause ventricular fibrillation if the anterior descending coronary artery is occluded but not in the absence of occlusion (Verrier *et al.* 1975). Such findings highlight myocardial vulnerability to adrenergic stimulation during ischaemia and suggest that the presence of myocardial ischaemia renders the heart susceptible to its action. Further evidence of this is provided by studies in which left stellate nerve stimulation in the cat produced greater electrophysiological responses during ischaemia than during normal perfusion (Sheridan *et al.* 1980).

It is generally accepted that β-adrenoceptor stimulation increases myocardial excitability. There are few studies of the effect of α-adrenoceptor stimulation in ischaemic myocardium. α-adrenoceptor stimulation of normal myocardium causes a weak positive inotropic effect and slight prolongation of action potential duration. α-adrenoceptor stimulation of normally perfused hearts with methoxamine (10^{-6} M) has no arrhythmogenic action but increases the incidence of ventricular tachycardia and fibrillation in hearts subjected to ischaemia and reperfusion. That such responses are mediated via α-adrenoceptors is indicated by the failure of β-blockade or histamine-receptor blockade to prevent them (Fig. 7.4). These observations were made in isolated perfused hearts devoid of central neuronal connections so that the altered sensitivity observed must have arisen at the level of nerve endings or within the myocytes. Much still needs to be discovered about the metabolic basis of such responses and it is likely that the ability of disease states to alter end-organ responsiveness to autonomic stimulation may be of great importance.

Vagal activity and arrhythmias

Increased vagal activity in patients following myocardial infarction is common, particularly following inferior infarction. Similar changes have been observed in experimental animals and there is evidence that it may

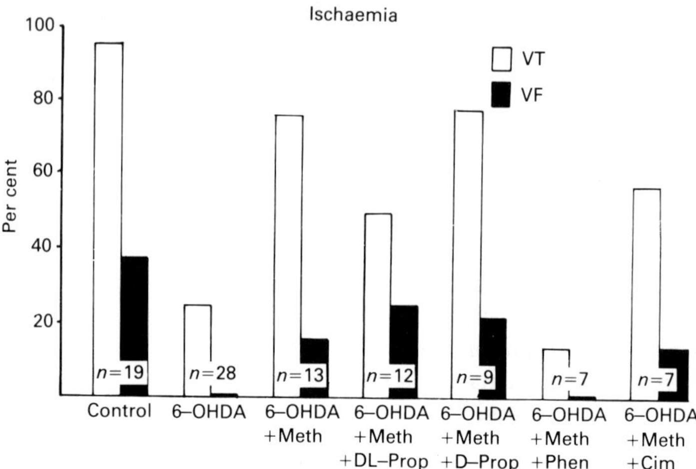

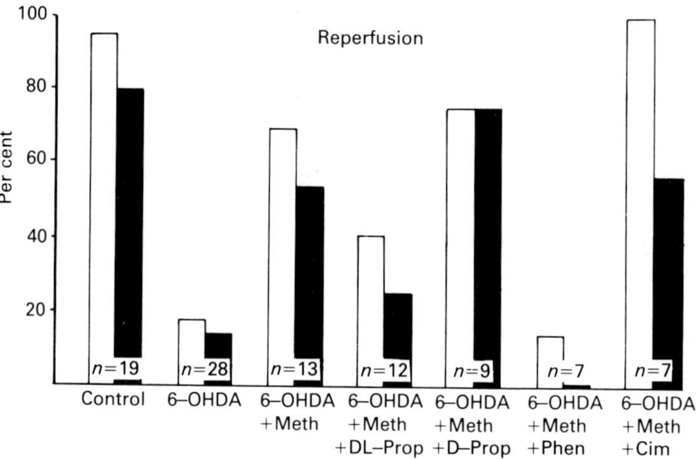

Fig. 7.4. Incidence of ventricular tachycardia (VT) and ventricular fibrillation (VF) during ischaemia and reperfusion in Langendorf-perfused guinea pig hearts. Catecholamine depletion by pre-treatment with 6-hydroxydopamine (6-OHDA) reduced VT and VF during ischaemia and reperfusion. Addition of methoxamine (Meth) reversed this. This arrhythmogenic effect was abolished by phentolamine (Phen), but not by propanolol (Prop) or cimetidine (Cim).

have an anti-arrhythmic action. In the cat, for example, vagotomy or administration of atropine increases the incidence of ventricular fibrillation (Corr and Gillis 1974). In some patients the bradycardia associated with such vagal tone may be extreme and cause hypotension, which in turn may adversely effect coronary perfusion pressure and thereby provoke further arrhythmias. In practice, bradycardia or heart block which is causing clinically significant hypotension should be treated with atropine (or pacing if appropriate), but the possibility of provoking ventricular arrhythmias, although remote, should be remembered.

CONCLUSION

Alteration in heart rate provides an efficient and simple means of altering cardiac output to meet varying needs. The autonomic nervous system has the greatest control of its modulation. Under its influence, cardiac performance is elegantly balanced to meet the demands of the body, whether in conditions of tranquillity or in the ultimate defence of its existence. Although its purpose is relatively simple, the mechanisms involved are complex and have evolved essentially for regulating physiological activity. Faced with disease within its own divisions or in the cardiac tissues upon which it acts, disturbances in heart rhythm are inevitable. Such disturbances can vary from mild inconvenience to sudden cardiac death. By learning more about its activity in such pathological conditions, we may be better able to assist its efforts to maintain a normal cardiac rhythm.

REFERENCES

Box, G. E. P. and Cox, D. R. (1964). An analysis of transformations. *J. R. statist. Soc.* **26**, 211–52.

Corr, P. B. and Gillis, R. A. (1974). Role of the vagus nerve in the cardiovascular changes induced by coronary occlusion. *Circulation* **49**, 86–97.

Culling, W., Penny, W. J., Lewis, M. J., Middleton, K., and Sheridan, D. J. (1984). Effects of myocardial catecholamine depletion on cellular electrophysiology and arrhythmias during ischaemia and reperfusion. *Cardiovasc. Res.* **18**, 675–82.

Ebert, P. E., Vanderbeck, R. B., Allgood, R. J., and Sabiston, D. C. (1970). Effect of chronic cardiac denervation on arrhythmias after coronary artery ligation. *Cardiovasc. Res.* **4**, 141–7.

Ewing, D. J., Campbell, I. W., Murray, A., Neilson, J. M. M., and Clarke, B. F. (1978). Immediate heart rate response to standing: simple test for autonomic neuropathy in diabetes. *Br. med. J.* **1**, 145–7.

Fitzgerald, J. D. (1982). The effects of beta-adrenoceptor blocking drugs on early arrhythmias in experimental and clinical myocardial ischaemia. In *Early arrhythmias resulting from myocardial ischaemia* (ed. J. R. Parratt), p. 295. MacMillan Press, London.

Gauduel, Y., Karagueuzian, H. S., and De Leiris, J. (1979). Deleterious effects of endogenous catecholamines on hypoxic myocardia cells following re-oxygenation. *J. mol. cell. Cardiol.* **11**, 717–31.

Geesbreght, J. M. and Randall, W. C. (1971). Area localisation of shifting cardiac pacemakers during sympathetic stimulation. *Am. J. Physiol.* **22**, 1522–7.

Gillis, R. A. (1971). Role of the nervous system in the arrhythmias produced by coronary occlusion in the cat. *Am. Heart J.* **81**, 677–84.

Gould, L., Reddy, C. V. R., Weinstein, T., and Gomprecht, R. F. (1975). Anti-arrhythmic prophylaxis with phentolamine in acute myocardial infarction. *J. clin. Pharmacol.* **51**, 191–7.

Hamilton Dougherty, A., Rinkenberger, R. L., and Naccarelli, G. V. (1986). Effect of pharmacologic autonomic blockade on ventriculoatrial conduction. *Am. J. Cardiol.* **57**, 1274–9.

Hutter, O. F. and Trautwein, W. (1956). Vagal and sympathetic effects on the pacemaker fibres of the sinus venosus of the heart. *J. gen. Physiol.* **39**, 715–33.

Mathes, P. and Gudbjarnason, S. (1971). Changes in norepinephrine stores in the canine heart following experimental myocardial infarction. *Am. Heart J.* **81**, 211–19.

Meek, W. J. and Eyster, J. A. E. (1914). Experiments on the origin and propagation of the impulse in the heart. IV. The effect of vagal stimulation and of cooling on the location of the pacemaker within the sino-auricular node. *Am. J. Physiol.* **34**, 368–83.

O'Brien, I. A. D., O'Hare, P., and Corrall, R. J. M. (1986). Heart rate variability in healthy subjects: effect of age and derivation of normal ranges for tests of autonomic function. *Br. Heart J.* **55**, 348–54.

Penny, W. J., Culling, W., Lewis, M. J., and Sheridan, D. J. (1985). Antiarrhythmic and electrophysiological effects of alpha-adrenoceptor blockade during myocardial ischaemia and reperfusion in isolated guinea pig heart. *J. mol. cell. Cardiol.* **17**, 399–409.

Rosen, M. R., Gelband, H., and Hoffman, B. F. (1971). Effects of phentolamine on electrophysiologic properties of isolated canine Purkinje fibres. *J. Pharmacol. exp. Ther.* **179**, 586–93.

Rowe, J. W. and Troen, B. R. (1980). Sympathetic nervous system and ageing in man. *Endocrinol. Rev.* **1**, 167–79.

Schuessler, R. B., Boineau, J. P., Whylds, A. C., Hill, D. A., Miller, C. B., and Roeske, W. R. (1986). Effect of canine cardiac nerves on heart rate, rhythm and pacemaker location. *Am. J. Physiol.* **250**, H630–H644.

Sheridan, D. J., Penkoske, P. A., Sobel, B. E., and Corr, P. B. (1980). Alpha adrenergic contributions to dysrrhythmia during myocardial ischaemia and reperfusion in cats. *J. clin. Invest.* **65**, 161–71.

Stewart, J. R., Burmeister, W. E., Burmeister, J., and Lucchesi, B. R. (1980). Electrophysiologic and antiarrhythmic effects of phentolamine in experimental coronary occlusion and reperfusion in the dog. *J. cardiovasc. Pharmacol.* **2**, 77–91.

Strang, R. C., Vetter, N., Rowe, N. J., and Oliver, M. F. (1974). Plasma cyclic AMP and total catecholamines during acute myocardial infarction in man. *Eur. J. clin. Invest.* **4**, 115–19.

Verrier, R. L., Calvert, A., and Lown, B. (1975). Effect of posterior hypothalamic stimulation on ventricular fibrillation threshold. *Am. J. Physiol.* **228**, 923–7.

Warner, H. R. and Cox, A. (1962). A mathematical model of heart rate controlled by sympathetic and vagus efferent information. *J. appl. Physiol.* **17**, 349–55.

Wollenberger, A. and Shahab, L. (1965). Anoxia-induced release of noradrenaline from the isolated perfused heart. *Nature, London* **207**, 88–9.

8. Cardiovascular baroreflex control in man

John Vann Jones

INTRODUCTION

The isolation and blocking techniques used to study cardiovascular reflexes in animals are largely inapplicable to man. In human beings it is difficult to study any one reflex in isolation as secondary reflexes from other sets of receptors soon come into play to modify any primary evoked response. Accepting these limitations a number of techniques have been developed to 'get at' the cardiovascular reflex responses in man. These include the Valsalva manoeuvre, lower-body negative pressure, cold pressor tests, and a variety of other physical and mental stimuli. In a discussion limited to baroreflex mechanisms the two principal techniques used have been injections of pressor substances or the application, by means of specially designed collars, of negative or positive pressures directly to the neck to stimulate the receptors located in the carotid sinuses. Low-pressure receptors, sometimes referred to as baroreceptors, have been well localized to the cardiopulmonary area and special techniques devised to study them. They are described in Chapters 5 and 11 and, therefore, this chapter will be limited to a description of the investigation and relevance of the systemic arterial baroreceptors in man.

BAROREFLEX MEASUREMENT TECHNIQUES IN MAN

Carotid-sinus massage can be used to stimulate the baroreceptors located there. The technique is crude and cannot be quantified but has its uses in such situations as attempting to revert abnormal supraventricular tachycardias back to normal sinus rhythm or to determine the possible presence of carotid-sinus hypersensitivity in patients with transient losses of consciousness. Other methods used have included carotid occlusion, sinus-nerve stimulation, and sinus-nerve block. All these will alter heart rate and blood pressure but cannot be used to quantify the baroreceptor reflex.

Vasoactive drugs

It was noticed that during sleep not only did blood pressure fall but so also did the heart rate. This implied that there must be diminished or reset baroreceptor function during sleep. In order to investigate this Smyth *et al.* (1969) developed a method for assessing baroreflex sensitivity. They measured the reflex slowing of the heart rate that occurred in response to small injections of the pressor agent angiotensin. It soon became clear that angiotensin also caused a tachycardia shortly after the bradycardia, presumably due to a central action, and angiotensin was soon abandoned in favour of the pure α-adrenergic stimulating agent phenylephrine. Others have since used other pressor agents but the principle remains the same. The use of this technique requires insertion of both indwelling venous and arterial lines. A small dose of phenylephrine (50–150 μg) is injected intravenously, usually out of sight of the subject, in a small volume of saline. The relationship between the evoked rise in blood pressure (usually 20–30 mm Hg) and the consequent slowing of heart rate (more usually expressed as lengthening of the R–R interval) is plotted and the least squares regression equation used to fit a linear regression line through these points. The slope of this line is taken as a measure of the individual's baroreflex sensitivity (Fig. 8.1). The steeper the slope the greater the baroreflex sensitivity. Approximately six such estimations are made in each individual at 3–5 minute intervals to allow blood pressure and heart rate to return to baseline between estimations. Obviously, there will be some variation from injection to injection in the scatter of the points around the regression line and accordingly the '*r*' value will vary. This can be corrected for by statistically weighting the results depending on the degree of variance around the regression line. After weighting, the mean of the results can be taken as the baroreflex sensitivity for that particular subject. This relationship appears to be reproducible and to be independent of the resting heart rate or systemic pressure.

The other half of the reflex arc can be studied by determining the heart-rate or pulse-interval response to a fall in blood pressure. This is usually done using one of the intravenous nitrates but nitroprusside and amylnitrate have also been used. A reflex tachycardia is produced but it tends to be less than the equivalent bradycardia evoked by phenylephrine and it is the latter which has evolved as the standard technique.

The bolus injections of phenylephrine produce 'ramp-like' effects but 'steady-state' techniques have also been used (Korner 1979) to determine baroreflex function during more sustained and steady changes in blood

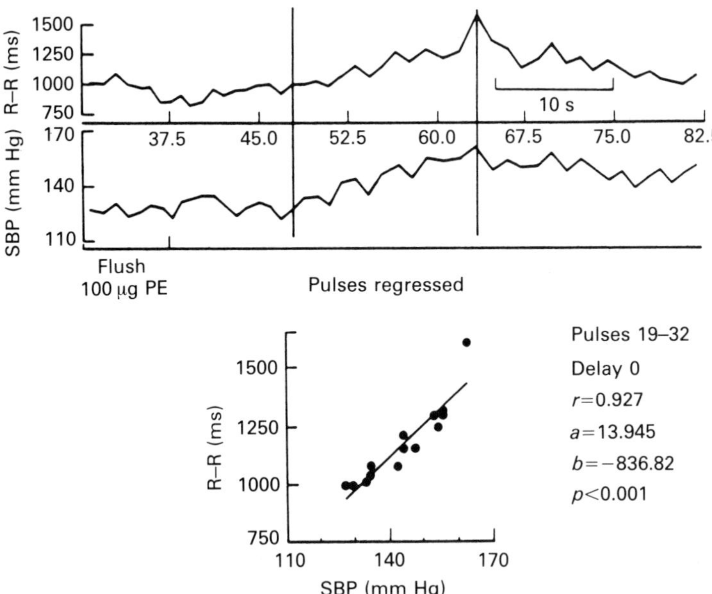

Fig. 8.1. The effect of phenylephrine (PE) injection on blood pressure and R–R interval. The pulse interval is regressed against the systolic blood pressure (SBP) and the regression line gives a measure of the slope of baroreflex sensitivity.

pressure. A brief infusion is used and the baroreflex sensitivity determined towards the end of the infusion period. The changes in pulse interval are usually less marked than with the ramp technique and are probably due much more to changes in sympathetic nervous activity than is the case with the bolus injection where the bradycardia produced is virtually totally due to vagal stimulation.

Neck chamber devices

The phenylephrine technique is invasive, involving as it does the insertion of an intra-arterial pressure line. This fact alone restricts its application while its use must necessarily only be limited to assessment of baroreflex control of heart rate. Therefore another technique has been widely used that is non-invasive and also can allow blood-pressure responses to be assessed. It involves the application of an airtight collar either partially or totally round the neck but embracing both carotid sinuses. By changing the pressure in the collar the degree of stimulus to the baroreceptors in the carotid sinuses can be changed. Neck suction slows the heart rate and causes a fall in blood pressure. This suction is, of course, 'seen' by the carotid sinuses as an increase in transmural pressure which is the same as an increase in blood pressure and hence the appropriate reflex response. Ernsting and Parry (1957) were the first to use this technique but Eckberg in particular and Mancia and his colleagues have been responsible for most of the information obtained using it. Another considerable advantage of this technique is that the carotid-sinus baroreflex can be studied almost in isolation while the effect on vascular resistance can also be determined. Not all of the externally applied pressure change is transmitted to the receptor site. There is a pressure gradient between the outside and the carotid sinus internally. It does seem however that most of the pressure change is transmitted.

Comparison of the drug-injection and neck-collar techniques

It is not always easy to successfully apply the neck collar and to obtain the necessary airtight seal. Moreover, necks vary and the loss of stimulus down the pressure gradient from outside to inside is also variable from subject to subject. Quantitative estimates of reflex activity are therefore less exact. It is obvious that the reflex changes evoked and the information conveyed from the carotid sinuses will be at variance with those from the aortic arch. Nevertheless, the initial responses obtained do seem to parallel those with the vasoactive-drug technique where at least the information being conveyed to the brain from both major baroreflex zones is in agreement. Steady-state information with the neck collar is probably less valuable and certainly the heart-rate responses are poorly sustained. The application of pressure or suction to the neck is not always comfortable especially with larger degrees of change. One considerable advantage that the vasoactive-drug method enjoys, therefore, is that it can and should be done with the patient oblivious to the fact that his reflex is being measured. This is not possible with the neck collar device and alerting or defence reactions may interfere with the reflex under study.

PHYSIOLOGICAL OBSERVATIONS IN MAN

The original stimulus for developing the phenylephrine-injection technique was to study baroreflex activity during sleep. Rather surprisingly, it was found that the reflex had reset to operate round the lower pressure at night and, if anything, the sensitivity of the reflex was increased. There is still some debate as to whether baroreflex sensitivity is increased in sleep but Conway *et al.* (1983) found this and also that, with increasing mental arousal as the subjects wakened from sleep, there was a progressive rise in blood pressure but also a progressive decrease in baroreflex sensitivity. This was interesting, suggesting as it does an ongoing buffering effect of the reflex rather than just the short sharp buffering effect that has often been suggested to be the principal role of the baroreflexes, that is acute rather than chronic blood-pressure determinants. With sleep the reflex seems to be at its most sensitive during rapid eye movement (REM) sleep. These observations have, of course, been made on heart-rate responses only as it is not possible to carry out neck-pressure studies and have the subjects remain asleep.

It is important not to assume invariably that what is true of the heart-rate response will also be so of the blood pressure. In exercise, both dynamic and static, the heart-rate response is progressively diminished until at rates of above 150 beats/min no bradycardia can be evoked by carotid-sinus activation. This does not appear to be the case with blood-pressure responses as neck suction still evokes a blood-pressure fall during static exercise. Mental arithmetic also diminishes baroreflex sensitivity when measured by the phenylephrine-injection method.

Baroreflex heart-rate responses have also been measured following exercise to see whether they could explain the persistent fall in blood pressure that occurs at this time (Somers *et al.* 1985). It was concluded that baroreflex sensitivity recovered slowly after exercise but eventually reached higher levels than pre-exercise and could contribute to the post-exercise drop in blood pressure.

Exercise programmes have a long-term effect on heart rate (slower) and blood pressure (lower). It has been shown that baroreflex sensitivity does not seem to bear any relationship to the level of physical fitness so that it would seem that changes in blood pressure and heart rate in well trained individuals are not due to changes in the reflex.

Eckberg, in the United States, has performed a long series of physiological experiments using his neck-collar device. With his collar he can change pressure very rapidly, almost in square-wave form, and is therefore able to perform experiments at different times in the cardiac cycle. In this way he has shown that the time within the cardiac cycle at which the stimulus is applied affects the magnitude of the pulse interval change and also its duration. Surprisingly, the rate of change of the stimulus was of little importance within the physiological range (Eckberg 1976, 1977*a*). Eckberg (1977*b*) also carried out a series of experiments where he applied suction to the collar, achieved a steady state with a new heart rate, and then applied more suction. In this way he was able to show that baroreflex sensitivity was independent of the pulse interval at pressures less than 160 mm Hg. This is important because it had earlier been shown by Pickering and colleagues, using the vasoactive-drug method, that there was a strong inverse correlation between resting heart rate and baroreflex sensitivity. Eckberg showed that the slower heart rate was probably a manifestation of greater baroreflex sensitivity in such subjects rather than its cause.

EFFECT OF DRUGS ON THE BAROREFLEX

General anaesthetics have profound acute effects on heart rate and blood pressure, and baroreflex sensitivity has been assessed in patients given a wide variety of these agents. Generally this has been assessed by vasoactive drugs measuring the heart-rate response. Thiopentone decreases baroreflex sensitivity and increases the heart rate. Halothane has been much studied. It results in resetting of the reflex and loss of baroreflex sensitivity. This has been assessed at up to 50 per cent loss but some investigators claim the loss of sensitivity as mild. Baroreflex activity recovers rapidly and at least with halothane seems to be restored to normal values before the patient has fully regained consciousness. Other anaesthetics that have been studied include methohexitone, fentanyl, and nitrous oxide. This latter is very similar to halothane causing resetting and loss of baroreflex sensitivity.

Many of the commonly used antihypertensive agents have been assessed with regard to their effects on the baroreflex. It is possible that propranolol, for instance, increases baroreflex sensitivity. This has been seen in several studies and could be a local effect on the receptors themselves. No such effect, however, has been seen with the few other β-blocking agents studied. Results tend to be conflicting both between studies with the same drug (for example, captopril has been claimed to increase baroreflex sensitivity while another study has shown no effect) and between drugs of the same class (for example, possible increased sensitivity with the calcium antagonist nifedipine but no effect with nicardipine).

One antihypertensive agent that does seem to have part of its mode of action via increasing baroreflex sensitivity which it appears to do centrally, is clonidine. This has been demonstrated in both animals and man (Sleight *et al.* 1975). In man there appears to be a dose-related effect with increasing baroreflex sensitivity with increasing doses. The importance of this observation is the implication that changes in baroreflex sensitivity can exert long-term blood-pressure effects.

BAROREFLEXES IN HYPERTENSION

Using the phenylephrine-injection technique Gribbin and co-workers (1971) showed that there was a linear relationship between blood pressure and baroreflex sensitivity and also between age and baroreflex sensitivity. Sensitivity declined with both increasing age (Fig. 8.2) and increasing blood pressure (Fig. 8.3). Others have found slight variations in these results; for example, Shimada *et al.* (1986) studied the relationship between age, baroreflex sensitivity, and systolic blood pressure in normotensive and hypertensive subjects. In the hypertensive subjects

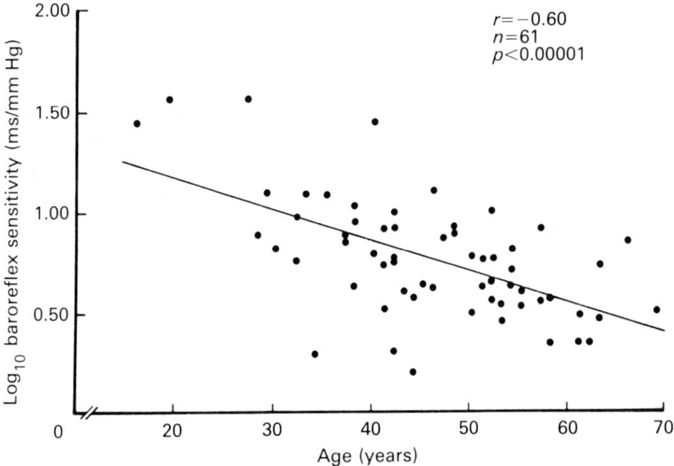

Fig. 8.2. The relationship between baroreflex sensitivity and age.

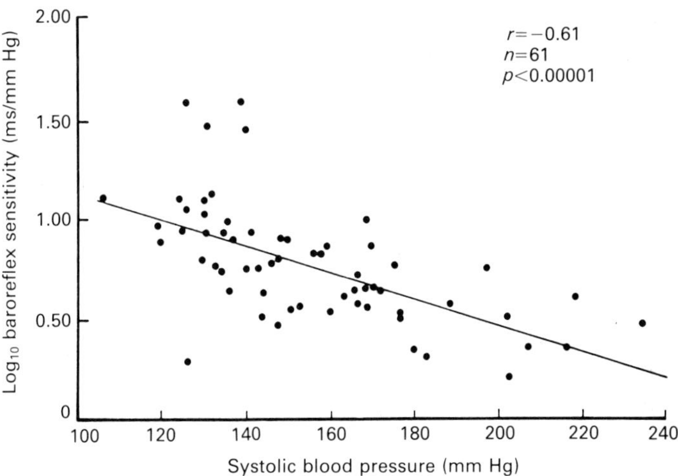

Fig. 8.3. The relationship between baroreflex sensitivity and systolic blood pressure.

baroreflex sensitivity was independently related to both age and systolic blood pressure. In the normotensive group, after correcting for age, baroreflex sensitivity was not correlated with systolic pressure. When all the subjects were grouped together, however, the relationship held for both age and systolic pressure.

Baroreflex sensitivity has been shown to be depressed in young people with very borderline elevations of pressure. It has also been found that the reflex is impaired in young normotensive subjects who have a family history of hypertension when compared to people of the same age and blood pressure in whom there is no such family history. This tends to suggest that the defect in baroreflex sensitivity is inherited rather than acquired. There have been no studies of young children, apart from neonates, although it is known that children with higher pressures tend to develop into adults with hypertension. The study on neonates was to demonstrate whether the reflex was fully developed at birth—apparently it is not.

Mancia and co-workers carried out extensive studies on heart-rate and blood-pressure responses using a neck-collar device in both normotensive and hypertensive patients (Mancia *et al.* 1977). They divided their hypertensive subjects into moderate or severe depending upon whether the mean blood pressure was above or below 145 mm Hg (Mancia *et al.* 1978). Their results differ somewhat from what might be expected from animal studies or on the basis of heart-rate responses induced by phenylephrine but this is the only group that has studied blood-pressure responses to neck-pressure changes in any great depth. They found that in hypertensive subjects reflex changes in blood pressure were greater when baroreceptor activity was increased. Exactly the opposite was seen in the normotensive subjects. Thus carotid-sinus suction produced a modest reflex fall in blood pressure in normotensive subjects but a more progressive response the more severe the hypertension. The opposite was seen when the pressure applied to the carotid sinus was a positive one.

The conclusion, therefore, is that the baroreceptors reset in hypertension but tend to overdo it so that the hypertensive subject is operating on the lower end of his reflex curve with the result that, when the pressure increases, more baroreceptor afferents are recruited than normal—hence more marked reflex effects. In normotensives the opposite is the case. These are interesting observations, carefully done, but they need to be confirmed. Mancia and colleagues also found that there did not seem to be a loss of baroreflex sensitivity, with regard to blood-pressure responses, in their hypertensive subjects.

Baroreflexes and blood-pressure variability

Watson *et al.* (1979) looked at the factors affecting blood-pressure variability and concluded that baroreflex sensitivity was important. They reported similar findings in a second series of studies comparing young hypertensive subjects with elderly normotensive and hypertensive groups. Using many thousands of blood-pressure measurements obtained by means of direct indwelling arterial cannulae, others have confirmed these findings using the phenylephrine technique, in groups of fully ambulant hypertensive patients (Sleight 1983) (Fig. 8.4). It would seem that the baroreflex exerts its control over blood pressure by means of the sympathetic nervous system and correlations have been shown between baroreflex sensitivity and noradrenalin release during

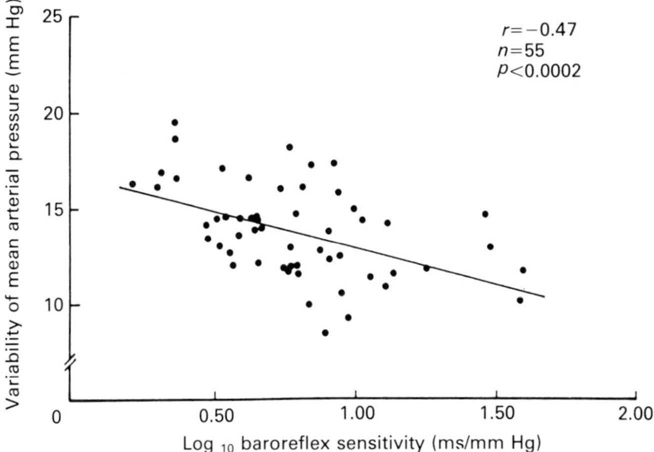

Fig. 8.4. The relationship between the variability of ambulatory waking mean arterial pressure and baroreflex sensitivity.

such manoeuvres as bicycling. Indeed it has even been advocated that measuring changes in plasma noradrenalin levels in response to step-wise reductions in blood pressure may be a good method of assessing baroreflex function.

Unfortunately, the opposite is less true—increasing blood pressure by phenylephrine infusions less predictably decreases plasma noradrenalin levels. This would be predictable from what is known about the kinetics of noradrenalin turnover. Phillipp *et al.* (1978) performed elegant experiments on the individual sensitivity, or rather reactivity, to infused and circulating noradrenalin. In both normotensive and hypertensive subjects an inverse relationship was seen between exercising plasma noradrenalin levels and the reactivity to infused noradrenalin. Thus the situation is more complex than initially suspected and actual levels of circulating noradrenalin are only a relatively crude measure of the vascular response itself.

The efferent limb of the reflex arc

The experiments of Wallin and associates on efferent sympathetic activity are described in Chapter 11. In summary, they have shown that sympathetic activity is independent of blood pressure in normotensive subjects and that there is a wide range of discharge frequencies. Despite this variation there seems to be inappropriate sympathetic activity in hypertension. Using the neck-collar technique Wallin and Eckberg (1982) showed that changes in carotid transmural pressure and hence baroreflex activity had marked transient effects on sympathetic nerve discharge. These responses occurred rapidly but disappeared almost as quickly. On the other hand, changes in pulse interval occurred quickly but persisted for as long as neck suction was applied. The conclusion from this study was that a common baroreceptor stimulus evoked a differential response in vagal and sympathetic outputs. The former was sustained and influenced by the change in carotid-sinus transmural pressure while the latter was transient and seemed more related to changes in transmural pressure rather than to absolute values.

BAROREFLEX STUDIES IN CONDITIONS WITH ASSOCIATED AUTONOMIC DYSFUNCTION

There have been relatively few studies of baroreflex function in diabetics despite the well known dysfunction of the autonomic nervous system in this condition. In a detailed study of 12 diabetics Eckberg *et al.* (1986) found considerable derangement of baroreflex function. Resting noradrenalin levels were subnormal and did not change with changes in blood pressure. Phenylephrine injections produced abnormally large pressor responses but little change in pulse interval occurred either spontaneously or in response to the injection. In diabetic patients with hypertension, including four with orthostatic hypotension Olshan *et al.* (1983) found evidence of significant baroreflex abnormality consistent with both vagal and sympathetic efferent damage. They also found that the degree of baroreflex sensitivity loss was inversely related to the degree of orthostatic hypotension. When supine, of course, these patients were hypertensive but no correlation could be found under these circumstances between baroreflex function and the height of the pressure.

OTHER MEDICAL CONDITIONS AFFECTING BAROREFLEX SENSITIVITY IN MAN

Studies of baroreflex sensitivity have been performed on patients with a wide variety of medical conditions. These include studies in patients after repair of coarctation of the aorta, in patients a few days after myocardial infarction, in renal dialysis patients, in people with chronic left ventricular dysfunction, in patients with Chagas' disease, and in cases of excess alcohol consumption. Almost invariably, the reflex has been found to be depressed to a variable extent in these conditions.

CAROTID-SINUS HYPERSENSITIVITY SYNDROME

Normally as people become older their baroreflexes become less sensitive (Gribbin *et al.* 1971). This is particularly so in elderly hypertensives and may be one reason why the systolic pressure is so variable in these elderly subjects. Somewhat parodoxically there are people, mostly elderly, whose carotid-sinus baroreflexes are hypersensitive and in whom relatively mild stimulation to the neck (for example with a tight collar or with shaving) results in a marked bradycardia and fall in blood pressure. If pronounced enough, this leads to carotid-sinus syncope and is one cause of transient loss of consciousness in the elderly. Until recently this was regarded as a relatively rare condition but Murphy *et al.* (1986) found evidence of its presence in 14 per cent of elderly people in nursing homes. They found that carotid-sinus hypersensitivity appeared to be a potent contributory factor to unexplained 'falls' in the elderly as well as to syncopal episodes.

The natural history of the condition, again surprisingly, is quite variable and a large percentage of patients seem to spontaneously remit. The mechanism of the hypersensitivity is unknown and there are no readily obvious differences between elderly people with depressed baroreflexes compared to those with hypersensitive reflexes.

A variety of treatments have been advocated and pacemaker insertion is now usual in these people although anticholinergic drugs have also had some success. The syndrome itself is classified as cardioinhibitory, where the principal effects of the reflex seem to be on heart rate (Type I) or vasodepressor where the reflex has less pronounced effects on heart rate but causes a peripheral vasodilatation and therefore drop in blood pressure (Type II). Peretz and Abdulla (1985) further subdivided these subjects into Type IA where predominantly sinus-node inhibition occurs or Type IB where the atrioventricular node is more affected. The importance of knowing whether the syncope is cardioinhibitory or vasodepressor is because of possible pacemaker therapy. Where the syndrome is predominantly cardioinhibitory, pacemaker insertion is very effective in abolishing the symptoms but is much less helpful, predictably, in the vasodepressor type. Fortunately, cardioinhibitory carotid-sinus hypersensitivity is far the commoner of the two types and pacemaker insertion is usually curative. There can be, of course, a mixed picture where pacing is partially successful only, but this too, surprisingly, is not as common as the cardioinhibitory type. It is possible, however, that the newer physiological or dual chamber pacemakers (DDI) may be of help in vasodepressor syncope.

The carotid hypersensitivity syndrome is more common in males. It does not seem to affect both sinuses equally and indeed may only be present on one side, more commonly the right carotid sinus.

CONCLUSION

In conclusion, there are two major techniques of assessing baroreflex activity in man. The vasoactive-drug method or the use of variable-pressure neck-collar devices. Each has its advantages and disadvantages. These methods have been used to assess baroreflex contribution to a variety of physiological and pathophysiological states. Naturally enough, however, most attention has focused on the possible role of these receptors in the pathogenesis of high blood pressure and its treatment.

REFERENCES

Conway, J., Boon, N., Jones, J. V., and Sleight, P. (1983). Involvement of the baroreceptor reflexes in the changes in blood pressure with sleep and mental arousal. *Hypertension* **5**, 746–8.

Eckberg, D. L. (1976). Temporal response patterns of the human sinus node to brief carotid baroreceptor stimuli. *J. Physiol., London* **258**, 769–82.

Eckberg, D. L. (1977*a*). Baroreflex inhibition of the human sinus node: importance of stimulus intensity, duration and rate of pressure change. *J. Physiol., London* **269**, 561–78.

Eckberg, D. L. (1977*b*). Adaptation of the human carotid baroreceptor–cardiac reflex. *J. Physiol., London* **269**, 579–90.

Eckberg, D. L., Harkins, S. W., Fritsch, J. M., Musgrave, G. E., and Gardner, D. F. (1986). Baroreflex control of plasma norepinephrine and heart period of healthy subjects and diabetic patients. *J. clin. Invest.* **78**, 366–74.

Ernsting, J. and Parry, D. J. (1957). Some observations on the effects of stimulating the stretch receptors in the carotid artery of man. *J. Physiol., London* **137**, 45–6.

Gribbin, B., Pickering, T. G., Sleight, P., and Peto, R. (1971). The effect of age and high blood pressure on baroreflex sensitivity in man. *Circulation Res.* **29**, 424–31.

Korner, P. I. (1979). Central nervous control of autonomic cardiovascular function. In *Handbook of physiology. The cardiovascular system* (ed. R. M. Berne), pp. 691–739. American Physiological Society, Washington, DC.

Mancia, G., Ferrari, A., Gregorini, L., Valentini, R., Ludbrook, J., and Zanchetti, A. (1977). Circulatory reflexes from carotid and extracarotid baroreceptor areas in man. *Circulation Res.* **41**, 309–15.

Mancia, G., Ludbrook, J., Ferrari, A., Gregorini, L., and Zanchetti, A. (1978). Baroreceptor reflexes in human hypertension. *Circulation Res.* **43**, 170–7.

Murphy, A. I., Rowbotham, B. J., Boyle, R. S., Thew, C. M., Fardoulys, J. A. and Wilson, K. (1986). Carotid sinus hypersensitivity in elderly nursing home patients. *Aust. NZ J. Med.* **16**, 24–7.

Olshan, A. R., O'Connor, D. T., Cohen, I. M., Mitas, J. A., and Stone, R. A. (1983). Baroreflex dysfunction in patients with adult-onset diabetes and hypertension. *Am. J. Med.* **74**, 233–42.

Peretz, D. I. and Abdulla, A. (1985). Management of cardioinhibitory hypersensitive carotid sinus syncope with permanent cardiac pacing—a seventeen year prospective study. *Can. J. Cardiol.* **1**, 86–91.

Phillipp, T., Distler, A., and Cordes, U. (1978). Sympathetic nervous system and blood pressure control in essential hypertension. *Lancet* **ii**, 959–63.

Shimada, K., Kitazumi, T., Ogura, H., Sadakane, N., and Ozawa, T. (1986). Differences in age-independent effects of blood pressure on baroreflex sensitivity between normal and hypertensive subjects. *Clin. Sci.* **70**, 489–94.

Sleight, P. (1983). The influence of arterial baroreceptors in man on the variability of blood pressure and plasma catecholamines in man. *Chest* **83** (Suppl. 2), 320–2.

Sleight, P., West, M. J., Korner, P. I., Oliver, J. R., Chalmers, J. P., and Robinson, J. L. (1975). The action of clonidine on the baroreflex control of heart rate in conscious animals and man, and on single aortic baroreceptor discharge in the rabbit. *Arch. int. Pharmacodyn. Ther.* **214**, 4–11.

Smyth, H. S., Sleight, P., and Pickering, G. W. (1969). Reflex regulation of arterial pressure during sleep in man: 'a quantitative method of assessing baroreflex sensitivity'. *Circulation Res.* **24**, 109–21.

Somers, V. K., Conway, J., Le Winter, M., and Sleight, P. (1985). The role of baroreflex sensitivity in post exercise hypotension. *J. Hypertension* **3** (Suppl. 3), S129–S130.

Wallin, B. G. and Eckberg, D. L. (1982). Sympathetic transients caused by abrupt alterations of carotid baroreceptor activity in humans. *Am. J. Physiol.* **242**, H185–H190.

Watson, R. D. S., Stallard, T. J., and Littler, W. A. (1979). Factors determining the variability of arterial pressure in hypertension. *Clin. Sci.* **57**, 283–5.

9. Fainting

Roger Hainsworth

INTRODUCTION

Fainting or syncope refers to a transient loss of consciousness resulting from an inadequate cerebral blood flow. A faint is frequently preceded by sweating, pallor, blurring of vision, dizziness, and nausea. It is much less common in supine subjects and subjects who become supine following a faint usually rapidly recover consciousness.

There is a wide variation in the susceptibility of individuals to fainting. The fainting of pregnant women or soldiers standing motionless in hot environments is well known. On the other hand, patients in heart failure rarely, if ever, faint. Factors which predispose to fainting include reduction in venous return, due to postural stress, blood loss, and straining (Valsalva manoeuvre). It can sometimes also be provoked by emotional stress. Some individuals may have abnormal reflex responses (for example, baroreceptor hypersensitivity or hyposensitivity) which increase the likelihood of fainting. Fainting does not usually point to organic disease, although it is clearly important to exclude diseases such as epilepsy, autonomic nervous disease, cerebrovascular disease, heart disease, particularly that involving the aortic valve, and various endocrine disorders. Most healthy individuals can precipitate at least presyncopal symptoms if, particularly in a warm environment (resulting in skin vasodilatation), they hyperventilate (to constrict cerebral blood vessels), suddenly stand from a crouching position (to allow abdominal blood vessels to fill with blood and to increase the height to which blood must be pumped to the brain), and perform a Valsalva manoeuvre (to impede the return of blood to the heart). This is a well known 'mess trick'.

The actual onset of the faint can be quite abrupt. Usually preceding the faint there is an increased activity of the sympathetic nervous system leading to a maintained or sometimes increased blood pressure accompanied by increases in heart rate and vascular resistance. Then, quite suddenly, heart rate drops and vascular resistance decreases, resulting in a profound fall in arterial blood pressure, inadequate cerebral perfusion, and loss of consciousness. This is the vasovagal attack, a term introduced in 1932 by Sir Thomas Lewis.

In this chapter I discuss the control of cerebral blood flow since inadequate flow causes fainting. I also discuss the factors leading to vasodilatation and to bradycardia and the consequences of these responses for the maintenance of blood pressure. The vasovagal syncope is described and I suggest a number of physiological mechanisms which may trigger this response.

CEREBRAL BLOOD FLOW

The blood flow to the human brain normally remains relatively constant. Unlike tissues, such as muscle or glands, in which large changes in blood flow result from changes in metabolic activity, changes in cerebral activity result in changes in flow which are usually too localized and too small overall to be apparent in estimates of total flow. Typical values of cerebral blood flow are 50–60 ml/min per 100 g brain tissue, about 15 per cent of the resting cardiac output.

The brain cannot withstand more than a few seconds of total interruption of flow without loss of consciousness; interruption for longer periods is liable to result in irreversible damage.

Regulation of cerebral blood flow

Cerebral blood flow shows marked autoregulation. That is, over a wide range of cerebral perfusion pressures, blood flow remains almost constant. The postulated mechanisms for maintaining a constant flow to a region when perfusion pressure decreases are a decrease in contraction of arteriolar smooth muscle in response to decreased stretch (the myogenic theory) and an increase in local concentrations of vasodilator metabolites following a transient decrease in flow (the metabolic theory). In the brain it seems likely that metabolic factors predominate although there may also be a myogenic component.

Cerebral blood flow can be altered by changes in activity in vasomotor nerves. However, the innervation is relatively sparse and the nervous control is thought to be relatively unimportant. Of much greater importance is the control by vasodilator metabolic products. Changes in the level of carbon dioxide in the arterial blood are particularly effective in causing changes in cerebral blood flow. At normal levels of arterial pressure an increase in P_{CO_2} to 7 kPa (52 mm Hg) would approximately double cerebral flow whereas a decrease to 4 kPa (30 mm Hg) would halve it. The level of CO_2 in the perfusing blood also influences the autoregulation of cerebral blood flow. Autoregulation is abolished during hypercapnia; during hypocapnia cerebral blood flow is markedly decreased at all perfusion pressures (Fig. 9.1).

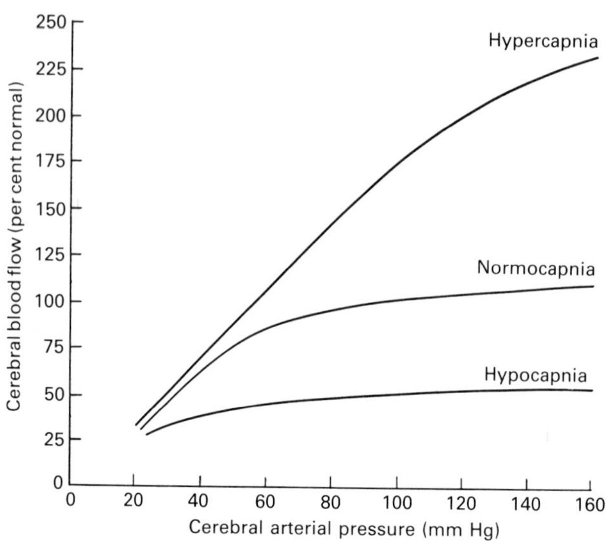

Fig. 9.1. Autoregulation of cerebral blood flow. The flow at normal cerebral perfusion pressure and normal arterial P_{CO_2} is taken as 100 per cent. Cerebral perfusion pressure (cerebral arterial pressure minus intracranial pressure) is 5–10 mm Hg less than cerebral arterial pressure. Above a pressure of about 60 mm Hg the flow is largely independent of pressure. During hypercapnia the autoregulation is largely lost. During hypocapnia blood flow is only about 50 per cent of the normal value, at all levels of CO_2.

The stimulus for vasodilatation is actually believed to be mediated through the hydrogen ion concentration in the cerebrospinal fluid (see Lassen 1974). Carbon dioxide crosses the blood–brain barrier and reacts with water to form hydrogen ions in the cerebrospinal fluid.

Cerebral blood flow during hypotension

It must first be appreciated that in the upright position cerebral arterial pressure is 15–30 mm Hg lower than that in the aortic arch and the difference is even greater compared with that in a dependent arm (Fig. 9.2). Consciousness starts to be lost when cerebral blood flow falls below about 25 ml/min/100 g, about half the normal flow. This level can be reached by severe hypocapnia ($P_{CO_2} < 3$ kPa) achieved by hyperventilation, or by cerebral arterial pressure falling below about 40 mm Hg (Fig. 9.1). Note that in the upright position the critical level of cerebral arterial pressure would correspond to a mean brachial arterial pressure of about 70 mm Hg; for example 90/60 mm Hg (mean pressure is approximately diastolic plus 1/3 pulse pressure). Fainting is much less likely to occur when subjects are supine because the cerebral arterial pressure is higher and there is less pooling of blood in dependent veins (Fig. 9.2).

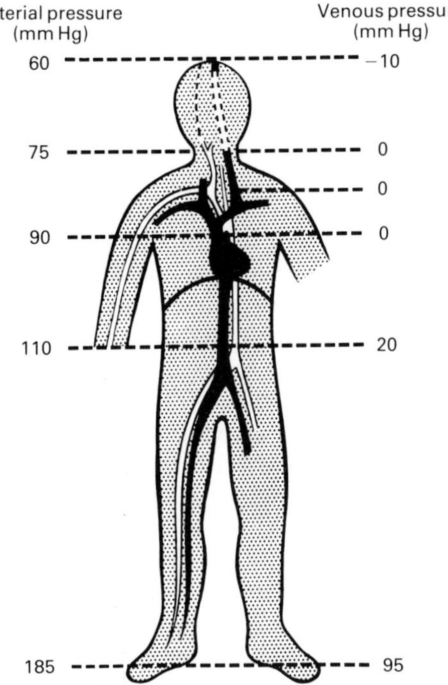

Fig. 9.2. Gravitational effects on arterial and venous blood pressures in erect motionless man. Arterial and venous pressures in the lower part of the body are increased and decreased in the upper part of the body. Note that cerebral arterial pressure is about 15 mm Hg lower than aortic root pressure. Because the brain is enclosed by rigid skull, the venous pressures may be below atmospheric. This results in a relatively constant arterial–venous pressure difference in different parts of the brain. (From Hainsworth (1985).)

VASODILATATION

According to Poiseuille's equation, if other variables including blood pressure remain constant, an increase in the radius of a vessel would lead to an increase in flow. Indeed, because radius is raised to the fourth power, a doubling of radius results in a 16-fold increase in flow. However, unless there is a response which prevents blood pressure from falling, vasodilatation also results in hypotension. By rearranging Poiseuille's equation, arterial pressure P can be seen to be dependent on cardiac output $\dot{Q}$ and a term r relating to the radius of resistance vessels

$$P \propto \dot{Q}/r^4.$$

Thus, the effect of vasodilatation on blood pressure depends on whether the change in r^4 is greater than the change in $\dot{Q}$.

Vasodilatation can be particularly pronounced in skeletal muscle. At rest in a comfortable environment, the cardiac output (typically about 5.5 l/min) is distributed so that less than 20 per cent of the total flow perfuses skeletal muscle even though this comprises nearly half the tissue mass. During severe muscular exercise total muscle blood flow may increase from 1 to 20 l/min and forms the major part of the cardiac output. This intense vasodilatation, however, does not normally lead to a fall in blood pressure but is actually usually associated with a moderate increase in pressure. The main reason for this is that the contracting muscles and increased respiratory activity pump blood back to the heart, and this increased venous return together with an increased activity in cardiac sympathetic nerves increases cardiac output.

The same effect does not occur when there is vasodilatation in the absence of increased muscular activity. Thus, administration of vasodilator drugs, such as sodium nitroprusside, or pharmacologically blocking sympathetic vasoconstrictor activity results in vasodilatation with little accompanying increase in cardiac output and this results in a decrease in blood pressure.

Cutaneous vasodilatation occurs in response to heat stress. This is caused partly by a direct effect on the skin blood vessels and partly through a decrease in the discharge of cutaneous sympathetic vasoconstrictor fibres resulting from warming the temperature-regulating centres in the hypothalamus. The range of cutaneous blood flow has been estimated to lie between as little as 20 ml/min for the entire skin during cooling of both skin and the body core to as much as 3 l/min during severe heat load (Folkow and Neil 1971). Thermally induced vasodilatation results in a decrease in total vascular resistance and an increased volume of blood in dependent vessels, particularly veins, which may decrease cardiac output and blood pressure and predispose to fainting.

Mechanisms of vasodilatation

The diameter of blood vessels can change in response to neural, chemical, or mechanical influences.

At rest, the degree of constriction of both resistance vessels (mainly arterioles) and capacitance vessels (mainly veins) is maintained by a tonic discharge in sympathetic vasoconstrictor (noradrenergic) nerves. A discharge frequency in these nerves of about 10 Hz results in near-maximal constriction of these vessels. However, at lower discharge frequencies (1–2 Hz) capacitance vessels are relatively more completely constricted than resistance vessels (Fig. 9.3). By determining the responses of resistance and capacitance to changes in carotid-sinus pressure and relating them to the responses in the same animals to direct

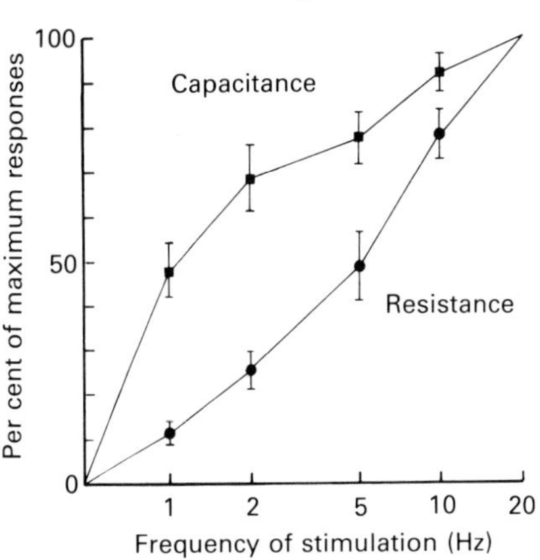

Fig. 9.3. Capacitance and resistance responses of abdominal circulation of anaesthetized dogs to stimulation of splanchnic nerves at various frequencies. Responses expressed as percentages of the changes at 20 Hz. Values are means +SE from 14 dogs. Note that at 1 Hz the capacitance response was nearly 50 per cent of maximal whereas the resistance response was only about 10 per cent of maximal. Above 2 Hz there was little further response of capacitance but larger responses of resistance. (Modified from Karim and Hainsworth (1976).)

stimulation of sympathetic nerves, it was possible to infer that changes in carotid-sinus pressure over the baroreceptor sensitivity range resulted in changes in sympathetic efferent discharge frequency between 0 and 5 Hz (Hainsworth and Karim 1976). Furthermore, there was no apparent difference in the discharge frequency to resistance and capacitance vessels which implies that, at most levels of pressure, capacitance vessels would be more completely constricted than resistance vessels. It should be noted that equating reflex responses to those occurring to regular stimulation of nerves may be an oversimplification since the spontaneous sympathetic discharge occurs irregularly in bursts (see Chapter 11).

At rest, sympathetic nerves are tonically active at a mean frequency of about 1 Hz. Inhibition of this tone results in dilatation of resistance vessels leading to a decrease in vascular resistance. There is also dilatation of capacitance vessels, at least those in the abdominal circulation (see Hainsworth 1985), leading to a decrease in cardiac output.

Vasodilatation in metabolically active tissues is largely brought about by locally produced chemical vasodilators. These are essentially the products of metabolic activity, so that the flow of blood through muscle, glands, etc. is directly related to their metabolism. Related to this is the phenomenon of autoregulation. This has already been mentioned in relation to the cerebral circulation but it is also observed to varying degrees in many other regions.

It is likely that blood flow to most regions is determined by a balance between neurally mediated vasoconstriction and metabolically mediated vasodilatation. Flow is thus normally less than it would be if solely under the influence of metabolic vasodilators. Abrupt removal of the neural vasoconstrictor activity may therefore result in a transient reactive hyperaemia. This is illustrated in Fig. 9.4 in which it can be seen that, during constant-pressure perfusion of a dog's hindlimb, stimulation of the efferent sympathetic nerves at 1 Hz decreased the blood flow by about 25 per cent. Immediately after switching off the stimulator, blood flow increased transiently with a peak of more than 30 per cent above the steady-state value.

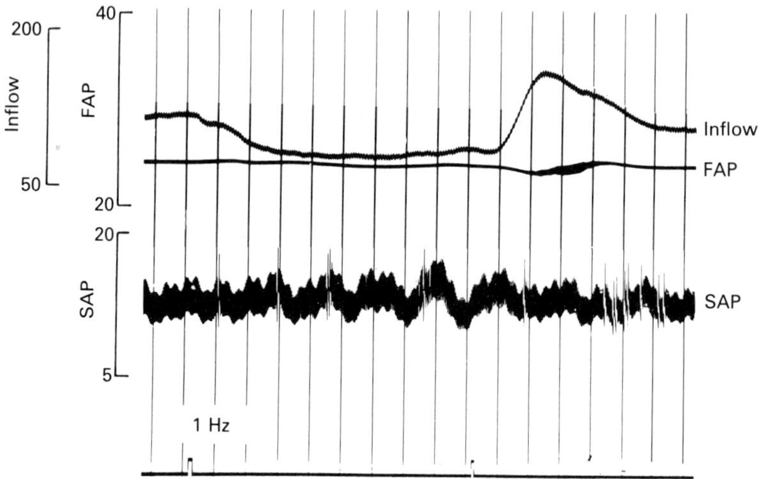

Fig. 9.4. Responses of blood flow, in a dog's hindlimb perfused at constant pressure, to electrical stimulation of the lumbar sympathetic trunk. Event marker shows start and end of stimulation. Traces are of flow (ml/min) and of femoral arterial perfusion pressure (FAP) and systemic arterial blood pressure (SAP) in kPa (1 kPa = 7.5 mm Hg). Note that flow is reduced during the period of stimulation and that it overshoots transiently on cessations of the stimulus. (Modified from Hainsworth *et al.* (1983).)

Active vasodilatation may occur in response to stimulation of vasodilator nerves. These nerves have been identified in glandular tissue and appear to be peptidergic. In some species cholinergic sympathetic vasodilator nerves have been identified in skeletal muscle. The existence of these fibres has been demonstrated either by pharmacologically blocking the vasoconstrictor fibres and then stimulating the efferent sympathetic nerves or by stimulating a region in the hypothalamus (the so-called defence area) and observing vasodilatation in skeletal muscle which could be blocked by atropine. In this way evidence of cholinergic sympathetic vasodilator fibres to skeletal muscle has been demonstrated in the cat, dog, fox, jackal, and mongoose, but not in the rabbit, hare, badger, polecat, or in seven species of primate (Uvnas 1966).

Do sympathetic vasodilator nerves occur in man?

It is widely assumed that man, like the dog and the cat, possesses cholinergic sympathetic vasodilator nerves to his skeletal muscle. The evidence in support of this comes largely from experiments, by Barcroft, Edholm, and Greenfield, on the responses of humans to decreasing circulating blood volume and emotional stress. Barcroft *et al.* (1944) and Barcroft and Edholm (1945) induced fainting by withdrawing blood and applying tourniquets to the thighs. Fainting was preceded by an abrupt increase in forearm blood flow which was prevented by sympathectomy or nerve block. Because the flow in the unblocked limb increased to become greater than that in the blocked limb, *active* vasodilatation was assumed. Blair *et al.* (1959) devised a number of ingenious stressful procedures for medical students, including mental arithmetic, physiology tests, simulated haemorrhage, and offering a dead rabbit's blood and stomach contents for drinking! These procedures resulted in muscle vasodilatation. The evidence for active vasodilatation was that it was usually smaller following sympathetic blockade or administration of atropine.

The evidence against the existence of cholinergic vasodilator nerves in man seems to be stronger. First, Uvnas (1966) obtained evidence for these nerves only in some subprimate species and not in any of several primates studied. So this reduces the likelihood of their existence in man. Second, the observation that a stressful stimulus results in an increase in flow in an innervated limb which is transiently greater than that in a sympathectomized limb does not prove active vasodilatation. This is because, following sympathectomy, blood flow, although initially high, decreases towards normal levels so that flow to the innervated limb could transiently be greater following abrupt withdrawal of sympathetic tone. It can be seen from the results of Blair *et al.* (1959) that, during stress, blood flow to an unblocked forearm did not exceed that in the other limb in which the nerves had been *acutely* blocked. This could thus be a form of reactive hyperaemia following inhibition of vasoconstrictor nerve activity (Fig. 9.4). The evidence in support of active cholinergic vasodilatation provided by the administration of atropine is also not conclusive because, although it blocked the bradycardia occurring during a vasovagal attack, the fall in blood pressure was not prevented (Lewis 1932). Also, intra-arterial atropine failed to block completely the limb vasodilatation in response to stress (Blair *et al.* 1959). A final piece of evidence against active vasodilatation was provided by Wallin and Sundlöf (1982) who recorded activity in efferent sympathetic nerves in humans during vasovagal fainting. They observed an abrupt cessation of nervous activity with the onset of the hypotension, but there was no suggestion of any increase in any nervous activity which would have been expected if vasodilator nerves had become active.

BRADYCARDIA

In resting subjects, heart rate tends to vary inversely with arterial blood pressure. This is Marey's law and it is dependent on the arterial baroreceptor reflex. In circumstances in which there is a widespread increase in the level of sympathetic activity, such as during exercise, heart rate and blood pressure would both increase.

Heart rate is controlled mainly by the activity in the vagus and sympathetic nerves, although it is also influenced by body temperature and the concentration of various hormones, particularly catecholamines. At rest there is a tonic vagal activity which tends to be less during inspiration leading to sinus arrhythmia. Intense vagal activity results in profound bradycardia and can even result in a period of asystole. However, during prolonged vagal stimulation there is usually vagal 'escape' which prevents a potentially dangerous prolonged asystole.

Effect of heart rate on cardiac output

Every student knows the relationship between cardiac output $\dot{Q}$, heart rate HR, and stroke volume SV to be $\dot{Q}=HR\times SV$. This equation is mathematically unarguable but can be physiologically misleading. It is undeniable that a profound bradycardia with periods of asystole results in a low cardiac output. If a heart is distended, cardiac output is directly proportional to heart rate. However, in resting subjects a change in heart rate between about 60 and 120 beats/min has a relatively small effect on cardiac output and above about 120 beats/min output decreases. The reason for this apparent anomaly is that an increase in rate is offset by a decrease in stroke volume. Linden (1968) suggested that the main effect of an increase in heart rate would be to *permit* an increase in output to occur. Thus, an increase in venous return could not increase cardiac output to the same extent if heart rate remained unchanged, but an increase in rate without an increase in venous return would have little effect. The effect of a change in heart rate on cardiac output is explained by Fig. 9.5. A decrease in heart rate from 80 to 60 beats/min lengthens diastolic filling time and the output per minute is little changed. At slower heart rates, there would be a prolonged period of diastasis during which filling would not increase and so output would fall. At fast heart rates, although systole is slightly shortened, most of the shortening is at the expense of diastolic filling time and cardiac output again falls.

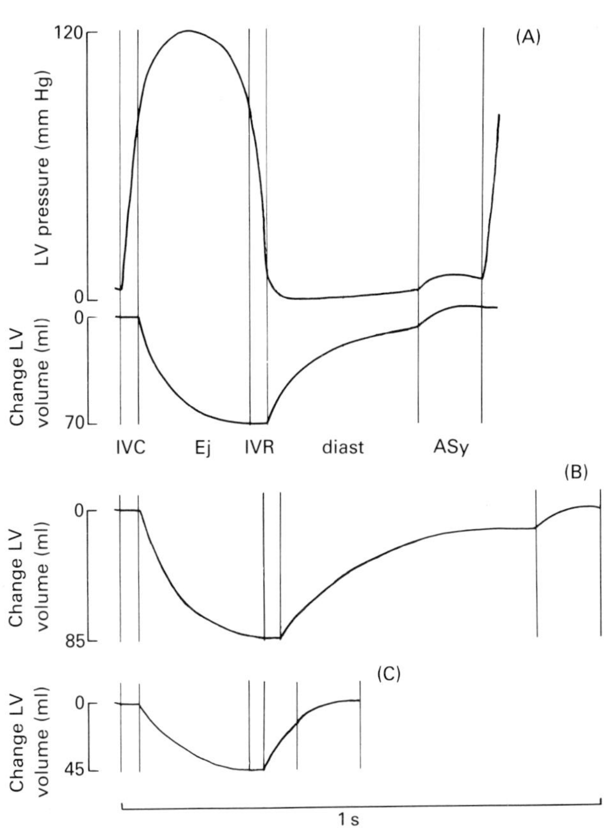

Fig. 9.5. Diagrammatic representation of left ventricular (LV) pressures and volumes during the cardiac cycle and the influence of heart rate. IVC, isovolumnic contraction phase; E, ejection phase; IVR, isovolumnic relaxation phase; diast, ventricular and atrial diastole; ASy, atrial systole. (A) Pressure and volume changes at a heart rate of 80 beat/min (cycle length 0.75 s). Note the rapid ventricular filling during early diastole and the contribution of atrial systole. Stroke volume is 70 ml and cardiac output is 5.6 l/min. (B) Volume changes at a heart rate of 60 beat/min (cycle length 1.0 s). Diastole is prolonged and there is a period of diastasis during which ventricular filling virtually ceases. Stroke volume increases to 85 ml and cardiac output is only slightly reduced at 5.1 l/min. (C) Volume changes at a heart rate of 120 beat/min (cycle length 0.5 s). The shortening is mainly at the expense of diastole which is greatly reduced. Atrial systole now makes a major contribution to ventricular filling. Stroke volume decreases to 45 ml and cardiac output remains almost unchanged at 5.4 l/min.

The effect of a change in heart rate on cardiac output is dependent on the rate of venous filling and whether it is accompanied by a change in the inotropic state. During exercise, an increase in heart rate is accompanied by a positive inotropic change which causes a reduction in the duration of systole. Venous return is high and this results in a large increase in output. On the other hand during fainting, due to hypovolaemia or peripheral vasodilatation, it is likely that venous filling pressure would be low and changes in heart rate would have little effect on cardiac output. This implies that, except in cases in which the bradycardia is profound (< 50 beats/min), it is unlikely to make a major contribution to a fall in arterial blood pressure.

THE VASOVAGAL SYNCOPE

Lewis (1932) described fainting attacks as being vasovagal because they were accompanied by hypotension and bradycardia. He considered that bradycardia usually was not the main cause of the faint since heart rate rarely fell to very low levels (< 50 beats/min) and the hypotension was little affected by the administration of atropine which prevented the bradycardia. More recently, Sander-Jensen *et al.* (1986) reported that the heart rate in patients admitted in haemorrhagic shock, although lower than expected, was seldom less than 60 beats/min.

Barcroft *et al.* (1944) performed an illuminating study in which they induced fainting in healthy subjects by bleeding and application of tourniquets to the legs. They observed that, before the onset of the faint, heart rate increased and there was also an increase in vascular resistance shown by blood pressure being relatively little changed despite a decrease in cardiac output. During the faint, blood pressure decreased abruptly, accompanied by decreases in heart rate and vascular resistance but no further fall and sometimes even a small increase in cardiac output. Similar observations, of a fall in vascular resistance but no further fall in cardiac output during fainting, were also made by Weissler *et al.* (1957) and Glick and Yu (1963).

Barcroft and Edholm (1945) reported an increase in forearm blood flow during fainting (Fig. 9.6) and suggested that the hypotension was due mainly to dilatation of vessels in skeletal muscle. However, more recent work has suggested that vasodilatation in hypotensive haemorrhage may be more widespread (Vatner and Morita 1987).

Emotional stress usually leads to increases in heart rate and blood pressure with little change in total vascular resistance. However, if a vasovagal faint occurs, blood pressure, heart rate, and forearm vascular resistance decrease abruptly.

Thus, a vasovagal attack is usually preceded by evidence of increased sympathetic and decreased vagal activity. During this stage blood pressure is maintained or, particularly in emotional faints, increased. The vasovagal attack is characterized by sudden onset of hypotension and bradycardia. The main cause of the hypotension is usually vasodilatation in skeletal muscle and probably elsewhere, due to inhibition of

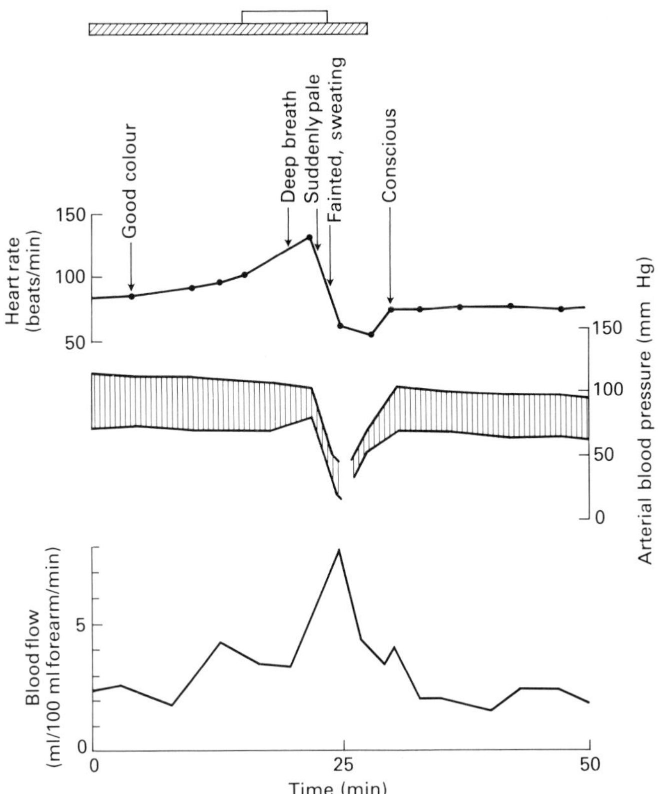

Fig. 9.6. Heart rate, arterial blood pressure, and forearm blood flow in a human subject during a haemorrhagic faint. Shaded bar: venous return impeded by application of tourniquets to both thighs; open bar: venesection. Note that initially blood pressure was relatively well maintained but that heart rate increased. Then heart rate slowed and blood pressure fell. This was accompanied by an increase in forearm blood flow. (Modified from Barcroft and Edholm (1945).)

sympathetic vasoconstrictor activity. The bradycardia is usually relatively unimportant because heart rate is seldom greatly slowed and cardiac output does not usually decrease with the onset of the faint.

Possible physiological mechanisms precipitating vasovagal attacks

Although much is known of the factors predisposing to fainting attacks and there have been several analyses of the haemodynamic changes which occur before and during the faint, the mechanism responsible for suddenly switching a response of tachycardia and vasoconstriction to one of bradycardia and vasodilatation remains a matter for speculation. A number of possibilities have been suggested.

An abnormal baroreceptor reflex

Glick and Yu (1963) suggested that the 'trigger' for a vasovagal attack was a transient increase in the stimulation of arterial baroreceptors. This effect might occur in emotional fainting which is accompanied by an initial increase in blood pressure. It is also conceivable that the gain of the baroreceptor reflex might be increased in some circumstances and there is some evidence that angiotensin and vasopressin may act on the central nervous pathways to have this effect (Bishop and Hasser 1987).

In the so-called carotid-sinus syndrome, syncope can result from an exaggerated baroreceptor reflex. In the original classical case, syncope was precipitated by pressure from a stiff winged collar. Usually, however, the precipitating cause is unknown. Attacks are characterized by bradycardia and hypotension. The bradycardia can be prevented by cardiac pacing or administration of atropine but this may not prevent the fall in blood pressure (Almquist *et al.* 1985).

Emotional stress

Electrical stimulation of a region within the hypothalamus of anaesthetized cats, the 'defence area', results in vasodilatation in skeletal muscle, which is blocked by atropine, and increases in heart rate and blood pressure (Eliasson *et al.* 1951). Similar responses were also observed in conscious cats during electrical stimulation of the same area or in response to the application of certain auditory, visual, or cutaneous stimuli (Abrahams *et al.* 1964). This is the 'defence reaction'.

Emotional stress in humans can also result in quite marked cardiovascular changes, including tachycardia, hypertension, and muscle vasodilatation. Barcroft *et al.* (1960) considered that these responses were comparable to the defence reaction in animals. However, in humans the vasodilator responses were only slightly reduced after atropine and can be attributed to increases in circulating adrenalin and reduction of vasoconstrictor activity.

In susceptible subjects, severe emotional stress can lead to a vasovagal syncope. The tachycardia and hypertension abruptly give way to bradycardia and hypotension. This response does not occur in animals during hypothalamic stimulation.

Stimulation of cardiac receptors

Activation of cardiac ventricular afferent nerves gives rise to a pattern of responses similar to that seen in vasovagal attacks. This is the Bezold–Jarisch reflex and it can be elicited by injection of chemical stimulants into the coronary circulation (Fig. 9.7). Stimulation of cardiac receptors also dilates resistance and capacitance vessels in the abdomen (Hainsworth *et al.* 1986).

Similar responses may also occur in humans following injection of

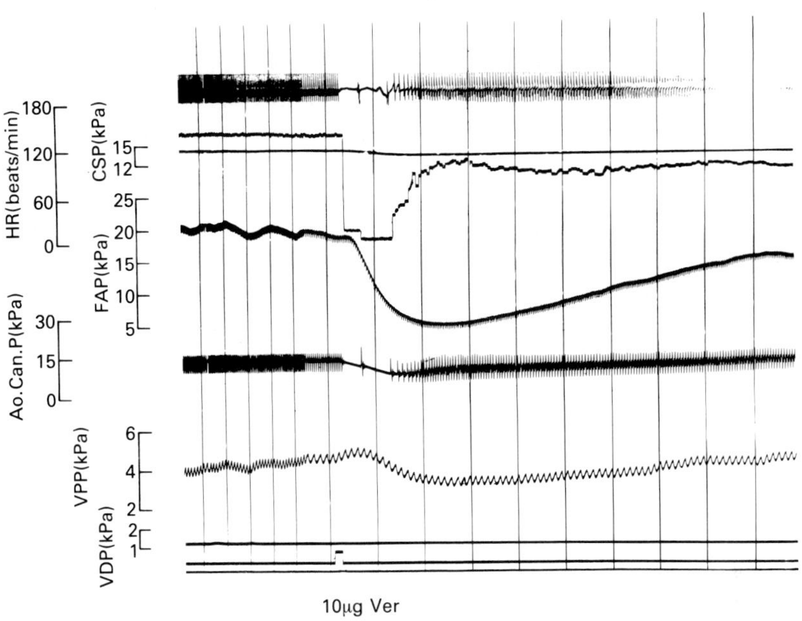

Fig. 9.7. Responses in the vascularly isolated perfused hindlimb of a dog to injection of veratridine into the aortic root. The femoral artery and a cutaneous vein were perfused at constant flows so that changes in arterial and venous perfusion pressures denote changes in arterial and venous resistance. Traces are of ECG, heart rate (HR), carotid-sinus pressure (CSP), femoral arterial perfusion pressure (FAP), aortic root pressure (Ao.Can.P., controlled), venous perfusion pressure (VPP), and venous draining pressure (VDP). Note that immediately following veratridine (Ver) (which was prevented from reaching reflexogenic areas other than those in the coronary circulation), there was a profound bradycardia and arterial and venous dilatation. Note that 1 kPa = 7.5 mm Hg. (From McGregor *et al.* (1986).)

contrast medium into the coronary circulation or during periods of myocardial ischaemia (see Hainsworth and McGregor 1987). It seems unlikely that such a powerful reflex would be elicited only following injections of toxic chemicals or during pathological conditions. Thorén (1987) summarized the evidence that unmyelinated ventricular afferent nerves are excited during haemorrhage. He suggested that the mechanism of excitation is probably an increased force of ventricular contraction, brought about by an increased activity in cardiac sympathetic nerves, accompanied by a reduced ventricular filling. In addition to bradycardia and vasodilatation, stimulation of ventricular receptors also results in a reflex relaxation of the stomach which could explain the feeling of nausea in some patients.

Initiation of a powerful depressor reflex by stimulation of cardiac ventricular receptors offers a plausible explanation for the vasovagal attack since this is usually preceded by tachycardia, reduced cardiac output, and increased cardiac sympathetic stimulation. However, if this is a simple reflex response, it is not clear why it should start so abruptly and persist after the stimulus has ceased; i.e. the bradycardia and hypotension should immediately remove the stimulus to the receptors. Furthermore, Vatner and Morita (1987) reported that, in unanaesthetized animals during hypotensive haemorrhage, there was a decrease in efferent renal-nerve activity but this was not prevented by vagal denervation, which would block afferent activity from cardiac receptors. They also made the interesting observations that blockade of opiate receptors by naloxone, while it did not affect the initial increase in renal nerve activity during non-hypotensive haemorrhage, did prevent the decrease during hypotensive haemorrhage.

SUMMARY AND CONCLUSIONS

Fainting refers to a transient loss of consciousness when cerebral blood flow is impaired. The critical level of cerebral arterial pressure is about 40 mm Hg and this is reached more readily in the upright subject than when supine. Usually, before the faint there is evidence of an increased activity in the sympathetic nerves. At the onset of the faint there is a sudden vasodilatation in skeletal muscle (and probably in other regions) and bradycardia. In most faints the major factor is probably vasodilatation, which results from inhibition of sympathetic vasoconstrictor activity and leads to a decrease in vascular resistance and therefore blood pressure. However, in some individuals, in whom the heart rate decreases below about 50 beats/min, bradycardia is also likely to be of importance.

The mechanism responsible for initiating a vasovagal attack is still unknown. It is likely to be preceded by a decrease in the circulating blood volume, as in postural stress or haemorrhage, and rarely occurs in hypervolaemic individuals, such as those in heart failure. It may also occur in susceptible individuals following emotional stress. Several trigger mechanisms have been proposed. These include transient stimulation of arterial baroreceptors the responses to which may be abnormally sensitive, as in the so-called carotid-sinus syndrome, or as the result of chemical action on the central nervous pathways. The defence reaction of animals, in which there is tachycardia, hypertension, and muscle vasodilatation in response to hypothalamic stimulation or emotional stress, may have a counterpart in the human. However, in animals this response does not develop into a vasovagal attack. There have also been suggestions that the vasovagal attack may be caused by the Bezold–Jarisch reflex in which stimulation of cardiac ventricular receptors, by powerful contraction on a nearly empty ventricle, may initiate a profound depressor response. However, the evidence on this too is as yet incomplete and the mechanism responsible for inducing the vasodilatation and bradycardia remains to be discovered.

The physiological advantages to a subject or to the species of a vasovagal attack can be speculated upon. It is certainly true that the maintenance of an adequate blood flow, particularly to the cerebral circulation, is infinitely more important than the control of arterial blood pressure. Since fainting is much more likely to occur when subjects are upright than when supine, a response which renders a subject supine and thereby assists venous return and cerebral perfusion, could be argued to be beneficial. However, there is no evidence that the response has evolved for this purpose, particularly since the actual stimulus is unknown, and it may simply be a coincidental response the real function of which is concerned with some entirely different purpose.

REFERENCES

Abrahams, V. C., Hilton, S. M., and Zbrozyna, A. W. (1964). The role of active muscle vasodilatation in the alerting stage of the defence reaction. *J. Physiol.* **171**, 189–202.

Almquist, A., Gornick, C., Benson, D. W. Jr., Dunnigan, A., and Benditt, D. G. (1985). Carotid sinus hypersensitivity: evaluation of the vasodepressor component. *Circulation* **71**, 927–36.

Barcroft, H., Brod, J., Heijl, Z., Hirsjarvi, E. A., and Kitchen, A. H. (1960). The mechanism of the vasodilatation in the forearm muscle during stress (mental arithmetic). *Clin. Sci.* **19**, 577–86.

Barcroft, H. and Edholm, O. G. (1945). On the vasodilatation in human skeletal muscle during post-haemorrhagic fainting. *J. Physiol.* **104**, 161–75.

Barcroft, H., Edholm, O. G., McMichael, J., and Sharpey-Schafer, E. P. (1944). Posthaemorrhagic fainting. Study by cardiac output and forearm flow. *Lancet* **i**, 489–91.

Bishop, V. S. and Hasser, E. M. (1987). Physiological role of ventricular receptors. In *Cardiogenic reflexes* (ed. R. Hainsworth, P. N. McWilliam, and D. A. S. G. Mary), pp. 62–73. Oxford University Press, Oxford.

Blair, D. A., Glover, W. E., Greenfield, A. D. M., and Roddie, I. C. (1959). Excitation of cholinergic vasodilator nerves to human skeletal muscles during emotional stress. *J. Physiol.* **148**, 633–47.

Eliasson, S., Folkow, B., Lindgren, P., and Uvnas, B. (1951). Activation of sympathetic vasodilator nerves to the skeletal muscles in the cat by hypothalamic stimulation. *Acta physiolog. scand.* **23**, 333–51.

Folkow, B. and Neil, E. (1971). *Circulation.* Oxford University Press, Oxford.

Glick, G. and Yu, P. N. (1963). Hemodynamic changes during spontaneous vasovagal reactions. *Am. J. Med.* **34**, 42–50.

Hainsworth, R. (1985). Arterial blood pressure. In *Hypotensive anaesthesia* (ed. G. E. H. Enderby), pp. 3–29. Churchill Livingstone, Edinburgh.

Hainsworth, R. and Karim, F. (1976). Responses of abdominal vascular capacitance in the anaesthetized dog to changes in carotid sinus pressure. *J. Physiol.* **262**, 659–77.

Hainsworth, R., Karim, F., McGregor, K. H., and Wood, L. M. (1983). Hind-limb vascular-capacitance responses in anaesthetized dogs. *J. Physiol.* **337**, 417–28.

Hainsworth, R. and McGregor, K. H. (1987). Reflex vascular responses to stimulation of cardiac ventricular receptors. In *Cardiogenic reflexes* (ed. R. Hainsworth, P. N. McWilliam, and D. A. S. G. Mary), pp. 44–61. Oxford University Press, Oxford.

Hainsworth, R., McGregor, K. H., and Ford, R. (1986). Effect of veratridine injected into the aortic root on resistance and capacitance in the abdominal circulation in anaesthetized dogs. *Quart. J. exp. Physiol.* **71**, 589–98.

Karim, F. and Hainsworth, R. (1976). Responses of abdominal vascular capacitance to stimulation of splanchnic nerves. *Am. J. Physiol.* **231**, 434–40.

Lassen, N. A. (1974). Control of cerebral circulation in health and disease. *Circulation Res.* **34**, 749–60.

Lewis, T. (1932). Vasovagal syncope and the carotid sinus mechanism. *Br. med. J.* **1**, 873–6.

Linden, R. J. (1968). The heart-ventricular function. *Anaesthesia* **23**, 566–84.

McGregor, K. H., Hainsworth, R., and Ford, R. (1986). Hind-limb vascular responses in anaesthetized dogs to aortic root injections of veratridine. *Quart. J. exp. Physiol.* **71**, 577–87.

Sander-Jensen, K., Secher, N. H., Bie, P., Warberg, J., and Schwartz, T. W. (1986). Vagal slowing of the heart during haemorrhage: observations from 20 consecutive hypotensive patients. *Br. med. J.* **292**, 364–6.

Thorén, P. (1987). Depressor reflexes from the heart during severe haemorrhage. In *Cardiogenic reflexes* (ed. R. Hainsworth, P. N. McWilliam, and D. A. S. G. Mary), pp. 389–401. Oxford University Press, Oxford.

Uvnas, B. (1966). Cholinergic vasodilator nerves. *Fed. Proc.* **25**, 1618–22.

Vatner, S. F. and Morita, H. (1987). Biphasic response of renal nerve activity to haemorrhage in the conscious animal. In *Cardiogenic reflexes* (ed. R. Hainsworth, P. N. McWilliam, and D. A. S. G. Mary), pp. 402–10. Oxford University Press, Oxford.

Wallin, B. G. and Sundlöf, G. (1982). Sympathetic outflow to muscle during vasovagal syncope. *J. autonom. nerv. Syst.* **6**, 287–91.

Weissler, A. M., Warren, J. V., Estes, E. H., McIntosh, H. D., and Leonard, J. J. (1957). Vasodepressor syncope. Factors influencing cardiac output. *Circulation* **15**, 875–82.

10. Pathophysiology of the vagus

P. M. Satchell

INTRODUCTION

The traditional approach to understanding autonomic failure consists of making deductions about the pathophysiology of a disease process from observations obtained by clinical investigation and pharmacological study. Unfortunately, it has rarely been possible to relate the results of these types of studies to one of the disease processes known to specifically affect neurons. There is no evidence which suggests that autonomic neurons are different from other neurons in their susceptibility to disease processes nor in the way in which they react to them. Thus, the determination of the effects of a disease process on the autonomic nervous system has some obvious advantages, particularly as the constraints of clinical investigations are different from those which must be observed with experimental studies in animals. The approach that has been employed in the studies described here uses a disease process as a tool to produce autonomic dysfunction.

The simplest division of the pathological processes which affect neurons is into those which result in axonal damage and those which result in damage to myelin. In this chapter the consequences of these processes in the vagus nerve alone will be considered. The vagus nerve embodies all the features that are characteristic of the autonomic division of the nervous system. As an introduction, the little that is known about the pathophysiological nature of vagal dysfunction in the various forms of clinical autonomic failure will be considered.

Autonomic failure and vagal function

Clinical vagal dysfunction is associated with a loss of cells in the dorsal vagal nuclei in autonomic failure (AF) (Chapter 25A) and in its variants. The process responsible is ill defined as is the nature of the vagal abnormalities that precede cell loss. In acute and subacute autonomic neuropathy, clinical vagal involvement is often prominent but the mechanism is obscure. A proportion of these neuropathies are of the axonopathy type. In these disorders, the evidence that the vagus is damaged is strong but the site of the damage in the vagus is almost always unknown in man. In many of these disorders the metabolic machinery of neurons is disturbed, but the nature of the different metabolic abnormalities is poorly understood.

An experimental approach: advantages and disadvantages

Unfortunately, both invasive and non-invasive clinical methods can only establish that there is or there is not an abnormality in the human parasympathetic nervous system. None of these clinical methods can tell us anything about the site at which the abnormality is located, its nature, or its consequences. An abnormal heart rate response produced by some manoeuvre, whether it be respiratory or postural, can result from a disease process affecting receptors, their afferent nerve fibres, the central processing structures, efferent nerve fibres, peripheral ganglia, postganglionic nerve fibres, their end-plate structures, or the heart itself. Thus, we are faced with a plethora of targets in which a disease process might produce significant pathophysiological changes as well as with clinical methods which, at best, can only detect abnormality in an overall reflex loop. In the studies to be described, a neuropathy of a specific type has been induced in animals and the changes in the vagus nerve determined. These studies examine vagal function in the intact conscious animal as well as the performance of individual parts of the vagal reflex loops in anaesthetized animals. As might be expected, this approach markedly reduces the chaos inherent in many of the clinical studies of autonomic dysfunction. This advantage is balanced by some important disadvantages.

One disadvantage is the propensity for all to equate the disease induced in an animal with that in man, a practice that is usually doomed because of the complexities of disease production, particularly of chronic disease in man. Direct modelling of human disease in animals ignores the significant variation that exists between species, particularly in organ structure, function, innervation, and susceptibility to external agents. The only way in which the study of a disease induced in an animal can be useful is if the disturbance of the physiology of that species by the pathological process is fully appreciated. It is from this position that predictions can be made about similar processes in man, providing that the relevant human physiology is itself understood. Another disadvantage is that our understanding of any disease process, even those which might be used as tools for investigating the nervous system, is far from complete. Some of these advantages and disadvantages will be illustrated by the studies carried out on the effects of a distal axonopathy on the vagus.

AXONAL NEUROPATHY AND THE VAGUS

Axonal neuropathy

The largest patient group exposed to autonomic studies is likely to be patients with peripheral neuropathy. In the majority of these patients, the predominant site of damage is the axon. A large proportion of these patients have diabetes and diabetic neuropathy, which can be considered as an axonal disorder (Sumner 1980).

The archetypal axonal disease is acrylamide neuropathy. Acrylamide produces pathological changes in the central and peripheral nervous system which are the same across a wide range of species including man (LeQuesne 1980). Acrylamide at low doses produces a distal axonopathy in the peripheral nervous system with relatively little involvement of the central nervous system. In this axonopathy, the distal portions of sensory nerve fibres and their end organs are the most vulnerable structures. Nerve fibres have a graded susceptibility, the longest and largest being the most vulnerable. When motor fibres are involved, it is the terminal portions of the fibres and the end-plates that are damaged first. Unmyelinated nerve fibres are only involved in peripheral nerves when the neuropathy is severe.

Acrylamide neuropathy has many features that are similar to the distal axonopathies of alcohol, vitamin deficiency, and drug intoxication, all diseases in which the metabolic machinery of the neuron is disturbed. It provides a clinical mimic of the common symmetrical sensorimotor neuropathy of diabetes. It lacks the seemingly unpredictable involvement of unmyelinated fibres which is a feature of a proportion of diabetic patients. At this stage it is worth repeating that acrylamide neuropathy does not provide us with an exact model of any specific clinical entity except human acrylamide neuropathy. Rather, it allows an appreciation of the pathophysiological consequences that a distal axonopathy produces on the nervous system.

In the studies described here, acrylamide neuropathy has been induced in a variety of species. In almost all cases the dose of acrylamide given, usually over months, has been 30 to 50 per cent less than that used by others, and almost all animals have been studied when they have only had a mild neuropathy. At this stage, hindlimb weakness has only just been present, and proprioceptive deficits have been the principal features of the symmetrical sensorimotor neuropathy. Peripheral nerve damage, assessed histologically and electrophysiologically, has been consistent with this clinical picture.

The vagus

The vagus is a nerve of the most delightful complexity. The vagus is a pathway for a myriad of control systems which have widely varying properties. In the following discussion, three control systems, which have a varying proportion of their peripheral nerve components within the vagus, are considered. First, in the blood-pressure control system, the vagus is the pathway for all thoracic baroreceptor nerve fibres in all species except the rabbit. The vagus also contains cardiomotor fibres, but a proportion of these and the vasomotor fibres lie outside the vagus. Second, in the respiratory control system, the vagus contains the complete afferent innervation of the lung as well as the motor innervation of the airways and secretory apparatus. The vagus contains some of the skeletomotor innervation of respiratory muscles but none of the innervation destined for the respiratory pump. Third, the vagus contains both the afferent and efferent innervation of the oesophagus. The consequences of a distal axonopathy on each control system, the relevant organ, the specific vagal nerve fibres, and nerve terminals will now be considered.

Thoracic baroreceptors

Blood pressure and heart rate are not altered in anaesthetized dogs, cats, and rabbits with mild acrylamide neuropathy. Anaesthesia impairs vagal function which reduces the value of measuring heart-rate variation. While it is not possible to mimic the Valsalva manoeuvre in anaesthetized animals, a transient reduction in venous return produces the same fluctuations in blood pressure and heart rate in normal dogs as it does in dogs with mild acrylamide neuropathy (Satchell 1981). Blood-pressure levels and baroreceptor sensitivity do not change in the conscious rabbit as a mild axonal neuropathy develops (unpublished observations). All these results suggest that the overall ability of baroreceptors to buffer changes in arterial pressure is little changed in mild axonal neuropathy.

In all the situations described above, carotid-sinus and aortic-arch baroreceptors are working in concert and the buffering ability of baroreceptors whose afferent fibres run in the vagus nerve cannot be separated out. Isolation and perfusion of both carotid sinuses from the arterial circulation allows the buffering ability of these and thoracic baroreceptors to be appreciated separately in animals in which the vagi are left untouched (Satchell 1984*a*). In this preparation, a step increase in carotid-sinus pressure in normal animals produces a reflex reduction in vagomotor and sympathetic vasomotor tone (Fig. 10.1). Because the resulting fall in arterial pressure is detected by thoracic baroreceptors, but not by the isolated carotid-sinus baroreceptors, the initial reflex effects are buffered after some delay. This preparation has produced the totally artificial situation in which the thoracic baroreceptors buffer or oppose the reflex changes produced by alterations in carotid-sinus

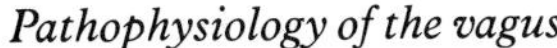

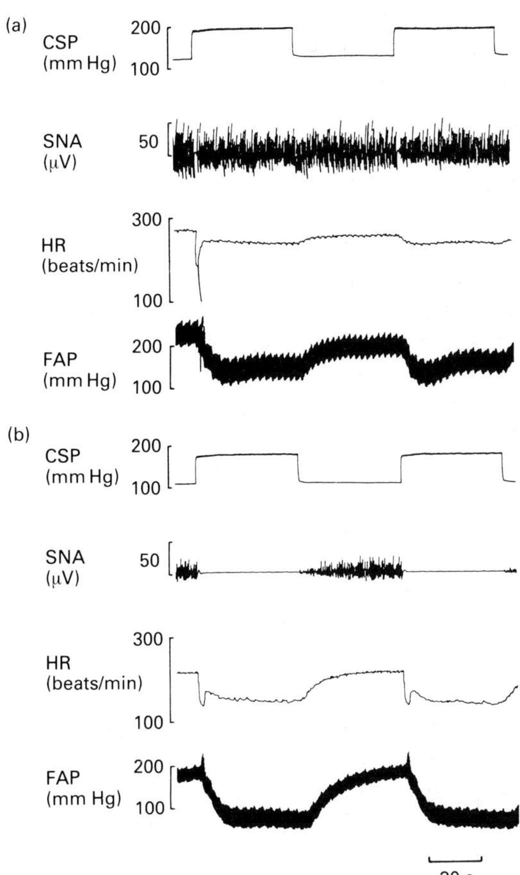

Fig. 10.1. The responses of renal sympathetic nerve activity (SNA), heart rate (HR), and femoral arterial pressure (FAP) to a step increase in carotid-sinus pressure (CSP) in a control animal (a) and an animal (b) with acrylamide neuropathy. In both dogs, which are anaesthetized with chloralose urethane, both carotid sinuses are isolated from the systemic circulation and the vagi are intact. In normal animals reflex effects of carotid-sinus baroreceptors are buffered by thoracic baroreceptors but in the animals with neuropathy this secondary buffering is lost (Satchell 1984*a*).

pressure. In animals with axonal neuropathy, the secondary buffering is lost and all the reflex effects from the carotid sinus baroreceptors appear exaggerated (Fig. 10.1). There are two possible explanations for these results. Either the carotid sinus baroreceptors produce an abnormal, sustained, exaggerated discharge, which can be shown to be untrue by direct recording from the carotid-sinus nerve (Satchell 1981), or the buffering ability of thoracic baroreceptors is reduced. The increased gain of the carotid-sinus baroreceptors observed in the artificial situation of this preparation (Satchell 1984*a*) has also been observed in identical preparations in which a vagotomy has been carried out (Schmidt *et al.* 1971). In contrast with these previous studies, vagal cardiomotor function appears unaffected in animals with acrylamide neuropathy (Fig. 10.1).

It can be proposed from these results that baroreceptor afferents running in the vagus but not in the carotid-sinus nerve are affected early in an axonal neuropathy and that vagal cardiomotor efferent fibres function normally. The first part of this proposition has been examined in a preliminary manner by recording simultaneously from the carotid-sinus nerve and the aortic depressor nerve in anaesthetized rabbits with mild acrylamide neuropathy. When the activity in one nerve is compared with the activity in the other, there is virtually no difference as systemic arterial pressure is lowered by haemorrhage in normal animals. In animals with mild neuropathy there is a comparative reduction in nerve activity in the depressor nerve at lower levels of arterial pressure (Fig. 10.2). This relative reduction in thoracic-baroreceptor activity is consistent with damage to the baroreceptors themselves, or to the terminal portions of baroreceptor nerve fibres, or both. The relatively greater vulnerability in axonal disease of the depressor nerve fibres compared with the carotid-sinus nerve fibres presumably reflects their different lengths.

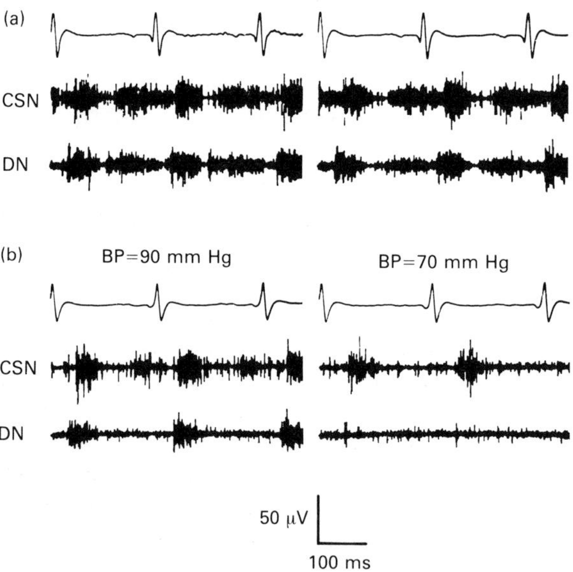

Fig. 10.2. In (a) carotid-sinus nerve activity (CSN) is very similar to depressor nerve activity (DN) at mean arterial blood pressures (BP) of 90 and 70 mm Hg in a control anaesthetized rabbit. This similarity has been observed by others (Irisawa and Ninomiya 1967). In contrast, in (b) the discharge pattern of the two baroreceptor nerves is dissimilar in an animal with acrylamide neuropathy.

In summary, thoracic baroreceptors whose afferent nerve fibres run in the vagus nerve are damaged in an axonal neuropathy, and the ability of these baroreceptors to induce reflex changes in the vagal cardiomotor and sympathetic vasoconstrictor outflows is reduced. In the intact animal, this decrease in the baroreceptor buffering ability is not apparent because the carotid-sinus baroreceptors, which are innervated by much shorter nerve fibres, are spared and can make up for the decreased thoracic baroreceptor drive. It has been shown that the four baroreceptor groups combine their signals in a non-additive manner and that a single baroreceptor nerve can take on 50 per cent of the overall buffering ability in the absence of the other three baroreceptor nerves (Stegemann and Müller-Bütow 1966).

Respiratory control system

Although the studies in conscious animals have so far provided little extra information on the changes in the cardiovascular control system in an axonal neuropathy, a full appreciation of the consequences of such a process on the respiratory control system makes studies in this state mandatory. Again these studies have been conducted in different species.

The Hering–Breuer reflex is the inhibition of the inspiration and the promotion of expiration produced by lung inflation. Slowly adapting pulmonary stretch receptors innervated by relatively large myelinated vagal nerve fibres constitute the afferent components of this reflex system. Rabbits under pentobarbitone anaesthesia suffer a reversible reduction in the strength of their Hering–Breuer reflex as they develop and recover from mild acrylamide neuropathy (Satchell 1985). Conscious dogs with a chronic side-hole tracheostomy show the same effect. The advantage of this latter preparation is that animals can be studied repeatedly while fully awake or in different sleep states. As these animals develop an axonopathy, their Hering–Breuer reflex becomes weaker, their respiration slows and deepens and they lose the broncho-dilatation which normally accompanies lung inflation (Fig. 10.3). These changes recover to a large degree (Hersch *et al.* 1986*a*). Of particular interest is the observation that there is a significant reduction in the strength of the Hering–Breuer reflex at the time that the first signs of peripheral neuropathy become apparent. Thus, there is a major disturbance in some components of the respiratory control system, particularly in those structures involved in transmitting information to the brainstem about lung dimensions. Other parts of the respiratory control system are also affected for rabbits become easier to intubate (Satchell 1985) and conscious dogs lose their cough reflexes as the neuropathy evolves (Hersch *et al.* 1985*b*).

These whole-animal studies suggest that a significant portion of the

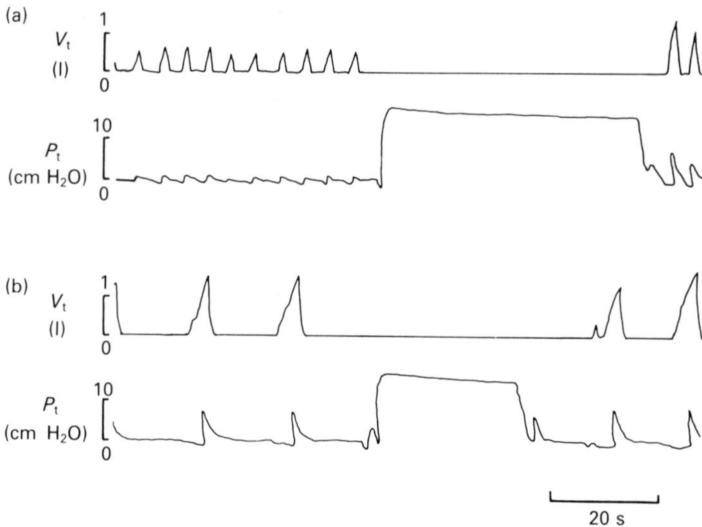

Fig. 10.3. The changes in tidal volume (V_t) and tracheal pressure (P_t) in a single conscious dog (a) before and (b) after acrylamide administration when a moderate neuropathy is present. Lung inflation of one litre via the chronic side-hole tracheostomy initially produces sustained inhibition of respiration. Later, when the neuropathy has evolved, this inspiratory inhibition becomes attenuated. At that time the respiratory pattern has also changed, becoming slower and deeper (Hersch *et al.* 1986*a*).

pulmonary vagal afferent inflow to the brainstem is damaged and that it is the larger vagal nerve fibres which are affected in an axonal neuropathy. The selective nature of the vagal damage is confirmed by the observation of a normal pulmonary chemoreflex in dogs and rabbits which have been exposed to capsaicin, a relatively specific stimulant of unmyelinated afferent fibres (unpublished observations).

The vagus is the pathway for bronchomotor efferent fibres and their function can be tested in the conscious dog which has a side-hole tracheostomy by measuring endotracheal-tube cuff pressure. This provides a measure of bronchomotor tone. Reflex fluctuations in bronchomotor tone produced by lung inflation are reduced in animals with axonal neuropathy, but this is to be expected in the light of the damage to the vagal afferent structures. However, changes in bronchomotor tone induced centrally or by stimulation of unmyelinated afferent nerve fibre endings are not altered as the animals develop neuropathy (Hersch *et al.* 1986*a*). In summary, the whole-animal studies have suggested that nerve fibres important in lung proprioception and defence are damaged in an axonal neuropathy. Other vagal pulmonary nerve fibres, such as unmyelinated afferent fibres and bronchomotor efferent fibres, appear relatively unimpaired.

Whole-animal studies can point to where lesions may exist, but confirmation of the site and identification of the abnormality require a more invasive approach. In dogs similar to those described in the above studies, a detailed examination of the pathophysiology within the vagus has been carried out by recording from single vagal afferent nerve fibres in anaesthetized animals with neuropathy (Hersch *et al.* 1986*b*). Nerve fibres innervating slowly adapting pulmonary stretch receptors have been selected and their firing rates compared in control animals and animals with neuropathy during reproducible deformations of the lung. There are four significant abnormalities. First, slowly adapting pulmonary stretch receptors have an abnormally elevated threshold. Second, these same units have significantly reduced firing rates at any given level of lung inflation, and, third, some pulmonary stretch receptors occasionally have grossly abnormal discharge patterns. It is likely that these three abnormalities represent damage to the receptor itself. Finally, a comparison of conduction velocities of the units in the two groups of animals suggests that there is a group of pulmonary stretch receptors innervated by the fastest conducting nerve fibres that are not transmitting impulses at all. In this case it is likely that there is damage to the distal portions of the afferent nerve fibre itself as well as to the receptor.

In summary, a distal axonopathy of the extrinsic innervation of the lung produces a selective afferent vagotomy. Only the larger myelinated fibres are damaged and it is the distal extremities of these fibres and their receptors that are most affected. Not all the respiratory control system components that travel in the vagus have been studied. It is unknown whether thoracic chemoreceptors are damaged in a distal axonopathy. The studies on carotid-sinus and thoracic baroreceptors suggest that the redundancy within the blood-pressure control system is sufficient to cope with the loss of a proportion of the baroreceptors. A similar argument can be developed for carotid-body and thoracic chemoreceptors. Preliminary studies suggest that overall chemosensitivity is not altered in a distal axonopathy (Hersch *et al.* 1985*a*).

Oesophagomotor control system

Studies on the changes in oesophageal motility and the oesophagomotor control system in a distal axonopathy have only been carried out in the dog. When dogs have moderate acrylamide neuropathy with mild but definite hindlimb weakness, they develop a feeding disorder which is due to the presence of megaoesophagus (Satchell and McLeod 1981). Vagotomy also produces megaoesophagus (Hwang *et al.* 1947). This type of oesophageal motility disorder also occurs in association with some naturally occurring neuropathies in the dog. These observations suggest that the extrinsic innervation of the oesophagus, which travels exclusively within the vagus, is damaged in a distal axonopathy. In animals with acrylamide neuropathy the oesophageal electromyogram remains normal even within the first week that megaoesophagus is present, and supramaximal stimulation of the distal vagal stump in anaesthetized animals with recently developed megaoesophagus results in normal contractions. At this stage the conduction velocity of oesophageal motor fibres is not altered (Satchell *et al.* 1982). The results of all these studies suggest that the motor innervation of the oesophagus is relatively intact.

If the motor innervation appears intact, two other pathophysiological possibilities must be considered: (1) there are significant changes in the intermyenteric plexus and the components of the oesophageal wall; and (2) there is a change in the afferent innervation of the oesophagus. The mechanical properties of the oesophageal wall, as measured by the wall compliance, do not change before the development of megaoesophagus but do so once it is established. The intermyenteric plexus appears histologically normal, even at the ultrastructural level (unpublished observations). However, the performance of oesophageal mechanoreceptors is altered in a distal axonopathy. These mechanoreceptors have been studied by recording from single oesophageal afferent-nerve fibres with the oesophagus surgically isolated *in vivo*. In this preparation, the firing rate of slowly adapting mechanoreceptors can be related to controlled deformations of the oesophagus (Satchell 1984*b*). In animals with early axonal neuropathy and without megaoesophagus, abnormalities can be observed in oesophageal mechanoreceptors that are identical to those found in pulmonary stretch receptors. In particular, the threshold of this type of receptor is elevated and the firing rate at set levels of distension is reduced (Satchell and McLeod 1984). It is also likely that the mechanoreceptors innervated by the fastest afferent fibres are not able to excite the distal axon, or that the distal axon is not able to transmit the impulses, or both. These non-conducting fibres are very much smaller than the equivalent non-conducting group in the pulmonary innervation as they have a maximum conduction velocity of only 28 m/s (Fig. 10.4). Very abnormal mechanoreceptor discharge patterns have not been observed but some instability in impulse transmission does occur (Satchell and McLeod 1984).

In summary, these results confirm that, as with the lung, the oesophagus becomes deafferented in a distal axonopathy. These changes are a primary defect and are not themselves due to oesophageal distension. In the larger oesophageal afferent-nerve fibres, the distal extremities of fibres and the receptors that they innervate are damaged.

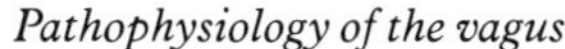

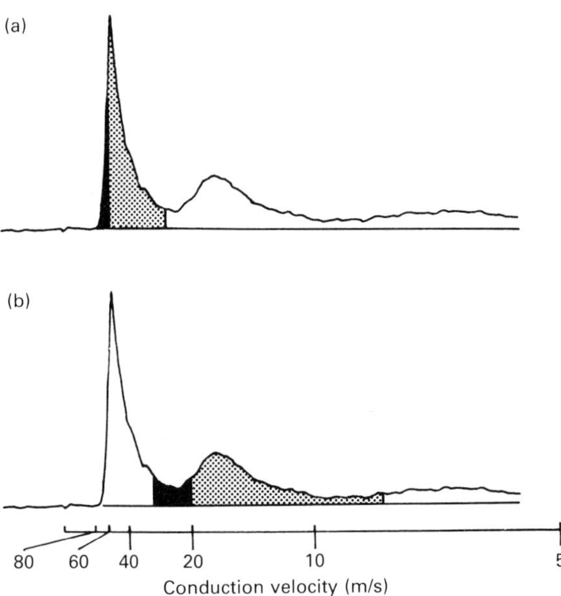

Fig. 10.4. (a) The spectrum of conduction velocities of single vagal nerve fibres innervating slowly adapting pulmonary stretch receptors is displayed (stippled and shaded areas) on the vagal compound-nerve action potential recorded in the upper cervical vagus of the dog. The nerve fibres innervating these receptors which have the fastest conduction velocities (shaded area) fail to transmit naturally produced impulses in the acrylamide animals. (b) Similarly, a group of nerve fibres with the fastest conduction velocities innervating slowly adapting oesophageal mechanoreceptors fail to transmit impulses produced by oesophageal distension in acrylamide-affected animals. Conduction velocity in m/s.

Major pathophysiological features

Several pathophysiological features occur repeatedly in the studies described. They occur independent of species and organ and are likely to be applicable to man. Slowly adapting mechanoreceptors, which are an integral part of a variety of control systems important in the 'internal homeostasis', lose their resting discharge in a distal axonopathy. This probably applies to more control systems than have been examined so far, as multifibre nerve recordings from the vagus, obtained when the nerve is being prepared for single-unit recordings, are quite abnormal. The normal 'roar' from a multitude of fibres discharging in concert and at random is completely lost. Under resting conditions, this normally busy nerve falls totally silent in an axonal neuropathy. Division of the vagus into finer strands rarely alters this observation, and deformation of innervated structures is required to produce any afferent discharge. When spontaneous discharges have been observed, the units involved have had conduction velocities in the unmyelinated range. The other major pathophysiological change is that those nerve fibres that can discharge have firing rates that are relatively very reduced.

Major histological features

Histological studies on the vagus trunk are remarkably unrewarding in the axonal neuropathy described above. There are no significant changes in the density or size distribution of myelinated fibres in the cervical, midthoracic, or supradiaphragmatic vagus (Satchell *et al.* 1982). At an ultrastructural level, nerve fibres in the midthoracic vagal trunk can occasionally be observed undergoing axonal degeneration (Fig. 10.5). When the thoracic vagus of an animal with neuropathy has been divided into one-centimetre sections and teased-fibre preparations of each of these sections examined, myelin beading, a feature of axonal degeneration, has only been observed in nerve segments just proximal to where the pulmonary vagal branches leave the vagus trunk (Fig. 10.6). Axonal degeneration has been observed in transverse section and with teased-fibre preparations in the pulmonary branch of the vagus nerve (Hersch *et al.* 1986*b*).

Consequences for man

As far as is known, the role of the baroreceptors in the circulatory control system is similar in animals and man. In predicting the changes in this control system in human distal axonopathies, it is probably legitimate to project the findings from affected animals to man in the absence of any relevant human studies. It is likely that patients with a chronic axonal neuropathy have non-functioning thoracic baroreceptors. It is just as likely that the carotid-sinus baroreceptors are relatively unaffected and that these provide enough baroreceptor buffering ability to cope with normal postural and exertional stresses.

When the respiratory control system is considered, it is less easy to project the findings from animals to man. In animals, axonal neuropathy markedly interferes with the respiratory pattern and with lung protective reflexes. Pneumonia after an anaesthetic is a significant hazard (Satchell 1985). In contrast, respiratory symptoms and signs are not described in human axonal neuropathy. There is an important lack of overlap here between the human pathophysiology, which is probably similar to that described in animals, and the lack of any observed consequences in man. This incongruence is less likely to be due to species variation in properties, such as the strength of the Hering–Breuer reflex, and is more probably due to the complexities of respiratory control in conscious humans. In the human respiratory control system there are multiple powerful inputs into the basic brainstem

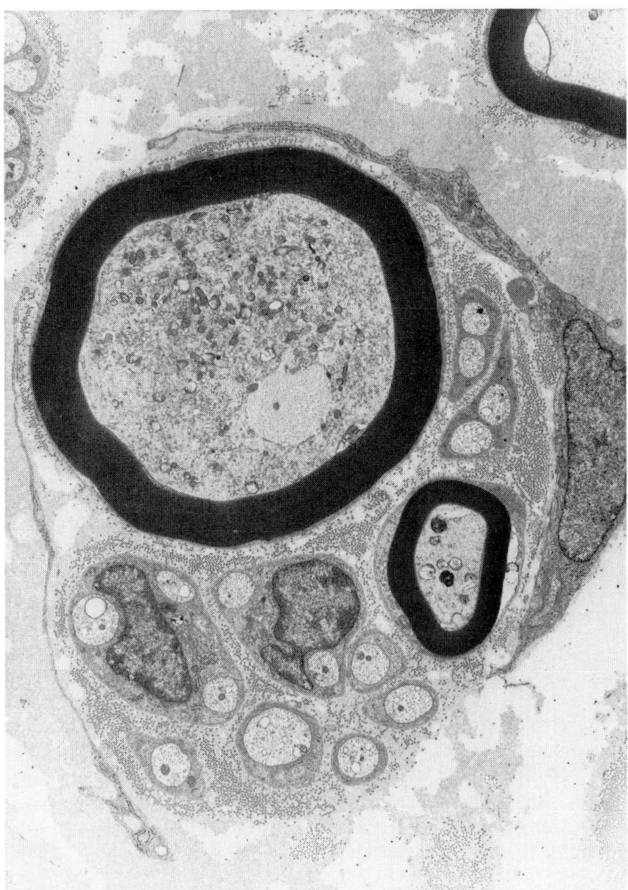

Fig. 10.5. Acrylamide neuropathy in the dog. Cross-section of the vagus at the level of the aortic arch in a dog with a sensorimotor neuropathy. An enlarged axon with a disproportionately thin myelin sheath is packed with mitochondria, electron dense bodies, and neurofilaments (×6000). These changes are the characteristic pathological alterations of a distal axonopathy. Unmyelinated fibres appear normal.

circuits that dominate and override the lower-order control loops during wakefulness. It is only when these inputs are quiescent that defects in the more basic control loops may become significant.

There is an increased mortality in patients with diabetic autonomic neuropathy (Chapter 36). Some of these deaths have occurred in situations, such as post-anaesthesia, where the respiratory drive is reduced (Page and Watkins 1978). Vagal abnormalities which interfere with the regulation of the rate and depth of respiration may contribute significantly to this dysfunction of the respiratory control system. This example illustrates well the problems of projecting animal findings to

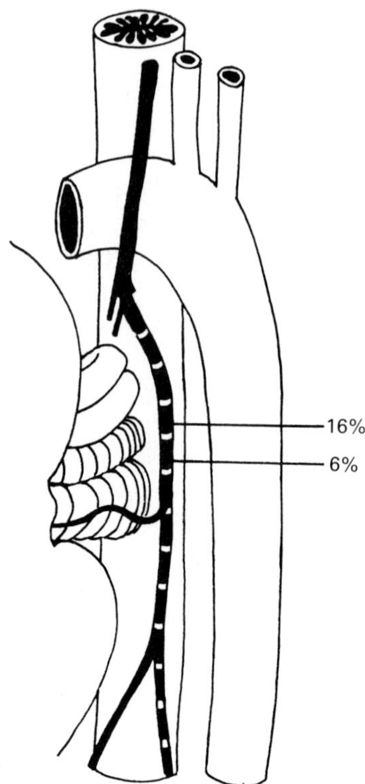

Fig. 10.6. The site and extent of fibres undergoing axonal degeneration in the vagal trunk in a single dog with acrylamide neuropathy. Teased-fibre preparations of the myelinated fibres in one-centimetre lengths of the vagus are devoid of degenerating fibres except where the percentage incidence is shown.

man. The factors important in the maintenance of respiratory rhythm when respiratory drive is reduced are ill understood in all species. An associated defect, which may be more important in this situation and which is even less understood, centres on the mechanisms essential for initiating respiration after a period of apnoea. These are only partially understood in animals (Sears *et al.* 1982) and are only just being investigated in man (Berssenbrugge *et al.* 1983). Disturbances in the initiation of rhythm are important, because another clinical situation where vagal abnormalities may be contributing to respiratory-control dysfunction is in sleep apnoea. This not only applies to the apnoea observed in diabetics (Rees *et al.* 1981), but also to those groups that are exposed to axonopathy-producing agents such as alcohol, for the animal studies suggest that vagal abnormalities in the respiratory-control system can be detected at a time when the signs of neuropathy are equivocal. Normally, the transition into and out of apnoea of limited duration occurs with absolute safety during sleep. This transition may be less secure in humans with axonal neuropathy if the vagus has a significant role in initiating respiration in humans. Until these mechanisms are understood in man, it is not possible to attribute any definite pathological role to the abnormalities that have been proposed from the animals with axonal neuropathy. At this stage it is unwise to attach great significance to the presence of grossly abnormal discharges in some pulmonary stretch receptors (Hersch *et al.* 1986*b*), because this type of abnormality has not been observed in other afferent nerves in acrylamide neuropathy. The observation of ectopic discharges in visceral afferent nerves in future studies would be important for our understanding of sudden death in some diabetics.

Even greater caution must be exercised in extrapolating the vagal pathophysiology of animals to man with axonal neuropathy when the extrinsic innervation of the oesophagus is considered. The species differences are considerable. The human oesophagus is a predominantly smooth-muscle structure which is functionally assisted by the force of gravity while the canine oesophagus is a predominantly skeletal-muscle structure whose activities are usually opposed by the force of gravity. In species with skeletal-muscle oesophagi, such as the dog and the rabbit, only the dog requires the sensory reinforcement provided by the presence of a bolus for efficient peristalsis (Janssens 1978). This dependence in the dog on the sensory information from the oesophagus almost certainly underlies the reason why this species develops megaoesophagus in the presence of naturally occurring or artificially produced axonal neuropathy. The uniqueness of the dog in the animal kingdom and the gross structural differences between the human and canine oesophagus suggest that alterations in oesophageal mechanoreceptor discharge patterns are unlikely to cause oesophageal dysfunction in man. This is not to say that oesophageal mechanoreceptors are not damaged in human distal axonopathy. They probably are, but these alterations cannot be assumed to be responsible for the oesophageal dysfunction observed in human axonal neuropathy until the role of the extrinsic innervation of the oesophagus is better understood in man.

DEMYELINATING NEUROPATHY AND THE VAGUS

Demyelinating neuropathy

The clinical spectrum of autonomic disturbances in demyelinating neuropathy has been reviewed in Chapter 34. There is little doubt that autonomic disturbances are mild and an inconstant feature in chronic demyelinating disease (McLeod and Tuck 1987). Vagal abnormalities, if present, are insignificant. The redundancy of the control systems that use the vagus, coupled with the probable scattered and non-uniform nature of the areas of demyelination suggest that clinical abnormalities should not be expected. As such, the process of chronic demyelination is a poor probe or tool for studying the pathophysiology of the autonomic nervous system in autonomic failure.

In contrast, acute demyelination is occasionally associated with profound and life-threatening autonomic dysfunction. While any experimental approach which uses acute demyelination as a probe for understanding autonomic dysfunction must be bedevilled by the comparatively random targeting of different structures in the vagus, the need for such studies is unquestioned. Only one study has confirmed histologically and electrophysiologically that the vagus suffers segmental demyelination and some coexistent axonal degeneration in acute demyelinating disease (Tuck *et al.* 1981). No studies have examined the pathophysiological consequences of these lesions. In particular, the role of acute conduction block in reflex systems, which have both myelinated and unmyelinated afferent and efferent fibres, has not been examined. Nor have the consequences of indirect damage to unmyelinated fibres by nearby foci of myelin destruction been studied. It is likely that some of the pathophysiological mechanisms underlying the rare but significant autonomic disturbances in acute demyelinating disease in man will be understood when studies of the type detailed in this chapter are employed.

CONCLUSIONS

Our understanding of the pathophysiology of autonomic failure can be enhanced by studying the autonomic dysfunction which results from an identified disease process. This experimental approach has provided some new concepts concerning vagal dysfunction in man. In the distal axonopathies, vagal afferent-nerve endings and their receptors are damaged at a stage when the clinical manifestations of peripheral neuropathy are few. The relative paucity of clinical autonomic abnormalities at this stage and at more advanced stages of disease reflect, at least in part, the redundancy provided by nerve fibres functionally similar to those damaged in the vagus but which have much shorter axons.

In the somatic nervous system there is a disparity in the vulnerability of sensory and motor fibres in the distal axonopathy process and this has been attributed to different neuronal cell volumes. This disparity appears exaggerated when the extent of afferent- and efferent-fibre dysfunction is studied in the vagus. This may only reflect the very great differences in nerve-fibre diameter that exist in the afferent and efferent innervation of the thoracic organs. A most striking abnormality in the receptors innervated by some vagal myelinated nerve fibres is the elevation of the threshold of the slowly adapting type of mechanoreceptor. The long-term clinical consequences of this loss of a resting discharge are surprisingly few. They await a clearer understanding of the role of this type of input in autonomic control systems and of the sequelae of a sustained absence of this type of activity in visceral afferent pathways.

REFERENCES

Berssenbrugge, A., Dempsey, J., Iber, C., Skatrud, J., and Wilson, P. (1983). Mechanisms of hypoxia-induced periodic breathing during sleep in humans. *J. Physiol., London* **343**, 507–24.

Hersch, M. I., McLeod, J. G., and Sullivan, C. E. (1985*a*). Ventilatory, arousal and cardiac responses to normocapnic hypoxia in acrylamide neuropathy. *Neurosci. Lett.* **19**, S70.

Hersch, M. I., Satchell, P. M., Sullivan, C. E., and McLeod, J. G. (1986*a*). Effect of canine acrylamide neuropathy on slowly adapting lung stretch receptors (SARs) and respiratory reflexes. *Proc. Int. Union physiol. Sci.* **30**, 297.

Hersch, M. I., Satchell, P. M., Sullivan, C. E., and McLeod, J. G. (1986*b*). Abnormal pulmonary slowly adapting receptors in canine acrylamide neuropathy. *J. appl. Physiol.* **60**, 376–84.

Hersch, M. I., Sullivan, C. E., and McLeod, J. G. (1985*b*). Abnormal cough reflexes in acrylamide neuropathy. *Proc. Aust. physiol. pharmacol. Soc.* **16**, 182P.

Hwang, K., Essex, H. E., and Mann, F. C. (1947). A study of certain problems resulting from vagotomy in dogs with special reference to emisis. *Am. J. Physiol.* **149**, 429–48.

Irisawa, H. and Ninomiya, I. (1967). Comparison of the averaged nervous activities of aortic and carotid sinus nerves. *Am. J. Physiol.* **213**, 504–10.

Janssens, J. (1978). The peristaltic mechanism of the oesophagus. Thesis, University of Leuven, Belgium.

LeQuesne, P. M. (1980). Acrylamide. In *Experimental and clinical neurotoxicology* (ed. P. S. Spencer and H. H. Schaumburg), pp. 309–25. Williams and Wilkins, Baltimore.

McLeod, J. G. and Tuck, R. R. (1987). Disorders of the autonomic nervous system. *Ann. Neurol.* **21**, 419–31, 519–30.

Page, M. McB. and Watkins, P. J. (1978). Cardiorespiratory arrest and diabetic autonomic neuropathy. *Lancet* **i**, 14–16.

Rees, P. J., Prior, J. G., Cochrane, G. M., and Clark, T. J. H. (1981). Sleep apnoea in diabetic patients with autonomic neuropathy. *J. R. Soc. Med.* **74**, 192–5.

Satchell, P. M. (1981). Autonomic dysfunction in canine acrylamide neuropathy. PhD thesis, University of Sydney.

Satchell, P. M. (1984*a*). Circulatory control in canine acrylamide neuropathy. *J. aut. nerv. Syst.* **10**, 93–106.

Satchell, P. M. (1984*b*). Canine oesophageal mechanoreceptors. *J. Physiol., London* **346**, 287–300.

Satchell, P. M. (1985). Reversible abnormalities of the Hering Breuer reflex in acrylamide neuropathy. *J. Neurol. Neurosurg. Psychiat.* **48**, 670–5.

Satchell, P. M. and McLeod, J. G. (1981). Megaoesophagus due to acrylamide neuropathy. *J. Neurol. Neurosurg. Psychiat.* **44**, 906–13.

Satchell, P. M. and McLeod, J. G. (1984). Abnormalities of oesophageal mechanoreceptors in canine acrylamide neuropathy. *J. Neurol. Neurosurg. Psychiat.* **47**, 692–8.

Satchell, P. M., McLeod, J. G., Harper, B., and Goodman, A. H. (1982). Abnormalities in the vagus nerve in canine acrylamide neuropathy. *J. Neurol. Neurosurg. Psychiat.* **45**, 609–19.

Schmidt, R. M., Kumada, M., and Sagawa, K. (1971). Cardiac output and total peripheral resistance in the carotid sinus reflex. *Am. J. Physiol.* **221**, 480–7.

Sears, T. A., Berger, A. J., and Phillipson, E. A. (1982). Reciprocal tonic activation of inspiratory and expiratory motoneurones by chemical drives. *Nature* **299**, 728–30.

Stegemann, J. and Müller-Bütow, H. (1966). Zur regeltheoretischen Analyse des Blutkreislaufes. *Pflüger's Arch. ges. Physiol.* **287**, 247–56.

Sumner, A. J. (1980). Axonal polyneuropathies. In *The physiology of peripheral nerve disease* (ed. A. J. Sumner), pp. 340–57. Saunders, Philadelphia.

Tuck, R. R., Pollard, J. D., and McLeod, J. G. (1981). Autonomic neuropathy in experimental allergic neuritis: an electrophysiological and histological study. *Brain* **104**, 187–208.

11. Intraneural recordings of normal and abnormal sympathetic activity in man

B. Gunnar Wallin

INTRODUCTION

Sympathetic neural functions are difficult to evaluate in man. The most common method has been to record sympathetic effector-organ activities, such as heart rate, blood flow, blood pressure, and sweat production, and use the data to draw conclusions about the neural drive. With such recordings a battery of clinical tests have been developed for detecting autonomic dysfunction (see Chapters 16 and 38). The main drawback with this approach is that data are difficult to interpret, both because effector organs react slowly to variations in sympathetic neural drive and because they also react to hormonal, local chemical, and mechanical stimuli. For the same reason our understanding of neurophysiological mechanisms underlying different autonomic reflexes is still incomplete. It was therefore an important methodological advancement when a technique was developed for microelectrode recordings of sympathetic action potentials in limb nerves of awake, unanaesthetized human subjects. With the new technique it became possible to get direct information about sympathetic neural outflow to skin and muscle in man both at rest and during various manoeuvres. Visceral sympathetic activity (and parasympathetic activity) is still inaccessible, but data obtained with the method has, nevertheless, provided new insights into the functional organization of the sympathetic system and a better understanding of the relationship between sympathetic activity and plasma levels of noradrenalin. The technique is too complex for routine diagnostic work but several studies on the pathophysiology of sympathetic failure have been published. This chapter will review first the characteristics of normal sympathetic outflow to skin and muscle and then the abnormalities found in certain diseases which have been investigated with the microneurographic technique. Specific references will be given only to recent work and pathophysiological findings. Other references can be found in Vallbo *et al.* (1979) and Wallin and Fagius (1986).

METHODS

Nerve recordings are made with tungsten microelectrodes with tip diameters of a few micrometres. The recording electrode is inserted manually through intact skin, into an underlying nerve with a reference electrode placed subcutaneously 1–2 cm away. Usually, multiunit activity is obtained but occasionally single units may be recorded. Most recordings are made in large nerves such as the peroneal, median, or tibial nerves but sometimes small cutaneous arm and leg nerves have been used. In man, peripheral nerves are composed of a varying number of fascicles, each of which is surrounded by a barrier of connective tissue. With the electrodes used, action potentials can be recorded only when the tip has penetrated a fascicle and then there is no cross-talk from neighbouring fascicles. Fascicles are most numerous distally where each contains fibres connected only to skin or only to a muscle, but in the proximal part of an extremity all fascicles are composed of a mixture of skin and muscle nerve fibres. For this reason mixed nerves are impaled as far distally as possible in order to obtain recordings from relatively 'pure' muscle or skin nerve fascicles. In some experiments, blood pressure was recorded in the brachial artery; in others, electrical skin resistance and a finger or toe plethysmogram (photoelectric) were monitored. Usually nerve recordings cause minimal discomfort. Detailed descriptions of the technique as well as evidence for the sympathetic nature of the recorded impulses were given previously (Vallbo *et al.* 1979).

Intraneural stimulation

In addition to its use for *recording* nerve impulses, the microelectrode can also be used for *evoking* action potentials by means of intraneural electrical stimulation (Wallin *et al.* 1983). All types of nerve fibres can be stimulated; weak pulses activate preferentially large-diamater axons but, with higher stimulus strength, action potentials are induced also in thin (A-delta and unmyelinated) fibres. Stimulation-induced cutaneous effector responses can be detected by monitoring blood flow and/or skin resistance. Local anaesthetic blocks of the nerve proximal or distal to the stimulation site can be used to differentiate between effector responses caused by reflexes and by centrifugally conducted impulses (see Blumberg and Wallin 1987).

NORMAL SYMPATHETIC OUTFLOW

Sympathetic skin nerve activity

The two most important sympathetic effector organs in the human skin, blood vessels and sweat glands, are innervated by separate sympathetic fibres with different conduction velocities. In nerves supplying the feet and the palms of the hands, vasoconstrictor and sudomotor impulses can be recorded from the same electrode site, suggesting that the fibres are intermingled. At rest at normal room temperature, spontaneous skin sympathetic activity consists of irregular bursts of impulses, varying in strength and duration and often occurring in the respiratory rhythm. Some spontaneous bursts are followed by both transient changes of skin resistance and plethysmographic signs of vasoconstriction indicating that they contain a mixture of vasoconstrictor and sudomotor impulses. Other bursts probably contain only vasoconstrictor impulses (i.e. they are followed by transient vasoconstriction but not by skin-resistance changes), whereas pure sudomotor bursts are unusual at normal room temperature. Arterial baroreceptor modulation of the outflow of vasoconstrictor impulses is weak or absent. Recently sudomotor impulses were found to be time-locked to the cardiac cycle but the significance of this is unclear. In addition to vasoconstrictor and sudomotor impulses, spontaneous skin sympathetic activity may contain pilomotor and possibly vasodilator impulses.

Recordings of cutaneous effector-organ responses have shown that spontaneous electrodermal and plethysmographic activity occurs in parallel in hands and feet and a similar parallelism in the underlying sympathetic discharges has also been demonstrated. This parallelism does not apply to all skin areas, however, and, during exposure to different temperatures, there are differences in sympathetic drives between the median nerve innervating the palm of the hand and the dorsal cutaneous nerve of the forearm.

Thermoregulatory effects

As expected, spontaneous skin sympathetic activity is affected by thermal stimuli, and body cooling leads to an increased outflow of impulses to the palm of the hand and the foot. At the same time, plethysmographically recorded pulse amplitudes in the digits are reduced, suggesting that the activity contains an increased number of vasoconstrictor impulses. During moderate warming, sympathetic activity is reduced to a minimum. With prolonged body heating there is again an increase of skin sympathetic activity, but this time associated with electrodermal signs of sweating, suggesting activation of sudomotor impulses. The results show that, by changing environmental temperature, one can activate selectively either the vasoconstrictor or the sudomotor neural system with suppression of activity in the other system.

The effects of mental stimuli

In agreement with the fact that stimuli with emotional effects may change skin colour and moisture, such stimuli, pleasant or unpleasant, regularly cause an increase of spontaneous skin sympathetic activity. Any unexpected stimulus, such as a sudden sound, touch, or pain stimulus anywhere on the skin surface, regularly evokes a single burst of impulses. Similar discharges are evoked by deep breaths. The latency to the start of the burst is 0.5–1.0 s, depending on the recording site and the subject's height. The latency differences are due mainly to differences in conduction time in postganglionic C fibres and reflex latencies can be used as an indirect measure of sympathetic conduction velocity. At intermediate or warm skin temperatures, bursts evoked by arousal or respiratory stimuli are followed by both vasoconstrictor and electrodermal responses. This simultaneous activation of vasoconstrictor and sudomotor fibres constitutes the basis for 'cold sweat'. In cooled subjects, however, the same manoeuvres may cause vasodilatation, i.e. vasodilator impulses may also be activated (Oberle *et al.*, unpublished).

Emotional excitement, brought on by a stressed conversation or a sudden request to solve an arithmetic problem, usually leads to an increase of skin sympathetic activity which is more long-lasting than that caused by arousal stimuli. Such an increase may occasionally last for several minutes after the end of the stimulus. In warm subjects the vascular response in glabrous skin evoked by stress is vasoconstriction, but it has recently been found that, in cooled subjects, vasodilatation often occurs (Elam and Wallin 1987). The mechanisms behind these opposing reactions are unclear. The results show, however, that there is complex interaction between neurally mediated thermoregulatory and emotional vascular responses in the human skin.

Neurally mediated cutaneous vasodilatation

Recently, the microneurography electrode has been used to stimulate skin nerves electrically while recording electrical resistance and blood flow in the skin (Wallin *et al.* 1983). With this approach painful intraneural stimulation was found to evoke a short-lasting sympathetic vasodilatory reflex in the skin on the dorsal side of the foot (Blumberg and Wallin 1987). Thin myelinated (A-delta) nerve fibres probably constitute the afferent limb of the reflex arc but whether the flow increase is due to inhibition of impulse traffic in vasoconstrictor fibres or increased activity in sudomotor or vasodilator fibres is not known. In glabrous skin flow responses to intraneural stimulation are more complex with vasodilatation in cold (< 25°C) and reflex vasoconstriction in warm (> 30°C) skin (Oberle *et al.*, unpublished). The underlying mechanisms are unclear but, since similar effects are evoked by mental stress (Elam and Wallin 1987), it is possible that the responses to intraneural stimulation are related to the stress of the induced pain.

After local anaesthesia of the nerve proximal to the stimulation site, high-intensity intraneural stimulation gave rise to a more long-lasting flow increase restricted to the innervation zone of the stimulated nerve fascicle. Probably this response was caused by antidromic stimulation of afferent C-fibres and may correspond to Lewis's classical axon reflex (Blumberg and Wallin 1987).

At present both the mechanisms behind these newly discovered blood flow responses and their physiological importance are unclear. The results demonstrate, however, that neural control of skin blood flow is complex; they also point to the possibility that abnormalities of skin circulation may comprise defects of either vasoconstriction or vasodilatation.

Sympathetic muscle nerve activity

Arterial baroreceptor influence

The temporal pattern of sympathetic discharges occurring in muscle nerve fascicles differs from that found in skin fascicles. The bursts are grouped in the cardiac rhythm; they occur most frequently during transient reductions of blood pressure and disappear when blood pressure goes up. Electrical stimulation of the carotid sinus nerves inhibits muscle sympathetic activity. In contrast, temporary baroreceptor denervation achieved by bilateral local anaesthetic blocks of glossopharyngeal and vagus nerves in the neck increases muscle sympathetic activity and eliminates its cardiac rhythmicity (Fagius *et al.* 1985). These findings suggest that the bursts are composed of vasoconstrictor impulses, the outflow of which is modulated by arterial baroreceptors. According to this view, bursts correspond to diastolic blood-pressure reductions whereas pauses between successive bursts correspond to systolic blood-pressure peaks. In agreement with this, there was a close correlation between beat-to-beat blood-pressure variations in patients with cardiac arrhythmias and the occurrence of sympathetic bursts, and also a linear relationship between the duration of the R–R-interval and the duration of corresponding sympathetic burst.

A detailed study of the quantitative relationship between muscle sympathetic activity and blood pressure showed that the variations of muscle sympathetic activity are determined by fluctuations of diastolic blood pressure, whereas other blood-pressure parameters seem to be of lesser importance. The findings are logical: the arterial baroreflex is inhibitory and, since the systolic inhibition is always complete, one expects activity to be determined by diastolic-pressure variations. Strength of activity is also dependent on the direction of an ongoing blood-pressure change and, for a given blood-pressure level, more bursts occur during falling than during rising pressure. When blood pressure changes were induced by intravenous infusions of vasoactive substances (phenylephrine or sodium nitroprusside), a blood-pressure reduction led to an increase and a blood-pressure increase to a reduction of the strength of muscle sympathetic activity (Eckberg *et al.* 1986). In contrast to this intimate relationship between dynamic variations of blood pressure and sympathetic activity (present in all individuals), no systemic correlation was found when subjects were compared with regard to their mean levels of diastolic blood pressure and sympathetic activity. This suggests that muscle sympathetic activity is important for buffering acute changes of blood pressure but has less importance for setting the long-term blood-pressure level.

Other evidence strengthens the idea that muscle sympathetic activity is primarily affected by *changes* of blood pressure. Application of sub-atmospheric pressure in a collar around the neck (neck suction) leads to an increased transmural carotid pressure (i.e. increased arterial baro-receptor firing) and one would therefore expect sympathetic outflow to become inhibited. However, with continuous neck suction at −40 mm Hg there was only an initial inhibition corresponding to application of suction and the sustained effects were minor. In another study neck suction or neck pressure was applied very rapidly and maintained for 5 seconds. Again, with application of the stimuli, there were clear changes of nerve activity but adaptation was almost complete within 1–2 seconds. Cardiac responses, on the other hand, showed much less adaptation suggesting that the stimulus induced maintained changes of afferent baroreceptor-nerve traffic and, therefore, adaptation of muscle sympathetic activity was to a large extent of central origin. However, since only carotid baroreceptors are affected directly by this type of stimulus, carotid and extracarotid arterial baroreceptors will convey different messages to the brainstem and we do not know whether there would be an equally pronounced adaptation if firing in all high-pressure receptors were changed at the same time. In conclusion, available evidence indicate that: (1) rapid changes of arterial baroreceptor activity effectively modulate sympathetic outflow to muscles; (2) it is uncertain to what extent static changes of baroreceptor activity lasting more than a few seconds induce static changes of sympathetic activity in muscle nerves; (3) interindividual differences in arterial blood pressure are not related to interindividual differences in the level of muscle-nerve sympathetic activity.

In patients with essential hypertension the findings were similar, i.e. the general character of muscle sympathetic activity was normal and there was no increase of the level of muscle sympathetic activity in the patients related to the blood-pressure level (Wallin and Fagius 1986; Wallin *et al.* 1987).

Influence from cardiopulmonary receptors

Apart from arterial baroreceptors, cardiopulmonary (sometimes called low-pressure) receptors also influence muscle sympathetic activity. These receptors are volume receptors located primarily in the heart and large vessels entering the heart. A reduction of intrathoracic blood volume, brought about by applying subatmospheric pressure around the lower body, caused an increase of muscle sympathetic activity which could not be explained as an arterial-baroreceptor effect and therefore presumably was elicited from the cardiopulmonary receptors. The increase in sympathetic activity did not wear off during several minutes and probably, therefore, such receptors exert a more static influence on muscle sympathetic activity than arterial baroreceptors.

The effect of various manoeuvres

In contrast to spontaneous skin sympathetic activity, the outflow of sympathetic impulses to muscles is not easily affected by minor disturbances such as arousal stimuli which do not themselves affect blood pressure. Any manoeuvre or situation associated with a change in blood pressure and/or central blood volume is, however, likely to produce a change of muscle sympathetic activity. For example, the modulation of muscle sympathetic activity in the respiratory rhythm may be secondary to respiration-induced variations of arterial blood pressure (Eckberg *et al.* 1985). A Valsalva manoeuvre, which causes transient reductions of both blood pressure and central blood volume is a reliable way of bringing about a short-lasting increase in muscle sympathetic activity. *Changes in posture* from lying to sitting to standing induce progressive increases of muscle sympathetic activity which presumably are due to unloading of both arterial and cardiopulmonary receptors. Similarly, the infusions of sodium nitroprusside and phenylephrine mentioned above also influence both arterial and cardiopulmonary baroreceptors and presumably both receptor stations contributed to the changes of muscle sympathetic activity (Eckberg *et al.* 1986).

There are, however, other receptor stations that may influence muscle sympathetic activity. *Hypoxia, hypercapnea* (Blumberg, personal communication); simulated *diving* (Fagius and Sundlöf 1986), and *the cold-pressor test* (Victor *et al.* 1987) all increase muscle sympathetic activity in spite of unchanged or increasing blood pressure. Emotional stress and isometric muscle contractions (e.g. handgrips) are also examples of complex manoeuvres usually associated with blood-pressure increases. Emotional stress induced by mental arithmetic causes no change of muscle sympathetic activity in the radial nerve but after 1–2 min sympathetic activity in the peroneal nerve increases (Anderson *et al.* 1987). *Isometric handgrips* at 30 per cent of maximal power cause a generalized increase of muscle sympathetic activity which is triggered from the contracting muscles, presumably because intramuscular chemosensitive nerve endings are activated by contraction-induced accumulation of metabolites (Mark *et al.* 1985). Changes of muscle sympathetic activity can be evoked also by hormones: both the reduction of activity caused by arginine vasopressin (Floras *et al.*, personal communication) and the increase caused by insulin (Fagius *et al.* 1986) may be due partly to direct effects on the central nervous system.

SYMPATHETIC TONE

Functional organization of sympathetic outflow

Traditionally, sympathetic reactions were thought to be slow and protracted and to occur in parallel in different parts of the body. This view of a diffusely acting system led to the term 'sympathetic tone' to describe the strength of a presumed global level of activity in sympathetic nerves. Clinically, subjects are often classified as having 'high sympathetic tone'. Unfortunately, the concept is not tenable. Direct nerve recordings both in animal and man reveal clear differences between the activity in one nerve and that in another as would be expected with differentiated regional control of sympathetic outflow. For example, when comparing spontaneous skin and muscle sympathetic activity in man, the temporal patterns of resting activity are different and various manoeuvres affect these activities differently. In contrast to such evidence for differences between sympathetic outflows to skin and muscle, there is a remarkable parallelism between the two neurograms when sympathetic activity is recorded simultaneously in different muscles nerves at rest. In a corresponding way, double recordings of sympathetic activity from skin nerves innervating the palm of the hands and the feet reveal a similar close parallelism between both neurograms. These findings show that there are different populations of sympathetic neurons, each of which is subjected to its own homogeneous supraspinal drive which may be different from that of other populations. Consequently, there is no common 'sympathetic tone'; if the term is to be retained, it should be used only when considering the sympathetic drive in specified nerves supplying well-defined effector organs.

Relationship between sympathetic muscle nerve activity and plasma noradrenalin

The plasma level of noradrenalin is often used as an index of sympathetic activity. This is partly based on the fact that noradrenalin is the principal transmitter released from postganglionic sympathetic neurons and partly on physiological studies showing that plasma levels of noradrenalin increase when sympathetic nerves to specific organs are stimulated electrically or when human subjects perform manoeuvres known to increase activity in some sympathetic nerves. Nevertheless, to which extent different sympathetic nerves contribute to the plasma concentration of noradrenalin was for long unknown.

Recently, however, a series of studies have shown that impulse traffic in sympathetic muscle nerves is an important (perhaps the most important) determinant of forearm venous plasma concentrations of noradrenalin. There are positive correlations between the frequency of sympathetic bursts in muscle nerves and plasma concentrations of noradrenalin in forearm venous blood in resting supine normotensive and hypertensive subjects. The relationship was present also in patients with cardiac failure who had increased mean levels of muscle sympathetic activity and plasma noradrenalin (Leimbach *et al.* 1986). Also changes of muscle sympathetic activity and plasma noradrenalin are related to each other during infusion of sodium nitroprusside and phenylephrine (Eckberg *et al.* 1986), the cold pressor test (Victor *et al.* 1987), and isometric handgrip (Wallin *et al.* 1987). In addition, when changes of muscle sympathetic activity are small as during mental stress (see above), plasma noradrenalin concentrations do not change much despite probable increases of sympathetic nerve traffic to other vascular beds.

How can these findings be explained? One contributing factor is that muscle is a large organ responsible for about 20 per cent of the total spill-over of noradrenalin to the blood. A second reason is that the contribution of noradrenalin from muscle is disproportionately high in forearm venous plasma. A third factor is that there is net extraction of noradrenalin in the liver and, therefore, the contribution of the plasma concentration from the splanchnic region is low.

If plasma concentrations of noradrenalin at rest to a large extent are determined by sympathetic outflow in muscle nerves, it becomes understandable why many authors find no relationship between plasma noradrenalin levels and blood-pressure levels in normotensive subjects at rest. Muscle sympathetic activity is modulated by dynamic arterial-baroreceptor mechanisms and there is no relationship between mean levels of sympathetic activity and blood pressure, either in normotensive or in hypertensive subjects. Consequently, we are left with a situation where an important determinant of the plasma level of noradrenalin may be impulse activity in sympathetic nerves supplying a vascular bed which is relatively unimportant for setting the long-term blood-pressure level.

ABNORMAL SYMPATHETIC OUTFLOW

A variety of lesions in different parts of the nervous system may result in pathological sympathetic activity which should be possible to detect in microneurographic recordings. The recording technique is inappropriate, however, for abnormalities which arise distal to the recording site, i.e. in the most distal parts of the postganglionic sympathetic neurons or in the neuroeffector junction. In such cases intraneural stimulation of sympathetic fibres combined with effector recordings may sometimes provide a methodological alternative. In principle, sympathetic abnormalities may be quantitative or qualitative. *Quantitative* abnormalities arise if the number of sympathetic action potentials reaching the effectors is reduced (or increased) resulting in weakened (or exaggerated) but qualitatively normal reflex responses. Such effects may be induced either from the afferent or efferent limb of a reflex arc (see below). A *qualitative* abnormality implies that reflex effects are evoked from a stimulus which normally is ineffective, or that the 'sign' of a reflex effect is reversed, e.g. if a normally exitatory response is turned into an inhibitory one.

An example of how qualitative abnormalities may arise has been demonstrated recently. As mentioned above Fagius *et al.* (1985) found that temporary baroreceptor deafferentation in normal humans eliminated cardiac rhythmicity of muscle sympathetic activity. When this occurred the integrated neurogram from the muscle nerve became fairly similar to that obtained from a skin nerve, i.e. many sympathetic bursts occurred in parallel in the two records. During the same period arousal stimuli gave rise to clear sympathetic reflex responses both in the skin and the muscle nerve. Normally such responses occur only in skin nerves and the muscle-nerve responses also disappeared as the anaesthesia wore off. Consequently, it appears that afferent-baroreceptor activity, in addition to being involved in blood-pressure homeostasis also serves as a powerful brake on reflex effects in muscle sympathetic activity from other types of afferent inputs; therefore, when baroreceptor inhibition was eliminated by the anaesthesia, such reflexes were unmasked. Another example was reported by Blumberg and Jänig (1983) following chronic lesions of cat extremity nerves. Some time after a peripheral nerve had been cut, the normal differences between muscle and skin vasoconstrictor activity were reduced and reflex effects became more similar in both types of nerves (proximal to the lesion). These findings show that interruption of various afferent pathways may result in abnormal sympathetic reflex patterns. If such effects would occur during the course of a disease, it seems likely that clinical symptoms would arise. This hypothesis would be in accordance with other examples of lesions in the nervous system revealing patterns which normally are concealed due to inhibitory regulation, e.g. the Babinski sign and reflex grasping.

Our knowledge about the precise mechanisms underlying pathological sympathetic reactions is limited but the character of an abnormality should depend on which reflex(es) and where in the reflex arc(s) the pathological influence occurs. In the conditions described below an attempt has been made to classify sympathetic abnormalities according to the anatomical site of the lesion.

Peripheral efferent lesions: polyneuropathy

Generalized neuropathies are due to toxic or metabolic disturbance and occur with many diseases, most commonly diabetes. In all polyneuropathies the peripheral nerve membrane becomes damaged and finally the fibres cease to conduct. In most cases symptoms such as weakness and sensory disturbances dominate but some patients have symptoms suggesting autonomic involvement (such as orthostatism, impotence, bladder dysfunction, dryness of hands and feet).

In somatic myelinated fibres there is usually lowered conduction velocity (which is an important way of diagnosing the disease) but until recently it was not known if conduction velocity was low also in sympathetic fibres. When sympathetic outflows to skin and muscle were recorded in patients with polyneuropathy of different aetiology, the character of the activity was found to be normal in most subjects (Fagius and Wallin 1980). Conduction velocity in sympathetic fibres was estimated indirectly from determination of sympathetic reflex latencies and all values were normal, even if patients had autonomic symptoms and marked slowing of skeletomotor conduction velocity (Fig. 11.1). The only difference between patients and normal subjects was that failure to find sympathetic activity was significantly more common in the patients. Failures were especially numerous in patients with diabetic polyneuropathy (Fagius 1982) and the lower their motor conduction velocity the

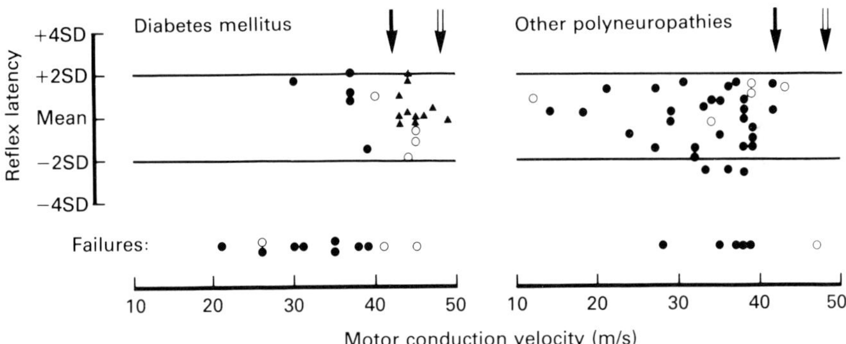

Fig. 11.1. Sympathetic reflex latencies (proportional to conduction velocity in postganglionic sympathetic fibres) expressed as standard deviations from normal and related to motor conduction velocity of the nerve recorded from in patients with polyneuropathy. The reflexes used were the arterial baroreflex (for muscle sympathetic activity) and an arousal reflex (for skin sympathetic activity). (○ and ●) patients with polyneuropathy, peroneal and median nerve, respectively, and (▲) diabetic patients without polyneuropathy, peroneal nerve. Failures, motor conduction velocity of the nerves in which no sympathetic activity could be found. Lower normal limit for motor conduction velocity in the peroneal and median nerve indicated by filled and open arrows, respectively. SD, standard deviation. (Taken with permission from Fagius (1982).)

greater the possibility of failure. The findings suggest that, in polyneuropathy, sympathetic outflow and conduction velocity are normal as long as the fibres conduct. With sympathetic involvement in the disease, postganglionic fibres probably cease to conduct one after the other until multiunit sympathetic activity can no longer be recorded (microneurographic failure). Thus, in most cases clinical symptoms arise because the number of functioning fibres is reduced, i.e. too few sympathetic action potentials reach the effector organs. It cannot be excluded, however, that in occasional cases fibres on the afferent side of various reflex arcs are also engaged in the disease. If so, symptoms due to failure of conduction in postganglionic sympathetic fibres may be mixed with symptoms due to the afferent lesion.

Peripheral afferent lesions

If peripheral nerve fibres on the afferent side of a sympathetic reflex arc are damaged, different effects will arise if the reflex is excitatory or inhibitory. The following diseases involve defects in arterial and/or cardiopulmonary baroreflexes which both have inhibitory effects on muscle sympathetic activity.

Decreased afferent activity: The Guillain–Barré syndrome

If afferent nerve traffic from arterial and cardiopulmonary baroreceptors should decrease, one would expect increases of sympathetic activity, heart rate, and blood pressure. This may occur in the Guillain–Barré syndrome, which is an acute inflammatory neuropathy causing paralysis and sensory disturbances. The severity and duration of the disease varies but most patients recover more or less completely within weeks or months. Two types of autonomic symptoms may develop, one suggestive or reduced and the other of exaggerated sympathetic activity. The first type has not been investigated microneurographically but it seems likely that the reason for the symptoms is similar to that in polyneuropathy, i.e. failure of conduction in postganglionic fibres. The other type of patient develops tachycardia, or heart arrhythmia and hypertension. Muscle sympathetic activity was recorded in three such patients both during the acute phase when they had their autonomic symptoms and twice after recovery (Fagius and Wallin 1983). The character of the activity was qualitatively similar throughout the disease, i.e. except for two brief episodes in the acute recording in one subject, pulse synchrony was preserved. Quantitatively, however, there were differences between repeated recordings. Whereas in normal subjects the incidence of sympathetic bursts is reproducible from day to day over many months, all patients had much higher numbers of sympathetic bursts during the acute phase than after recovery. This is illustrated in Fig. 11.2 in which the number of sympathetic bursts in recording one is plotted against

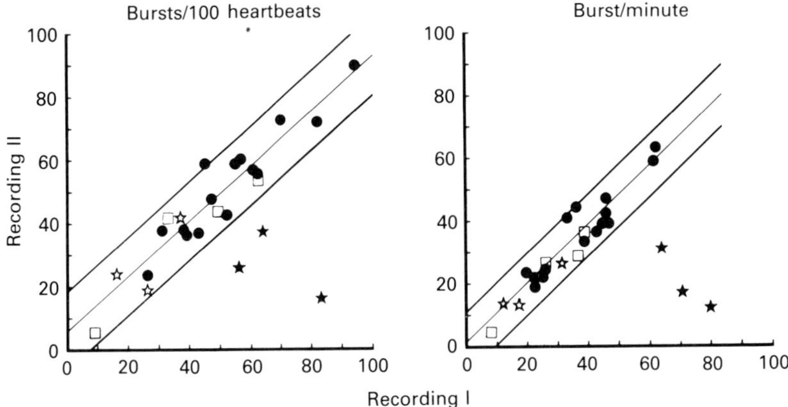

Fig. 11.2. Quantity of sympathetic bursts at two consecutive recordings plotted against each other. ★, Guillain–Barré syndrome with tachycardia and hypertension; acute and first follow-up recording. ☆, Guillain–Barré syndrome with tachycardia and hypertension; both recordings after recovery. □, Guillain–Barré syndrome without autonomic involvement. ●, Healthy subjects. Thick lines indicate 2 standard deviations (SD) from the regression line. $r=0.94$ for both graphs. Note clear aberration of the three Guillain-Barré syndrome patients with hypertension and tachycardia at the recording during their acute illness. (Taken with permission from Fagius and Wallin (1983).)

corresponding number in recording two. Normal subjects are centred around the 45° line, whereas the Guillain–Barré patients fall well outside the normal range. Note also that in the two recordings after recovery the incidence of sympathetic bursts were reproducible in the patients: in other words when the symptoms disappeared, results of repeated sympathetic recordings became normal.

The most reasonable explanation for the increase of muscle sympathetic activity is that peripheral afferent baroreceptor fibres were affected by the neuropathy and that this led to reduced inhibition of brainstem vasomotor centres. As mentioned above, afferent impulses from both arterial and cardiopulmonary baroreceptors inhibit muscle sympathetic activity but arterial baroreceptor influence is mainly dynamic, whereas influence from low-pressure receptors is more static. In view of these reflex properties, a decreased afferent inflow from cardiopulmonary receptors with preserved arterial-baroreceptor function may explain the findings in the patients.

Increased afferent activity: syncope

Increased afferent nerve traffic from baroreceptors should be expected to inhibit sympathetic activity, decrease heart rate, and lower blood pressure. Physiologically, this occurs as part of normal homeostatic blood-pressure regulation, whenever a transient blood-pressure increase in buffered by baroreceptor mechanisms. If buffering reactions become exaggerated, they will cause more pronounced blood-pressure falls and ultimately syncope. A syncopal reaction can probably be induced by increased activity both from arterial and cardiopulmonary receptors. One knows that, with a sufficiently large reduction of circulating blood volume in cats, compensatory mechanisms suddenly fail and a precipitous fall in blood pressure occurs. It has been suggested that this is a reflex effect of increased afferent activity from cardiac ventricular receptors, triggered by the mechanical stress of strong ventricular contractions around successively smaller stroke volumes. Activation of sympathetic vasodilator fibres has also been suggested to be part of the syncopal reaction.

Muscle sympathetic activity was recorded in two subjects during *vasovagal syncope* (Wallin and Sundlöf 1982) and in both cases sympathetic activity disappeared suddenly when syncope occurred. This does not exclude activation of vasodilator fibres but it shows that withdrawal of vasoconstrictor activity contributes importantly to muscle vasodilatation during syncope. The sympathetic withdrawal may well be due to influence from cardiac ventricular receptors as outlined above.

Presumably, pathological activity in afferent nerve fibres from arterial baroreceptors causes sympathetic inhibition and syncope in patients with so-called hypersensitive carotid-sinus baroreceptors but no direct evidence from human nerve recordings is available. Recently, however, a case of *glossopharyngeal neuralgia with syncope* was studied (Wallin *et al.* 1984) in whom each syncope was found to be associated with cessation of muscle sympathetic activity (Fig. 11.3). In glossopharyngeal neuralgia the patient gets short-lasting severe pain attacks in the throat evoked by

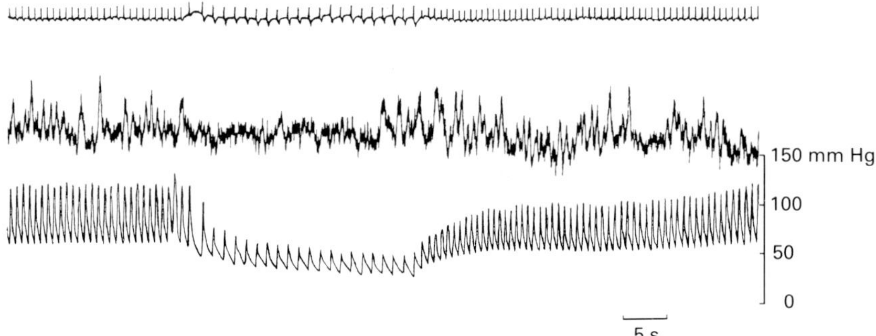

Fig. 11.3. Recordings of ECG (upper trace), muscle sympathetic activity (middle trace), and intra-arterial blood pressure (bottom trace) during attack of glossopharyngeal neuralgia associated with syncope. Sympathetic activity displayed in mean voltage neurogram (time constant 0.1 s). Horizontal bar indicates period when cardiac pacemaker was activated. (Taken with permission from Wallin *et al.* (1984).)

chewing, swallowing, coughing, etc. Occasionally, fainting is precipitated simultaneously with the pain. Figure 11.3 illustrates that a functioning cardiac pacemaker did not prevent blood-pressure fall and syncope, probably because of simultaneous inhibition of sympathetic outflow to the periphery.

How can the combination of throat pain and cardiovascular inhibition with syncope be explained? It is well known that afferent fibres from the mucous membrane of the throat and afferent fibres from carotid baroreceptors both run in the glossopharyngeal nerve. It has been suggested that there is a pathological 'synapse', a so-called ephapse, in the glossopharyngeal nerve at which pain impulses are misdirected and jump over to baroreceptor fibres. When this barrage of afferent impulses reaches brainstem vasomotor centres, there is profound inhibition and fainting occurs. Our data agree with this hypothesis.

Central lesions: spinal-cord injury

So far, sympathetic outflow in man has been recorded only after one type of central nervous lesion, namely traumatic spinal-cord injury (Wallin and Stjernberg 1984; Stjernberg *et al.* 1986). In this condition supraspinal influence can no longer reach spinal sympathetic motoneurons below the lesion which leads to loss of many sympathetic reflex mechanisms. Impaired blood-pressure and temperature regulation are the most obvious clinical consequences of such physiological defects. In addition, patients with spinal-cord lesions sometimes develop attacks of increased blood pressure together with headache, sweating, piloerection, and a general uncomfortable feeling. The symptoms may be evoked by various external stimuli, internal stimuli such as a full bladder, or they may occur spontaneously. There is good evidence that the attacks are sympathetically mediated and the term sympathetic hyperreflexia, which is sometimes used, reflects the hypothesis that the attacks are due to sympathetic overactivity. Recently, a group of patients with, in most cases, complete traumatic spinal-cord lesions (the majority at the cervical level) were studied with sympathetic recordings from nerves leaving the spinal cord caudal to the lesion. The aims were: (1) to monitor spinal sympathetic outflow as it appears without influence from baroreceptors, chemoreceptors, central thermoreceptors, etc.; (2) to search for evidence for or against the hypothesis that the attacks of increased blood pressure are due to sympathetic overactivity.

In the patients the activity was found to differ in two important respects from the normal: (1) both in skin and muscle fascicles there was much less spontaneous sympathetic activity than in intact subjects and when spontaneous activity occurred in muscle fascicles there was no cardiac rhythmicity; (2) sympathetic reflex discharges were more difficult to evoke than in normal man. A stimulus usually evoked only one sympathetic burst and prolonged discharges were very rare. These findings give no indication that excitability in decentralized spinal sympathetic motoneurons is increased; on the contrary, it seems to be lower than when supraspinal connections are intact. In addition, distension of the urinary bladder led to only weak or moderate increase of sympathetic activity; nevertheless, pronounced long-lasting blood-pressure increases occurred. Taken together the results suggest that attacks of high blood pressure in patients with spinal-cord lesions are not due to sympathetic hyperactivity; other mechanisms must contribute. The conclusion agrees with previous measurements of plasma concentrations of noradrenalin in such patients. At rest, the plasma levels are lower than normally and, although the concentration increases during blood-pressure increases, it usually does not exceed the level at rest in normal subjects.

A third difference between the patients and normal subjects was a qualitative abnormality which is of special interest with regard to the functional organization of sympathetic outflow. In intact subjects an arousal stimulus such as an electrical skin shock causes sympathetic excitation in skin nerves but no response in muscle nerves. Since in patients with spinal-cord lesions the same stimulus caused excitatory responses both in skin and muscle nerves (Fig. 11.4), the conclusion must be that in intact man there is powerful supraspinal inhibition of spinal sympathetic motoneurons to muscle. The source of inhibition may be afferent activity from arterial and/or cardiopulmonary baroreceptors since local anaesthetic block of nerve traffic from these receptors also had the effect that arousal stimuli induced sympathetic reflex responses in parallel in skin and muscle nerves (Fagius *et al.* 1985). The site of interaction between arousal and baroreceptor reflexes is not known, but the locus ceruleus is a possibility since it is known to participate in arousal reactions and also to be influenced by afferent activity from cardiopulmonary baroreceptors.

The finding that sympathetic reflex responses occurred in parallel in skin and muscle nerves means that there is vasoconstriction in a larger vascular region than normally. This may be one mechanism contributing to the episodes of hypertension in the patients. If spinal reflex responses are true mass responses, i.e. if they extend also to visceral sympathetic nerves, this factor would attain greater relative importance. Another contributing mechanism could be that sympathetic discharges induced in the patients vasoconstrictions which had significantly longer durations than in normal subjects (Wallin and Stjernberg 1984). Third, the absence of baroreflex compensation will contribute: once even minor increases of sympathetic activity are induced, the resulting pressure response will not be counteracted.

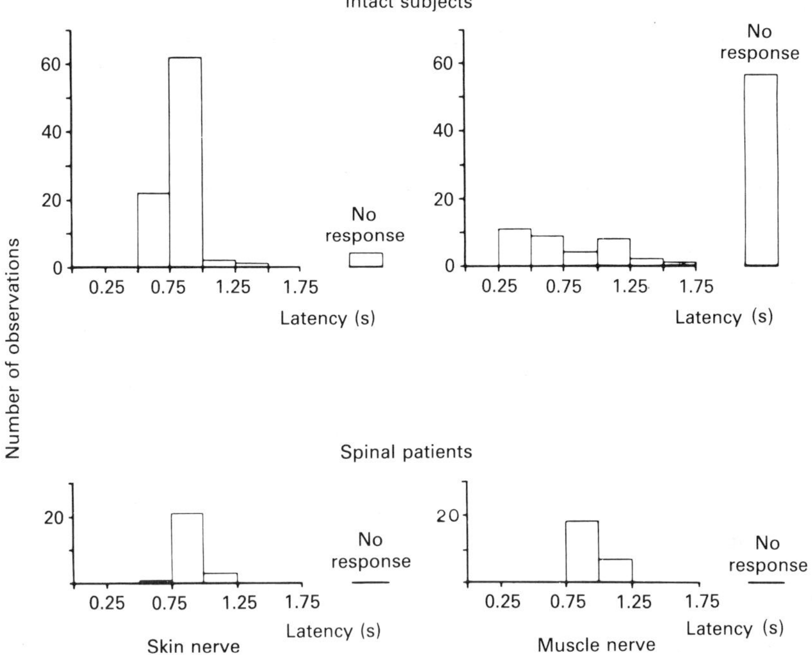

Fig. 11.4. Comparison of the occurrence of sympathetic reflex discharges evoked by electrical skin stimuli applied to the upper part of the thigh in five intact subjects and two patients with traumatic spinal-cord lesion at the C5 and T7 levels, respectively. Simultaneous recordings of sympathetic activity in skin and muscle fascicles (one in each peroneal nerve). In intact subjects 93 per cent of the stimuli evoked responses in the skin nerve after a latency of 0.5–1 second. In muscle-nerve fascicles no burst occurred after 61 per cent of the stimuli and the bursts recorded showed no systematic relationship to the stimuli. In contrast, in the patients all 26 stimuli evoked reflex discharges in both types of nerves. (Data from Stjernberg *et al.* (1986).)

CONCLUDING REMARKS

The microneurographic technique has unique advantages for studying sympathetic function in man. It is specific in the sense that postganglionic impulse traffic to well defined anatomical regions is recorded. Both resting activity and changes of activity induced by manoeuvres can be monitored and correlated to effector function, neurohormone levels, and the subject's experience. The technique also has limitations. Even if it is known to which region the impulses are conducted their exact target is undefined. At best, cutaneous vasomotor and sudomotor impulses may be distinguished in multiunit records but even with single-unit recordings in skin nerves one does not know if a vasomotor impulse reaches arterial or venous vessels, resistance vessels, or AV-shunts. The technique is not useful with abnormalities that lead to total absence of activity. In addition, if the activity is qualitatively abnormal, it may be difficult for the investigator to prove the sympathetic nature of the recorded activity.

Acknowledgements

This work was supported by the Swedish Medical Research Council, Grant No. B87-04-03546-16C. I thank Mrs Eva Guggenheim for expert secretarial help.

REFERENCES

Anderson, E. A., Wallin, B. G., and Mark, A. L. (1987). Dissociation of sympathetic nerve activity in arm and leg muscle during mental stress. *Hypertension* **9** (Suppl. III), 114–19.

Blumberg, H. and Jänig, W. (1983). Changes of reflexes in vasoconstrictor neurons supplying the cat hindlimb following chronic nerve lesions: A model for studying mechanisms of reflex sympathetic dystrophy? *J. auton. nerv. Syst.* **7**, 399–411.

Blumberg, H. and Wallin, B. G. (1987). Direct evidence of neurally mediated vasodilatation in hairy skin of the human foot. *J. Physiol., London* **382**, 105–21.

Eckberg, D. L., Andersson, O. K., Hedner, T., Rea, R. F., and Wallin, B. G. (1986). Baroreflex control of muscle sympathetic activity and plasma noradrenaline in man. *J. Hypertension* **4** (Suppl. 6), 5718–19.

Eckberg, D. L., Nerhed, C., and Wallin, B. G. (1985). Respiratory modulation of muscle sympathetic and vagal cardiac outflow in man. *J. Physiol., London* **365**, 181–96.

Elam, M. and Wallin, B. G. (1987). Skin blood flow responses to mental stress in man depend on body temperature. *Acta physiol. scand.* **129**, 429–31.

Fagius, J. (1982). Microneurographic findings in diabetic polyneuropathy with special reference to sympathetic nerve activity. *Diabetologia* **23**, 415–20.

Fagius, J., Niklasson, F., and Berne, C. (1986). Sympathetic outflow in human muscle nerves increases during hypoglycemia. *Diabetes* **35**, 1124–9.

Fagius, J. and Sundlöf, G. (1986). The diving response in man: Effects on sympathetic activity in muscle and skin nerve fascicles. *J. Physiol., London* **377**, 429–43.

Fagius, J. and Wallin B. G. (1980). Sympathetic reflex latencies and conduction velocities in patients with polyneuropathy. *J. neurol. Sci.* **47**, 449–61.

Fagius, J. and Wallin B. G. (1983). Microneurographic evidence of excessive sympathetic outflow in the Guillain–Barré syndrome. *Brain* **106**, 589–600.

Fagius, J., Wallin, B. G., Sundlöf, G., Nerhed, C., and Englesson, S. (1985). Sympathetic outflow in man after anaesthesia of the glossopharyngeal and vagus nerves. *Brain* **108**, 335–50.

Leimbach, W. N., Wallin, B. G., Victor, R. G., Aylward, P. E., Sundlöf, G., and Mark, A. L. (1986). Direct evidence from intraneural recordings for increased central sympathetic outflow in patients with heart failure. *Circulation* **73**, 913–19.

Mark, A. L., Victor, R. G., Nerhed, C., and Wallin, B. G. (1985). Microneurographic studies of the mechanisms of sympathetic nerve responses to static exercise in humans. *Circulation Res.* **57**, 461–9.

Stjernberg, L., Blumberg, H., and Wallin, B. G. (1986). Sympathetic activity in man after spinal cord injury. Outflow to muscle below the lesion. *Brain* **109**, 695–715.

Vallbo, Å, B., Hagbarth, K.-E., Torebjörk, H. E., and Wallin, B. G. (1979). Somatosensory, proprioceptive and sympathetic activity in human peripheral nerves. *Physiol. Rev.* **59**, 919–57.

Victor, R. G., Leimbach, W. N., Seals, D. R., Wallin, B. G., and Mark, A. L. (1987). Effects of the cold pressor test on muscle sympathetic nerve activity in humans. *Hypertension* **9**, 429–36.

Wallin, B. G., Blumberg, H., and Hynninen, P. (1983). Intraneural stimulation as a method to study sympathetic function in the human skin. *Neurosci. Lett.* **36**, 189–94.

Wallin, B. G. and Fagius, J. (1986). The sympathetic nervous system in man—aspects derived from microelectrode recordings. *Trends Neurosci.* **9**, 63–7.

Wallin, B. G., Mörlin, C., and Hjemdahl, P. (1987). Muscle sympathetic activity and venuous plasma noradrenaline concentrations during static exercise in normotensive and hypertensive subjects. *Acta physiol. scand.* **129**, 489–97.

Wallin, B. G. and Stjernberg, L. (1984). Sympathetic activity in man after spinal cord injury. Outflow to skin below the lesion. *Brain* **107**, 183–98.

Wallin, B. G. and Sundlöf, G. (1982). Sympathetic outflow to muscles during vasovagal syncope. *J. auton. nerv. Syst.* **6**, 373–9.

Wallin, B. G., Westerberg, C.-E., and Sundlöf, G. (1984). Syncope induced by glossopharyngeal neuralgia: sympathetic outflow to muscle. *Neurology* **24**, 522–4.

12. Neural control of the urinary bladder and sexual organs: experimental studies in animals

William C. de Groat and William D. Steers

INTRODUCTION

Various functions of the urogenital tract are controlled by extrinsic nervous pathways which involve neurons in the brain, spinal cord, and peripheral ganglia. Many of these functions are complex, requiring the participation of somatic as well as autonomic efferent mechanisms and the integration of neural and endocrine systems. Due to the complexities of the neurohumoral factors regulating the urogenital organs, the activities of these organs are sensitive to a wide variety of injuries, diseases, and chemicals which affect the nervous system. Thus, neurologic mechanisms are an important consideration in the diagnosis and treatment of disorders of the urogenital tract.

This chapter will review experimental studies in animals which have provided insights into the anatomical organization and the transmitters involved in the neural control of urogenital function.

INNERVATION OF THE LOWER URINARY TRACT

The storage and periodic elimination of urine is dependent upon the activity of two functional units in the lower urinary tract: (1) a reservoir (the urinary bladder); and (2) an outlet consisting of bladder neck, urethra, and striated muscles of the urethral sphincter. These structures are in turn controlled by three sets of peripheral nerves: sacral parasympathetic (pelvic nerves); thoracolumbar sympathetic (hypogastric nerves and sympathetic chain); and sacral somatic nerves (pudendal nerves) (Fig. 12.1) (Kuru 1965; de Groat and Kawatani 1985).

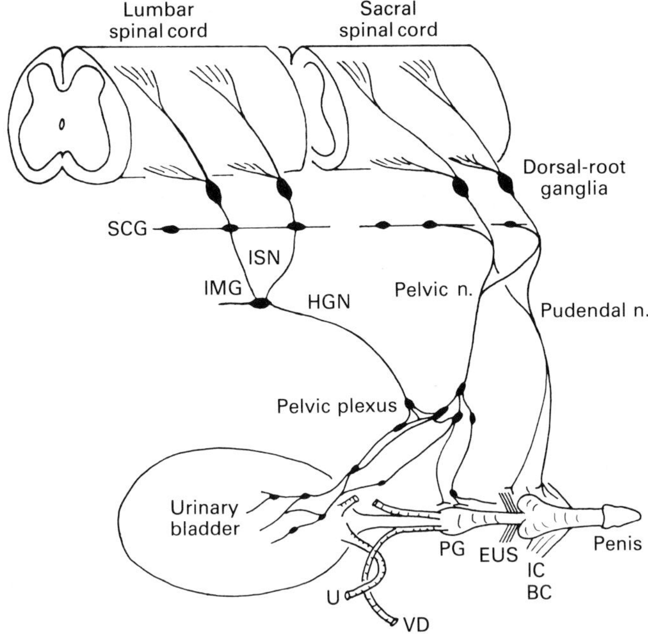

Fig. 12.1. Diagram showing the sympathetic, parasympathetic, and somatic innervation of the urogenital tract of the male cat. Sympathetic preganglionic pathways emerge from the lumbar spinal cord and pass to the sympathetic-chain ganglia (SCG) and then via the inferior splanchnic nerves (ISN) to the inferior mesenteric ganglia (IMG). Preganglionic and postganglionic sympathetic axons then travel in the hypogastric nerve (HGN) to the pelvic plexus and the urogenital organs. Parasympathetic preganglionic axons which originate in the sacral spinal cord pass in the pelvic nerve to ganglion cells in the pelvic plexus and to distal ganglia in the organs. Sacral somatic pathways are contained in the pudendal nerve, which provides an innervation to the penis, the ischiocavernosus (IC), bulbocavernosus (BC), and external urethral sphincter (EUS) muscles. The pudendal and pelvic nerves also receive postganglionic axons from the caudal sympathetic-chain ganglia. These three sets of nerves contain afferent axons from the lumbosacral dorsal-root ganglia. U, ureter; PG, prostate gland; VD, vas deferens.

Sacral parasympathetic pathways

The sacral parasympathetic outflow provides the major excitatory input to the urinary bladder. Cholinergic preganglionic neurons located in the intermediolateral region of the sacral spinal cord send axons via the pelvic nerves to ganglion cells in the pelvic plexus (inferior hypogastric plexus) and in the wall of the bladder. The ganglion cells in turn excite bladder smooth muscle via the release of cholinergic (acetylcholine) and, in some species, non-cholinergic–non-adrenergic transmitters. Cholinergic excitatory transmission is mediated by muscarinic receptors, which are blocked by atropine, whereas non-cholinergic transmission is thought to be mediated by the purinergic transmitter, adenosine

Table 12.1. Receptors for putative transmitters in the lower urinary tract

Tissue	*Cholinergic*	*Adrenergic*	*Other*
Bladder body	+ (M_2)	− (β_2)	+ Purinergic (P_2) − VIP + Substance P
Bladder base	+ (M_2)	+ (α_2)	0 Purinergic − VIP
Ganglia	+ (N) + (M_1)	− (α_2) + (β)	− Encephalinergic (δ) − Purinergic (P_1) + Substance P
Urethra	+ (M)	+ (α_1) ± (α_2) − (β_2)	± Purinergic − VIP + Neuropeptide Y
Sphincter striated muscle	+ (N)		

Letters in parentheses indicate receptor type, e.g. M (muscarinic) and N (nicotinic). +, −, and 0 indicate excitatory, inhibitory, and weak or no effects, respectively.

triphosphate (ATP), acting on P_2 purinergic receptors (Burnstock 1986) (Table 12.1).

A small percentage (10–15 per cent) of cholinergic bladder ganglion cells also contain vasoactive intestinal polypeptide (VIP) (Lundberg *et al.* 1980). This substance is released into the venous effluent from the bladder by electrical stimulation of the pelvic nerves and, when administered exogenously, depresses the activity of bladder smooth muscle. Thus, it has been speculated that VIP might be co-released with acetylcholine from cholinergic nerves and function as an inhibitory transmitter in the bladder.

Co-localization of excitatory and inhibitory substances in the same neuron also occurs in the parasympathetic preganglionic pathways to the urinary bladder of the cat. Cholinergic preganglionic neurons exhibit leucine encephalin immunoreactivity (L-ENK-IR) and L-ENK-IR is present in preganglionic terminals in bladder ganglia (de Groat and Kawatani 1985; de Groat *et al.* 1986). Various pharmacological experiments indicated that endogenous L-ENK is released by stimulation of preganglionic nerves and can act presynaptically on δ opiate receptors to inhibit cholinergic transmission in bladder ganglia. The inhibition is blocked by the administration of an opiate antagonist, naloxone. Based on these findings it has been proposed that encephalins are co-released with acetylcholine and may be involved in an autoinhibitory mechanism in bladder ganglia.

Thoracolumbar sympathetic pathways

Recent anatomical and physiological studies have shown that sympathetic pathways to the lower urinary tract of the cat originate in the lumbosacral sympathetic-chain ganglia as well as in the prevertebral ganglia (inferior mesenteric ganglia) (de Groat and Kawatani 1985). Input from the sacral-chain ganglia passes to the bladder via the pelvic nerves, whereas fibres from the upper lumbar and inferior mesenteric ganglia travel in the hypogastric nerves. Sympathetic efferent pathways in the hypogastric and pelvic nerves in the cat elicit similar effects in the bladder consisting of: (1) inhibition of detrusor muscle via β-adrenergic receptors; (2) excitation of the bladder base and urethra via α-receptors; and (3) inhibition and facilitation in bladder parasympathetic ganglia via α- and β-receptors, respectively (Table 12.1) (de Groat and Booth 1980*a*).

Somatic efferent pathways

The efferent innervation of the periurethral and external urethral striated muscles in various species originates from cells in a circumscribed region of the lateral ventral horn which is termed Onuf's nucleus or the sphincter motor nucleus. These cells send their axons into the pudendal nerve. The sphincter motor nucleus exhibits a number of morphological and histochemical characteristics which distinguishes it from other motor nuclei controlling the limb muscles. In regard to dendritic patterns and spectrum of peptidergic inputs, the sphincter motor nucleus closely resembles the sacral autonomic nucleus with which it has a close functional relationship (de Groat *et al.* 1986).

Afferent pathways

Afferent axons innervating the lower urinary tract are present in the three sets of nerves (de Groat 1986; Jänig and Morrisson 1986). The most important afferents for initiating micturition are those passing in the pelvic nerve to the sacral spinal cord (Kuru 1965). In the cat these afferents are small Aδ and C fibres which convey impulses from tension receptors in the bladder wall. Electrophysiological studies show that bladder afferents in the pelvic nerve respond in a graded manner to passive distension as well as active contraction of the bladder (Jänig and Morrisson 1986). The intravesical pressure thresholds for activation of these afferents in the cat range from 5 to 15 mm Hg which is consistent with pressures at which humans report the first sensation of filling during cystometry. High-threshold afferents have not been detected. Thus, noxious events in the bladder may be encoded by different patterns or high rates of firing in afferents which also transmit non-noxious information from the bladder.

Mechanoreceptor afferents from the bladder and urethra have also been identified in the sympathetic nerves (hypogastric and inferior splanchnic) passing to the lumbar spinal cord (Jänig and Morrisson

1986). These afferent pathways consist of myelinated as well as unmyelinated axons and respond in a similar manner as the afferents in the pelvic nerve. The function of sympathetic nerve afferents in the control of micturition is uncertain.

Afferent pathways from the urethra, which transmit the sensations of temperature, pain, and passage of urine, as well as afferents from the striated sphincter muscles travel in the pudendal nerve to the sacral spinal cord. These afferents are known to have a modulatory influence on the micturition reflex in the cat.

The central projections of pelvic, pudendal, and hypogastric nerve afferents have been studied in several species including the cat, rat, and monkey (de Groat *et al.* 1986; de Groat 1986). In the cat the general population of visceral afferents in the pelvic nerve (Fig. 12.2), including afferents from the bladder (Fig. 12.3(a)) project to restricted regions of the spinal cord. The afferent axons enter Lissauer's tract and then send collaterals through the marginal zone laterally and medially around the dorsal horn. Afferent terminals are heavily concentrated in lamina I particularly on the lateral side of the dorsal horn (termed the lateral collateral pathway, LCP) and in lateral laminae V–VII in the area of the sacral parasympathetic nucleus (SPN) as well as in the dorsal commissure. At upper lumbar levels hypogastric nerve afferents also terminate primarily in lateral laminae I and V of the dorsal horn.

Pudendal afferent pathways from internal tissues such as the urethra and urethral sphincters exhibit a similar pattern of termination in the sacral spinal cord (Fig. 12.3(b)), whereas pudendal afferent pathways from cutaneous receptors have a prominent projection to the deeper layers of the dorsal horn and the dorsal commissure. The overlap of bladder and urethral afferents in the LCP and dorsal commissure indicates that this region is likely to be an important site of viscerosomatic integration and to be involved in co-ordinating bladder and sphincter activity during micturition.

Analysis of neurotransmitter mechanisms in afferent pathways to the lower urinary tract has focused primarily on neuropeptides, since a number of these substances, including VIP, substance P, cholecystokinin, calcitonin gene-related peptide (CGRP), and dynorphins are present in afferent projections to the lumbosacral spinal cord (de Groat 1987). The distribution of certain peptides such as VIP (Fig. 12.3(d)), substance P, and dynorphin are very similar to the distribution of bladder afferents in the LCP (Fig. 12.3(a)). This has been noted in various species including man (Fig. 12.3(e)). The use of immunocytochemical techniques in combination with axonal tracing techniques to label bladder afferent neurons in the dorsal-root ganglia shows that a large percentage of these cells exhibit peptide immunoreactivity: VIP (24 per cent), substance P (22 per cent), and leucine encephalin (5 per cent) being the most

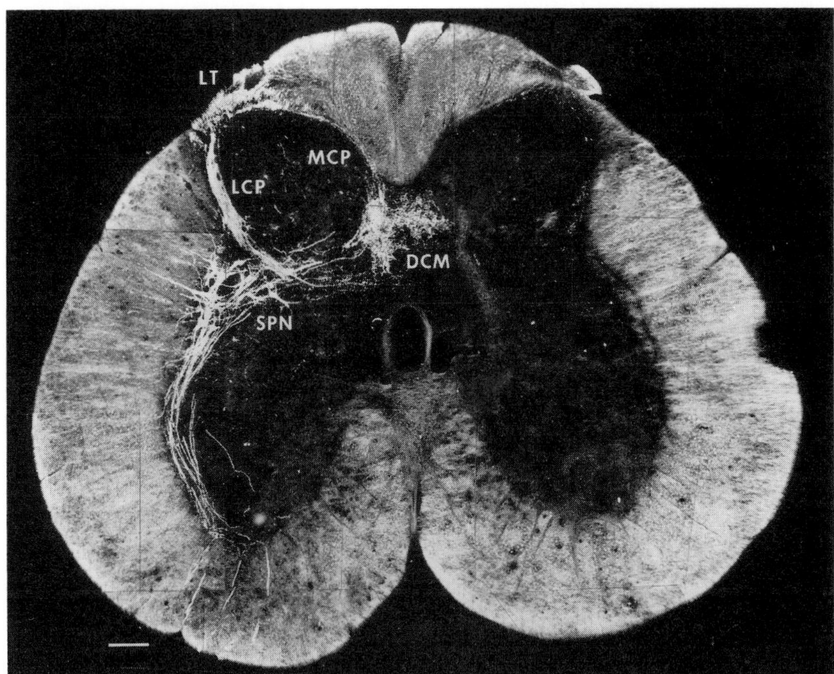

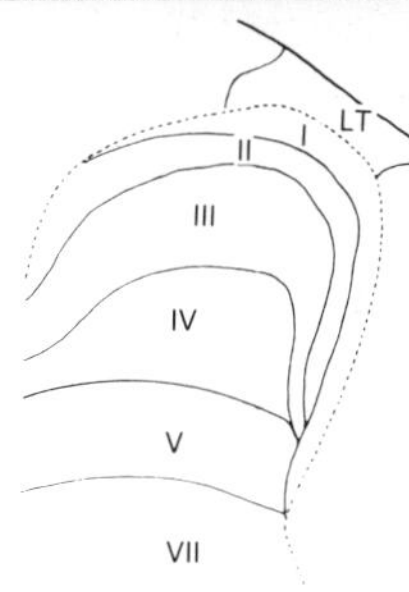

Fig. 12.2. Transverse section of S2 spinal cord showing labelling of primary afferents and preganglionic neurons after application of horseradish peroxidase (HRP) to the left pelvic nerve in the cat. Pelvic afferents enter Lissauer's tract (LT). Afferent collaterals enter lamina I and extend laterally in a large bundle, the lateral collateral pathway (LCP), into the area of the sacral parasympathetic nucleus (SPN). Collaterals also extend medially in a smaller group, the medial collaterial pathway (MCP), into the dorsal grey commissure (DCM), where they expand into a large terminal field ipsilaterally and contralaterally. Small numbers of afferents are also present in contralateral laminae I and V. This photomicrograph was made using darkfield illumination with polarized light. Bar represents 200 μm. Inset shows the laminar organization of the sacral dorsal horn according to Rexed. (From Morgan *et al.* (1981).)

common peptides in the cat (Fig. 12.3(c)). Substance P, VIP, and CGRP are also present in afferents from the rat urinary tract (Maggi and Meli 1986; de Groat 1987).

The large percentage of cells containing peptides suggests that some peptides may coexist in the same cells. This has been confirmed for bladder afferent cells using double-colour immunocytochemistry (Fig. 12.3(f)). For example, 50–60 per cent of VIP- or leucine encephalin-containing bladder afferent neurons exhibit substance P immunoreactivity. VIP and leucine encephalin as well as substance P and CGRP

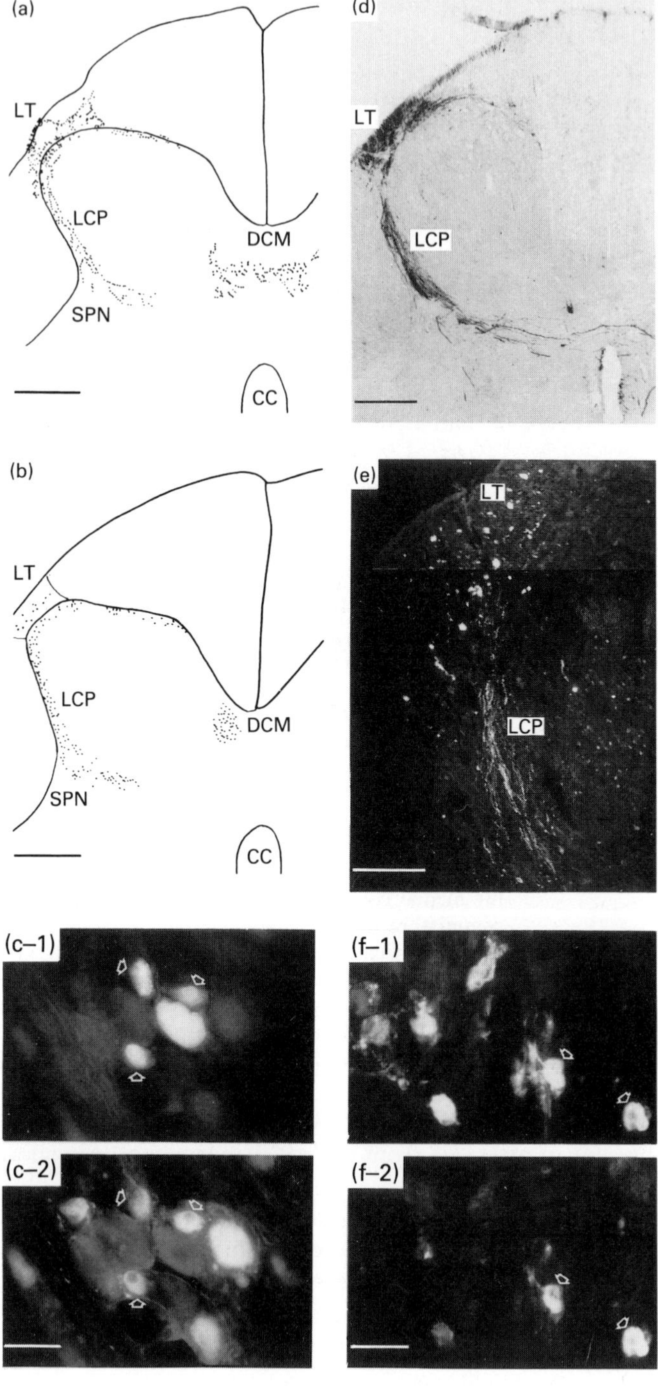
(a)
LT
LCP
DCM
SPN
CC
(d)
LT
LCP
(b)
LT
LCP
DCM
SPN
CC
(e)
LT
LCP
(c–1)
(f–1)
(c–2)
(f–2)

are also co-localized in a large percentage of cells (de Groat *et al.* 1986; de Groat 1987). A similar distribution of neuropeptides occurs in hypogastric afferent neurons in the lumbar dorsal-root ganglia of the cat, whereas pudendal-nerve afferent neurons in the sacral dorsal-root ganglia have a considerably lower percentage of certain peptidergic cells (e.g. VIP and encephalin).

The physiological significance of peptides and peptide-co-localization in urinary tract afferents is attracting considerable attention. In the rat, pharmacological studies with capsaicin indicate that peptides are important in the afferent limb of the micturition reflex (Maggi and Meli 1986; de Groat 1987). Capsaicin is an agent which in small doses acts on unmyelinated afferents to release substance P and related peptides, whereas in large doses it depletes peptide stores and destroys peptidergic afferents. The local administration of capsaicin to the urinary bladder releases substance P from afferent nerves and produces an initial stimulation of the activity of the vesical smooth muscle and a facilitation of the micturition reflex (Maggi and Meli 1986). In large doses administered systemically to neonatal rats or to adult rats, capsaicin depresses the micturition reflex. These findings raise the possibility that substance P or a related peptide may be an excitatory transmitter in the afferent pathway from the bladder. It has also been speculated that other

---

Fig. 12.3. Afferent pathways to the sacral spinal cord. (a) Camera lucida drawing of the central projections of bladder afferents in the sacral (S_2) dorsal horn (DH) of the cat. CC, central canal. Afferent terminals were labelled by transganglionic transport of HRP from nerves on the surface of the bladder. Labelled axons were present in Lissauer's tract (LT), the lateral collateral pathway (LCP), the sacral parasympathetic nucleus (SPN), and the dorsal commissure (DCM). (b) Afferent projections in the S_2 dorsal horn of the cat labelled by HRP injected into the external urethral sphincter. (c) Two photomicrographs of the same section through the S_2 dorsal-root ganglion showing bladder afferent cells (c-1) labelled by fast blue injected into the bladder wall. Several of these labelled cells (arrows in (c-1) and (c-2)) contain VIP-immunoreactivity (VIP-IR). Dye-labelled cells were blue when visualized with UV light at 340–80 nm excitation wavelength and VIP cells were green when visualized with UV light at 430–80 nm wavelength. (d) The distribution of VIP-IR in LT and LCP of the S_2 segment of the cat spinal cord. (e) VIP-IR in the sacral dorsal horn of the S_3 segment of the human spinal cord. Large bundles of VIP axons are present in LT and smaller numbers of axons are present in lamina I on the lateral edge of the dorsal horn. (f) Co-localization of substance P-IR and VIP-IR in sacral (S_2) dorsal root ganglion cells of the cat. Substance P-IR (f-1) stained with TRITC (red colour, at 530–60 nm excitation wavelength) and in (f-2) the same section showing VIP-IR in two of the same ganglion cells (arrows) stained with FITC (green colour at 430–80 nm excitation wavelength). VIP was detected with rabbit polyclonal antisera, whereas substance P was detected by rat monoclonal antisera. Calibration represents 250 m in (a) and (b), 50 m in (c), 300 m in (d), 220 m in (e), and 60 m in (f). (From de Groat *et al.* (1986).)

peptides (e.g. encephalins) co-localized with substance P may be inhibitory modulators in the afferent pathways (de Groat *et al.* 1986; de Groat 1987).

CENTRAL REFLEX PATHWAYS TO THE LOWER URINARY TRACT

The central pathways controlling lower urinary tract function have been examined in various species including the cat, dog, and rat (Kuru 1965; de Groat 1975; Satoh *et al.* 1978; McMahon and Spillane 1982; de Groat and Kawatani 1985; Thor *et al.* 1986). However, electrophysiological data have been obtained primarily in the cat. The neural mechanisms regulating micturition seem to be organized as simple on–off switching circuits, which maintain a reciprocal relationship between the bladder and the urethral outlet. During urine storage, a low level of afferent activity in the pelvic nerve and possibly also in proprioceptive afferents in the pudendal nerve initiates reflex efferent firing in sympathetic and somatic pathways to the bladder base and urethra, while the parasympathetic efferent outflow to the bladder body is quiescent (Table 12.2). During micturition a high level of vesical afferent activity reverses the pattern of efferent outflow, producing firing in the parasympathetic pathways and inhibition of the sympathetic and somatic pathways.

These basic reflex mechanisms require the integrative action of neuronal populations at various levels of the neuraxis (Fig. 12.4). Certain reflexes, for example, those mediating the excitatory outflow to the sphincters and the sympathetic inhibitory outflow to the bladder, are organized at the spinal level (Fig. 12.5), whereas the parasympathetic outflow to the detrusor has a more complicated central organization (Fig. 12.4).

Table 12.2. Reflexes to the lower urinary tract

Afferent pathway	*Efferent pathway*	*Central pathway*
Urine storage		
Low-level vesical afferent activity (pelvic nerve)	External sphincter contraction (somatic nerves) Internal sphincter contraction (sympathetic nerves) Detrusor inhibition (sympathetic nerves) Ganglionic inhibition (sympathetic nerves) Sacral parasympathetic outflow inactive	Spinal reflexes
Micturition		
High-level vesical afferent activity (pelvic nerve)	Inhibition of external sphincter activity Inhibition of sympathetic outflow Activation of parasympathetic outflow	Spinobulbospinal reflexes

From de Groat and Booth (1984).

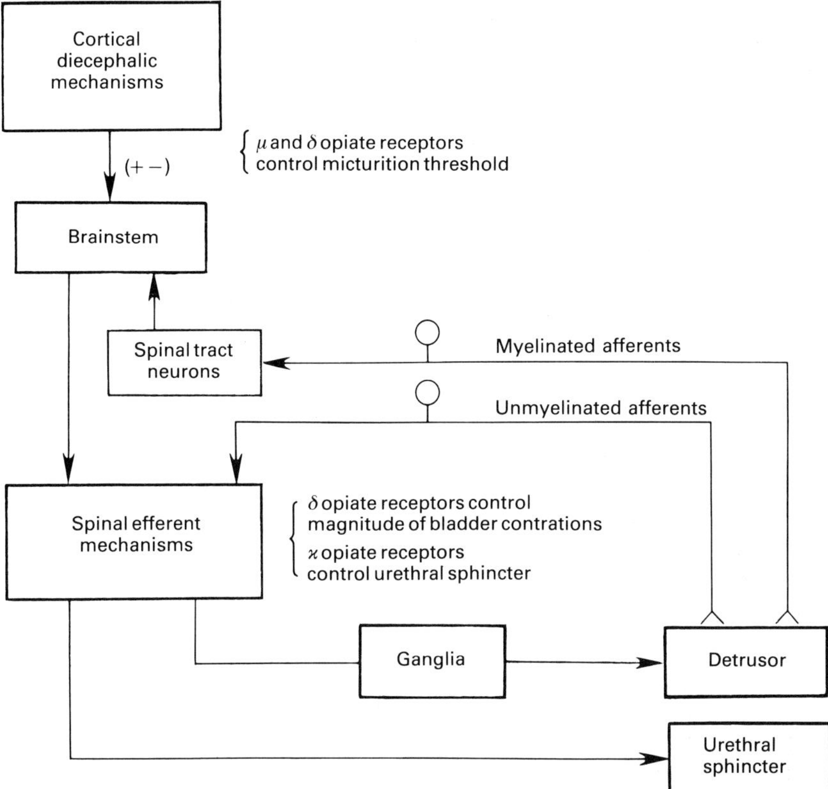

Fig. 12.4. Diagram of the central reflex pathways and encephalinergic mechanisms which regulate micturition in the cat. In animals with intact neuraxis, micturition is initiated by a supraspinal reflex pathway passing through a centre in the brainstem. The pathway is triggered by myelinated afferents (A-δ) connected to tension receptors in the bladder wall. In chronic spinal animals, connections between the brainstem and the sacral spinal cord are interrupted and micturition is initially blocked. However, in chronic spinal animals a spinal reflex mechanism emerges which is triggered by unmyelinated (C-fibre) vesical afferents. The C-fibre reflex pathway is usually weak or undetectable in animals with an intact nervous system. Pharmacological studies have shown that in the brain μ or δ opiate receptors control micturition threshold and bladder capacity, whereas in the spinal cord opiate receptors control the magnitude of bladder contractions. κ opiate receptors mediate a depression of the pudendal motor outflow to the external urethral spincter.

Parasympathetic pathways

Early studies in cats using brain-lesioning techniques revealed that neurons in the rostral brainstem at the level of the inferior colliculus had an essential role in the control of micturition (Kuru 1965). Removal of the brain areas above the inferior colliculus by intercollicular decerebration did not interfere with micturition. However, transection of the

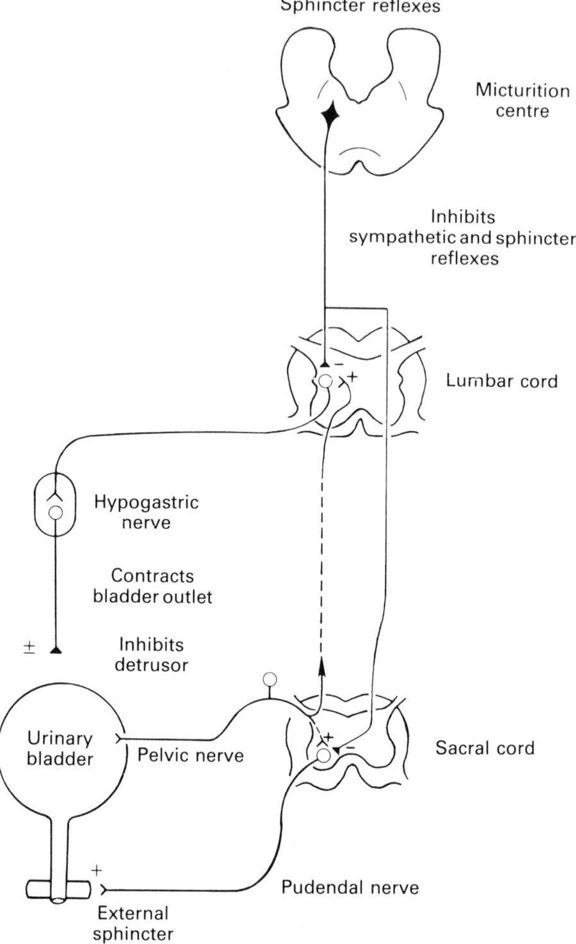

Fig. 12.5. Diagram showing detrusor–sphincter reflexes. During the storage of urine, distention of the bladder produces low-level vesical afferent firing, which in turn stimulates (1) the sympathetic outflow to the bladder outlet (base and urethra) and (2) pudendal outflow to the external urethral sphincter. These responses occur by spinal reflex pathways and represent 'guarding reflexes', which promote continence. Sympathetic firing also inhibits detrusor muscle and transmission in bladder ganglia. At the initiation of micturition, intense vesical afferent activity activates the brainstem micturition centre, which inhibits the spinal guarding reflexes.

neuraxis at any point below the colliculi abolished micturition. Bilateral lesions in the rostral pons in the region of the locus ceruleus also abolished micturition, whereas electrical stimulation at this site triggered bladder contractions and micturition (Kuru 1965; de Groat 1975; Satoh *et al.* 1978; McMahon and Spillane 1982). These observations led to the concept of a spinobulbospinal micturition-reflex pathway that passes through a centre in the pons. This pathway is in turn modulated by inhibitory and excitatory influences from areas of the brain rostral to the pons (e.g. diencephalon and cerebral cortex) (Fig. 12.4).

More recent electrophysiological and neuroanatomical studies in cats and rats provide further support for a spinobulbospinal micturition reflex, but demonstrate a spinal reflex as well (de Groat *et al.* 1986). In cats with an intact neuraxis the spinobulbospinal reflex pathway is the most prominent. Recordings from postganglionic nerves on the surface of the urinary bladder show that reflex firing occurs with a long latency (100 ms) following stimulation of myelinated (Aδ) vesical afferents in the pelvic nerve. Afferent stimulation also evokes negative field potentials in the rostral pons at latencies of 30–40 ms, whereas stimulation in the pons evokes firing on vesical postganglionic neurons at latencies of 70–85 ms. Thus, the sum of the latencies for the spinobulbar and bulbospinal components of the reflex pathway approximates the latency for the entire reflex. The spinobulbospinal reflex is present in decerebrate animals but is absent in acute or chronic spinal animals.

A second reflex, which is less prominent and present in only 60 per cent of cats with an intact neuraxis occurs with a considerably longer latency (180–200 ms) following stimulation of vesical afferents and only at intensities of stimulation that are sufficient to activate unmyelinated (C-fibre) afferents (de Groat *et al.* 1986; Thor *et al.* 1986). The reflex is abolished in acute spinal cats, but reappears in chronic spinal animals with the development of automatic micturition. Thus two distinct cental pathways (supraspinal and spinal) utilizing different peripheral afferent limbs (A and C fibre) exist for the mediation of detrusor to detrusor reflexes (Fig. 12.4). The supraspinal pathway seems to have the major role in the initiation of bladder contractions in animals with an intact neuraxis. While the function of the spinal reflex pathway in normal animals is uncertain, it is essential for the development of automatic micturition in paraplegic animals. Spinobulbospinal and spinal micturition reflexes have also been demonstrated in the rat. However, in this species both reflex pathways appear to utilize an afferent limb consisting of myelinated fibres.

Axonal tracing studies provide insights into the neural connections between the pontine micturition centre and the sacral spinal cord (Holstege *et al.* 1986). Neurons in the dorsomedial pons send direct projections to the sacral parasympathetic nucleus and to the lateral edge of the sacral dorsal horn (the LCP) which contains dendritic projections from the sacral preganglionic neurons and afferent inputs from the bladder. Thus, the sites of termination of descending projections from the pontine micturition centre are optimally located to regulate reflex mechanisms at the spinal level. A second area in the dorsolateral pons sends projections to the sphincter motor nucleus in the sacral spinal cord. Electric stimulation of this dorsolateral area elicits sphincter contractions, whereas stimulation of the medial pontine area inhibits sphincter activity and elicits bladder contractions.

The pons receives ascending projections from spinal-tract neurons located in lateral laminae I, V, and VII of the sacral cord. These spinal-tract neurons are located at sites receiving dense projections from bladder afferent pathways (Fig. 12.3(a)) and respond to distension or contraction of the bladder. Thus, a considerable body of neuro-anatomical and electrophysiological data support the concept of a spino-bulbospinal micturition reflex pathway as outlined in Fig. 12.4.

Sympathetic pathways

The integrity of the sympathetic input to the lower urinary tract is not essential for the performance of micturition. However, physiologic experiments in cats and rats indicate that, during bladder filling, the sympathetic system does provide a tonic inhibitory input to the bladder as well as an excitatory input to the urethra (de Groat and Kawatani 1985). This sympathetic input is physiologically significant since surgical interruption or pharmacologic blockade of the sympathetic innervation can reduce urethral outflow resistance, reduce bladder capacity, and increase the frequency and amplitude of bladder contractions recorded under constant volume conditions.

Sympathetic reflex activity is elicited by a sacrolumbar intersegmental spinal reflex pathway which is triggered by vesical afferent activity in the pelvic nerves (Fig. 12.5) (de Groat 1975). The reflex pathway is inhibited when bladder pressure is raised to the threshold for producing micturition. This inhibitory response is abolished by transection of the spinal cord at the lower thoracic level, indicating that it originates at a supraspinal site, possibly the pontine micturition centre. Thus, vesico-sympathetic reflexes represent a negative feedback mechanism whereby an increase in bladder pressure tends to increase inhibitory input to vesical ganglia and smooth muscle, thus allowing the bladder to accommodate large volumes (Fig. 12.5). Increased sympathetic excitatory input to the bladder base and urethra would complement these mechanisms by increasing outflow resistance. During micturition these reflexes are suppressed by supraspinal controls thereby facilitating bladder emptying.

Somatic pathways to the urethral sphincter

Motoneurons innervating the striated muscles of the urethral sphincter exhibit a tonic discharge which increases during bladder filling. This activity is mediated in part by low-level afferent input from the bladder.

During micturition the firing of sphincter motoneurons is inhibited (Kuru 1965). This inhibition is dependent in part on supraspinal mechanisms, since it is not as prominent in chronic spinal animals. Electrical stimulation of the pontine micturition centre induces sphincter relaxation suggesting that bulbospinal pathways from the pons may be responsible for maintaining the normal reciprocal relationship between bladder and sphincter.

NEUROTRANSMITTERS IN MICTURITION REFLEX PATHWAYS

Encephalins

Immunocytochemical and pharmacological experiments have focused attention on the role of central encephalinergic inhibitory mechanisms in the regulation of micturition. Encephalinergic varicosities are very prominent in the region of the sacral parasympathetic nucleus and the sphincter motor nucleus in the sacral spinal cord as well as in the region of the pontine micturition centre of various species.

Administration of exogenous encephalins or opiate drugs to the brain by intracerebroventricular injection or to sacral spinal cord by intrathecal injection in the cat and rat depresses micturition and sphincter reflexes (de Groat *et al.* 1986; Maggi and Meli 1986). Three types of opiate receptors mediate these depressant effects (μ, δ, and κ). In the cat spinal cord δ opiate receptors are primarily responsible for inhibition of micturition reflex, whereas both μ and δ opiate receptors mediate inhibition in the cat brain (Fig. 12.4). Sphincter reflexes are resistant to the actions of the μ and δ opiate agonists administered to the spinal cord, but are inhibited by the intrathecal administration of κ-receptor agonists. In the rat both μ- and δ-receptors are involved in the brain and spinal cord in the inhibition of bladder reflexes. The inhibitory effects of exogenous encephalins and opiate drugs are reversed by the systemic, intrathecal, or intracerebroventricular administration of the opiate antagonist, naloxone.

Intrathecal or epidural administration of various opiate drugs with actions on μ-receptors (e.g. morphine, methadone, fentanyl, and meperidine) also depress bladder function in humans, however the epidural administration of pentazocine which is a κ-receptor agonist produces analgesia but does elicit urinary retention (de Groat and Kawatani 1986). This is consistent with the results in animals indicating that κ-receptors are not involved in opioid depression of bladder reflexes.

The role of endogenous opioid peptides in the control of micturition in animals has been examined by administering drugs which enhance or antagonize the actions of opioid peptides. Thiorphan, a substance that inhibits the metabolism of encephalins, depresses bladder reflexes in the cat following intrathecal or intracerebroventricular injection. The inhibitory effect of thiorphan is antagonized by naloxone.

Naloxone also has direct effects on micturition in the absence of thiorphan indicating that endogenous opioid peptides have a role in controlling micturition (de Groat *et al.* 1986; Maggi and Meli 1986). The administration of naloxone systemically, intrathecally, intracerebroventricularly, or by microinjection into the pontine micturition centre facilitates the micturition reflex. In low doses naloxone reduces the bladder volume necessary to evoke micturition. Naloxone also increases the frequency and magnitude of low-amplitude pressure waves on the tonus limb of the cystometrogram in chloralose-anaesthetized cats. These pressure waves are similar to uninhibited contractions seen in patients with hyperactive bladder reflexes. Injections of small doses of naloxone into the pontine micturition centre of decerebrate cats also lowers the micturition threshold. In high doses the drug produces sustained contractions of the bladder and firing on bladder postganglionic nerves. The effect is noted in anaesthetized animals with an intact neuraxis or in decerebrate unanaesthetized animals, but not in acute spinal animals where the spinobulbospinal micturition reflex pathway is interrupted.

However, in chronic spinal (paraplegic) cats and rats which exhibit automatic micturition, naloxone administered systemically or injected intrathecally induces rhythmic bladder contractions, spontaneous urination, and facilitates the micturition reflex elicited by cutaneous stimulation in the lumbosacral dermatomes (Thor *et al.* 1986; de Groat *et al.* 1986). These data indicate that the spinal pathways involved in micturition are also under a tonic encephalinergic inhibitory control.

Naloxone also affects bladder function in man (de Groat and Kawatani 1985). In normal patients a significant rise in intravesical pressure (i.e. decreased bladder compliance) is noted during cystometry following naloxone. Bladder capacity is reduced and some patients who have stable bladders prior to the drug become unstable after naloxone. Naloxone increases the instability index during cystometry in patients with idiopathic detrusor instability. Naloxone also facilitates bladder activity in patients with incomplete suprasacral spinal cord lesions, reducing by approximately one-third the bladder volume necessary to induce micturition.

Inhibitory amino acids

Pharmacological experiments indicate that the inhibitory amino acids, glycine and gamma aminobutyric acid (GABA), are involved in the control bladder reflexes in the cat spinal cord and the brainstem, respectively. Strychnine, a glycine antagonist, reduces spinal inhibitory mechanisms in the sacral parasympathetic pathways to the bladder. On the other hand, bicuculline (a GABA antagonist) administered into the pontine micturition centre blocks the inhibitory effects of various GABA agonists and also decreases the bladder volume threshold for inducing micturition in decerebrate unanaesthetized cats. The latter data indicates that GABAergic inhibitory mechanisms in the pons are involved in regulating bladder capacity.

5-hydroxytryptamine (serotonin)

The lumbosacral sympathetic and parasympathetic autonomic centres receive a dense serotonergic input from the raphe nuclei in the caudal brainstem. Systemic administration of the serotonergic precursor, 5-hydroxytryptophan, inhibits the parasympathetic micturition reflex but facilitates vesicosympathetic reflexes. Since electrical stimulation of the serotonergic neurons in raphe nuclei also inhibits bladder activity, it is possible that bulbospinal serotonergic pathways are involved in inhibiting micturition.

INNERVATION OF SEXUAL ORGANS

In man the physiologic changes initiated by erotic stimuli are divided into four distinct phases (excitement, plateau, orgasm, and resolution) which are designated collectively the sexual response cycle (Levin 1980; de Groat and Booth 1984). Although anatomic differences obviously preclude identical responses in male and female during each phase of the cycle it is clear that similar secretory responses (vaginal lubrication, prostatic and bulbourethral gland secretion), vascular responses (penile and clitoral erection), and responses of smooth and striated muscles occur in both sexes (Table 12.3). This section will review experimental studies in animals which examined the neural mechanisms regulating these physiologic responses.

The sex organs like the lower urinary tract receive an innervation from three sets of nerves: sacral parasympathetic (pelvic), thoraco-lumbar sympathetic (hypogastric and lumbar sympathetic chain), and somatic (pudendal) nerves (Fig. 12.1) (Sjöstrand 1965; Bell 1972; Elbadawi and Goodman 1980; Hart and Leedy 1985; de Groat and Steers 1987).

Parasympathetic pathways

Preganglionic axons arising from neurons in the sacral spinal cord provide an excitatory input to parasympathetic ganglion cells (Fig. 12.1) in the pelvic plexus which in turn innervate: (1) erectile tissue in the

Table 12.3. Male sexual reflexes

Response	*Afferent nerves*	*Efferent nerves*	*Central pathway*	*Effector organ*
Penile erection				
Reflexogenic	Pudendal nerve	Sacral parasympathetic	Sacral spinal reflex	Dilatation of arterial supply to corpus cavernosum and corpus spongiosum
Psychogenic	Auditory, imaginative visual, olfactory	Sacral parasympathetic Lumbar sympathetic	Supraspinal origin	
Glandular secretion	Pudendal nerve	Sacral parasympathetic Lumbar sympathetic	Sacral spinal reflex	Seminal vesicles and prostate
Seminal emission	Pudendal nerve	Lumbar sympathetic	Intersegmental spinal reflex (sacrolumbar)	Contraction of vas deferens, ampulla, seminal vesicles, prostate; and closure of bladder neck
Ejaculation	Pudendal nerve	Somatic efferents in pudendal nerves	Sacral spinal reflex	Rhythmic contractions of bulbocavernosus and ischiocavernosus muscles

From de Groat and Booth (1980*b*).

penis clitoris; (2) smooth muscle and glandular tissue in the prostate, urethra, seminal vesicles, vagina, uterus; and (3) blood vessels and possibly secretory epithelia in various structures. Among the numerous sexual functions controlled by the sacral parasympathetic pathway, the one which has attracted the most research interest and for which there is the most detailed information is penile erection.

Since the initial observation by Eckhard in 1863 that electrical stimulation of the pelvic nerves in the dog produced penile erection, the mechanisms involved in erection have been investigated in various species. It is clear that parasympathetic neural activity induces vasodilatation in penile blood vessels and increases blood flow to the cavernous tissue (Bell 1972; Lue *et al.* 1983; Andersson *et al.* 1984; de Groat and Steers 1987). However, the mechanisms underlying the vasodilatation and the transmitters mediating the response are still being investigated.

Cholinergic mechanisms

Two putative transmitter mechanisms, cholinergic and peptidergic, are currently receiving the most attention. Although acetylcholine has been identified as a transmitter at many parasympathetic postganglionic neuroeffector junctions and acetylcholinesterase-containing nerves (presumably cholinergic) are present in the penis, the role of acetylcholine in the penile erection has been questioned. This is based on the lack of convincing and consistent pharmacological data. For example, in some species atropine, a muscarinic cholinergic antagonist, reduces but does not completely block penile erections, whereas in other species, including man, it has no effect on erections (Andersson *et al.* 1984; de Groat and Steers 1987). Furthermore, the local administration of exogenous acetylcholine increases penile volume in some species but has never been shown to induce complete erections.

In vitro studies on isolated cavernosal smooth muscle also provide some support for a cholinergic mechanism in erection. Studies in the rabbit reveal that acetylcholine relaxes cavernosal muscle strips first contracted by noradrenalin. The relaxation is blocked by atropine, indicating that muscarinic receptors can mediate a relaxation of penile smooth muscle. Acetylcholine-induced relaxation also occurs *in vitro* in human corpus cavernosal tissue. In addition, electrical-field stimulation of the tissue elicits a relaxation which is potentiated by physostigmine, an anticholinesterase drug, and which is partially blocked by atropine. These studies suggest that cholinergic neurotransmission plays an important though not exclusive role in the relaxation of corpus cavernosal smooth muscle.

The relaxant actions of exogenous acetylcholine on penile smooth muscle may be indirect via the release of endogenous substances which in turn activate second-messenger systems in the smooth-muscle cells (Burnstock 1986; de Groat and Steers 1987). It is known that the actions of exogenous acetylcholine on large arteries are dependent upon the release of endothelial-derived relaxing factor (EDRF) from endothelial cells. EDRF stimulates guanylate cyclase which increases the intracellular levels of cyclic guanosine monophosphate (cyclic GMP) leading to relaxation of the smooth muscle. Cyclic GMP has been implicated in neurally evoked relaxation of bovine and canine penile arteries as well as bovine penile smooth muscle.

Peptidergic mechanisms

The identification of neuropeptides as mediators of noncholinergic–nonadrenergic transmission at various sites in the mammalian peripheral nervous system (Burnstock 1986) has focused attention on the possible role of these agents in the vasodilator pathways to the penis. Several substances including VIP, substance P, and neuropeptide Y have been identified in nerves supplying the penile vasculature (Lundberg *et al.* 1980; Burnstock 1986). Among these peptides VIP is the most promising transmitter candidate. VIP immunoreactivity in penile nerves in human, monkey, and dog is associated with large dense-core vesicles which are located in varicosities containing small clear, presumably cholinergic vesicles (Burnstock 1986; de Groat and Steers 1987). These findings are consistent with immunocytochemical results in the rat demonstrating that cholinergic pelvic ganglionic cells projecting to the penis contain VIP. Additional evidence for a role of VIP in penile erection includes experiments, in which local administration of VIP to man, monkey, or dog increased penile volume (Andersson *et al.* 1984). VIP also induces relaxation of *in vitro* preparations of corpus cavernosum, corpus spongiosum, smooth muscle, and penile blood vessels from many species. Finally, an increase in VIP concentration occurs in the venous effluent of the penis of man and dog during psychogenic, drug, or electrically-induced erections.

The effect of VIP in penile erectile tissue may involve several mechanisms. Direct relaxation of smooth muscle may be mediated by increased levels of cyclic adenosine monophosphate. In addition, VIP could facilitate muscarinic cholinergic transmission in the penis as it does in other organs, such as the salivary gland and autonomic ganglia. Since VIP and acetylcholine are co-localized in the penile nerves, it is possible that a synergistic interaction between these two transmitters occurs during erection.

Sympathetic pathways

Sympathetic pathways to the reproductive organs follow three routes: (1) the hypogastric nerves; (2) the pelvic nerves; and (3) the pudendal nerves (Fig. 12.1). The sympathetic nerves provide an input to penile and clitoral erectile tissue and to blood vessels throughout the reproductive organs as well as to smooth muscle of the ductus deferens, seminal vesicles, prostate, vagina, and uterus (Sjöstrand 1965; Bell 1972; Elbadawi and Goodman 1980).

Sympathetic postganglionic neurons are thought to release primarily noradrenalin; however, other substances, such as acetylcholine, adenosine triphosphate (ATP), and neuropeptides have also been identified as transmitters in these neurons (Burnstock 1986).

Sympathetic inputs to the erectile tissue can initiate tumescence as well as detumescence by release of different transmitters (de Groat and Steers 1987). Inputs from the caudal sympathetic ganglia which contain noradrenalin and possibly neuropeptide Y produce vasoconstriction of penile blood vessels and detumescence via actions on α-adrenergic and peptide receptors. On the other hand, inputs from the hypogastric nerve which pass through ganglionic relay stations in the pelvic plexus can produce vasodilatation and penile erection as well as detumescence. Pharmacological experiments indicate that acetylcholine and non-cholinergic transmitters, such as VIP, mediate the erectile response.

Sympathetic nerves provide excitatory inputs to the ductus deferens, seminal vesicles, prostate, vaginal and uterine smooth muscle (Sjöstrand 1965; Bell 1972; Elbadawi and Goodman 1980). These excitatory responses are mediated by an action of noradrenalin on α-adrenergic receptors. In the ductus deferens and seminal vesicles a second excitatory transmitter, ATP, is co-released with noradrenalin and acts on non-adrenergic, purinergic receptors (Burnstock 1986).

Somatic pathways

The pudendal nerves arising from the lumbosacral segments of the spinal cord provide efferent excitatory input to the bulbocavernosus and ischiocavernosus muscles (Fig. 12.1). These muscles are responsible for ejaculation in male and contribute to the rhythmic perineal contractions during orgasm in the female (Levin 1980; Hart and Leedy 1985). In many species, including cat, monkey, and man, the motoneurons innervating these muscles are located in Onuf's nucleus, whereas in the rat they are located in a separate nucleus in the medial part of the ventral horn.

In rat, dog, and man the bulbocavernosus nucleus is sexually dimorphic, males having a considerably larger number of motoneurons than females (de Groat and Steers 1987). This sexual dimorphism has been attributed to the trophic influence of androgens during neonatal development. Androgens also have an influence in adult animals. For example, castration in the adult rat and dog produces a dramatic decrease in somal size and dendritic length of bulbocavernosus motoneurons. The changes are reversed by the administration of testosterone. These data are consistent with behavioural studies in the rat which show that sexual reflexes in rats are influenced by the actions of androgen on neural elements in the spinal cord.

Afferent pathways

Afferent pathways to the penis, clitoris, and vagina are present in the pudendal nerves (Levin 1980; Hart and Leedy 1985). Afferent pathways to deeper structures such as the uterine cervix and uterine horns are present in the pelvic and hypogastric nerves, respectively. Cervical afferent neurons are located primarily in the sacral dorsal-root ganglia whereas uterine horn afferent neurons are located primarily in the upper lumbar dorsal-root ganglia. Electrophysiological studies have shown that afferents from the penis respond to tactile stimuli whereas the great majority of afferents from the uterus are of the polymodal type which respond to non-noxious and noxious mechanical and chemical stimuli.

Substance P and CGRP are present in a considerable proportion of the afferent neurons innervating the genital organs (de Groat 1987). For example, it has been estimated that 45–80 per cent of the lumbosacral dorsal-root ganglia cells innervating the female genital tract contain CGRP. At many sites the two peptides are co-localized in the same neuron and therefore, may function as co-transmitters in afferent pathways in the genital organs.

Peptidergic axons are associated with blood vessels, non-vascular smooth muscle, squamous and glandular epithelium. In the female the most prominent substance P–CGRP innervation occurs in the vagina. In the male, where substance P and CGRP fibres are less dense, they are located in the glans penis, ductus deferens, seminal vesicles, and epididymides (de Groat 1987).

CENTRAL REFLEX MECHANISMS CONTROLLING THE SEXUAL ORGANS

Erection

Penile erection is primarily an involuntary or reflex phenomenon that can be elicited by a variety of reflexogenic and psychogenic stimuli and by at least two distinct central mechanisms (i.e. spinal and supraspinal) (Table 12.3) which probably act synergistically (de Groat and Booth 1984; de Groat and Steers 1987). The central control of clitoral erection is likely to be mediated by similar mechanisms but has not been studied in detail (Levin 1980).

Reflexogenic erections

Reflexogenic penile erections which are elicited by exteroceptive stimulation of the genital regions are mediated by a sacral spinal reflex pathway having an afferent limb in the pudendal nerve and an efferent limb in the sacral parasympathetic nerves (Fig. 12.6) (Hart and Leedy 1985; de Groat and Steers 1987).

The central organization of the reflex pathway has been studied in several species of animals. Axonal tracing techniques have revealed that pudendal afferent pathways from the penis of the cat and rat terminate in the medial dorsal horn and dorsal commissure (Fig. 12.6). Interneurons in these regions are activated by tactile stimulation of the penis and are presumably involved in transmitting sensations to the brain in

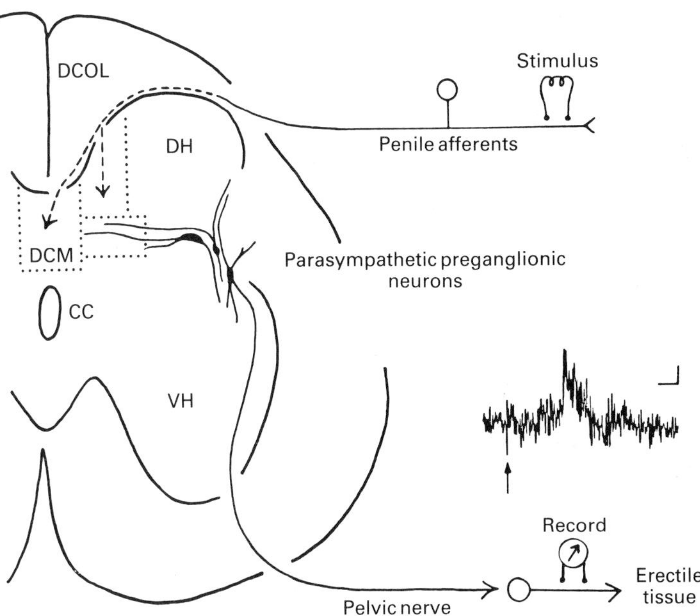

Fig. 12.6. Diagram showing the reflex pathway for inducing penile erection. Horseradish peroxidase axonal tracing studies in the cat have shown the relationship between sacral parasympathetic preganglionic neurons and afferent projections from the penis. Penile afferents in the pudendal nerve project to the medial side of the dorsal horn (DH) and the dorsal commissure (DCM) in the S_2 segment of the spinal cord. Preganglionic neurons send dendrites into regions of afferent termination. Dorsal column (DCOL), ventral horn (VH), and central canal (CC). In the rat electrical stimulation of the penile afferents in the dorsal nerve of the penis elicits reflex firing in efferent pathways to the penis. Inset is an example of a reflex discharge in parasympathetic postganglionic axons in penile nerves. The reflexes which occur at a long latency (mean 75 ms) are present in normal and chronic spinal rats and are blocked by section of the pelvic nerve. Stimulus marked by arrow. Horizontal calibration 20 ms, vertical calibration 10 μV.

addition to activating parasympathetic preganglionic neurons which induce erection. The preganglionic neurons are located in the intermediolateral nucleus of the sacral spinal cord and send dendritic projections into areas of laminae V–VII and the dorsal commissure which receive afferent input from the penis (Fig. 12.6) (de Groat *et al.* 1986). Thus the afferent and efferent components of the reflex pathway are in close proximity.

In the rat electrical stimulation of the dorsal nerve of the penis evokes several long-latency (mean 75 ms) reflex discharges in postganglionic axons passing from the major pelvic ganglion into the penile nerves (Fig. 12.6). Since some of these reflexes are obtained in both normal and chronic spinal rats and are eliminated by transection of the pelvic nerves, it is clear that they are mediated by a polysynaptic spinal reflex pathway involving efferent neurons in the sacral autonomic outflow.

In the rat penile afferents also project into the ventral horn and appear to make contacts with the soma and dendrites of motoneurons. These connections could be involved in the somatic reflex mechanisms involved in copulation.

Psychogenic erections

Psychogenic erections are initiated by supraspinal centres in response to auditory, visual, olfactory, and imaginative stimuli. The efferent limb of the reflex pathway traverses both the thoracolumbar and the sacral autonomic outflow (Table 12.3). Studies conducted in monkeys and rats indicate that hypothalamic and limbic pathways play a key role in erection and that the medial preoptic-anterior hypothalamic area is an important integrating centre (Hart and Leedy 1985; de Groat and Steers 1987). Electrical stimulation at this site produces full erections in the anaesthetized and unanaesthetized animals, whereas lesions at the same site generally suppress sexual behaviour.

Efferent pathways from the medial preoptic area enter the medial forebrain bundle and then pass caudally into the midbrain tegmental region near the lateral part of the substantia nigra. Caudal to the midbrain the efferent pathway for erection travels in the ventrolateral pons and medulla and then in the lateral funiculus of the spinal cord. Descending projections from the hypothalamic nuclei terminate in lumbosacral spinal autonomic and somatic centres involved in erection.

Secretion

During the first and second phases of the sexual response cycle, activity in parasympathetic and sympathetic pathways in the male stimulates mucus secretion from the bulbourethral and Littré glands and secretion from the seminal vesicles and prostate gland (Table 12.3).

Acetylcholine has been implicated as an efferent transmitter since cholinomimetic agents mimic neurally evoked secretion from some glands (de Groat and Booth 1984).

In the female, erotic stimuli elicit vaginal lubrication and mucus secretion from Bartholin's glands (Levin 1980). Vaginal lubrication is thought to be secondary to increased vaginal blood and, possibly, changes in capillary permeability leading to increased formation of plasma transudate which passes through the epithelium to the vaginal surface. An active secretory mechanism is unlikely since the vaginal epithelium is devoid of glands. VIP has been implicated as the efferent transmitter in vaginal lubrication and increased vaginal blood flow (Ottesen 1983).

Emission–ejaculation

The third phase of the sexual act (orgasm) which is accompanied by emission and ejaculation of semen involves the co-ordination of autonomic and somatic reflex mechanisms at different levels of the lumbosacral spinal cord (de Groat and Booth 1984; Hart and Leedy 1985). During the first step in the process (emission), reflex activity in the thoracolumbar sympathetic outflow elicits rhythmic contractions of the smooth muscle of the seminal vesicles, prostate, ductus deferens, and ampulla resulting in the ejection of sperm and glandular secretions into the urethra and at the same time closure of the vesical neck to prevent backflow of semen into the bladder. Pharmacological studies have shown that these responses are mediated by the adrenergic transmitter noradrenalin acting on α-adrenergic receptors and the purinergic transmitter, ATP. Seminal emission may be modulated also by cholinergic nerves which can block the release of adrenergic transmitters (Burnstock 1986).

After emission of semen into the proximal urethra, rhythmic contractions of the bulbocavernosus, ischiocavernosus, and periurethral striated muscles result in ejaculation. The afferent and efferent limbs of the ejaculatory reflex are contained in the pudendal nerve. The sensations accompanying ejaculation, or rhythmic vaginal contractions in the female, represent a major component of the orgasmic response (Levin 1980).

NEUROTRANSMITTERS IN SEXUAL REFLEX PATHWAYS

Pharmacological studies in animals have implicated many neurotransmitter systems in the central control of sexual function. The literature relevant to this topic is extensive (see review by Crowley and Zelman 1981) and will be summarized very briefly in this section.

Monoamines

The monoaminergic transmitters (5-hydroxytryptamine, dopamine, and noradrenalin) appear to have varied roles in the central mechanisms underlying sexual behaviour. For example, pharmacological blockade or destruction of the 5-hydroxytryptamine (5-HT) containing pathways in the brain facilitates sexual activity in male rats and rabbits, whereas the administration of a 5-HT precursor decreases sexual activity (Crowley and Zelman 1981). These data indicate that 5-HT pathways in the brain exert a general depressant effect on sexual motivation. However, other studies imply that at the level of the spinal cord 5-HT mechanisms facilitate seminal emission, but diminish penile erections in the rat.

Noradrenergic pathways exert an inhibitory influence on sexual function. Clonidine, a centrally acting α_2-adrenergic receptor agonist, inhibits erections and copulatory activity in rats. The inhibitory effects of clonidine are reversed by yohimbine, an α_2-adrenergic receptor antagonist. The administration of yohimbine alone increases sexual motivation suggesting that sexual activity is tonically inhibited by a noradrenergic pathway.

Dopaminergic pathways have a facilitatory effect on male copulatory behaviour in the rat. Administration of L-dopa, a precursor of dopamine, or the administration of dopamine receptor agonists increases mounting, intromissions, and ejaculations in male rats. On the other hand, lesions of the dopamine system depress copulatory behaviour.

Neuropeptides and GABA

Oxytocin, a neuropeptide which is present in efferent pathways from the hypothalamus to spinal autonomic centres, facilitates penile erectile mechanisms in the rat when administered in nanogram quantities into the cerebral ventricles. On the other hand, the opioid peptides and GABA inhibit copulatory behaviour when administered into the brain of male rats, whereas the administration of receptor antagonists for either type of transmitter facilitate copulatory behaviour.

Thus a broad spectrum of neurotransmitters seem to be involved in the control of sexual behaviour in the rodent. It is uncertain whether these findings are generally applicable to man. However, the susceptibility of human sexual function to a broad range of drugs suggests that sexual behaviour in humans, as in rodents, depends on a variety of neurochemical mechanisms.

REFERENCES

Andersson, P-O., Bloom, S. R., and Mellander, S. (1984). Haemodynamics of pelvic nerve induced penile erection in the dog: Possible mediation by vasoactive intestinal polypeptide. *J. Physiol., London* **350**, 209–24.

Bell, C. (1972). Autonomic nervous control of reproduction: Circulatory and other factors. *Pharmacol. Rev.* **24**, 657–736.

Burnstock, G. (1986). The changing face of autonomic neurotransmission. *Acta physiol. scand.* **126**, 67–91.

Crowley, W. R. and Zelman, F. P. (1981). The neurochemical control of mating behavior. In *Neuroendocrinology of reproduction, physiology and behavior* (ed. N. T. Adler), pp. 451–84. Plenum Press, New York.

de Groat, W. C. (1975). Nervous control of the urinary bladder of the cat. *Brain Res.* **87**, 201–11.

de Groat, W. C. (1986). Spinal cord projections and neuropeptides in visceral afferent neurons. In *Visceral sensation, progress in brain research* (ed. F. Cervero and J. F. B. Morrison), Vol. 67, pp. 165–87. Elsevier, Holland.

de Groat, W. C. (1987). Neuropeptides in pelvic afferent pathways. *Experientia* **43**, 801–13.

de Groat, W. C. and Booth, A. M. (1980*a*). Inhibition and facilitation in parasympathetic ganglia of the urinary bladder. *Fed. Proc.* **39**, 2990–6.

de Groat, W. C. and Booth, A. M. (1980*b*). Physiology of male sexual function. *Ann. intern. Med.* **92**, 329.

de Groat, W. C. and Booth, A. M. (1984). Autonomic systems to urinary bladder and sexual organs. In *Peripheral neuropathy* (ed. P. J. Dyck, P. K. Thomas, E. H. Lambert, and R. Bunge), Vol. 1, pp. 285–99. W. B. Saunders, Philadelphia.

de Groat, W. C. and Kawatani, M. (1985). Neural control of the urinary bladder: possible relationship between peptidergic inhibitory mechanisms and detrusor instability. *Neurol. Urodynam.* **4**, 285–300.

de Groat, W. C., Kawatani, M., Hisamitsu, T., Booth, A. M., Roppolo, J. R., Thor, K., Tuttle, P., and Nagel, J. (1986). Neural control of micturition: the role of neuropeptides. *J. auton. nerv. Syst.* Suppl. 369–87.

de Groat, W. C. and Steers, W. D. (1987). The neuroanatomy and neurophysiology of penile erection. In *Contemporary management of impotence and infertility* (ed. E. A. Tanagho, T. F. Lue, and D. D. McClure). Williams and Wilkins, Baltimore. (In press.)

Elbadawi, A. and Goodman, D. C. (1980). Autonomic innervation of accessory male genital glands. In *Male accessory sex glands* (ed. E. Spring-Mills and E. S. E. Hafez), pp. 101–28. Elsevier, Holland.

Hart, B. L. and Leedy, M. G. (1985). Neurological basis of male sexual behavior: a comparative analysis. In *Handbook of behavioral neurobiology*, pp. 373–422. Plenum, New York.

Holstege, G., Griffiths, D., DeWall, H., and Dalm, E. (1986). Anatomical and physiological observations in supraspinal control of bladder and urethral sphincter muscles in the cat. *J. comp. Neurol.* **250**, 449–61.

Jänig, W. and Morrisson, J. F. B. (1986). Functional properties of spinal visceral afferents supplying abdominal and pelvic organs, with special emphasis on visceral nociception. In *Visceral sensation, progress in brain research* (ed. F. Cervero and J. F. B. Morrisson), Vol. 67, pp. 87–114. Elsevier, Holland.

Kuru, M. (1965). Nervous control of micturition. *Physiol. Rev.* **45**, 425–94.

Levin, R. J. (1980). The physiology of sexual function in women. *Clin. Obstet. Gynecol.* **7**, 213–52.

Lue, T. F., Takamura, T., Schmidt, R. A., Palubinshos, A. J., and Tanagho, E. A. (1983). Hemodynamics of erection in the monkey. *J. Urol.* **130**, 1237–41.

Lundberg, J. M., Hokfelt, T., Anggard, A., Uvnas-Wallensten, K., Brimijoin, S., Brodin, E., and Fahrenkrug, J. (1980). Peripheral peptide neurons: Distribution, axonal transport, and some aspects on possible function. In *Neural peptides and neuronal communication* (ed. E. Costa and M. Trabucchi), pp. 25–36. Raven Press, New York.

Maggi, C. A. and Meli, A. (1986). The role of neuropeptides in the regulation of the micturition reflex. *J. auton. Pharmacol.* **6**, 133–62.

McMahon, S. B. and Spillane, R. (1982). Brain stem influences on the parasympathetic supply to the urinary bladder of the cat. *Brain Res.* **235**, 237–49.

Morgan, C., Nadelhaft, I., and de Groat, W. C. (1981). The distribution of visceral primary afferents from the pelvic nerve within Lissauer's tract and the spinal gray matter and its relationship to the sacral parasympathetic nucleus. *J. comp. neurol.* **201**, 415–40.

Ottesen, B. (1983). Vasoactive intestinal polypeptide as a neurotransmitter in the female genital tract. *Am. J. Obstet. Gynecol.* **147**, 208–23.

Satoh, K., Shimizu, M., Tohyama, M., and Maeda, T. (1978). Localization of the micturition reflex center at dorsolateral pontine tegmentum of the rat. *Neurosci. Lett.* **8**, 27–33.

Sjöstrand, N. O. (1965). The adrenergic innervation of the vas deferens and the accessory male genital glands. *Acta. physiol. scand. Suppl.* **257**, 1–70.

Thor, K., Kawatani, M., and de Groat, W. C. (1986). Plasticity in the reflex pathways to the lower urinary tract of the cat during postnatal development and following spinal cord injury. In *Development and plasticity of the mammalian spinal cord* (ed. M. E. Goldberger, A. Gorio, and M. Murray), Vol. 3, pp. 65–80. Liviana Press, Padua.

13. Autonomic control of the pelvic organs

G. S. Brindley

INTRODUCTION

All pelvic organs receive a sympathetic efferent supply. This consists of: (1) myelinated preganglionic nerve fibres, which leave the spinal cord by lower thoracic and upper lumbar anterior roots; (2) ganglion cells, of which some lie in the sympathetic chains, but many lie in or near the pelvic organs supplied; and (3) the axons of these ganglion cells, called postganglionic fibres, of which most are unmyelinated, but a few are myelinated. The pelvic sympathetic fibres enter the pelvis from above. The greatest number run in the hypogastric plexus, which descends in front of the lower abdominal aorta and its bifurcation, and the left common iliac vein. Smaller numbers run in the right and left sympathetic chains.

Some pelvic organs also receive a parasympathetic efferent autonomic supply. Like the sympathetic pathway, it has a ganglionic relay. Its preganglionic fibres leave the spinal cord by the second, third, and fourth sacral anterior roots. They pass through the corresponding anterior sacral foramina in the anterior primary rami. Small branches of these rami then combine to form, for a short distance, a compact plexus, the pelvic splanchnic plexus or pelvic splanchnic nerve, on the upper surface of the levator ani muscle. This plexus probably contains nearly all the preganglionic pelvic parasympathetic fibres. They are mixed with afferent fibres and a few somatic motor fibres, which innervate part of the levator ani muscle and perhaps part of the intrinsic striated sphincter of the urethra. The pelvic parasympathetic ganglion cells lie in small ganglia near the organs supplied, and also scattered within these organs.

It has long been suspected for various autonomic ganglia, and is now established beyond doubt for the inferior mesenteric ganglion of the guinea-pig (Kreulen and Peters 1986), that afferent fibres (probably collateral branches of fibres that also have endings in the spinal cord) synapse with ganglion cells and can influence them. Such synapses provide a possible mechanism for local reflexes independent of the spinal cord. These reflexes may be important in the intestine, where loss of the preganglionic excitatory (parasympathetic) supply does not abolish motor activity. In pelvic and abdominal organs other than the intestine there is little evidence to suggest significant local reflex function in man.

It has also long been suspected that synaptic connections between one autonomic ganglion cell and another exist. I can find no firm evidence in favour of such cross-connections, but no evidence at all against them.

For preganglionic fibres, the distinction between sympathetic and parasympathetic is by definition absolutely clear: if they run in thoracic or lumbar anterior roots they are sympathetic, and if in sacral roots they are parasympathetic. For ganglion cells and the postganglionic fibres that arise from them, the distinction may be blurred because some ganglion cells may receive synaptic contacts from both sympathetic and parasympathetic preganglionic fibres (El Badawi and Schenk 1966). However, the distinction remains useful in practice. A ganglion cell should be called sympathetic if its excitatory input is wholly or mainly thoracolumbar, and parasympathetic if it is excited wholly or mainly by fibres of sacral segmental nerves or (outside the pelvis) cranial nerves.

The cells of origin of the preganglionic sympathetic and parasympathetic fibres that supply pelvic organs lie in the intermediolateral part of the grey matter of the T10 to L2 (sometimes L3) and S2 to S4 segments of the spinal cord. They are accessible to spinal reflex and cerebral influences of many kinds, some consistent and well known, some variable or obscure, and doubtless some not yet guessed at. The pathways by which spinal reflex and cerebral influences act on autonomic outflow cells are mainly unknown, though a few relevant facts have been gleaned from clinical observations. The present chapter will deal only with peripheral mechanisms, and will say nothing about the brain or spinal cord.

URINARY TRACT

Ureter

During extreme diuresis, the lumen of the ureter is continuously open over its whole length, and it must act merely as a pipe. At average and low rates of urine production, the urine is propelled in discrete boluses by peristaltic waves which run along the ureter. When a kidney is transplanted with its ureter, these waves occur (and transport urine efficiently) from the day of transplantation. They are thus not dependent on nervous connections with the spinal cord. Nor do they need local nervous connections: application of tetrodotoxin does not block them. The renal pelvis normally acts as pacemaker for the waves, and usually each wave passes along the whole length of the ureter, though at high pacemaker frequencies conduction failure can occur (1:2, 1:3, or irregular block) at any point on the ureter, so that the frequency of waves can be lower at the vesical end of the ureter than at the renal pelvis. There is no inbuilt directionality in the ureter; a segment transplanted with reverse polarity functions normally (Melick *et al.* 1962), and, if a uretero–ureterostomy (artificial Y ureter) is made as treatment for disease or injury of the lower part of one ureter, waves can sometimes be seen to run down one ureter to the junction, and then up to the opposite pelvis. All segments of the ureter are capable of pacemaker activity, as well as of conduction in either direction. The frequency of pacemaker activity is increased by distension, and this functionally appropriate response is independent of nerves.

The intrinsic ureteric smooth-muscle activity is probably modifiable to a small extent by the autonomic system. There is no known parasympathetic supply. Sympathetic fibres are present, but stimulation of the hypogastric plexus (Gruber 1933) has only very small effects on motor activity of the ureter other than at its outlet, and even the small effects seen have not been controlled for the possibility that they are secondary to changes in urine flow. However, drugs that stimulate α- and β-adrenoceptors have demonstrable effects on the ureter, both isolated (Morita and Tsuchida 1983) and *in situ* (Morita *et al.* 1986), and it seems likely that the adrenoceptors responsible are innervated by sympathetic fibres. α-adrenoceptor stimulation increases the frequency of pacemaker activity slightly, abolishes conduction block if this was previously present, and increases the resistance of the ureter to flow, greatly at low flows and slightly at high flows. β-adrenoceptor stimulation promotes conduction block and decreases the resistance to flow. The functional significance of these changes, whether they are driven by nerves or only by blood-borne catecholamines, is very obscure.

It seems that muscarinic transmission to ureteric smooth muscle is absent or negligible: carbachol, in concentrations up to 100 times that which makes the bladder contract, does not influence the motor activity of the isolated human ureter (Thomiak *et al.* 1985). Thus the use of antimuscarinic drugs in treating renal colic is irrational.

In contrast to the rest of the ureter, the ureterovesical junction has, in man, a clear and conspicuous response to sympathetic stimulation. Learmonth (1931) observed by cystoscopy that, when the hypogastric plexus was stimulated, the orifices of the ureters contracted, the detrusor remaining relaxed.

The ureter resembles the internal anal sphincter, and differs from most other pelvic organs, in containing no ganglion cells (Notley 1971).

Detrusor muscle of the bladder

The excitatory motor supply to the detrusor muscle is parasympathetic. Its preganglionic fibres leave the spinal cord in the second, third, and fourth sacral anterior roots, but not always in all three of these pairs of roots. The most common pattern is for the main supply to be from S3, with small contributions from S2 and S4. In some people either S2 or S4 contributes nothing, and in a few either the S2 or the S4 innervation exceeds that from S3 (Brindley *et al.* 1986). In all mammalian species examined, including primates, if sacral roots of one side only are stimulated electrically, the detrusor contraction is mainly restricted to that side (Gruber 1933).

Impulse frequencies in the preganglionic parasympathetic fibres to the bladder seem to be higher than the 1 to 5 impulses per second observed in most preganglionic autonomic fibres: to achieve by electrical stimulation a speed of rise of bladder pressure as great as occurs in a reflex detrusor contraction, at least 12 and sometimes 18 electrical pulses per second must be delivered to the sacral roots (Brindley *et al.* 1982).

In most or all non-primate mammals, the parasympathetic excitatory action on the detrusor is mainly non-cholinergic. Attempts to discover the transmitter (Callahan and Creed 1986) have not yet been successful. In man, non-cholinergic mechanisms have been reported in isolated bladder strips, but also denied (Sibley 1987). If real, they seem to be of little importance. The intact bladder of man and other old-world primates behaves as if its postganglionic parasympathetic endings are wholly cholinergic (muscarinic) (Craggs *et al.* 1986). Large doses of antimuscarinic drugs block its contractions completely. However, doses that patients will tolerate for long-term administration probably weaken these contractions only by a small percentage. Although the detrusor muscle is sensitive to antimuscarinic drugs, it is no more so than the sinoatrial node, the salivary glands, and the ciliary muscle of the eye, and the effects on these organs limit the dose.

The detrusor muscle, in man as in other mammals, has a sympathetic supply. In the cat and rhesus monkey, but not in the dog or rabbit, this supply has been found to be inhibitory: stimulation of the hypogastric plexus relaxes the detrusor and diminishes the motor response to simultaneous parasympathetic stimulation (Elliot 1907). I can find no published evidence for an inhibitory action in man. In the ferret, guinea-pig, and male goat, hypogastric stimulation has a strong excitatory action on the detrusor (Elliot 1907). There is certainly no strong excitatory action in man, (Learmonth 1931; Brindley 1986*a*), and probably no excitatory action at all.

Surgical removal of para-aortic lymph nodes (for example in the treatment of testicular carcinoma) often damages the hypogastric plexus, and it seems that the damage is often a total interruption. Patients with this lesion rarely become incontinent of urine. In a few of them, cystometry has been done, and has not revealed any detrusor instability. Thus hypogastric inhibition of the detrusor, if it occurs at all in man, is not important for continence.

It will soon be known whether electrical stimulation of the hypogastric plexus in man has any action, inhibitory or excitatory, on the detrusor muscle, because implanted stimulators of the hypogastric plexus are now in regular use as a means of achieving fertility in men with spinal injuries (Brindley 1986*a*). Some of these men also have sacral anterior root stimulators to control their bladders, so it will be possible to test whether hypogastric stimulation alone affects bladder pressure, and also whether it modifies the effect of parasympathetic stimulation. Informal observations already show that there are no large effects, but time will be needed to establish whether there are small ones.

Trigone, bladder neck, and upper urethra

The smooth muscle of the upper urethra contracts in response to stimulation of the hypogastric plexus in all mammals yet tested, including old-world monkeys of both sexes (Gruber 1933), and man (Learmonth 1931).

In many mammalian species, including man, the trigone has been described as contracting under hypogastric stimulation, though the detrusor seemed to be unaffected (Gruber 1933; Learmonth 1931). The function of the smooth muscle of the trigone is obscure.

The smooth muscle of the upper urethra is obviously sphincteric, and forms part of the normal mechanism of urinary continence. The bladder neck evidently acts with it as part of the same mechanism. In most normal people the bladder neck can be seen by X-ray screening to remain closed at any tolerated fullness of the bladder, despite coughing, straining, or landing from a jump, and to open when voiding is voluntarily initiated. It follows that in most people the bladder neck suffices for continence, provided that its anatomical position and support are such that the abdominal pressure acts almost without attenuation on its outside.

Many fully continent women have permanently open bladder necks radiologically (Versi *et al.* 1986). Their urethral pressure profiles show the proximal shortening that one would expect from this radiological appearance. In these women, and in men after prostatectomy, continence depends on urethral smooth and striated muscle. It is almost certain that the smooth muscle alone can suffice, since continence is usually preserved after bilateral pudendal neurectomy or pudendal block, and sometimes preserved in patients who have cauda equina lesions that interrupt all sacral roots, and therefore paralyse all pelvic striated muscle.

The sympathetic excitatory action on urethral smooth muscle appears to be wholly or mainly α-adrenergic. α_1-adrenoceptor blockers relax urethral smooth muscle, producing large decreases in intraurethral pressure in both men and women (Awad *et al.* 1976). However, there is a difference between men and women in the innervation of the proximal urethra (Gosling *et al.* 1977). In men, nerve fibres containing catecholamines are very abundant in urethral smooth muscle, and nerve fibres containing acetylcholinesterase are very scarce. In women these proportions are reversed. This sex difference has doubtless some relation to the function of the male upper urethra in preventing retrograde ejaculation, but is obscure. It is not certain that the fibres that contain acetylcholinesterase are involved in muscarinic transmission to smooth muscle, and it is unknown whether they are excitatory or inhibitory, sympathetic or parasympathetic.

α_1-adrenoceptor stimulants (ephedrine, phenylpropanolamine) cause bladder neck and urethral smooth muscle to contract, as do noradrenalin re-uptake blockers (maprotilene, desipramine, imipramine). Both groups of excitatory drugs are useful in some forms of urinary incontinence. Their use in treating retrograde ejaculation will be considered in the section on the male genital tract.

Electrical stimulation of the sacral parasympathetic pathway, either at the anterior spinal roots or at the pelvic splanchnic plexus, inhibits the smooth muscle of the urethra in male and female cats (Elliot 1907) and baboons (Brindley, unpublished) by a non-muscarinic action. It has been observed to do so in one woman, in whom the S4 roots innervated the urethral smooth muscle but not the detrusor, so that pure urethral effects could be observed (Torrens 1978). Stimulation of sacral anterior roots by an implanted (bladder-controlling) stimulator regularly causes opening of the bladder neck, but the bladder pressure rises simultaneously, so this does not constitute clear confirmation of Torrens's single observation that there is direct inhibitory action on sphincteric smooth muscle. The question can and will be settled (if the inhibition is non-muscarinic in man as in the baboon) by stimulating the sacral anterior roots when the patient has been given a dose of an antimuscarinic drug so large as to prevent all detrusor contraction.

Besides its function in maintaining continence, the smooth muscle of the male upper urethra and bladder neck prevents retrograde ejaculation. If it is weakened by surgical interference, autonomic neuropathy, or an incomplete lesion of the hypogastric plexus, retrograde ejaculation commonly occurs. It is likely, though unproved, that during ejaculation the sympathetic drive to the upper urethral and bladder neck smooth muscle (and hence the force that it exerts) is temporarily increased.

The urethra is acted on by striated muscle of two kinds. The extrinsic rhabdosphincter lies outside the wall of the urethra and forms part of the urogenital diaphragm. It resembles other pelvic muscles histologically. It is innervated, as they are, by the pudendal nerve, and probably contracts synchronously with them in all or nearly all circumstances. The intrinsic rhabdosphincter lies within the wall of the urethra, partly distal to the urethral smooth muscle, but overlapping it. The intrinsic rhabdosphincter is histologically different from other pelvic muscles (Gosling 1979). It is probably not wholly innervated by the pudendal nerve, but receives some motor fibres which, though somatic, run with the pelvic splanchnic plexus (Gosling 1979). There are widespread suspicions that the contractions of the intrinsic rhabdosphincter may not be synchronous with those of the pelvic floor, but I have seen no good published evidence that they are not.

The two rhabdosphincters are the only means by which micturition can be interrupted quickly. They form an important back-up to the smooth-muscle mechanism in some people who have detrusor instability accompanied by episodes of involuntary opening of the bladder neck, but nevertheless remain continent. They achieve continence by contracting the striated sphincter during the episodes of bladder neck opening.

It is likely, but not certain, that the rhabdosphincters can maintain continence when all smooth muscle of the bladder neck and urethra is inactivated. The uncertainty arises because lesions (hypogastric plexus) and drugs (α_1-adrenoceptor blockers) which relax urethral and bladder neck smooth muscle but spare continence do not necessarily inactivate the smooth muscle totally.

By analogy with other skeletal muscle, it is unlikely that the autonomic system has any important action, other than vasomotor, on either rhabdosphincter.

GONADS

Ovary

No parasympathetic supply is known. The abundant sympathetic supply enters the ovary (at least in the rat) as two well-defined bundles, one accompanying the ovarian artery and veins ('ovarian plexus') and the other lying in the suspensory ligament ('superior ovarian nerve') (Lawrence and Burden 1980). Cutting both removes almost all noradrenalin fluorescence from the ovary. Examination of the distribution of fluorescence after cutting each bundle separately shows that the ovarian plexus innervates mainly blood vessels, and the superior ovarian nerve innervates both blood vessels and interstitial tissue.

Electrical stimulation of one superior ovarian nerve in anaesthetized dioestrous rats depletes the ipsilateral ovary of progesterone. If the rats are pre-treated with phentolamine, this effect is not merely abolished, but reversed (Weiss *et al.* 1982). Thus there is an α-adrenergic mechanism which either augments the release of progesterone or (more likely) suppresses its synthesis, and a non-α-adrenergic mechanism which does the opposite. It is not likely that these effects are merely secondary to vasomotor changes, because noradrenalin has been shown to influence the production of steroid hormones by ovarian cells in culture (Dyer and Erickson 1985; Aguado and Ojeda 1986). There is suggestive evidence that, besides these α-adrenergic mechanisms, there may be vasoactive intestinal polypeptide (VIP)-ergic sympathetic fibres that influence steroid output, in this case oestradiol (Ahmed *et al.* 1986).

Ovarian follicles contain smooth muscle, and strips cut from them contract if they are stimulated electrically or if noradrenalin is added to the suspending medium. The responses to electrical stimulation are abolished by tetrodotoxin and greatly diminished by phentolamine (Kannisto *et al.* 1986). They therefore almost certainly involve α-noradrenergic nerve fibres. These fibres may play some part in ovulation, at least in the cow, the species on which these experiments were done.

Despite all the above, it does not seem likely that the sympathetic supply plays a necessary or major part in controlling ovarian function. Transplanted or denervated rat ovaries ovulate and produce hormones nearly normally (Wylie *et al.* 1985). Complete loss of sympathetic supply to the ovaries in women is uncommon and difficult to prove, so probably no indubitable case of it has been reported. However, extensive injury or disease affecting the lower thoracic and upper lumbar cord must destroy many of the pelvic preganglionic sympathetic fibres and greatly alter the way in which the rest function; yet it seems to leave menstrual cycles and ovulation largely unchanged.

Testis

No parasympathetic supply to the testis is known. There is a sympathetic supply. Testes examined after lumbar sympathectomy in cats, dogs, and guinea-pigs show severe depression of spermatogenesis at one week but partial recovery after 3 months (King and Langworthy 1940). The depression is doubtless at least partly due to vasomotor changes. Effects on transport of liquid along the epididymis may also play a part. I can find no direct evidence as to whether the sympathetic supply also influences spermatogenesis or androgen production. It is certainly not essential for either, since both have been observed to continue after transplantation of testes in several mammalian species. However, in view of the evidence strongly suggesting autonomic influences on hormone production in the ovary, it would not be surprising if such influences were discovered in the testis.

LOWER GENITAL TRACT

Epididymis

The whole length of the epididymis contains smooth muscle, and it is likely that this assists the movement of spermatozoa along it. At least in the cauda epididymidis of the rabbit, this motor activity seems to be under adrenergic control, either hormonal or nervous, since α-adrenoceptor blockers cause great accumulation of spermatozoa in the cauda epididymidis (Zankl and Leidl 1969). In man, nerve fibres containing noradrenalin are present along the whole length of the epididymis (Baumgarten *et al.* 1971).

It is not known whether there are autonomic influences on the secretory activity of the epididymis.

Vas deferens, seminal vesicle, and prostate

The abundant smooth muscle of the seminal vesicle and prostate becomes strongly active during ejaculation. So probably does that of the vas deferens.

The three organs have no known parasympathetic supply (Gruber 1933), and in the cat and baboon stimulation of sacral roots has no obvious effect (Brindley, unpublished). They have a sympathetic supply whose preganglionic fibres run in the hypogastric plexus. Electrical stimulation of this plexus causes powerful synchronous activation of all their smooth muscle, and emission of semen. Stimulation by radio-linked implant is practicable, and effective in achieving fertility in some men who cannot ejaculate (Brindley 1986*a*).

It is sometimes asserted that there is peristalsis in the vas deferens during ejaculation. This assertion seems to be based on observations made by Budge in 1858 on rabbits under electrical stimulation of lumbar spinal roots. I can find no published confirmation of them except a tentative statement ('appeared to undergo a peristaltic movement') for the cat (Semans and Langworthy 1938). If, in an anaesthetized rhesus monkey or baboon with electrodes on its hypogastric plexus, one vas deferens is exposed from epididymis to bladder, and the abdomen and scrotum positioned so that almost all the vas deferens lies bent into a series of waves, it is easy to observe the effect of sympathetic stimulation (Brindley, unpublished). Within 1 or 2 seconds nearly all the waves disappear, so that the vas runs straight except where it is constrained by some strong anatomical structure. The total shortening appears to be about 25 per cent. Within a few seconds of ceasing to stimulate, the waves reappear as the vas resumes its normal length. At no time is any peristalsis visible to the naked eye. Nevertheless, peristalsis may occur in the vas deferens at ejaculation or (perhaps more appropriately) at other times. Budge's old observation of peristalsis is made easier to believe by the fact that the vas deferens of many species, including man, contracts rhythmically when isolated in an organ bath (Anton *et al.* 1977).

The sympathetic supply to the vas deferens, seminal vesicle, and prostate resembles that to the urethral smooth muscle in being α-adrenergic, and all four organs are affected similarly by drugs that influence α_1-adrenergic transmission. *Suppression* of the activity of their smooth muscle is not therapeutically useful. *Augmentation* is useful in retrograde ejaculation or non-ejaculation with preserved organism, when these conditions are due to nerve damage. The damage may be an incomplete hypogastric plexus lesion, of which the commonest cause is diabetic neuropathy, or a lesion that destroys part but not all of the T10 to L2 region of the spinal cord. α_1-adrenergic agonists have been used with some success for this purpose, but noradrenalin re-uptake blockers are much better (Brooks *et al.* 1980; Brindley 1985*a*). Their use in treating ejaculatory failure is analogous to the use of neostigmine in treating myasthenia gravis: by slowing the removal of the scarce chemical transmitter they should strengthen the smooth-muscle contractions *at orgasm*, without having much effect at other times. Maprotilene and desipramine are theoretically preferable to imipramine because they are more specific. If the lesion of the hypogastric plexus is complete, all these drugs must presumably fail.

In the dog, hypogastric stimulation augments secretion from the prostate, as well as causing contraction of smooth muscle. The effects on secretion, unlike those on smooth muscle, are blocked by atropine and imitated by pilocarpine (Farrell and Lyman 1937).

Erectile tissue

Firm knowledge about the physiology of erection comes mainly from observations on the penis, but it is likely that most of it is applicable to the erectile tissue of the clitoris, labia minora, and vagina.

Erection of the spongy erectile tissue of the glans and corpus spongiosum, and probably of all erectile tissue in women, depends on opening up the arterial supply to it and relaxing the trabecular smooth muscle in it. Venous drainage remains free during erection, and there is probably no special mechanism to restrict it.

Erection of the corpora cavernosa differs from that of spongy erectile tissue in that, besides the opening of arteries and relaxation of trabeculae, there is a closure of venous drainage. The outlets from the corpora cavernosa into the draining veins are opened and closed by a mechanism that is unique in known physiology. The muscular action that closes them is not the contraction of smooth muscle, as in other known vasomotor mechanisms, but its relaxation (Brindley 1985*b*). Appropriate signals from the autonomic nervous system can cause the venous outlets to open or close even if the pressure in the corpus cavernosum is artificially maintained constant at above the systolic blood pressure (Brindley 1983). Structures have been seen by electron microscopy that seem likely to be those responsible for this reversal of the usual action of smooth muscle on blood vessels (Lue *et al.* 1985).

The opening up of arterial supply that also occurs in erection depends, as one would expect, on relaxation of the muscular coats of arteries. For the corpus cavernosum, it is arteries within this structure (i.e. the cavernosal artery and its helicine branches) that are mainly responsible, as is shown by the fact that in most men intracavernosal injection of drugs that relax smooth muscle (papaverine, phenoxybenzamine) in doses too small to have any action outside that structure, causes *full* cavernosal erection. However, there are some men whose pattern of response to smooth-muscle relaxants strongly suggests that, at least in them, arteries outside the corpus cavernosum (penile artery and the first part of the cavernosal artery) take part in the vasodilator response to sexual arousal. In these men small intracavernosal doses of papaverine cause incomplete erection; increasing the dose does not increase the action, but sexual arousal, with intracavernosal papaverine or sometimes even without it, causes full erection (Brindley, unpublished). The probable interpretation is that the drug dilates the intracavernosal vessels fully, but does not affect the extracavernosal supply vessels; sexual arousal adds the extracavernosal vasodilatation that is needed in these men (though not in most men) to achieve full erection.

The penis has three distinct autonomic nerve supplies: parasympathetic erectile, sympathetic erectile, and sympathetic anti-erectile. The first of these has been well known for over a century (Eckhardt 1863). The second and third, though not recent discoveries, have only recently emerged from obscurity and controversy.

The parasympathetic erectile fibres in man leave the spinal cord by the second and third sacral anterior roots. Erection can be produced by electrical stimulation of these roots. Better responses are usually obtained from S2 than from S3. Stimulation of S4 rarely causes any swelling of the penis.

From branches of the sacral segmental nerves the parasympathetic erectile fibres enter the pelvic splanchnic plexus, where they are presumably mixed with parasympathetic fibres that innervate the bladder. The next part of their course is not exactly known, but a combination of fairly recent anatomical and surgical evidence (Walsh and Donker 1982) shows that they, together with the sympathetic erectile fibres, run close to the prostate and membranous urethra. Here they were often damaged in the older techniques of prostatectomy and urethral sphincterotomy. Current techniques, using the new anatomical knowledge, allow them to be spared.

The preganglionic fibres of the sympathetic erectile and anti-erectile pathways leave the cord by lower thoracic and upper lumbar anterior roots; the exact segments are unknown. At the level of the bifurcation of the aorta, the erectile and anti-erectile fibres are anatomically separate in the rabbit (Sjöstrand and Klinge 1979), the erectile fibres running in the hypogastric plexus and the anti-erectile in the sympathetic chains. In the cat and baboon, the hypogastric plexus contains both erectile and anti-erectile fibres, and stimulating it electrically can cause either erection or shrinkage of the penis, the effect varying with the pulse frequency. Small doses of α_1-adrenoceptor blockers convert the response to a purely erectile one. In man, only erectile responses have yet been observed on stimulating the hypogastric plexus (Brindley 1986*a*), but by analogy with the baboon it is likely that some anti-erectile fibres are also present. Penile responses to stimulation of the lower parts of the sympathetic chains have not yet been studied in any primate. It seems likely that, as in the rabbit, anti-erectile effects would be found.

The autonomic plexuses of the pelvis are anatomically complex, and little is known about the course by which the sympathetic erectile and anti-erectile fibres reach the erectile tissue. However, these plexuses can be stimulated electrically through the rectum. This is regularly done to obtain semen from men with spinal injuries (Brindley 1984) and to test the efferent innervation of the bladder. It could be used to make a rough map of the erectile, anti-erectile, or detrusor-activating autonomic fibres in a given patient, if this information were needed.

The excitatory transmission from postganglionic fibres to smooth-muscle cells in the sympathetic anti-erectile pathway is α_1-adrenergic. Blocking the α_1-adrenoceptors with intracavernosal phenoxybenzamine, phentolamine, or thymoxamine causes full erection in most normal men; blocking the release of noradrenalin from the sympathetic anti-erectile terminals with intracavernosal guanethidine causes very conspicuous enlargement of the penis, but not full erection (Brindley 1986*b*). The difference between these two states doubtless depends on the stimulation of α_1-adrenoceptors by circulating catecholamines when local noradrenalin release is prevented by guanethidine but the adrenoceptors are not blocked.

The mechanism of inhibitory transmission from postganglionic fibres to smooth muscle cells in the parasympathetic and sympathetic erectile pathways is unknown. It is clearly not muscarinic, since erection is unaffected by as much as 1.8 mg of atropine given intravenously

(Brindley, unpublished), and by intracavernosal doses that should give even higher local concentrations (Brindley 1986*b*). Nor is it β-adrenergic (Brindley 1986*b*). VIP is a candidate for consideration as possible transmitter, since it is present at appropriate sites in the penis (Polak *et al.* 1981) and has appropriate actions on penile smooth muscle (Adaikan *et al.* 1986).

Editor's note. Space prevents inclusion of a review of the fallopian tubes and uterus. The colon, rectum, and anal canal are reviewed in Chapter 14 and there is a recent review by Gonella *et al.* (1986).

REFERENCES

Adaikan, P. G., Kottegoda, S. R., and Ratnam, S. S. (1986). Is vasoactive intestinal polypeptide the principal transmitter involved in human penile erection? *J. Urol.* **135**, 638–40.

Aguado, L. and Ojeda, S. R. (1986). Prepubertal rat ovary: hormonal modulation of beta-adrenergic receptors and of progesterone response to adrenergic stimulation. *Biol. Reprod.* **34**, 45–50.

Ahmed, C. E., Dees, W. L., and Ojeda, S. R. (1986). The immature rat ovary is innervated by VIP-containing fibers and responds to VIP with steroid secretion. *Endocrinology* **118**, 1882–9.

Anton, P. G., Duncan, M. E., and McGrath, J. C. (1977). An analysis of the anatomical basis for the mechanical response to motor nerve stimulation of the rat vas deferens. *J. Physiol.* **272**, 23–43; **273**, 45.

Awad, S. A., Downie, J. W., and Lywood, D. W. (1976). Sympathetic activity in the proximal urethra in patients with urinary obstruction. *J. Urol.* **115**, 545–7.

Baumgarten, H. G., Holstein, A. F., and Rosengren, E. (1971). Arrangement, ultrastructure and adrenergic innervation of smooth musculature of the ductuli efferentes, ductus epididymis and ductus deferens of man. *Z. Zellforsch. Mikroskop. Anat.* **120**, 37–79.

Brindley, G. S. (1983). Physiology of erection and management of paraplegic infertility. In *Male infertility* (ed. T. B. Hargreave). Springer, Berlin.

Brindley, G. S. (1984). The fertility of men with spinal injuries. *Paraplegia* **22**, 337–48.

Brindley, G. S. (1985*a*). Pathophysiology of erection and ejaculation. In *Textbook of genito-urinary surgery* (ed. H. N. Whitfield and W. F. Hendry) Vol. 2, pp. 1083–94. Churchill Livingstone, Edinburgh.

Brindley, G. S. (1985*b*). The neurophysiology of erection. *First World Meeting on Impotence*, pp. 39–45. Centre d'Etudes et de Recherche de l'Impuissance, Paris.

Brindley, G. S. (1986*a*). Sacral root and hypogastric plexus stimulators and what these implants tell us about autonomic actions on the bladder and urethra. *Clin. Sci.* **70**, 415–45.

Brindley, G. S. (1986*b*). Pilot experiments on the actions of drugs injected into the human corpus cavernosum penis. *Br. J. Pharmacol.* **87**, 495–500.

Brindley, G. S., Polkey, C. E., and Rushton, D. N. (1982). Sacral anterior root stimulators for bladder control in paraplegia. *Paraplegia* **20**, 365–81.

Brindley, G. S., Polkey, C. E., Rushton, D. N., and Cardozo, L. (1986). Sacral anterior root stimulators for bladder control in paraplegia: the first 50 cases. *J. Neurol. Neurosurg. Psychiat.* **49**, 1104–14.

Brooks, M. E., Berezin, M., and Braf, Z. (1980). Treatment of retrograde ejaculation with imipramine. *Urology* **15**, 353–5.

Budge, J. (1858). Ueber das Centrum genitospinale des N sympathicus. *Virchow's Arch.* **15**, 115–26.

Callahan, S. M. and Creed, K. E. (1986). Non-cholinergic neurotransmission and the effects of peptides on the urinary bladder of guinea-pigs and rabbits. *J. Physiol.* **374**, 103–5.

Craggs, M. D., Rushton, D. N., and Stephenson, J. D. (1986). A putative non-cholinergic mechanism in urinary bladders of new but not old world primates. *J. Urol.* **136**, 1348–50.

Dyer, C. A. and Erickson, G. F. (1985). Norepinephrine amplifies HCG-stimulated androgen biosynthesis by ovarian theca-interstitial cells. *Endocrinology* **116**, 1645–52.

Eckhardt, C. (1863). Untersuchungen über die Erektion des Penis beim Hunde. *Beitr. Anat. Physiol.* **3**, 123–66.

El Badawi, A. and Schenk, E. A. (1966). Dual innervation of the mammalian urinary bladder. *Am. J. Anat.* **119**, 405–27.

Elliot, J. (1907). The innervation of the bladder and urethra. *J. Physiol.* **35**, 367–445.

Farrell, J. I. and Lyman, Y. (1937). A study of the secretory nerves of, and the action of certain drugs on, the prostate gland. *Am. J. Physiol.* **118**, 64–70.

Gonella, J., Blanquet, F., Grimand, J. C., and Bouvier, M. (1986). La commande nerveuse extrinsèque de colon et du sphincter anal interne. *Gastroenterol. clin. Biol.* **10**, 158–76.

Gosling, J. A. (1979). The structure of the bladder and urethra in relation to function. *Urol. Clin. N. Am.* **6**, 31–8.

Gosling, J. A., Dixon, J. S., and Lendon, R. G. (1977). The autonomic innervation of the human male and female bladder neck and proximal urethra. *J. Urol.* **118**, 302.

Gruber, C. M. (1933). The autonomic innervation of the genito-urinary system. *Physiol. Rev.* **13**, 497–509.

Kannisto, P. Owman, C., Schmidt, G., and Walles, B. (1986). Evidence for pre-junctional GABA receptors mediating inhibition of ovarian follicle contraction induced by nerve stimulation (cattle). *Eur. J. Pharmacol.* **122**, 123–9.

King, A. B. and Langworthy, O. R. (1940). Testicular degeneration following interruption of the sympathetic pathways. *J. Urol.* **44**, 74–82.

Kreulen, D. L. and Peters, S. (1986). Non-cholinergic transmission in a sympathetic ganglion of the guinea-pig elicited by colonic distension. *J. Physiol.* **374**, 315–34.

Lawrence, J. E. and Burden, H. W. (1980). The origin of the extrinsic adrenergic innervation to the rat ovary. *Anat. Rec.* **196**, 51–9.

Learmonth, J. R. (1931). A contribution to the neurophysiology of the urinary bladder in man. *Brain* **54**, 147–76.

Lue, T., Schmidt, R. A., and Tanagho, E. A. (1985). Histologic basis of venous constriction during erection induced by the intracorporeal injection of papaverine in dogs. *1st World Meeting on Impotence* 120–4.

Melick, W. F., Maryka, J. J., and Schmidt, J. H. (1962). Experimental studies of ureteral peristaltic pattern in the pig. 2. Myogenic activity of the pig ureter. *J. Urol.* **86**, 46–50.

Morita, T. and Tsuchida, S. (1983). Roles of adrenergic drugs in the renal pacemaker control of ureteral peristalsis. *Urol. int.* **38**, 285–92.

Morita, T., Wheeler, M. A., and Weiss, R. M. (1986). Effects of noradrenaline, isoproterenol and acetylcholine on ureteral resistance. *J. Urol.* **135**, 1296–8.

Notley, R. G. (1971). The innervation and musculature of the human ureter. *Ann. R. Coll. Surg. Engl.* **49**, 250–67.

Polak, J. M., Gu, J., Mina, S., and Bloom, S. R. (1981). Vipergic nerves in the penis. *Lancet* **ii**, 217–19.

Semans, J. H. and Langworthy, O. R. (1938). Observations on the neurophysiology of sexual function in the male cat. *J. Urol.* **40**, 836–46.

Sibley, G. N. A. (1984). A comparison of spontaneous and nerve-mediated activity in bladder muscle from man, pig and rabbit. *J. Physiol.* **354**, 431–43.

Sjöstrand, N. O. and Klinge, E. (1979). Principal mechanisms controlling penile retraction and protrusion in rabbits. *Acta physiol. scand.* **106**, 199–214.

Thomiak, R. H. H., Barlow, R. B., and Smith, P. J. B. (1985). Are there valid reasons for using anti-muscarinic drugs in the management of renal colic? *Br. J. Urol.* **57**, 498–9.

Torrens, M. J. (1978). Urethral sphincteric responses to stimulation of the sacral nerves in the human female. *Urol. int.* **33**, 22–6.

Versi, E., Cardozo, L. D., Studd, J. W., Brincat, M., O'Dowd, T. M., and Cooper, D. J. (1986). Internal urinary sphincter in maintenance of female continence. *Br. med. J.* **292**, 166–7.

Walsh, P. C. and Donker, P. J. (1982). Impotence following radical prostatectomy: insight into etiology and prevention. *J. Urol.* **128**, 492–7.

Weiss, G. K., Dail, W. G., and Ratner, A. (1982). Evidence for direct neural control of ovarian steroidogenesis in rats. *J. Reprod. Fertil.* **65**, 507–11.

Wylie, S. N., Roche, P. J., and Gibson, W. R. (1985). Ovulation after sympathetic denervation of the rat ovary produced by freezing its nerve supply. *J. Reprod. Fertil.* **75**, 369–73.

Zankl, H. and Leidl, W. (1969). Effect of vasoligation and a sympatholytic agent on the number of sperm cells in the epididymis in rabbits. *J. Reprod. Fertil.* **18**, 181–2.

14. The enteric nervous system: structure and pathology

N. D. Heaton, J. R. Garrett, and E. R. Howard

INTRODUCTION

The autonomic innervation of the gastrointestinal tract and the wide variety of pathological processes which may affect it are the subjects of increasing interest and investigation. In 1898 Langley coined the term 'autonomic nervous system' to express the idea of 'local autonomy' which exists to a limited extent in the sympathetic and parasympathetic nervous systems. He included the enteric nervous system as a separate and distinct division as it appeared to have a greater degree of independence from the central nervous system (and was therefore more deserving of the description 'autonomic') and its nerve cells had histologically distinct characteristics.

The enteric nervous system may be affected by a wide variety of pathological processes which include congenital, degenerative, inflammatory, metabolic, and parasitic disease. However, some well defined disorders of the gut may be caused by abnormal function of the intrinsic nerves without obvious histological change—examples of these include diffuse oesophageal spasm and some forms of intestinal pseudo-obstruction.

Abnormalities of gut innervation have to be distinguished from disorders of smooth muscle function, myoelectrical activity, or hormonal control. The end result of damage to intrinsic nerves is a loss of co-ordinated peristalsis in the affected segment, proximal smooth-muscle hypertrophy, and dilatation. The involvement of adjacent sphincters and particularly the loss of reflex relaxation results in further proximal hypertrophy and dilatation.

The degree of independence of function enjoyed by the enteric nervous system in the small and large bowel is shown by the relatively minor incidence of side-effects of extrinsic denervation such as truncal vagotomy. This contrasts, for example, with the severe loss of function in aganglionosis (Hirschsprung's disease) and the absence of the normal intrinsic innervation. The presence of intact intrinsic neurons rather than intact higher centres are critical for normal bowel motility.

THE NORMAL INNERVATION

The intrinsic innervation

The enteric nervous system consists of two ganglionic plexuses which run without interruption from the oesophagus to the anus. There is wide variation in neuronal shape and density in both plexuses in different regions of the gut. Striated muscle sphincters which are under a degree of voluntary control are present at either end of the gastrointestinal tract. In 1840 Remak observed ganglion cells in the wall of the pharynx and stomach; Meissner later described neurons within the submucosa, a finding confirmed by Lister who believed that the plexus regulated muscle contraction. In 1864 Auerbach described the myenteric plexus lying between the circular and longitudinal muscle layers consisting of ganglion cells interconnected by unmyelinated nerve fibres. Myelinated fibres are rarely found within the enteric plexus. The submucosal nerve plexuses are subdivided into Henle's plexus which lies adjacent to the inner aspect of the circular muscle and Meissner's plexus which is closer to the mucosa. These divisions are purely anatomical and no functional difference has yet been ascribed to them. A subserosal plexus has also been described in the stomach and small bowel of some animals, but there is no convincing evidence for its existence in man. The submucosal and myenteric plexuses are interconnected and innervate the mucosa, muscle layers, and blood vessels. No morphological distinction can be made between afferent and efferent nerves at present, but attempts are being made to unravel the complexity of the enteric nervous system by histological, histochemical, ultrastructural, and immunocytochemical investigation.

Histological appearance

Early attempts were made by Dogiel to classify enteric neurons into three types by their morphological appearance with methylene blue staining. Type 1 cells were multipolar with short branching dendrites which anastomosed with other similar cells and had single axons which he believed were motor to smooth muscle. Type 2 neurons had long dendritic endings in the mucosa (probably sensory), and type 3 cells were identified by short non-anastomosing dendrites. This method was not practical for the study of human bowel and was superseded by silver staining (Schofield 1968; Smith 1972). Using this method the myenteric plexus appears as a mesh of nerve fibres containing 20–30 axons of varying thickness. Ganglion cells are found at the corners of this mesh.

Some intrinsic nerves are thick and clearly stained in comparison to finer fibres which are a mixture of intrinsic and extrinsic nerves. Only a small proportion of intrinsic ganglion cells are argyrophilic, particularly in the small bowel although their numbers increase in the colon. The axons of argyrophilic neurons pass to neighbouring ganglia, while their dendrites end on argyrophobe neurons. However, the use of silver staining is limited by the relatively small proportion of neurons which stain positively; axons may not be distinguished from dendrites and no distinction may be made between motor, sensory, or interneurons.

Cholinesterase activity

Most intrinsic neurons in the myenteric plexus show strong cholinesterase activity (Fig. 14.1), although there is variation in the size and structure of ganglia and the intensity of cholinesterase staining. Individual ganglion cells also vary in size and cholinesterase activity; those with the strongest activity appear to be 'cholinergic' and account for the majority of intrinsic neurons and may correspond to argyrophobe cells identified by silver staining techniques.

Fine cholinesterase-positive nerves are present in the circular muscle

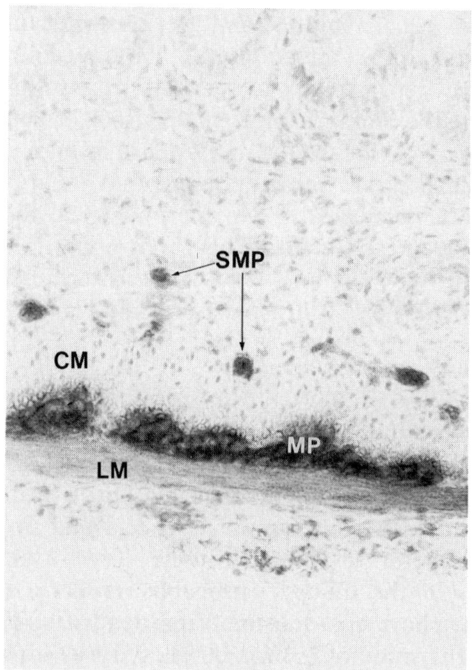

Fig. 14.1. Normal human fetal colon at 16 weeks stained for acetylcholinesterase activity, showing the developing myenteric (MP) and submucous plexuses (SMP). CM, circular muscle; LM, longitudinal muscle. Magnification ×250.

and larger trunks may be seen passing from the myenteric to the submucous plexuses. There are fewer nerves in the longitudinal muscle layer, but the number of nerves in both muscle layers appears to be relatively constant throughout the small and large bowel.

Ganglia within the submucosa often show less cholinesterase activity than those in the myenteric plexus, but have many positive nerves in close association.

Ultrastructural appearance

Studies of the myenteric plexus using the electron microscope reveal a complex structure resembling primitive central nervous tissue. The myenteric plexus lacks intraganglionic collagen, a feature that contrasts markedly with other peripheral autonomic ganglia and may relate to the unique mechanical stresses that ganglion cells are exposed to during peristalsis (Gabella 1979). The myenteric ganglia are compact, and the neurons reveal a wide variation in both size and cytoplasmic inclusions. Occasional neurons are seen with a particularly dense cytoplasm which suggest there are at least two types of cells relating perhaps to the argyrophobe and argyrophil cells described previously (Smith 1972). Another feature of the myenteric plexus is the peripheral position neurons occupy in ganglia with parts of their surface exposed to the basal lamina and the underlying circular and longitudinal muscle cells. There are large numbers of predominantly unmyelinated axons, dendrites, and supporting cells. The supporting cells have features in common with both the astroglial cells of the central nervous system and Schwann cells.

The basal lamina and supporting glial cells form a sheath around the myenteric plexus separating it from the extracellular space. The sheath excludes intraganglionic capillaries which therefore lie outside the glial covering. They are non-fenestrated and thick-walled resembling cerebral capillaries and possibly represent a 'blood–myenteric plexus barrier'. However, small molecules appear to have no difficulty in penetrating the ganglia and this may expose the autonomic nerves of the gut to injury from a wide variety of drug and metabolic insults from which the central nervous system is protected.

Many different enteric neurons have been recognized by their ultrastructural appearance and vesicle content (Furness and Costa 1980). Relatively few axons are found within the muscle layers and each axon appears to innervate several muscle fibres. Neurotransmitters are stored within vesicles along the course of these axons, particularly within varicosities which are often adjacent to muscle fibres (Howard and Garrett 1970). There are few recognizable pre- or postsynaptic structures and the axons simply run in close proximity to smooth muscle cells (Figs. 14.2 and 14.3).

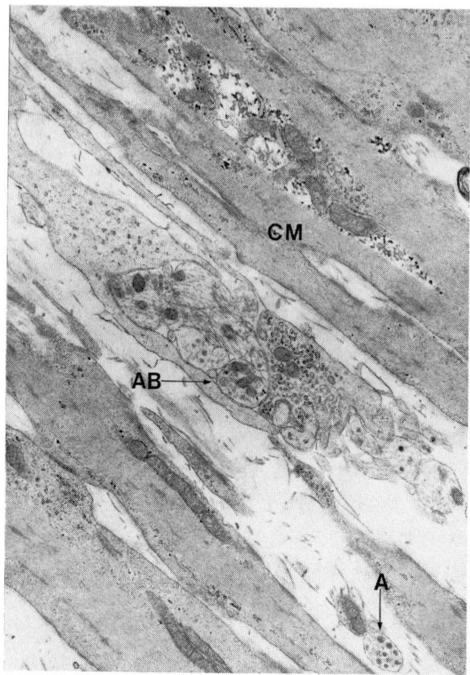

Fig. 14.2. Electron micrograph of axon bundle (AB) passing through circular muscle (CM). Individual axon (A) containing neurosecretory vesicles in close proximity to smooth muscle. Magnification ×8200.

The extrinsic innervation

This may be subdivided into parasympathetic, sympathetic, and sensory (afferent) nerves. The striking feature is the relative independence of the enteric nervous system from the central nervous system. Disruption of the extrinsic nerve supply leads to little or no impairment of function in the small and large bowel. The oesophagus and stomach, however, are dependent on the extrinsic innervation for normal function. This contrasts with lesions involving the intrinsic innervation which interrupt reflex pathways between sensory and inter- and motor neurons and lead to significant bowel dysfunction.

Parasympathetic innervation: the vagus nerve and the sacral parasympathetic nerves

The vagus is often considered an efferent nerve, but up to 80 per cent of its nerve fibres are afferent. The cells bodies of vagal fibres are present in the medulla and the jugular and nodose ganglia. The majority of vagal fibres are unmyelinated cholinergic axons, but adrenergic and non-cholinergic inhibitory nerves are also present. Recently, peptides

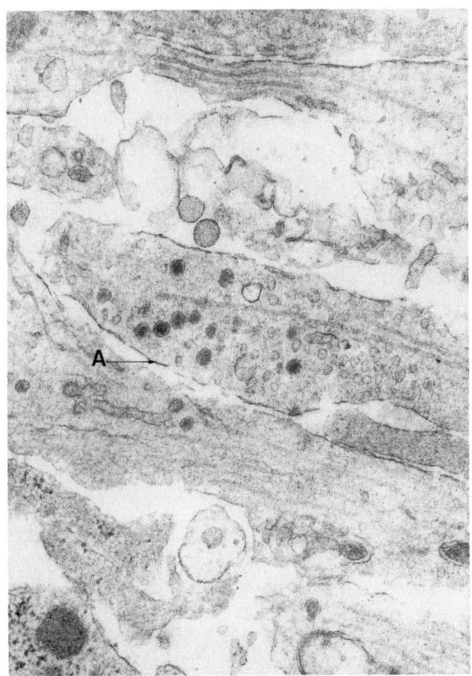

Fig. 14.3. Electron micrograph. Myenteric axon containing a mixed population of neurosecretory vesicles. A, individual axon. Magnification ×17 500.

including substance P, vasoactive intestinal polypeptide (VIP), somatostatin, and encephalin have been identified and appear to be involved in sensory pathways. The vagal innervation extends from the oesophagus to the transverse colon. The large area supplied by the vagus means that relatively few vagal fibres control a large number of intrinsic neurons. Smith (1972) showed that in the mouse one parasympathetic fibre innervated at least 48 intrinsic neurons.

The distal hindgut receives a parasympathetic supply from the second, third, and fourth sacral segments via the pelvic nerves. The parasympathetic nerves acting via the enteric ganglia are motor to the gut, but appear to have very little effect on smooth muscle of the internal anal sphincter.

Sympathetic innervation

Stimulation of the splanchnic or mesenteric nerves from the thoracolumbar outflow of the spinal cord inhibits gastrointestinal motility. In man as in most other mammals all adrenergic nerve-cell bodies are extrinsic to the gut (guinea-pig proximal colon is an exception). Adrenergic nerves enter the bowel in association with mesenteric blood vessels and are arranged around the myenteric and submucous ganglia

(Furness and Costa 1974). There is only a sparse supply to the smooth muscle layers including the muscularis mucosae (Fig. 14.4), which increases in the distal colo-rectum. There are, however, differences between species and various regions of the gut.

The cell bodies of the postganglionic fibres lie in the prevertebral ganglia of the coeliac, superior mesenteric, inferior mesenteric, and pelvic plexuses. The preganglionic nerves originate from the thoraco-lumbar spinal cord. T2–7 supply the oesophagus via the stellate ganglia and thoracic sympathetic chain, and segments T6–9 innervate stomach through the greater splanchnic nerves and coeliac ganglia. T6–11 and T12–L2 supply the small and large bowel, respectively. Adrenergic nerves decrease gut motility by acting indirectly on excitatory intrinsic cholinergic neurons to inhibit acetylcholine release, and only have a minor direct inhibitory action on smooth muscle. At rest adrenergic nerves innervating the myenteric plexus are inactive; activity is stimulated by reflex pathways from various levels including intrinsic, prevertebral ganglia, thoracolumbar spinal cord, and more centrally (Furness and Costa 1974).

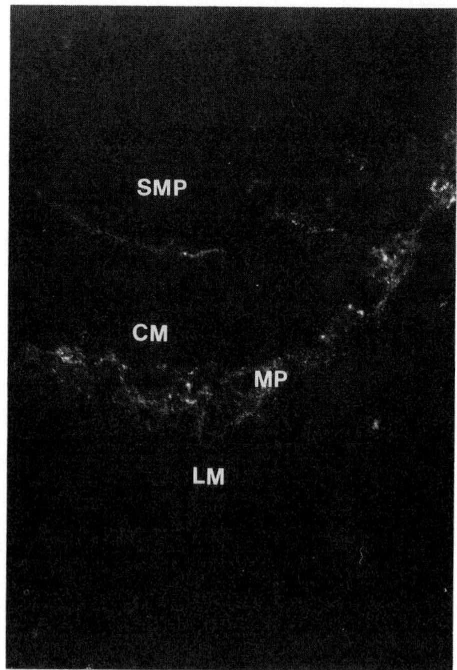

Fig. 14.4. Catecholamine fluorescence. Normal distribution of adrenergic nerves in human fetal colon at 16 weeks. Nerves arranged around myenteric (MP) and submucous plexuses (SMP). Note the sparse supply to circular (CM) and longitudinal muscles (LM). Magnification ×275.

Afferent innervation

Little is known of these nerves in man. Morphologically, the sensory endings are difficult to identify but may be small unmyelinated fibres ending in the mucosa and muscle. Some nerves are extrinsic; the majority, however, are intrinsic passing either to other enteric neurons or to the prevertebral ganglia. Receptors have been identified which respond to mechanical stimulation, particularly tension and stretch, to chemical stimuli such as intraluminal pH, glucose, and amino acids. Intestinal vagal receptors to glucose and heat have also been described (Rozé 1981).

Other intrinsic nerves

The existence of non-adrenergic, non-cholinergic inhibitory nerves was recognized by Langley in 1898 when he described gastric relaxation after vagal stimulation. Enteric nerves without the ultrastructural characteristics of adrenergic or cholinergic vesicles were later recognized and the large electron-dense cored vesicles were classified as 'P'-type. The development of immunocytochemistry, radioimmunoassay, and radioceptor assay techniques have revealed the presence of many substances other than the classical neurotransmitters acetylcholine and noradrenalin. The idea of one neurotransmitter per axon has been revised; each axon may contain several neurotransmitters capable of different actions. The largest group investigated are the peptide-hormones which have been identified in endocrine cells and enteric neurons. Some of these putative transmitters are present in both the gastrointestinal tract and the central nervous system.

Substance P, vasoactive intestinal polypeptide (VIP), encephalin, gastrin/cholecystokinin, neurotensin, somatostatin, calcitonin gene related peptide (CGRP), galanin, and neuropeptide Y (NPY) are some that have been identified in the enteric plexuses. Substance P-, VIP-, and encephalin-like immunoreactivity have also been identified in the human vagus.

5-Hydroxytryptamine seems established as a neurotransmitter in mammalian myenteric plexus; dopamine, gama-aminobutyric acid (GABA), histamine, and purine derivatives, including adenosine-5-triphosphate (ATP), have also been proposed as neurotransmitters.

As peristalsis depends on co-ordinated waves of descending inhibition followed by descending excitation, interest has focused on possible intrinsic inhibitory nerves. ATP or VIP have been proposed as the neurotransmitter in these nerves, whereas the excitatory wave is associated with cholinergic nerves. The roles of many peptides in the control of gut motility are still unknown, although some act by enhancing or antagonizing the release of acetylcholine.

Circulating intestinal hormones (gastrin, secretin, CCK, pancreatic polypeptide, motilin, enteroglucagon, etc.) may modify bowel activity by their influence on the autonomous activity of intestinal smooth muscle. Smooth-muscle cells have receptors for both classical neurotransmitters and gastrointestinal peptides; at least 16 have now been identified, for example, on the muscle of the lower oesophageal sphincter (LOS) (Goyal and Rattan 1975). Neuronal activity may also be modified by circulating peptides and catecholamines. An example is the activation of excitatory cholinergic nerves in the LOS by circulating motilin.

Thus the neural control of gastrointestinal motility is mediated through a series of complex references involving the intrinsic plexus, pelvic and sympathetic ganglia, spinal cord, and the central nervous system. Intrinsic neural activity may be modified by the action of extrinsic nerves, circulating hormones, and the central nervous system. Pathological processes which interfere with any part of this control system will alter gastrointestinal function.

THE DEVELOPMENT OF THE ENTERIC NERVOUS SYSTEM

Enteric ganglia are derived from 'vagal' neural-crest cells which migrate into the area of the branchial arches, before becoming incorporated into the developing foregut. These neural-crest cells colonize the gut at an early stage of development well before the ingrowth of extrinsic nerves. As the bowel elongates, these precursor cells become distributed throughout its length. The chick–quail chimera marker system has been used to determine the migration and development of neural crest cells (Cochard and Le Douarin 1982). Distinct morphological differences exist between the neural crest of the chick and quail, but transplantation of neural-crest cells between the two species results in apparently normal migration and development of both transplanted and host tissues which remain readily identifiable.

Studies in the chick have confirmed that the vagal neural crest is the major source of enteric neurons, although there is a relatively minor contribution of neurons to the postumbilical gut from the lumbosacral neural crest. It seems likely that man is similar to the rabbit and mouse in having a single source of enteric neurons migrating from the vagal neural crest (Okamoto and Ueda 1967). The sacral parasympathetic nerves (S2, 3, 4) innervating the distal hindgut develop from sacral neural crest, but there is no evidence of neurons migrating from this source to the distal bowel in man. Le Douarin (Cochard and Le Douarin 1982) also confirmed the potential of all levels of the neural crest to develop into enteric neurons when transplanted. This suggests that environmental influences may be more important in determining the neuronal characteristics than any initial premigration programming.

The use of explants of the gut tube of the chick embryo and its growth on chorio-allantoic membrane has confirmed that neural-crest cells from all levels are able to form enteric neurons. However, there does appear to be a long delay between the arrival of neuronal precursors and their development into morphologically recognizable ganglion cells (Gershon *et al.* 1983). This may explain the varying descriptions in the appearance of ganglion cells along craniocaudal gradients. During migration neural crest cells initially become committed to a neuronal type, then to either an autonomic or a sensory role, and finally to a particular neurotransmitter. A normal migratory and enteric microenvironment are necessary for the normal development of the enteric nervous system.

PATHOLOGY OF THE ENTERIC NERVOUS SYSTEM

Oesophagus

The elderly

Oesophageal motor dysfunction which includes loss of tone, loss of stripping waves, and tertiary contractions is common in the elderly. A loss of ganglion cells in the myenteric plexus in association with a round-cell infiltrate has been described. However, diseases which impair the neuromuscular pathways controlling swallowing such as cerebrovascular disease, parkinsonism, pseudobulbar palsy, and diabetes mellitus are more commonly the cause.

Lower oesophageal sphincter (LOS) incompetence (gastrooesophageal reflux)

Gastrooesophageal reflux presents with heartburn, oesophagitis, and occasionally with oesophageal stricture. The primary abnormality is a loss of LOS tone and its failure to respond to increased intra-abdominal pressure. This pressure-rise reflex is also reduced after truncal vagotomy and there is evidence of abnormal vagal function in at least 25 per cent of these patients.

Achalasia

Achalasia is an unusual neuromuscular disorder of the oesophagus characterized by the absence of normal oesophageal peristalsis and the failure of the lower oesophageal sphincter to relax reflexly after swallowing. Clinically it presents with dysphagia for liquids and solids, pain, oesophageal regurgitation, and, in the elderly, with aspiration pneumonia (Fig. 14.6). Radiological features include the loss of normal oesophageal peristalsis, dilatation, and a smooth tapering appearance of the distal oesophagus (Fig. 14.5). Oesophageal manometry confirms the loss of normal peristalsis, the failure of lower oesophageal relaxation,

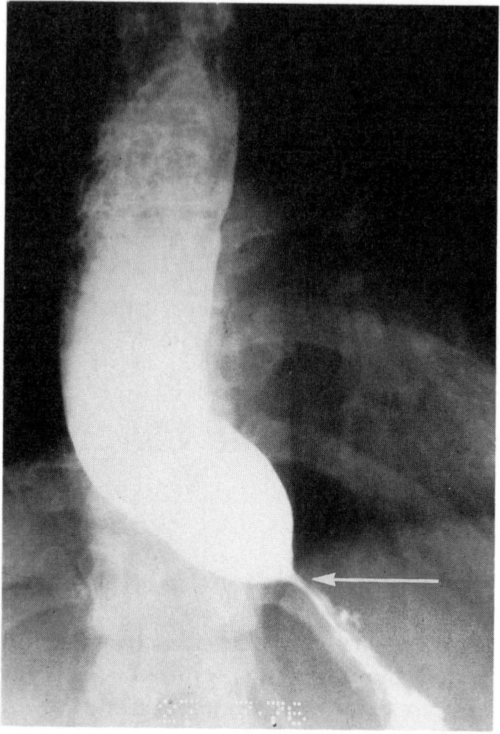

Fig. 14.5. Achalasia. Barium swallow showing a narrowed lower oesophageal segment (arrowed). Dilated proximal oesophagus filled with barium.

and an elevated resting LOS pressure. Symptoms may be relieved by either sphincter dilatation or cardiomyotomy.

Achalasia occurs at all ages, including infants, but presents most frequently between the fifth and sixth decades. Fewer than a fifth of patients present within one year of the onset of symptoms.

Rake first reported the absence of myenteric neurons in two cases of achalasia examined at post-mortem in association with a lymphocytic infiltration which was most marked in the cardia and less marked proximally. Hurst and Rake (1930) drew attention to the marked dilatation and circular smooth-muscle hypertrophy found in achalasia, but which was absent from longstanding organic oesophageal strictures. He drew a parallel to Hirschsprung's disease and suggested that both might have a similar pathology, and confirmed the absence of ganglion cells in the myenteric plexus of the cardia. However, the loss of neurons in the cardia appears to be rather more variable than in the body of the oesophagus. Degenerative changes in the dorsal vagal nucleus in the medulla and vagus nerves have been described, but many investigators

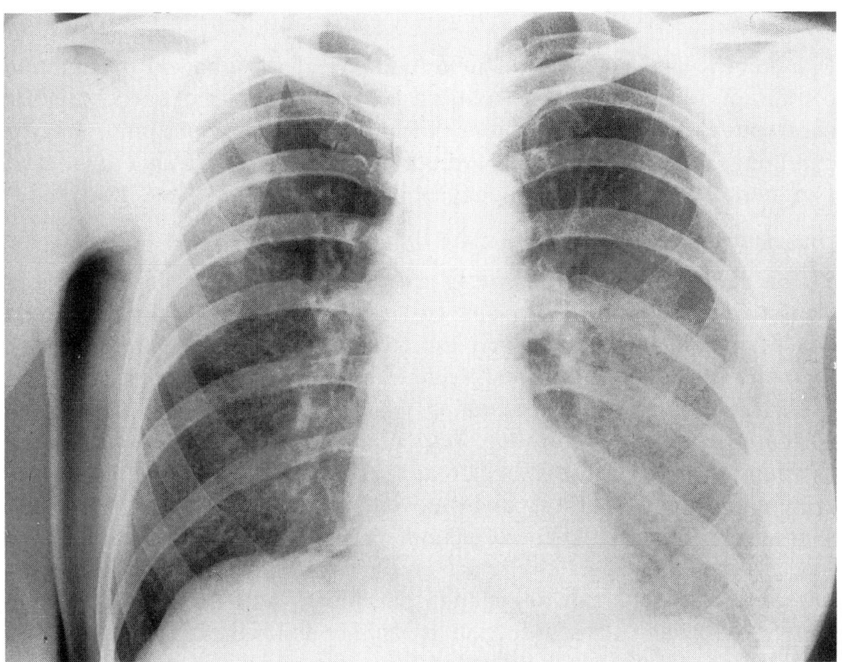

Fig. 14.6. Achalasia. Plain chest X-ray. Aspiration pneumonia secondary to achalasia.

have found no abnormality. However, as many of the nerve fibres in the vagus are unmyelinated (and do not undergo Wallerian degeneration), relatively major abnormalities can be missed. Clinical evidence of vagal involvement in achalasia is provided by the insulin stress test in which gastric acid secretion is stimulated by insulin-induced hypoglycaemia. This requires intact vagal nerves and approximately half the patients with achalasia have abnormal responses.

VIP immunoreactive nerve fibres in the lower oesophagus are reduced in number and content in achalasia. This could be secondary to neuronal degeneration, although substance P levels are unaffected. VIP relaxes oesophageal smooth muscle *in vitro* and the LOS *in vivo* and may be the neurotransmitter involved in reflex relaxation.

Achalasia secondary to adenocarcinoma of the oesophagus, cardia, bronchus, and pancreas, in close proximity to or invading the myenteric plexus of the oesophagus has been reported. Reversible achalasia has been described following treatment of a lymphoma in the distal oesophagus. The mechanism may be secondary to direct myenteric plexus invasion, or indirectly as part of a peripheral neuropathy induced by malignancy, or represent a non-specific oesophageal response to distal obstruction.

Diabetes

Manometric and radiological investigations of oesophageal dysfunction commonly reveal absent or reduced primary peristaltic waves, tertiary contractions, loss of LOS tone with associated reflux, and delayed emptying, although clinical symptoms such as dysphagia are rare. Degenerative changes in oesophageal nerve trunks have been described.

American trypanosomiasis (Chagas' disease)

This is caused by *Trypanosomiasis cruzi*, a protozoal parasite endemic in Central and South America and carried by the blood-sucking reduviid bug, *Triatoma infestons*, which excretes the trypanosome in its faeces. Human infection results from trypanosomes entering through abrasions of the face and mucous membranes.

There is a brisk immune response which eliminates circulating trypanosomes from the bloodstream. A visible granuloma is usually present at the site of trypanosome entry and the initial infection is characterized by fever, hepatosplenomegaly, and local lymphadenopathy. The parasite lodges in the heart and nervous plexuses of the gastrointestinal tract; the salivary glands, the biliary and urinary tracts may also be affected. Acute infection is usually followed by a long-lasting quiescent phase before the development of cardiac and gastrointestinal complications. Koberle (1963) initially suggested that dead parasites release a neurotoxin which injures autonomic nerves, but more recently an autoimmune mechanism has been recognized. *T. cruzi* shares common antigenic components with heart muscle cells and enteric ganglion cells. The presence of an antiparasympathetic-neuron IgG has been described in 83 per cent of patients. Vagal ganglion cells are also destroyed and replaced with lymphocytic infiltrates. Specific treatment is indicated for the acute phase, but there is no evidence that it benefits the chronic phase of the illness.

The oesophagus, colo-rectum, and duodenum are most frequently involved and present with slowly progressive dysphagia and constipation. The severity of dysfunction is related to the degree of destruction of neurons and Schwann cells in the myenteric plexus which are replaced by connective tissue. Hypertrophy and possibly hyperplasia of circular smooth muscle occurs in the early phase of the disease, but, as dilatation progresses, the muscle becomes thin.

The initial involvement is confined to the body of the oesophagus and the lower oesophageal sphincter is only affected later. Abnormal oesophageal motility occurs with destruction of 50 per cent of the myenteric-plexus neurons and dilatation when 90 per cent are destroyed. The motility disorder is similar to achalasia and barium examination reveals tertiary waves, stasis of contrast, spastic oesophageal contractions, and failure of the LOS to relax. Oesophageal dilatation is gradually progressive and may reach 8–10 cm in diameter. The oesophageal smooth muscle is hypersensitive to cholinergic drugs, and the response is ascribed to a denervation hypersensitivity. Carcinoma is a late complication in 5–10 per cent of patients with megaoesophagus.

Balloon dilatation of the lower oesophagus or cardiomyotomy (Heller's procedure) can give long-term remission of symptoms. The long-term prognosis is dependent on the severity of myocardial involvement.

Stomach

Diabetes

Patients with acute gastric dilatation secondary to diabetic ketoacidosis present with abdominal pain and vomiting which is relieved by nasogastric aspiration and good diabetic control.

Prolonged gastric dilatation with reduced peristalsis and delayed emptying (gastroparesis diabeticorum) is a feature of diabetic autonomic neuropathy but it is an uncommon complication. Symptoms of gastric-outlet obstruction, if severe, are difficult to treat satisfactorily. Small, frequent meals, drugs such as metoclopramide, and surgical drainage procedures are usually of limited benefit. Gastric vagal denervation is thought to cause the gastroparesis and electron microscopic studies of the vagus have shown a marked reduction in the number of unmyelinated fibres.

Gastric vagal denervation may also explain a reported decrease in gastric-acid production and incidence of duodenal (but not gastric) ulcers in diabetics (Hosking *et al.* 1978).

Hypertrophic pyloric stenosis of infancy

This is characterized by hypertrophy and hyperplasia of pyloric circular muscle causing gastric-outlet obstruction. Hirschsprung's description in 1888 established infantile pyloric stenosis as a recognizable clinical entity. The mean incidence in the United Kingdom is 2.5 per 1000 live births and may be increasing. Symptoms start most commonly at 3 weeks, but occur at any time up to 3 months of age. It is four times more common in boys and associated with a strong hereditary influence with a polygenic mode of inheritance. Clinically, patients present with forceful projectile vomiting and constipation. Visible gastric peristalsis and a palpable pyloric 'tumour' confirm the diagnosis. The radiological features include delayed gastric emptying and an elongated pyloric canal. A true congenital origin seems unlikely as five out of 1000 newborn male infants with normal barium meals later developed pyloric stenosis.

Many abnormalities of the enteric innervation have been reported, but there is disagreement over their significance and as to whether the changes are primary or secondary to compression by circular smooth muscle hypertrophy. Degenerating myenteric ganglia and reduced numbers of ganglion cells and nerve trunks prompted suggestions that excessive vagal stimulation might cause neuronal 'exhaustion'.

Delayed development of the myenteric plexus and associated motor overactivity was proposed to explain the development of circular muscle hypertrophy and mechanical obstruction. However, there is no increase in the incidence of pyloric stenosis in premature infants. The absence of argyrophil neurons (co-ordinating peristalsis) without degenerative changes was reported in a small number of patients, and a similar deficiency of these cells was described in a familial syndrome of short small bowel, malrotation, and pyloric hypertrophy with an absence of peristalsis. There was also overgrowth of extrinsic axons and increased numbers of often immature neurons per ganglion.

The conflict between possible developmental and degenerative aetiologies has not resolved with the study of the peptidergic innervation. Decreased numbers of substance-P, encephalin, VIP, and neuropeptide-Y immunoreactive nerves have been described in the hypertrophied pyloric circular muscle. There is no agreement, however, over the presence or absence of degenerative changes in the remaining nerves.

Surgical division of the pyloric circular muscle leads to resolution of the muscle hypertrophy and the pylorus becomes macroscopically normal within months. Bypass procedures surprisingly lead to the persistence of muscle hypertrophy into adult life.

Primary hypertrophic pyloric stenosis of adults

Primary hypertrophic stenosis presents most commonly in the fifth decade with symptoms of gastric-outlet obstruction and is often complicated by gastritis or gastric ulceration. Hypertrophy and hyperplasia of the circular muscle is most marked at the pyloroduodenal junction. Smith described two cases with absent argyrophil neurons and an increase in the number of Schwann cells, but other studies have found no abnormality in either the number or appearance of ganglion cells.

Duodenum

Idiopathic megaduodenum

Hypertrophy and dilatation of the duodenum was first ascribed to mechanical obstruction by the superior mesenteric blood vessels. However, two cases were described with non-rotation of the colon where the superior mesenteric vessels did not cross the duodenum and bypass operations in other patients have not led to a decrease in duodenal size. An isolated absence of duodenal ganglion cells with a normal jejunal myenteric plexus has been recognized. Although megaduodenum is considered to be a separate entity, it is becoming apparent that many cases form part of the spectrum of chronic intestinal pseudo-obstruction. These patients present with vomiting and abdominal pain; investigation of family members may reveal asymptomatic megaduodenum. Systemic sclerosis may also affect the duodenum causing dilatation and obstruction. Surgical treatment is often disappointing and should be reserved for patients with severe symptoms and apparently localized disease. Side-to-side duodeno–jejunostomy has been most widely used to relieve symptoms.

Chagas' disease

Megaduodenum is usually associated with the presence of megaoesophagus and megacolon. Smooth-muscle hypertrophy and dilatation follow increasing neuronal destruction in the myenteric plexus (Koberle 1963).

Jejunum and ileum

Jejunal diverticulosis

Jejunal diverticula are usually multiple, occurring on the mesenteric border of the small bowel, are thought to be acquired, and present in adult life. Only 10–40 per cent are believed to present with intestinal pseudo-obstruction, blind-loop syndrome, volvulus, or with complications of diverticula (abscess, perforation, haemorrhage). In a group of patients with jejunal diverticulosis and intestinal pseudo-obstruction Krishnamurthy *et al.* (1983) described neuronal and axonal degeneration with intranuclear inclusions typical of a visceral neuropathy in one patient. Two patients had a visceral myopathy and four others had smooth-muscle fibrosis and degeneration characteristic of systemic sclerosis. In contrast to other forms of intestinal pseudo-obstruction, there is less involvement of the oesophagus, stomach, and colon. Because of the diffuse nature of the underlying disorder, surgical resection of the bowel containing diverticula seldom provides long-term relief.

Intestinal pseudo-obstruction

Intestinal pseudo-obstruction presents clinically with the symptoms and signs of intestinal obstruction with no underlying mechanical cause. Plain abdominal X-rays suggest mechanical obstruction, but barium studies show disordered motility. Isolated segments of small or large bowel or the entire gastrointestinal tract may be involved. It may be present as an acute (paralytic or adynamic ileus) or as a chronic (continuous or recurring) disorder. Chronic pseudo-obstruction is often secondary to diseases such as scleroderma, systemic lupus erythematosus, dermatomyositis, amyloidosis, and neurological disorders which include Parkinson's disease, multiple sclerosis, myotonia dystrophica, and a number of drug-induced disorders.

Adynamic or paralytic ileus

Small-bowel motility may be altered by a wide range of conditions. Sepsis, electrolyte imbalance, brain injury, abdominal surgery, and major organ failure may all be associated with ileus. Transient bowel dysfunction in the neonatal period may occur with hypothyroidism, hypermagnesaemia, maternal ingestion of psychotrophic drugs, heroin, and ganglion-blocking agents. Recovery follows treatment with intravenous fluids, but surgical causes may prove difficult to exclude if there is severe or long-lasting intestinal obstruction.

The intestinal obstruction is characterized by a loss of effective peristalsis although myogenic contractility and responses to electrical and chemical stimuli are normal. Furness and Costa (1974) identified peripheral, prevertebral ganglionic, and spinal pathways involved in ileus. Possible underlying mechanisms include increased sympathetic nervous activity, non-cholinergic non-adrenergic inhibitory nerves, increased circulating catecholamines and gastrointestinal hormones.

It has been suggested that ileus has a protective function directing blood away from the gut to increase cardiac output. It is significant that noradrenergic nerves innervate both the gut vasculature and myenteric neurons. Stimulation of these nerves reduces the blood supply to the bowel and decreases neuronal activity in the myenteric plexus thus indirectly reducing peristalsic activity.

Ileus invariably resolves with the correction of the underlying cause. The treatment of prolonged postoperative ileus with drugs which block noradrenalin release or α-adrenergic receptor sites on myenteric ganglia have proved successful in clinical practice (Neely and Catchpole 1971). Direct stimulation of bowel motility by increasing 'parasympathetic drive' using choline esters, such as carbachol, or by the anticholinesterase neostigmine has also been effective either alone or in combination with adrenergic blockers. More recently the peptides, caerulin and motilin, have been used with moderate success.

Chronic idiopathic intestinal pseudo-obstruction

This disorder is characterized by the clinical features of mechanical bowel obstruction; barium studies, however, reveal abnormal gastrointestinal motility and no organic obstruction. The diagnosis should be reserved for cases with normal smooth-muscle and ganglion-cell morphology. Theoretically, abnormalities of intrinsic neurons, smooth muscle, and intestinal hormones must be responsible for the disordered motility and subsequent functional bowel obstruction. Many conditions previously grouped under this title have been distinguished by the use of physiological, histochemical, and ultrastructural investigations and divisions into neuronal (visceral neuropathy) or myogenic (visceral myopathy) abnormalities or combinations of the two are now feasible.

Clinical symptoms of intermittent abdominal pain, distension, vomiting, and diarrhoea or constipation usually begin during adolescence, and a family history of pesudo-obstruction is present in a third of patients.

Visceral myopathies present with oesophageal dysfunction (low-amplitude simultaneous contractions after swallowing), gross megaduodenum, decreased small-bowel motility, and bladder involvement is common. A familial incidence indicates a dominant mode of inheritance with incomplete penetration. Systemic sclerosis primarily affecting small bowel presents with a very similar appearance. Abnormalities described in visceral neuropathies using silver stains include the loss of argyrophobe and argyrophil neurons, axonal damage and degeneration with increased numbers of Schwann cells (Schuffler *et al.* 1981). In contrast to visceral myopathies, there are continuous spontaneous oesophageal contractions, more modest duodenal dilatation, and hyperactive small-bowel contractions which are associated with poor propulsion.

Degenerative changes of myenteric argyrophobe neurons have been described in association with mental retardation and basal ganglia calcification in a postmeasles encephalitis syndrome. The loss of myenteric ganglion cells, Schwann-cell proliferation, and intranuclear inclusions in neurons and glial cells of the myenteric plexus, spinal-cord, dorsal-root, and coeliac-plexus ganglia resulted in hyperactive, unco-ordinated gastrointestinal muscle activity.

Some disease processes appear to be purely functional and no structural abnormalities are identifiable. Defective muscarinic receptors and a lack of response to cholinergic and anticholinesterase drugs have been described in a patient with chronic intestinal pseudo-obstruction and an autoimmune mechanism with the production of an antibody to muscarinic receptors was thought to be responsible (Bannister and Hoyes 1981).

Colon and rectum

Diabetes

Diarrhoea may present in association with severe peripheral autonomic neuropathy. Typically, the diarrhoea is nocturnal, profuse, watery, provoked by meals, and associated with urgency and tenesmus. Treatment is symptomatic, spontaneous remissions occur, but recurrence is usual. Degenerative changes have been described in oesophageal and coeliac ganglia, and have been compared to postvagotomy diarrhoea.

Animal studies reveal abnormal enteric nerves with some features of progressive axonal dystrophy and regeneration.

Constipation is the commonest bowel disorder affecting approximately one-fifth of patients with diabetic neuropathy. Colonic motility is reduced and the postprandial gastrocolic reflex is absent.

Chagas' disease

Destruction of the myenteric plexus of the colon and rectum is common, resulting in a dilated and thickened colon, and presents with constipation or sigmoid volvulus. Colonic dilatation may regress after a defunctioning colostomy implying that anorectal dysfunction is important in the onset of intestinal obstruction.

Inflammatory bowel disease

Ulcerative colitis is a chronic inflammatory disease of the rectal mucosa which may extend to involve the rest of the large bowel. Increased numbers of ganglion cells have been described in chronic ulcerative colitis with Schwann cell and axon hyperplasia (Storsteen *et al.* 1953). With progressive inflammation, however, ganglion cell numbers decrease. Crohn's disease is a chronic inflammatory disorder involving all layers of the bowel wall and may affect any part of the gastrointestinal tract. Striking hyperplasia of mucosal VIP nerves and increases in the VIP content of affected bowel have been described in Crohn's, but not in ulcerative colitis or normal controls (Bishop *et al.* 1982). Ultrastructural studies have also revealed hyperplasia of nerves with degenerative changes in inflamed areas.

Familial dysautonomia

This is characterized by autonomic instability, impaired taste and pain sensation, hyporeflexia, fever, seizures, vomiting attacks, and a lack of normal lachrymation which occasionally responds dramatically to methacholine. Abnormalities of catecholamine metabolism, noradrenalin sensitivity, and response to intradermal histamine injection are present. A defect in the formation, storage, or release of acetylcholine has been postulated. Abnormal oesophageal motility, delayed relaxation of oesophageal sphincters associated with aspiration pneumonia, and mega-oesophagus are described. Patients may also present with diarrhoea or constipation and investigation has revealed jejunal distension, megacolon, and absent rectoanal reflexes with normal external anal sphincter responses.

Developmental anomalies

Aganglionosis

Hirschsprung described two patients with chronic constipation and congenital megacolon in 1887 and 6 years later Osler suggested that it was caused by a defect in the innervation of the colon which resulted in a failure of normal evacuation. The absence of ganglion cells in variable lengths of the rectum and colon was not recognized, however, for a further 50 years.

The incidence of congenital aganglionosis is one in 5000 live births; it has a sex-modified multifactorial mode of inheritance, although in some families an autosomal recessive inheritance is a possibility. There is a preponderance of males (4:1), which is most marked in short-segment disease. Children present with intestinal obstruction or chronic constipation. The severity of the presentation does not necessarily correlate to the length of aganglionic bowel. Enterocolitis is the major cause of death and is associated with a 30 per cent mortality (Fig. 14.7). The management of these children is colostomy (ileostomy for small-bowel involvement) and rectal biopsy followed by a definitive resection at approximately 6 months of age.

Aganglionic segments begin at the internal anal sphincter and extend proximally. The aganglionosis is limited to the rectosigmoid in 74 per cent of patients, 18 per cent involve more proximal colon, and 8 per cent extend throughout the colon and sometimes involve the small bowel.

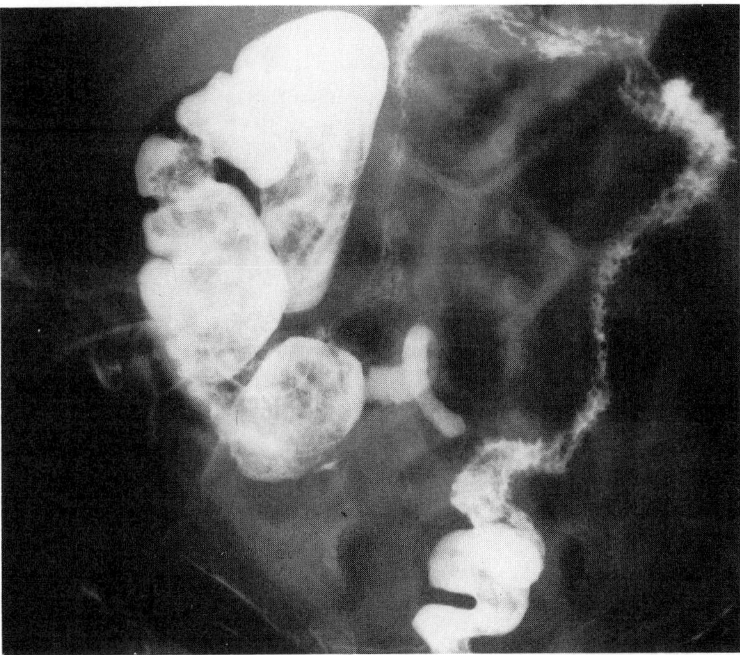

Fig. 14.7. Long-segment aganglionosis. Contrast enema outlining a contracted rectum and colon with dilated proximal bowel. Irregular mucosal pattern typical of enterocolitis.

The entire gastrointestinal tract is involved in rare cases (Kleinhaus *et al.* 1979).

The constant histological abnormality is the absence of ganglion cells in affected segments and the presence of large nerve trunks in the submucosal and myenteric plexuses (Howard and Garrett 1970). Histochemical studies show that these large nerve trunks are strongly positive for acetylcholinesterase activity and are thought to represent extrinsic cholinergic, parasympathetic nerves. Acetylcholinesterase-positive nerves within the lamina propria, muscularis mucosae, and circular muscle are increased in number (Fig. 14.8). The greatest number of acetylcholinesterase nerves in the circular muscle occur in the most distal aganglionic rectum and the severity of the clinical presentation relates to the number of nerves. Their numbers decrease proximally and the most proximal aganglionic and adjacent ganglionic tissues usually contain fewer nerves in the muscle layers than normal. Ultrastructurally, these predominantly unmyelinated nerves appear to be normal, and neuroeffector junctions within muscle are identifiable, suggesting that the

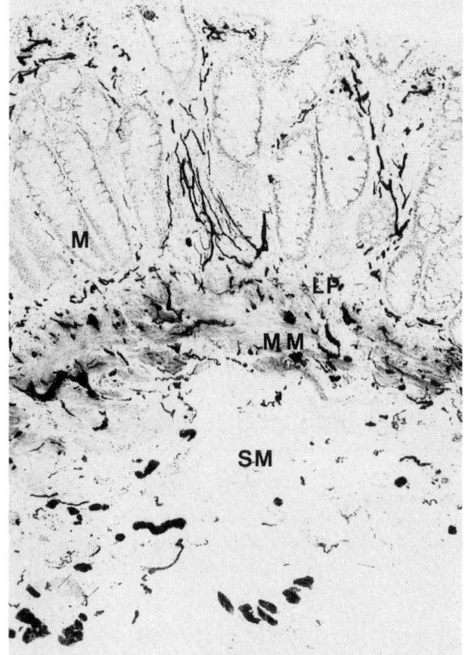

Fig. 14.8. Hirschsprung's disease. Stained for acetylcholinesterase activity. Increased numbers of strongly positive nerves in the lamina propria (LP) and muscularis mucosae (MM). Large strongly staining nerve trunks in the submucosa (SM). M, mucosa. Magnification ×75.

nerves are functional. This is supported by the observation that spinal anaesthesia causes relaxation of the aganglionic bowel.

In the absence of ganglia the adrenergic innervation is abnormal. There is a variable increase in the number of adrenergic nerves particularly in the smooth muscles layers. There are reduced numbers or complete absence of intrinsic peptide-containing nerves such as VIP, substance P, and serotonin. Increased numbers of extrinsic calcitonin gene-related peptide (CGRP)- and neuropeptide Y (NPY)-containing nerves have recently been described. CGRP occurs in sensory nerves implying that there is an overgrowth of all extrinsic nerves. A rare association of total colonic aganglionosis and failure of autonomic control of ventilation in infants has been ascribed to an absence of stem serotonergic nerves in the brain and gut.

There are several abnormalities in aganglionosis that contribute to the development of intestinal obstruction and megacolon. The absence of ganglion cells results in the failure of co-ordinated peristalsis. The uncoordinated contractions are dependent on the degree of cholinergic innervation to the circular muscle layer. The absence of peptidergic inhibitory nerves further enhances circular muscle excitation. Pressure studies of the anorectum have demonstrated an absent reflex relaxation of internal anal sphincter muscle which normally occurs with rectal distension and this adds a further obstructive element.

Associated congenital abnormalities include Down's syndrome, congenital deafness, and Waardenburg's syndrome (white forelock, widened epicanthic distance, broad nose root, and congenital deafness), hypoganglionosis, and multiple endocrine neoplasia type IIa.

Hypoganglionosis

The presence of reduced numbers of ganglion cells and nerves in the 'transitional' zone of Hirschsprung's disease is well recognized, but this appearance has been described in the absence of an aganglionic segment.

Hyperganglionosis

The presence of increased numbers of ganglion cells in some children presenting with severe bowel dysfunction is well recognized (Fadda *et al.* 1983). Symptoms vary from acute neonatal intestinal obstruction to chronic constipation. Fluid, electrolyte, and protein losses from the gut may be significant particularly if there is an associated enterocolitis. Uncoordinated segmental contractions with poor peristaltic activity are seen on barium enema and may be diagnostic. Hirschsprung's disease must be excluded by rectal biopsy. Anorectal inhibitory reflexes may be absent as they are in Hirschsprung's disease and thus cause confusion.

The pathological features of hyperganglionosis include hyperplasia of the submucosal and myenteric plexuses (Fig. 14.9), neurons within the

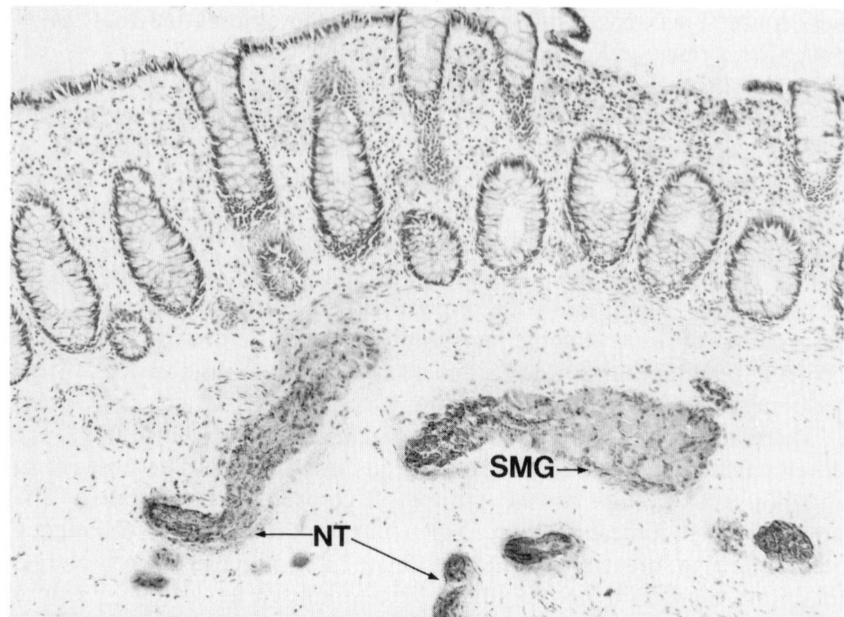

Fig. 14.9. Hyperganglionosis. Stained for acetylcholinesterase activity. Large submucosal ganglia (SMG) and nerve trunks (NT). Many neurons show weak acetylcholinesterase activity. Magnification ×150.

lamina propria, and increased numbers of cholinesterase-positive nerve fibres within the lamina propria and circular muscle (Meier-Ruge 1974). Ultrastructural studies reveal large numbers of axons containing many peptidergic vesicles (Fig. 14.10). Hyperganglionosis has been reported in association with distal aganglionosis which, if recognized, may cause persistent bowel dysfunction after a pullthrough operation. A diffuse form affecting the entire gastrointestinal tract is recognized as part of multiple endocrine adenomas type 2b (medullary-cell carcinoma of the thyroid, phaeochromocytoma, and mucosal neuromas). Gastrointestinal symptoms invariably precede the development of these neuroendocrine tumours.

Neurofibromatosis

Gastrointestinal neurofibromata may present in Von Recklinghausen's disease with constipation, intestinal obstruction, or intussusception. Diffuse areas of hyperplastic axons and normal numbers of ganglion cells have been reported in association with megacolon.

Immaturity of the myenteric plexus

Neonatal functional bowel obstruction has been associated with hypothyroidism, hypermagnesaemia, and maternal ingestion of psychotrophic

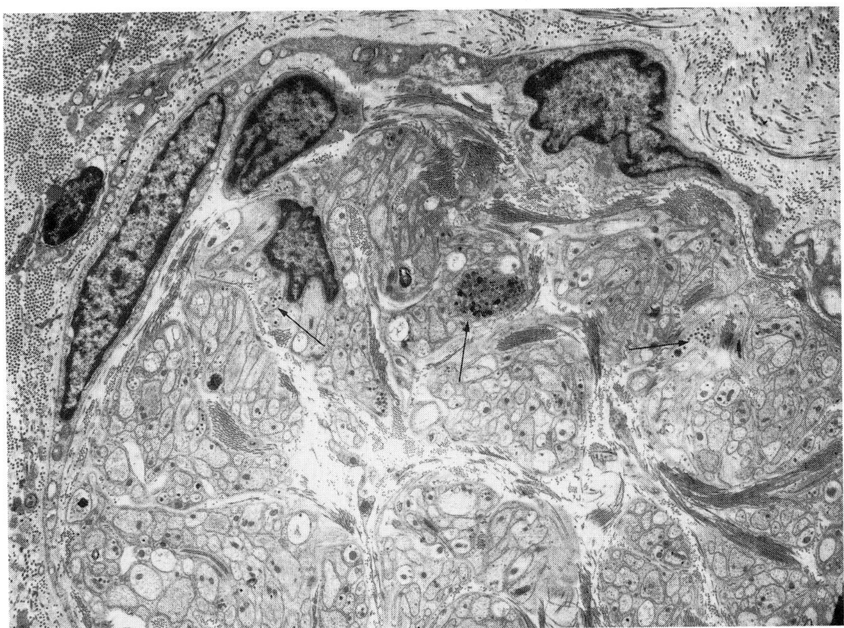

Fig. 14.10. Hyperganglionosis. Electron micrograph of giant submucosal nerve trunk. Several axons containing neurosecretory vesicles arrowed. Magnification ×4550.

or ganglion-blocking drugs. The clinical presentation varies in severity from meconium plug syndrome to complete bowel atony. Aganglionosis and cystic fibrosis have to be excluded. Immaturity of the distal myenteric plexus is a significant factor in determining the severity. Maturation may not occur in the most severe cases and this is associated with a poor prognosis.

Drugs

The autonomic nerves of the gut are affected by a wide range of drugs. Their effects may be temporary, such as constipation caused by anticholinergic action of tricyclic antidepressants or atropine. Constipation or ileus are also side-effects of vincristine and vinblastine, vinca alkaloids, used in the treatment of malignant disease. The side-effects are usually reversible and may form part of a more generalized small-fibre neuropathy. Ultrastructural examination reveals neurotubular injury.

The long-term effects of purgatives, particularly the anthraquinones (cascara, senna, rhubarb) which are stimulant cathartics, on the enteric have been studied by Smith (1972). Chronic purgation results in the thinning of the muscle coat, melanosis coli, and myenteric plexus damage. The loss of argyrophil neurons and Schwann-cell hyperplasia are more marked in the right colon. Ultrastructural changes include axonal swelling and degeneration and occur with the administration of both anthroquinones and bisacodyl.

The administration of drugs such as quinacrine, chlorpromazine, and mepacrine to mice and rats produces megacolon and irreversible damage to the myenteric plexus.

CONCLUSION

The application of physiological, histological, immunocytochemical, and ultrastructural techniques to the study of the autonomic innervation of the gut has revealed an immensely complex picture. The identification of normal patterns of development, morphology, and function has led to the recognition of morphological abnormalities which are associated with well defined clinical conditions and which have altered patient management. The use of more sophisticated investigative techniques may lead to the recognition of more subtle variations and abnormalities in the autonomic innervation of the gut.

REFERENCES

Bannister, R. and Hoyes, A. D. (1981). Generalized smooth-muscle disease with defective muscurinic receptor function. *Br. med. J.* **282**, 1015–18.

Bishop, A. E., Ferri, G. L., Probert, L., Bloom, S. R., and Polak, J. M. (1982). Peptidergic nerves. *Scand. J. Gastroenterol. Suppl.* **71**, 43–59.

Cochard, P. and Le Douarin, N. M. (1982). Development of the intrinsic innervation of the gut. *Scand. J. Gastroenterol. Suppl.* **71**, 1–14.

Fadda, B., Maier, W. A., Meier-Ruge, W., Scharli, A., and Daum, R. (1983). Eine Kritische 10-Jahres-Analyse Klinische und biophscher Diagnostik. *Z. Kinderchir.* **38**, 305–11.

Furness, J. B. and Costa, M. (1974). The adrenergic innervation of the gastrointestinal tract. *Review Physiol.* **69**, 1–51.

Furness, J. B. and Costa, M. (1980). Types of nerve in the enteric nervous system. *Neuroscience* **5**, 1–20.

Gabella, G. (1979). Innervation of the gastrointestinal tract. *Int. Rev. Cytol.* **59**, 129–93.

Garrett, J. R. and Howard, E. R. (1983). Myenteric plexus of the hindgut: developmental abnormalities in humans and experimental studies. *Development of the Autonomic Nervous System.* CIBA Foundation Symposium, pp. 326–54. Pitman Medical, London.

Gershon, M. D., Payette, R. F., and Rothman, T. P. (1983). Development of the enteric nervous system. *Fed. Proc.* **42**, 1620–5.

Goyal, R. K. and Rattan, S. (1975). Nature of vagal inhibitory innervation to the lower oesophageal sphincter. *J. clin. Invest.* **55**, 1119–26.

Hosking, D. J., Bennet, T., and Hampton, D. M. (1978). Diabetic autonomic neuropathy. *Diabetes* **27**, 1043–54.

Howard, E. R. and Garrett, J. R. (1970). Histochemistry and electron microscopy of rectum and colon in Hirschsprung's disease. *Proc. R. Soc. Med.* **63**, 20–2.

Hurst, A. F. and Rake, G. W. (1930). Achalasia of the cardia (so-called cardiospasm). *Quart. J. Med.* **23**, 491–509.

Kleinhaus, S., Boley, S. J., Sheran, M., and Sieber, W. K. (1979). Hirschsprung's disease. A survey of the members of the surgical section of the academy of Pediatrics. *J. pediatr. Surg.* **14**, 588–97.

Koberle, F. (1963). Enteromegaly and cardiomegaly in Chagas' disease. *Gut* **4**, 399–405.

Krishnamurthy, S., Kelly, M. M., Rohrmann, C. A., and Schuffler, M. D. (1983). Jejunal diverticulosis. A heterogeneous disorder caused by a variety of abnormalities of smooth muscle or myenteric plexus. *Gastroenterology* **85**, 538–47.

Meier-Ruge, W. (1974). Hirschsprung's disease: its aetiology, pathogenesis and differential diagnosis. *Curr. Top. Pathol.* **59**, 131–79.

Neely, J. and Catchpole, B. (1971). Ileus. The restoration of alimentary tract motility by pharmacological means. *Br. J. Surg.* **58**, 21–8.

Okamoto, E. and Ueda, T. (1967). Embryogenesis of intramural ganglia of the gut and its relation to Hirschsprung's disease. *J. pediatr. Surg.* **2**, 437–43.

Rozé, C. (1980). Neurohumoral control of gastrointestinal motility. *Reprod. nutr. Dev.* **20**, 1125–41.

Schofield, G. C. (1968). Anatomy of muscular and neural tissues in the alimentary canal. *Handbook of physiology, section 6, alimentary canal, volume IV, motility*, Vol. 80, pp. 1579–627. American Physiological Society, Washington, DC.

Schuffler, M. D., Rohrmann, C. A., Chaffee, R. G., Brand, D. L., Delaney, J. H., and Young, J. H. (1981). Chronic intestinal pseudo-obstruction. A report of 27 cases and review of the literature. *Medicine, Baltimore* **60**, 173–96.

Smith, B. (1972). *The neuropathology of the alimentary tract.* Edward Arnold, London.

Storsteen, K. A., Kernohan, J. W., and Bargen, J. A. (1953). The myenteric plexus in chronic ulcerative colitis. *Surg. Gynecol. Obstet.* **97**, 335–402.

Part II

Autonomic failure: clinical and pathophysiological studies

15. Clinical features of autonomic failure

A. Symptoms, signs, and special investigations

Roger Bannister

CLASSIFICATION

The clinical classification of primary autonomic failure adopted in this book (see Chapter 1) is as follows:

1. Patients with pure autonomic failure (PAF) without associated neurological disorders, formerly known as 'idiopathic orthostatic hypotension'.
2. Patients with autonomic failure (AF) associated with Parkinson's disease (PD).
3. Patients with autonomic failure (AF) and multiple system atrophy (MSA); MSA is a group of central neurological degenerations, often but not always including parkinsonism. The combination of AF and MSA is known as the Shy–Drager syndrome (Shy and Drager 1960). For brevity, in this book the use of the acronym MSA can be taken to mean MSA associated with AF.

GENERAL FEATURES

The particular autonomic functions affected differ in degree from case to case, but are remarkably similar in all these three groups. The patients are middle-aged or elderly, and males are affected more often than females. The patients with AF and PD are some five years older than patients with AF and MSA or PAF alone. Occasionally, there is a family history of a similar disorder (Lewis 1964). In men, impotence and loss of libido are commonly the first symptoms. Disturbances of micturition are common early symptoms in both sexes, and in men have often been wrongly diagnosed as evidence of prostatism. Indeed many patients have undergone prostate operations which have not led to clinical improvement (see Chapter 23). Patients living in hot climates may complain of inability to sweat which could lead to heat-stroke in the tropics but rarely causes problems in temperate countries. The most dramatic symptom, however, and the commonest reason for seeking medical advice, is postural dizziness, or even fainting, on standing erect especially in the morning or after meals or exercise.

One curious symptom of autonomic failure which presumably reflects a phase of denervation supersensitivity is that in some patients, over a few weeks or months, an autonomic function may appear hyperactive before failure occurs. This may in particular be noted in salivation or sweating and in sexual function in the male in which more frequent spontaneous erection may precede erectile failure.

Postural hypotension

The postural attacks may be 'drop' attacks resembling sudden brainstem vascular dysfunction, but more commonly there is a gradual fading of consciousness over half a minute or so while the patient is standing or walking. A neckache radiating to the occipital region of the skull and shoulders, often precedes actual loss of consciousness. The neckache may be due to ischaemia in chronically active neck and back muscles but no way has yet been devised to investigate this very common and virtually unique symptom of chronic postural hypotension.

Occasionally patients may complain of other symptoms suggesting muscle ischaemia. For example, some have described the classical symptoms of angina on exercise and others have described leg symptoms which have features suggestive of 'claudication' affecting the cauda equina. Perhaps surprisingly, despite a very low systolic blood pressure of under 60 mm Hg during exercise at the time anginal symptoms occur, the electrocardiogram usually fails to show T-wave inversion or other signs of ischaemia.

In the postural hypotensive attacks, usually after a visual disturbance or sensation of dizziness, the patient may then fall slowly to his knees; experience teaches him that, after lying flat, recovery and loss of all symptoms, including the neckache, will occur within a few minutes. The recovery from such transient neurological symptoms is usually complete and occlusive cerebrovascular incidents are rare, possibly because many patients, after years of postural hypotension, have preserved effective compensatory cerebral autoregulation (Thomas and Bannister 1980). The attacks of loss of consciousness also differ from normal fainting in that the patient usually cannot sweat, and there is no vagal cardiac slowing (see Chapter 9). Symptoms are strikingly worse in the mornings and also after meals, in hot weather and after exercise, all of which cause an unfavourable redistribution of blood volume. The disease is likely to be progressive for several years before significant incapacity occurs because autonomic compensatory mechanisms postpone overt failure. Some rare non-neurological presentations occur. A few patients if treated by bed rest for hypotensive symptoms develop persistent recumbent hypertension, mainly due to loss of baroreflexes, of such severity that they may develop papilloedema with retinal haemorrhages.

Visual disturbances

Sometimes there are transient visual disturbances, scotomata, positive hallucinations, or tunnel vision, suggesting occipital-lobe ischaemia. The symptoms of visual disturbance may be particularly striking in some patients with autonomic failure when standing or walking. One observant patient was able to classify the disturbances into three kinds. First, there was a disturbance of primary colours, but particularly yellow and red, in which they became brilliant, and secondary colours, or pastel shades, appeared non-existent. Second, objects might appear in a photo-negative form, that is dark shades being light and the light shades being dark, mostly in various shades of green. Finally if he did not lie down promptly and had developed a severe neckache and one of the previous disturbances of vision had been present for several minutes, he would then find that his central vision was blurred. On closing his eyes he would see a very clear oval orange or yellow shape filling the whole of the central field with a dark background outside it and in the very centre what appeared to be an irregularly shaped black hole. Once this particular disturbance had occurred it might take some 30 minutes to subside completely.

On occasions patients describe visual disturbances accompanied by neck and even lumbar aching, brought on by physical exertion while standing, particularly after a meal. In the male using the arms during washing up after meals and in the female using an ironing board appear, under conditions of critically reduced systolic pressure to imitate the effects of subclavian steal syndrome. Similar visual disturbances were described by Ross Russell and Page (1983) in patients with critical underperfusion of the brain and retina with extensive occlusive disease of the extracranial arteries. In patients with autonomic failure, however, such symptoms are relatively benign and patients simply use them as a warning sign that they must lie down quickly.

Defective sweating

When tested by increasing a patient's body temperature, partial or complete loss of thermoregulatory sweating is invariably present (Bannister *et al.* 1967) (see Fig. 15.1). Sweating occurs after pilocarpine or intracutaneous mecholyl in both PAF and AF with MSA, though more reduced in the former.

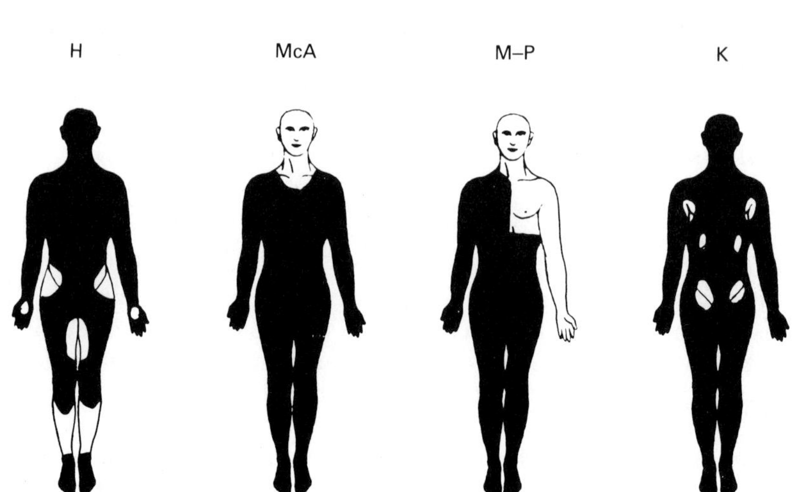

Fig. 15.1. Sweating response to 1°C rise in central body temperature in four patients with autonomic failure. (Taken with permission from Bannister *et al.* (1967).)

Sexual function

Sexual function in the male is lost early. Failure of erection occurs first and later is followed by disturbance of ejaculation consistent with a progressive sympathetic and parasympathetic failure. As discussed in Chapter 13, complex techniques using pharmacological agents or electrical stimulation may enable some sexual function to be achieved for a time.

Bladder function and management

Bladder symptoms are a combination of urgency, frequency, and nocturia due to uninhibited detrusor activity, or incontinence due to sphincter weakness, or, later, overflow incontinence due to an atonic bladder. During attempted evacuation there may be a weak or interrupted stream or incomplete evacuation, with residual urine. At its most severe there may be a complete inability to urinate. In autonomic failure there may be all combinations of upper and lower motor neuron lesions affecting the detrusor and internal and external sphincter muscles.

As described in Chapters 23 and 25A, the degeneration of sacral autonomic neurons (Onuf's nucleus) leads to the loss of both autonomic and somatic efferents as the nucleus has a status intermediate between ordinary somatic motorneurons and autonomic neurons. The anal and urethral sphincter impairment results from the loss of both innervations. Incontinence, usually without retention, is the result. There is in addition detrusor instability with lack of the capacity to initiate micturition in MSA which is probably the result of a lesion of the pontine centre for micturition. Very occasionally, reduction of the outflow resistance can be achieved surgically, although routine operations based on the common belief that the patient may have prostatism almost always make these patients worse. An appropriate operation, however, may postpone the need for the use of surgical drainage in the male. Expensive ureteric sphincter implants are as yet not available for general use. In younger females with good co-ordination, intermittent self-catheterization may sometimes be an acceptable management instead of continuous drainage or the use of incontinence pads.

Bowel function

Bowel control is sometimes affected, with rectal incontinence or intermittent diarrhoea as symptoms. A few cases of AF and MSA with predominant bowel disturbance and cholinergic dysfunction (including salivation) have been described (Khurana *et al.* 1980). A marked disturbance of bowel function suggests the possibility of amyloid.

CLINICAL FEATURES OF MULTIPLE SYSTEM ATROPHY

Pupils

Abnormalities recorded in patients with AF and MSA include Horner's syndrome, alternating anisocoria, and abnormal pupillary responses to drugs. Ponsford, Paul, and Bannister (unpublished observations) studied 16 patients with AF and MSA and compared them with patients with Parkinson's disease and age-matched controls. There was alternating anisocoria in five patients. This was variable and different from the alternating resting anisocoria which was noted in a single case of acute pandysautonomia. It was concluded that in MSA the disturbance was due to a central lesion rather than to unilateral hypersensitivity to cholinergic drugs on one side and to adrenergic drugs on the contralateral side. Alternating anisocoria differs from the variable but consistently lateralized anisocoria in the patients with pandysautonomia and the pupillotonia of the Holmes–Adie syndrome which reflects the different hypersensitivity of the two pupils to circulating cholinergic drugs.

In more than half the patients with multiple system atrophy or Parkinson's disease, with or without autonomic failure, there was an abnormal and excessive constrictor response to methacholine. The degree of constriction in the more sensitive pupils was in the same range as in the Holmes–Adie syndrome. More than half of the patients with autonomic failure, whether associated with MSA or PD, showed an abnormal sensitivity.

Disturbances of breathing

Rhythm and depth control (see Chapter 24)

The disturbance of breathing may occur during the day with involuntary inspiratory gasps (Bannister *et al.* 1967) or 'cluster' breathing (Lockwood 1976) which appear to have a central origin. At night the patients may develop the sleep apnoea syndrome. The sleep apnoea may be 'central' with cessation of respiratory motor activity or 'obstructive' in which there is a disturbance of the pharyngeal and laryngeal muscles. There is in addition evidence of an alteration of CO_2 sensitivity in patients with AF probably due to the brainstem lesion. The patient of Guilleminault *et al.* (1977) with AF and MSA also had a much-reduced amount of rapid eye movement (REM) sleep and had disturbed non-REM sleep. He had an average of 452 apnoeas (lasting 10 to 90 seconds) during the course of a night's sleep, which accounted for an average of 55 per cent of his total sleep time. This study showed that pulmonary arterial pressure rose progressively during sleep in direct association with each apnoeic episode and related hypoxaemia and hypocapnia, but without development of systemic hypertension, sinus arrhythmia, or extreme bradycardia which occurred in the REM sleep of patients who did not have autonomic failure.

Laryngeal function (see Chapter 24)

At night, stridor with consequent hypoxia may secondarily cause disturbances of brainstem function and apnoea. The laryngeal stridor is due to a bilateral defect of the laryngeal abductors (Williams *et al.* 1979; Guindi *et al.* 1980*b*) with changes of denervation on laryngeal electromyography (Guindi *et al.* 1981). At post-mortem an atrophy of the posterior cricoarytenoid muscles was found, due to an unusual form of denervation (Bannister *et al.* 1981). In the only case in which the laryngeal nerve was studied at post-mortem there appeared to be a reduced number of nerve fibres, although the nucleus ambiguus, thought to be the nucleus from which neurons innervating the laryngeal abductors arise, failed to show any selective neuronal loss. Once stridor and apnoea occur, tracheostomy cannot be long delayed. It is justified because such patients may manage well for several years before other symptoms become troublesome or incapacitating.

General neurological examination

The general neurological features only occur in patients with Parkinson's disease or multiple system atrophy. The symptoms and signs of Parkinson's disease need not be described further. The following forms of multiple system atrophy are recognized:

Striatonigral degeneration

In this disease there is a predominance of rigidity without much tremor, associated with progressive loss of facial expression and limb akinesis. Facial expression is often less affected than in Parkinson's disease. The patient has difficulty in standing, walking, or turning and has difficulty in feeding himself. As a result of akinesis the speech becomes faint and slurred (see Chapters 25 and 33).

Olivopontocerebellar atrophy

In this form of multiple system atrophy, not included in Shy and Drager's description, there is a prominent disturbance of gait with truncal ataxia which frequently makes it impossible for the patient to stand without support. In addition, marked slurring of speech occurs with irregularity of speed of diction. There may also be a mild or moderate intention tremor affecting the arms and legs (see Chapters 25 and 33).

Pyramidal lesion

In either of these forms of degeneration there may be a pyramidal increase in tone, together with impaired rapid hand and foot movements and exaggerated deep-tendon jerks and bilateral extensor plantar responses. It is of course difficult to detect a pyramidal disturbance of tone in the presence of the extrapyramidal disturbance. Primitive reflexes such as the palmomental reflex may also be present. Progressive muscle wasting not infrequently occurs (see Chapter 31B) though this is not as marked as in motor neuron disease. Fasciculation occurs rarely but on electromyographic examination there is usually some evidence of denervation with little evidence of any abnormality of peripheral-nerve motor conduction (see Chapter 30).

Intellectual state

Dementia is no commoner than might be expected on the basis of chance in patients of this age group. It is surprising to observe preserved intellectual function in a patient who is almost totally incapacitated in terms of motor control, orthostatic blood-pressure regulation, and bladder disturbance. This is of course in striking contrast to the neuronal degeneration of presenile dementia (Alzheimer's disease) in which the predominant degeneration affects cortical cholinergic neurons. It is also in contrast to the intellectual impairment which is a feature of many cases of Parkinson's disease.

Affect

There is no evidence of a mood defect when allowance is made for the considerable disability of patients with autonomic failure and multiple system atrophy (Robertson and Bannister, unpublished observations). This is surprising in view of the hypothesis that central catecholamine function plays a part in the preservation of normal mood and that patients with depression can be helped by augmenting central noradrenergic function.

Sensory function

In two cases out of a personal series of more than 150 patients with autonomic failure and multiple system atrophy, there was sensory loss in the legs, confirmed by loss of sural sensory action potentials in one and by post-mortem studies in the other (Bannister and Oppenheimer 1972). This suggests a possible link between sensory neuropathy, AF, and multiple system atrophy (Chapter 1). Low and Fealey (Chapter 30) review the evidence for a mild peripheral neuropathy in PAF and MSA.

Biochemical investigation

See Chapters 18 and 19.

CLINICAL DIAGNOSIS OF MULTIPLE SYSTEM ATROPHY

Clearly there are difficulties in distinguishing clinically the degree of striatonigral degeneration (SND) and olivopontocerebellar atrophy (OPCA) in patients with the features of both. In our experience careful attempts to elicit signs of striatonigral disease and cerebellar disease will usually give a correct diagnosis as judged by the only real criterion, the ultimate pathologically verification. The best picture of the relationship between these two forms of MSA comes from the clinicopathological correlations described by Oppenheimer and Lees (see Chapters 25A and 33). Of 56 cases of AF from our own studies and literature reports, with full clinical and pathological assessment, 10 had Lewy body disease, five of them without clinical parkinsonism and none with other neurological symptoms or signs. None of these at post-mortem had lesions of either SND or OPCA. Their mean age of death was 72 years. Of the remaining 46 cases with the clinical symptoms and signs of MSA, parkinsonism was recorded in 35 cases but not in the remainder. At post-mortem, however, all 46 had nigral lesions and 34 also had lesions of the putamen. Only 25 had the full pathological features of olivopontocerebellar atrophy but 21 of these also had the pathological changes of SND. There may be limited value in striving clinically to separate SND from OPCA though we have attempted to do so in Chapter 15B on the grounds of clinical signs at diagnosis. The association between autonomic failure is closer and more frequent with SND than with OPCA but, having stated that, both groups show considerable overlap in the ultimate pathology, even though in life one form only is present or predominates at diagnosis and through the early stages. The association with autonomic failure, however, marks out these patients from the other progressive cerebellar syndromes especially predominantly inherited cases, which have little relationship with SND or autonomic failure.

NEW TECHNIQUES OF INVESTIGATION OF MULTIPLE SYSTEM ATROPHY

CT scanning

Until the last few years, CT scans of the brainstem and cerebellum were obscured by artefact. With modern CT scanning the enlargement of the cisterna ambiens associated with brainstem atrophy is visible along with atrophy of the pons and cerebral peduncles. In olivopontocerebellar atrophy, atrophy of the vermis and cerebellar cortex is visible (Savoiardo *et al.* 1983; Huang and Plaitakis 1984).

Magnetic resonance imaging

The putaminal changes which are unique to multiple system atrophy can be identified by T1 weighted magnetic resonance imaging (MRI) (see Fig. 15.2 (Pastakia *et al.* 1987) as shown by Brown *et al.* (1987). They found that changes ranked with the severity of the rigidity but not the other parkinsonian features of tremor or bradykinesis. Decreased signal intensity was found in the posterolateral putamen on T2 weighted scans which corresponds to the cell loss seen pathologically in this area of the basal ganglia in MSA. No abnormality was seen in the scans of patients with pure autonomic failure.

Brainstem auditory evoked potentials in autonomic failure

The usefulness of brainstem auditory evoked responses in providing an easier non-invasive means of assessing the integrity of brainstem function in multiple sclerosis (Prasher and Gibson 1980) led us to investigate its use in patients with autonomic failure (Prasher and Bannister 1986). A group of patients with pure autonomic failure (PAF) and uncomplicated Parkinson's disease failed to show any abnormality. However, in nearly all the patients with multiple system atrophy (MSA)

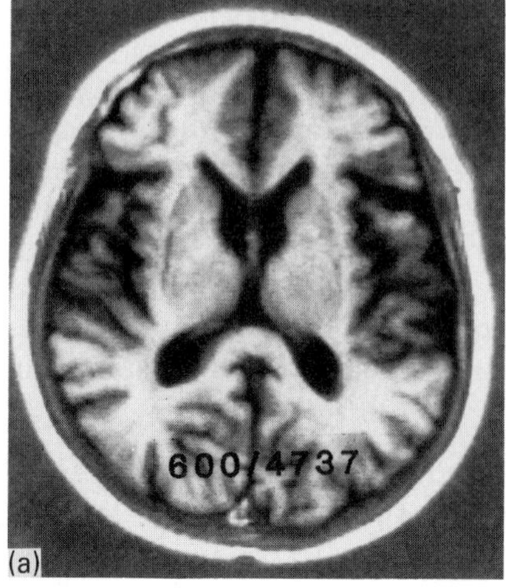

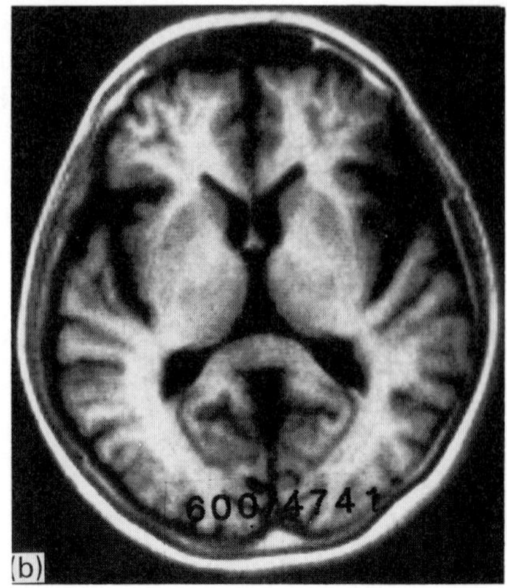

Fig. 15.2. MR imaging in (a) patient with multiple system atrophy which shows decreased signal density in the putamen in contrast with that of (b) a healthy age-matched control.

there was a disruption of the brainstem responses in the pontomedullary region with delay or reduction of components of the response generated beyond this region (Fig. 15.3). The brainstem auditory evoked potentials, which are now widely available, may be helpful in distinguishing at an early stage the patients developing multiple system atrophy from the patients with pure autonomic failure, in whom the prognosis is so much better and the management so much easier.

Positron emission tomography (PET)

A report of PET scanning in MSA is described on pp. 11–12 and another primary degenerative disease already studied in addition to Parkinson's disease is progressive supranuclear palsy. Clinically, this disease presents as an atypical parkinsonian-like syndrome which has some clinical features, particularly parkinsonian rigidity and a failure to respond to L-dopa, which resemble multiple system atrophy. Figure 15.4 (by courtesy of Baron *et al.* 1985) shows the mapping of dopamine D-2 receptors (76 Br-bromo-spiperone binding sites) *in vivo* by PET. This confirms the decrease in the number of striatal dopamine receptors. The defect is of particular interest in that D-1 receptors do not seem to be

---

Fig. 15.3. (a) Mean and standard deviation of absolute amplitude of Wave V for the groups tested. (PD, Parkinson's disease; PAF, pure autonomic failure; MSA with AF, multiple system atrophy with autonomic failure.) Note the major reduction in the mean and variance of the amplitude of Wave V in MSA with AF. (b) Brainstem

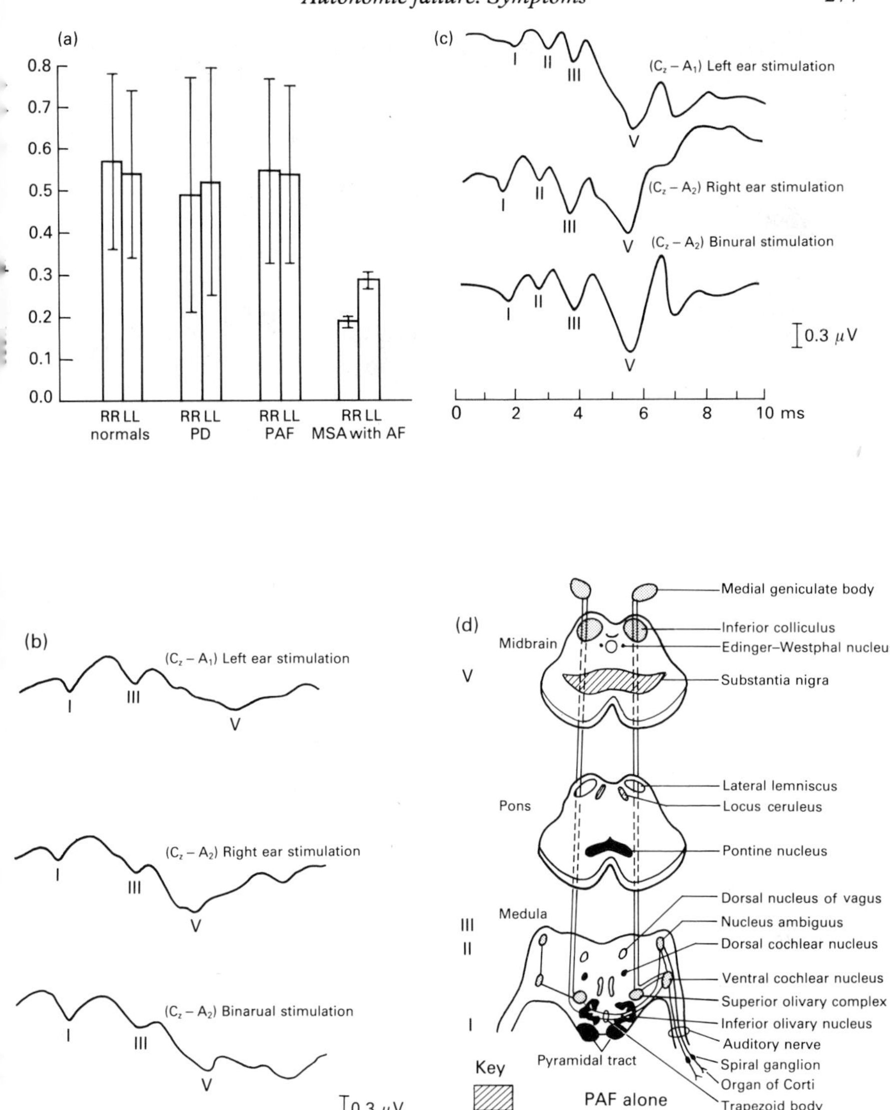

responses of multiple system atrophy: bilateral abnormalities more severe on the left. (c) Brainstem responses of PAF: normal in amplitude and latency. (d) This diagram shows sites involved in PAF alone which clearly do not affect the BAEP. As these sites, which involve central autonomic control, are also affected in AF with MSA it is necessary to exclude the sites common to both syndromes. Therefore, by subtraction, the remaining sites in which degeneration is exclusive to the MSA component of the syndrome may be obtained. The auditory pathways are also shown with the Roman numerals indicating the generator sites of the brainstem potentials.

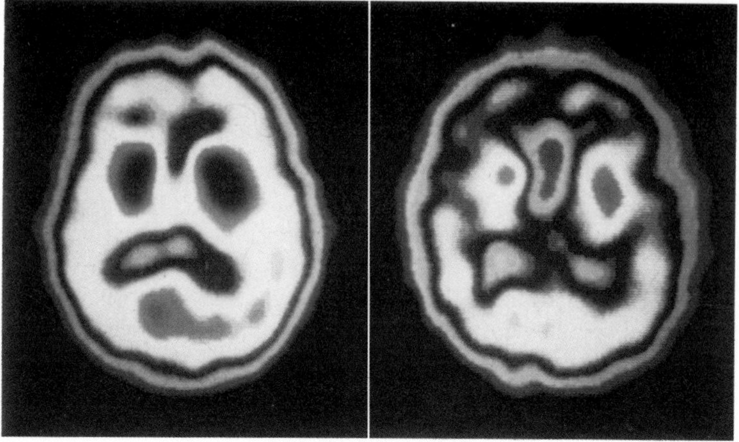

Fig. 15.4. Positron emission tomography at the level of the basal ganglia, revealing the distribution of 76 Br-bromo-spiperone, after i.v. injection in a control and a patient with progressive supranuclear palsy (PSP). Four to five hours after the injection of bromo-spiperone, a high concentration of radioactivity (dark area) is observed in the striatum of the control (left), whereas accumulation is low in the patient with PSP (right). (Taken with permission from Baron *et al.* (1985).)

affected. The application of PET scanning to MSA shows reduced storage of ^{18}F-dopa in the putamen.

PARKINSON'S DISEASE AND AUTONOMIC FAILURE

The question of whether, and to what degree, autonomic involvement occurs in Parkinson's disease has been disputed for many years. The problem has been confused by the clinical description of supposed minor autonomic disturbances in Parkinson's disease, whose significance is difficult to assess, like greasy skin or unequal pupils. Autonomic involvement may better be defined as a measurable sympathetic or parasympathetic dysfunction, assessed by physiological or biochemical means. Using these strict criteria, autonomic involvement in Parkinson's disease is uncommon.

If a battery of tests of the kind described in Chapter 16 is undertaken, it is possible to say with reasonable certainty whether a parkinsonian patient also has autonomic failure according to defined autonomic criteria. The autonomic failure syndrome associated with Parkinson's disease as defined by these tests is rare and less common than the association of autonomic failure with multiple system atrophy, which is itself also a rare syndrome. A problem arises with early cases of autonomic failure because in studying the autonomic nervous system there are compensatory mechanisms, both neurological and hormonal, which can mask the early stages of insufficiency. There have to be marked changes before autonomic failure becomes clinically manifest, but, taking account of the clinical picture and the other neurological signs, it is possible to fit patients with clinical parkinsonism into one of two diagnostic categories—either autonomic failure with Parkinson's disease or autonomic failure with multiple system atrophy.

The final verification of the correctness of the diagnosis in life lies in post-mortem pathological examination. Oppenheimer (see Chapter 25A) summarizes the cases of autonomic failure and Parkinson's disease in life in which there was loss of intermediolateral column cells and shows that the number of intermediolateral column cells in Parkinson's disease without autonomic failure was normal.

The vast majority of patients with Parkinson's disease do not have autonomic failure according to strict physiological and biochemical criteria. Some patients with classical Parkinson's disease do have mild orthostatic hypotension when compared with control groups. There have been reports that levels of plasma noradrenalin in these patients are in a lower range than in normal controls (Turkka 1986). However, such patients do not have the abnormalities of cardiovascular reflex control which are linked with baroreceptor defects and intermediolateral column cell loss which are characteristic of the autonomic failure syndrome. Gross *et al.* (1972) studied 20 patients with moderate Parkinson's disease, wishing to exclude abnormalities which occur with advanced parkinsonism and compared them with controls. The only abnormality was that on head up-tilt their blood pressures were significantly lower than matched controls. There was, therefore, some increased lability of cardiovascular control. The conclusion was drawn that, because the cardiovascular reflexes and Valsalva tests were normal, there may be changes in the midbrain or hypothalamus associated with classical Parkinson's disease pathology which affect the input to the autonomic nervous system and which might well be the reason for these relatively mild abnormalities.

In summary, there are three clinical presentations of autonomic failure: (1) pure autonomic failure; (2) autonomic failure with parkinsonism; and (3) autonomic failure with multiple system atrophy. Cases in the first two groups both have Lewy bodies, but not the striatonigral or olivopontocerebellar changes of multiple system atrophy. In all, there are changes in the brainstem pigmented nuclei which appear to be related to the autonomic degeneration. All of them have intermediolateral column cell loss.

However, there are only two groups of autonomic failure patients pathologically. The first have changes associated with Lewy bodies and often but not always with the clinicopathological features of Parkinson's disease. The second group have the more widespread neurological and neurochemical changes of multiple system atrophy. Both groups suffer from a similar primary, that is causally unknown, degeneration of the autonomic nervous system. There are no known provoking factors for this disorder, nor any metabolic or infective factors. Should we regard autonomic failure with Lewy bodies, but no nigral loss or clinical parkinsonism, as a form of Parkinson's disease? The time course is quite different from what we regard as Parkinson's disease but there clearly is some close link between these cases. What is the relationship between these cases and those with multiple system atrophy? Although there are some abnormalities which these patients share, there is not a continuum and they must be accepted as separate clinicopathological groups.

THE EFFECT OF AGEING ON DIAGNOSIS OF AUTONOMIC FAILURE

Since most patients with the autonomic failure syndromes are middle-aged or elderly, it is important to consider whether the symptoms of autonomic failure may sometimes be due to age alone. In one study (Johnson *et al.* 1965) 17 of 100 elderly patients in a geriatric hospital had orthostatic falls of more than 20 mm of systolic pressure and 5 falls in excess of 40 mm. Several had postural hypotensive symptoms. Without diagnosing the syndrome of autonomic failure several possible causes can be invoked. These include failure of cerebral autoregulation (Wollner *et al.* 1979), diminished β-adrenoceptor responsiveness in old age (see Chapter 19 and Van Brummelen *et al.* 1981), as well as reduced α_1-adrenoceptor responsiveness (Elliott *et al.* 1982), loss of elasticity of arterial walls with age (Gribbin *et al.* 1971), and the loss of baroreflex sensitivity with age (Collins *et al.* 1980), which may be the result of structural changes in the nerve endings in the wall of the human carotid sinus and aortic arch (Abraham 1967). Postural hypotension in the elderly does not appear to be the result of a failure of release of noradrenalin from sympathetic endings, as noradrenalin concentrations on standing did not differ between two groups of elderly subjects with and without orthostatic hypotension (Robinson *et al.* 1983). More research is needed into the relative contributions of these possible causes to hypotension in the elderly, but, when due allowance is made for this, autonomic failure as a syndrome is rarely mistaken for orthostatic hypotension of the elderly.

CLINICAL COURSE OF AUTONOMIC FAILURE

(see Chapter 15B)

The clinical progression of patients with pure autonomic failure is relatively benign since the hypotensive symptoms can usually be controlled by head-up tilt or fludrocortisone so that life expectancy is only a little reduced and sphincter disturbance may be minimal. Occasionally patients may survive from diagnosis for more than 20 years, raising the possibility that in some patients, non-progressive lesions occur. Patients with autonomic failure and Parkinson's disease fare less well than patients with uncomplicated Parkinson's disease but again may survive for many years.

Patients with autonomic failure associated with multiple system atrophy face a distressing progression of their disability, unmitigated by any loss of insight as their intelligence is almost always preserved. They often remain surprisingly cheerful, especially when attempts to help them with various drug regimes are pursued. These attempts are entirely justifiable since there is never any single drug regime that can be automatically applied to patients with such a variety of sites and extents of their lesions. But within 5 years the patients with autonomic failure are barely mobile, due to the extrapyramidal and pyramidal weakness and will have a sphincter disturbance that can be helped but not cured. The preterminal development is often sleep apnoea or stridor. Death in sleep may be due to stridor or apnoea and may sometimes be a providential release. The denervation supersensitivity of sympathetic α- and β-receptors of the heart may render these patients more liable to cardiac arrhythmias from which they may die, as in patients with diabetic autonomic neuropathy (Page and Watkins 1978).

B. Autonomic failure: a comparison between UK and US experience

Roger Bannister, Christopher Mathias, and Ronald Polinsky

A group of cases of pure autonomic failure (PAF) and of multiple system atrophy (MSA) in the UK and US were compared retrospectively using an agreed *pro forma* for analysis of clinical features. For the purposes of this analysis MSA means autonomic failure with multiple system atrophy. In general, a striking similarity of the clinical experience was found in the two countries.

Table 15.1 shows a strong male preponderance in both autonomic failure syndromes except for a female preponderance in the PAF group in the US. The sex ratios for the US patients differ from the general NIH patient population admitted during the same period which represents both sexes equally. Table 15.2 shows the frequency of autonomic symptoms at presentation. In the US the frequency of all autonomic symptoms at presentation in PAF is lower than in the UK series. This, taken in conjunction with the earlier age of onset in the US (Table 15.3) and the longer duration of the illness (Table 15.3) suggests that in the US, possibly because of the average hotter climate orthostatic symptoms are recognized sooner. It may be that US patients seek medical attention at an earlier stage of the disease. In neither the UK nor the US series of MSA was there much difference in the time of onset of the autonomic and other neurological symptoms. The earlier presentation of autonomic symptoms in MSA may help to differentiate these cases from Parkinson's disease with autonomic failure. In the UK analysis postural dizziness was twice as common as either loss of consciousness or transient impairment of vision at presentation. Bladder and sphincter symptoms were about twice as common at presentation in MSA as in PAF. Though impotence was common at onset in both series, it was present in due course in virtually all males with autonomic failure.

Table 15.3 shows that the age of onset of patients with MSA does not differ greatly though, as already commented, the PAF patients appear to be diagnosed when younger in the US. Table 15.4 shows that the extent of the postural fall in blood pressure on tilt or standing and the supine blood pressure were similar in PAF and MSA in the UK and the US.

A further comment is needed on the neurological symptoms and signs in MSA. In a study in the UK we attempted to separate the different types of MSA. Within this group there are some 20 per cent with only signs of olivopontocerebellar atrophy (OPCA), an equal number with only striatonigral degeneration, and the remaining 60 per cent with mixed symptoms and signs of both, usually with added pyramidal signs.

Table 15.1. Sex incidence

	UK	*US*
PAF		
Total number	24	22
Male:female	17:7	8:14
AF + MSA		
Total number	74	44
Male: female	47:26	29:15

Table 15.2. Frequency of autonomic symptoms at presentation

	UK	*US*
PAF		
Number of cases	24	22
Orthostatic hypotension (per cent)	92	73
Urinary (per cent)	27	0
Impotence (males only) (per cent)	94	55
AF + MSA		
Number of cases	73	44
Orthostatic hypotension (per cent)	74	30
Urinary (per cent)	52	18
Impotence (males only) (per cent)	83	48

Table 15.3. Age of onset and duration of illness

	UK	*US*
PAF		
Number	24 (10 dead)	22 (2 dead)
Age (years)	58±10	47±3
	(38–78)	25–68)
Duration	9±1	14±2
	(2–16)	(5–31)
AF + MSA		
Number	73 (56 dead)	44 (26 dead)
Age (years)	54±10	51±1
	(34–74)	(25–67)
Duration (years)	3±2	8±1
	(1–8)	(2–15)

Table 15.4. Supine and standing (US) or tilt (UK) blood pressure

	UK *Systolic*	*Diastolic*	*US* *Systolic*	*Diastolic*
PAF*				
Supine	142±31	74±17	143±7	85±4
Standing/tilt (45°)	93±34	53±15	80±57	51±4
AF + MSA†				
Supine	145±26	83±15	151±4	93±2
Standing/tilt (45°)	97±29	58±16	96±31	65±2

* There were, respectively, 24 and 22 cases of PAF in the UK and US studies.
† There were, respectively, 73 and 44 cases of AF + MSA in the UK and US studies.

The combination of pyramidal and extrapyramidal rigidity is probably the reason why rigidity is twice as common as the other parkinsonian symptoms of bradykinesis and tremor in MSA. In the UK cases with predominant OPCA the incidence of bladder symptoms was lower and the recumbent blood pressure higher than the group as a whole but the extent of the postural fall was as great. The survival of the OPCA group was no different. Overall in the UK no obvious differences in autonomic features were found in the different types of MSA; therefore, in this analysis we have not subdivided MSA into OPCA, SND, and mixed groups.

By comparison with MSA, PAF is a relatively benign disease. In both the UK and US two-thirds of the MSA cases died during follow-up whereas only 10 per cent of the US cases of PAF died during follow-up. In the UK three of the 10 patients with PAF are known to have died of a carcinoma but this appeared well after the onset of PAF so there is no evidence that PAF was mistaken for a paraneoplastic syndrome.

Table 15.5 shows the plasma noradrenalin (NA) values. There are no US standing values for comparison because most patients were unable to stand for the duration of the test. We are in agreement with regard to the low plasma noradrenalin level in PAF. A review of previous differences and their possible reasons is included in Chapters 16 and 17. However the differences in the MSA group require discussion. There are several factors that may affect the comparison.

1. The UK basal levels are higher in MSA (and also slightly higher in PAF). A number of factors, which include assay differences and variation in diet (sodium intake for instance), could affect the basal NA level and we do not have such data on each of our patients.
2. The range of basal NA in MSA appears to be greater than in normal individuals. In the US there was a small group of MSA patients with a low plasma noradrenalin and it was suggested that these patients might have transsynaptic degeneration. It will be recalled that the original UK plasma NA observations (Bannister *et al.* 1977) showed that the majority of cases of MSA had a low and sometimes a very low basal noradrenalin. This had also been the UK explanation of the low levels in MSA.
3. The occurrence of a high basal noradrenalin in some MSA patients, though at first perhaps confusing, is consistent with either the inability to switch off noradrenalin released by baroreflex mechanisms, or, as in all plasma noradrenalin measurements, may reflect some alteration of clearance.

In the UK we have also studied a series of 25 cases of Parkinson's disease (PD) with autonomic failure. This group has a strong male preponderance and differs from autonomic failure with multiple system

Table 15.5. Plasma noradrenalin in autonomic failure

	UK	*US*
PAF		
Number	19	20
Supine (pg/ml)	119±19	76±18
Tilt (pg/ml)	135±21	*
AF + MSA		
Number	15	37
Supine (pg/ml)	279±38	265±21
Tilt (pg/ml)	334±50	*

* No values in US because standing attempted for five minutes and, because many patients were unable to stand as long as this, measurements were unreliable and were not taken.

atrophy, as already described (Chapter 15A). The presenting autonomic symptoms were postural dizziness and impotence which was present in one-third of the males. Though the mean age of onset of the neurological symptoms of Parkinson's disease was 57, their parkinsonian symptoms preceded the autonomic failure symptoms by some 5 years whereas, in AF and MSA, the onset of both types of symptoms was within the same year. At the time of diagnosis of AF with PD the degree of postural fall was similar to that of the PAF and MSA patients, countering the suggestion that these patients merely had the mild postural fall which occurs in most parkinsonian patients (see Chapter 15A). The fact, however, that they were on average 5 years older means that the complicating effects of ageing itself and possibly the effect of L-dopa, to which unlike most MSA patients they respond, has to be considered.

In summary, there are obvious difficulties in comparing data from different centres in a retrospective fashion but from the study we conclude that our patients represent the same variants of autonomic failure. We hope that this comparison will reduce the degree of confusion that may still exist in some centres on both sides of the Atlantic. The slight change in terms used now for the variants of autonomic failure since the last edition of this book reflects an agreement to replace the term 'idiopathic orthostatic hypotension' (IOH) with 'pure autonomic failure' (PAF). The word 'pure' does not carry with its name the assumption that PAF is identical pathologically, which is, of course, the only ultimate diagnostic criterion, with AF with PD or AF with MSA. The term 'progressive' which was attached to all three groups has been dropped as it added no clear distinguishing feature between them. Moreover, some patients with pure autonomic failure can function well, with or without treatment, and appear clinically unchanged for several years and so the aspect of progression in PAF need not be stressed. On the other hand the fact that the syndrome must remain 'pure', that is uncontaminated by any non-autonomic neurological or other symptoms or signs, remains crucial to the diagnosis. In addition, PAF occurs in the absence of any identifiable cause for autonomic neuropathy.

Finally we agree that our initial clinical diagnosis, though strengthened by the physiological, biochemical, and pharmacological tests, can occasionally be proved wrong. This salutary fact should warn the clinician against giving too confident or optimistic a prognosis. For example, a lady of 68 whom we diagnosed as having PAF 4 years ago (though we were puzzled that her plasma noradrenalin level was in the normal range) had 3 years later developed tremor and a year later had clearly developed all the signs of MSA; she now has a tracheostomy.

Despite all the physiological, biochemical, and pharmacological characterization of the precise pathophysiology in autonomic failure, it still must be stressed that the diagnosis remains a clinical one in individual cases.

REFERENCES

Abraham, A., (1967). The structure of baroreceptors in pathological conditions in man. In *Baroreceptors and hypertension* (ed. P. Keydl), pp. 273–91. Pergamon Press, Oxford.

Bannister, R., Ardill, L., and Fentem, P. (1967). Defective autonomic control of blood vessels in idiopathic orthostatic hypotension. *Brain* **90**, 725–46.

Bannister, R., Gibson, W., Michaels, L., and Oppenheimer, D. R. (1981). Laryngeal abductor paralysis in multiple system atrophy. *Brain* **104**, 351–68.

Bannister, R. and Oppenheimer, D. R. (1972). Degenerative diseases of the nervous system associated with autonomic failure. *Brain* **95**, 457–74.

Bannister, R., Sever, P., and Gross, M. (1977). Cardiovascular reflexes and biochemical responses in progressive autonomic failure. *Brain* **100**, 327–44.

Baron, J. C., Mazière, B., Loc'h, C., Sgouropoulos, P., Bonnet, A. M., and Agid, Y. (1985). Progressive supranuclear palsy. Loss of striatonigral dopamine receptors demonstrated in vivo by positron tomography. *Lancet* **i**, 1163–4.

Brown, R. T., Polinsky, R. J., DiChiro, G., Pastakia, B., Wener, L., and Simmons, J. T. (1987). *J. Neurol. Neurosurg. Psychiat.* **50**, 913–14.

Collins, K. J., Exton-Smith, A. N., James, M. H., and Oliver, D. J. (1980). Functional changes in autonomic nervous responses with ageing. *Age Ageing* **9**, 17–24.

Elliott, H. L., Sumner, D. J., McLean, K., Rubin, P. C., and Reid, J. L. (1982). Effect of age on adrenoreceptor responsiveness in man. *Clin. Sci.* **63**, 305s–308s.

Gribbin, B., Pickering, T. G., Sleight, P., and Peto, R. (1971). Effect of age and high blood pressure on baroreflex sensitivity in man. *Circulation Res.* **29**, 424–31.

Gross, M., Bannister, R., and Godwin-Austen, R. (1972). Orthostatic hypotension in Parkinson's disease. *Lancet* **i**, 174–6.

Guilleminault, C., Tilkian, A., Lehrman, K., Forno, L., and Dement, W. C. (1977). Sleep apnoea syndrome: states of sleep and autonomic dysfunction. *J. Neurol. Neurosurg. Psychiat.* **40**, 718–25.

Guindi, G. M., Bannister, R., Gibson, W., and Payne, J. K. (1981). Laryngeal electromyography in multiple system atrophy with autonomic failure. *J. Neurol. Neurosurg. Psychiat.* **44**, 49–53.

Guindi, G. M., Michaels, M., Bannister, R., and Gibson, W. (1980). Pathology of the intrinsic muscles of the larynx. *Clin. Otolaryngol.* **6**, 101–9.

Huang, Y. O. and Plaitakis, A. (1984). Morphological changes of olivopontocerebellar atrophy in computed tomography and comments on its pathogenesis. *Adv. Neurol.* **41**, 39–85.

Johnson, R. H., Smith, A. C., Spalding, J. M. K., and Wollner, L. (1965). Effect of posture on blood pressure in elderly patients. *Lancet* **i**, 731–3.

Khurana, R. K., Nelson, E., Azzarelli, B., and Garcia, J. H. (1980). Shy–Drager syndrome: diagnosis and treatment of cholinergic dysfunction. *Neurology, Minneapolis* **30**, 805–9.

Lewis, P. (1964). Familial orthostatic hypotension. *Brain* **87**, 719–28.

Lockwood, A. H. (1976). The Shy–Drager syndrome with abnormal respiration and antidiuretic hormone release. *Arch. Neurol., Chicago* **33**, 292–5.

Page, M. McB. and Watkins, P. J. (1978). Cardiorespiratory arrest and diabetic autonomic neuropathy. *Lancet* **i**, 14–16.

Pastakia, B., Polinsky, R., DiChiro, G., Simmons, J. T., Brown, R., and Wener, L. (1987). Multiple system atrophy (Shy–Drager syndrome) MR imaging. *Radiology* **159**, 499–502.

Prasher, D. K. and Bannister, R. (1986). Brainstem auditory evoked potentials in patients with multiple system atrophy with progressive autonomic failure (Shy–Drager syndrome). *J. Neurol. Neurosurg. Psychiat.* **49**, 278–89.

Prasher, D. K. and Gibson, W. P. R. (1980). Brainstem auditory evoked potentials. A comparative study of monaural vs binaural stimulation in the detection of multiple sclerosis. *Clin. Neurophysiol.* **50**, 247–53.

Robinson, B. J., Johnson, R. H., Lambie, D. G., and Palmer, K. T. (1983). Do elderly patients with an excessive fall in blood pressure on standing have evidence of autonomic failure? *Clin. Sci.* **64**, 587–91.

Ross Russell, R. W., and Page, N. G. R. (1983). Critical perfusion of brain and retina. *Brain* **106**, 419–34.

Savoiardo, J. W., Bracchi, M., Passerini, A., Visciani, A., DiDonato, S., and Cocchinni, F. (1983). Computed tomography of olivopontocerebellar atrophy. *Am. J. Neuroradiol.* **4**, 509–12.

Schwartz, G. A. (1975). Idiopathic orthostatic hypotension (Shy–Drager syndrome) a form of multiple system atrophy. In *Handbook of clinical neurology* (ed. P. J. Vinken and G. W. Bruyn), Vol. 22, pp. 264–7. Elsevier/North Holland, Amsterdam.

Shy, G. M. and Drager, G. A. (1960). A neurological syndrome associated with orthostatic hypotension. *Arch. Neurol., Chicago* **3**, 511–27.

Thomas, D. J. and Bannister, R. (1980). Preservation of autoregulation of cerebral blood flow in autonomic failure. *J. neurol. Sci.* **44**, 205–12.

Turkka, J. (1986). Autonomic dysfunction in Parkinson's disease. *Acta Universitatis Ouluensis* **D142**, 15–66.

Van Brummelen, P., Buhler, F. R., Kiowsi, W., and Amman, F. W. (1981). Age-related decrease in cardiac and peripheral vascular responsiveness to isoprenaline: studies in normal subjects. *Clin. Sci.* **60**, 571–7.

Williams, A., Hanson, D., and Calne, D. B. (1979). Vocal cord paralysis in the Shy–Drager syndrome. *J. Neurol. Neurosurg. Psychiat.* **42**, 151–3.

Wollner, L., McCarthy, S. T., Soper, N. D. W., and Macy, D. T. (1979). Failure of cerebral autoregulation as a cause of brain dysfunction in the elderly. *Br. med. J.* **i**, 1117–18.

16. Testing autonomic reflexes

Roger Bannister and Christopher Mathias

INTRODUCTION

In autonomic failure (AF) the homeostatic control of blood pressure is disturbed by lesions at several levels from the hypothalamus to the periphery. Figure 16.1 shows a much simplified diagram of some of the neurological pathways involved in the regulation of blood pressure. There are cortical, limbic, anterior, and posterior hypothalamic and medullary 'centres' at which the input from the carotid sinus and other afferents can be integrated and the output through the vagus and sympathetic system to the heart and blood vessels may be co-ordinated.

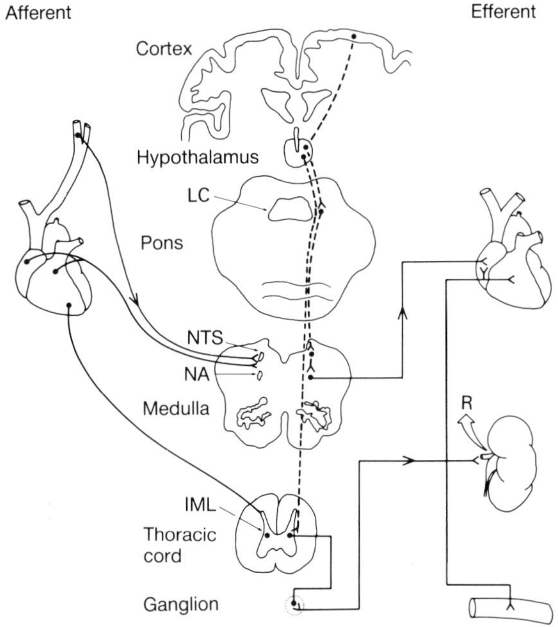

Fig. 16.1. Diagram of cardiovascular control mechanism. LC, locus ceruleus; NA, nucleus ambiguus; NTS, nucleus tractus solitarius; IML, intermediolateral column; R, renin. (Taken with permission from Bannister *et al.* (1979).)

Histochemical fluorescence and immunohistological techniques (Ungerstedt 1971) have localized monoaminergic transmitter pathways in the central nervous system of animals which play a major part in central cardiovascular control. In the cat the output from the baroreceptors passes to the nucleus tractus solitarius; the vagal output is through the nucleus ambiguus and the sympathetic output through the reticular paramedian nuclei (see Chapter 4). In autonomic failure in man, the baroreceptors, as feedback transducers in cybernetic terms, do not produce the required responses in the effectors, the resistance and capacity vessels, the heart, and the kidneys. This causes both a change in the 'set point' pressure and an instability in the response to various stresses. Defects in the cardiovascular reflexes affect short-term adjustment, but the long-term compensatory changes of blood volume, which are more difficult to study, are equally important.

The methods of investigation reviewed here are selected for their simplicity and practical usefulness from an obviously very much wider range of possible autonomic tests which are discussed more fully in Chapters 17, 37 and 38. Since autonomic function deteriorates with ageing, it is necessary to compare any defects in patients with results in control subjects of comparable age (Collins *et al.* 1980).

POSTURAL HYPOTENSION

When a fall of more than 20 mm systolic pressure on standing is found in a patient with symptoms, further investigation is justified, and a battery of equipment (Table 16.1) and tests (Table 16.2) are available. Sufficiently precise arterial pressure recording is difficult by conventional sphygomanometry and it then may be important to confirm precisely the extent of the postural fall by monitoring of blood pressure with an arterial catheter. Radial or brachial artery catheterization will show this precisely and also the fluctuations with various manoeuvres. The instability of blood pressure in autonomic failure is due partly to lack of baroreflex control, but probably also to supersensitivity of partially denervated vessels to the transmitter noradrenalin. This may cause recumbent hypertension, leading to hypertensive retinopathy or even cerebral haemorrhage. Investigation of cardiac function has shown that in autonomic failure cardiac output falls on head-up tilt as venous pressure is reduced due to pooling of blood in the legs, resembling the response in the Starling isolated heart–lung experimental preparation. Blood pressure falls during exercise even when the effect of gravity is eliminated when the patient is recumbent (Marshall *et al.* 1961). This is due to a lack of vasoconstriction which normally occurs in other vascular beds in exercise to compensate for the vasodilatation in the exercising muscles.

Table 16.1. Equipment at National Hospital autonomic unit

Measurement	*Equipment*
Forearm blood flow	Mercury in silastic strain gauge plethysmography*
Arterial blood pressure	Transducer*
Continuous heart rate	Beat-to-beat recorder*
Respiratory rate	Nasal thermister probe*
Finger plethysmography	Infra-red flow probe*
Palmar sweating	Skin resistance probe*
Cerebral EEG monitoring	EEG leads and filters*
Non-invasive blood pressure	Automated sphygmomanometer (Sentron)
Electrocardiography	Oscilloscope with printing facility
Non-invasive cardiac output	Doppler technique with computation (Exerdop)
Capillary blood flow	Laser Doppler flowmeter (Perimed PF2B)
Surface and deep temperature	Probes for continuous multiple temperature recordings†
Bladder and sphincter function	Cystometrogram (see Chapter 23); Medelec electromyographic recorder
Recording from autonomic fibres	Microneuronography (see Chapter 11)

* Used in conjunction with multichannel recorder (six-channel Ormed).
† Used in conjunction with Elab and PanLab recorders.

Table 16.2. Some useful clinical tests of autonomic failure

A. Cardiovascular reflexes

Tests performed and responses

1. *Change of posture:* BP and pulse rate monitored while subject is supine and then repeated measurements are made at 60° head-up tilt position: test of total baroreflex pathway. Pulse rate and plasma noradrenalin responses to standing. Lower-body negative pressure is an alternative to tilt or standing. For tests on standing see Chapters 17, 37, and 38.

2. *Deep breathing:* presence or absence of sinus arrhythmia: test of vagal efferent pathway.

3. *Carotid massage:* right and left sides, in turn monitoring cardiac rate and blood pressure; test of vagal efferent pathway. Caution in case of supersensitivity.

4. *Hyperventilation:* for 30 seconds, causing hypocapnia and fall in blood pressure; response suggests afferent lesion, if baroreflex block.

5. *Inspiratory gasp:* causing reflex vasoconstriction of hands; spinal-cord reflex.

6. *Stress:* causing hypertension and tachycardia; tests of sympathetic efferent pathway.
   (a) Handgrip, submaximal sustained for 90 s.
   (b) Sudden cortical arousal by unexpected noise.
   (c) Mental arithmetic (rapid serial subtraction of 7 from 100).
   (d) Cold pressor test—hand immersed in water at 4°C for 90 s.

7. *Breath holding:* test of central breathing control; prolonged if vagal afferent dysfunction.

Table 16.2. (*cont.*)

8. *Valsalva manoeuvre*
   After a deep inspiration the patient performs a forced expiration for 12 s through a tube connected to a mercury manometer. Most subjects can maintain a pressure of 30 mm Hg. In normal subjects there is an increased tachycardia for the 10 s of sustained forced expiration. Blood pressure falls initially but should cease to fall after the first few seconds if peripheral sympathetic vasoconstriction is normal. On release from blowing there is normally a BP overshoot and a compensatory reflex bradycardia.
9. *Pharmacological and biochemical tests*
   (*a*) Plasma noradrenalin at rest and after 5–10 minutes standing or tilt.
   (*b*) Pressor response and cardiac slowing to infusion of noradrenalin; test of baroreflex sensitivity.
   (*c*) Pressor response and noradrenalin response to infusion of tyramine; test of cytoplasmic stores of noradrenalin.
   (*d*) Cardiac rate response to isoprenaline infusion; test of β-receptor cardiac function.
   (*e*) Cardiac slowing to atropine; test of vagal function.
   (*f*) Adrenoceptor binding studies; α-adrenoceptors on platelets and β-adrenoceptors on lymphocytes (see Chapter 19).
   (*g*) Plasma dopamine and dopamine-β-hydroxylase to exclude dopamine-β-hydroxylase deficiency.
   (*h*) Hormonal responses: plasma vasopressin to tilt (see Chapter 21); pancreatic polypeptide to hypoglycaemia (see Chapter 18); growth hormone to clonidine or hypoglycaemia.

B. Sweating

1. Response to body heating in order to cause a rise of 1°C oral or rectal temperature in the course of 90 min. Record sweating and measure hand blood flow. Test of sympathetic pathway from hypothalamus to periphery.
2. Response to brief trunk heating with electric lamp source for 90 s; a reflex response, without involving change of blood temperature, utilizing same efferent pathway as response to body heating.
3. Responses to intramuscular pilocarpine; acts directly on sweat glands (see Chapter 42).
4. Pilomotor and sudomotor response to intradermal methacholine; absent with complete postganglionic lesion.
5. Sweating tests to study abnormal distribution of sweating; gustatory sweating.

C. Pupillary responses

1. Instillation of 1:1000 adrenalin. Response: dilatation after sympathetic postganglionic denervation; no effect on normal pupil.
2. Instillation of 4 per cent cocaine. Response: dilatation of normal pupil; no effect after sympathetic denervation.
3. Instillation of fresh 2.5 per cent methacholine. Response: constriction after parasympathetic denervation; no effect on normal pupil.

D. Skin responses

Intracutaneous injection of 0.05 ml of 1:1000 histamine phosphate causes a wheal surrounded by erythema and erythematous flare. The flare of this triple response is an axon reflex mediated by antidromic transmission along sensory fibres.

E. Bladder and sexual function (see Chapters 12, 13, and 23)

F. Intraneural recording (see Chapter 11)

SYMPATHETIC EFFERENT FIBRES TO VESSELS

There are three principal systems of autonomic fibres which protect against postural hypotension (see Table 16.3). The most important are the sympathetic efferent fibres to capacity and resistance vessels in muscles and the splanchnic area and also to the kidneys, affecting renin release. A lumbar sympathectomy has little effect on blood pressure, and even a combined lumbar and cervical sympathectomy has only a transient effect. The splanchnic area is of critical importance and loss of the major part of the total sympathetic outflow is probably necessary before postural hypotension occurs (Low *et al.* 1975). Less important are the sympathetic cardioaccelerator fibres and the parasympathetic efferent fibres to the heart.

Table 16.3. Selected tests of autonomic function

1. **Sympathetic efferent constrictor fibres to capacity and resistance vessels:**
   (*a*) Postural hypotension
   (*b*) Lack of overshoot after Valsalva test
   (*c*) Lack of blood pressure rise on stress
2. **Sympathetic efferent fibres to heart**
   (*a*) Lack of tachycardia during Valsalva, phase II
   (*b*) Lack of tachycardia on tilting
   (*c*) Lack of tachycardia on cortical arousal
   (*d*) Lack of tachycardia on isometric exercise
3. **Parasympathetic efferent fibres to heart**
   (*a*) Lack of sinus arrhythmia
   (*b*) Lack of effect of carotid massage
   (*c*) Lack of bradycardia after Valsalva, phase IV
   (*d*) Lack of rise of cardiac rate with atropine

Postural hypotension occurs with any major lesion of the sympathetic efferent fibres. There is no overshoot after the Valsalva manoeuvre, as in a normal subject. Figure 16.2 shows an intra-arterial recording with a beat-to-beat recording of cardiac rate (bottom). The tachycardia during the Valsalva manoeuvre is blocked by propranolol and unaffected by atropine, and is principally sympathetically mediated. When venous return falls and cardiac output drops as a result of the raised intra-thoracic pressure caused by the manoeuvre, arterial pressure falls steadily at first (phase II) but then recovers again as compensatory vaso-constriction and tachycardia occur. In autonomic failure, in addition to the decline in blood pressure in phase II, no overshoot occurs (phase IV) because there is a reduced vasoconstriction of the peripheral circulation into which the increased cardiac output is pumped (Fig. 16.2).

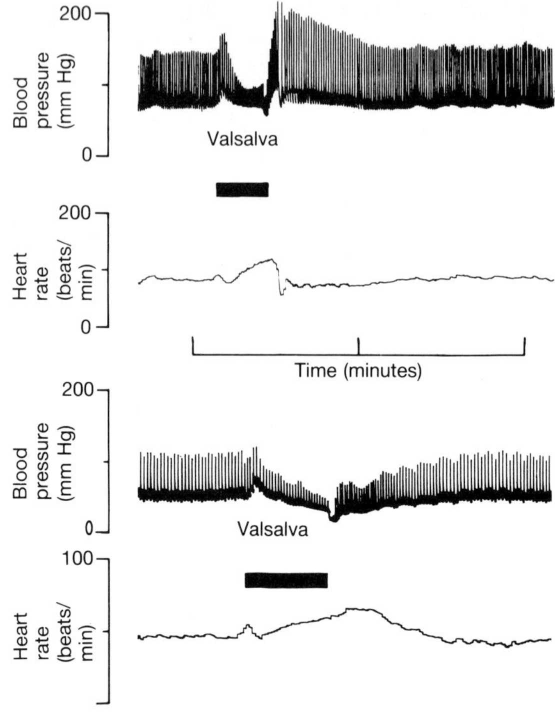

Fig. 16.2. Changes in blood pressure and heart rate before, during, and after the Valsalva manoeuvre, when intrathoracic pressure was raised to 40 mm Hg in a normal subject (*upper trace*) and in a patient (*lower trace*). In the normal subject release of intrathoracic pressure was accompanied by an increase in blood pressure and a reduction in heart rate below basal levels. In the patient there was a gradual increase in blood pressure implying impairment of sympathetic vasoconstrictor pathways. The heart-rate scale varies in the two subjects.

SYMPATHETIC EFFERENT FIBRES TO HEART

The second system protecting against postural hypotension, the sympathetic cardiac efferent fibres, are tested by tilting, cortical arousal, and isometric exercise. The tachycardia on tilting and on stress or exercise is probably mediated by similar sympathetic efferent pathways, though different vascular beds are involved and in some active vasodilatation may occur (Bannister *et al.* 1967).

PARASYMPATHETIC EFFERENT FIBRES TO HEART

The third relevant reflex system protecting against orthostatic hypotension is the parasympathetic rate control of the heart which is, in functional terms, not as important. Figure 16.3 shows a cardiac beat-to-beat recording during deep breathing. In a normal subject sinus arrythmia may be as great as 20–30 beats with deep breathing and is measurable during shallow breathing. The mechanism of sinus arrhythmia is uncertain (see Chapter 4) but the efferent path is the vagal parasympathetic supply to the heart (Wheeler and Watkins 1973). It is abolished by atropine and is absent in autonomic failure. Parasympathetic function may also be tested by the bradycardia on carotid massage. The response is usually absent in autonomic failure.

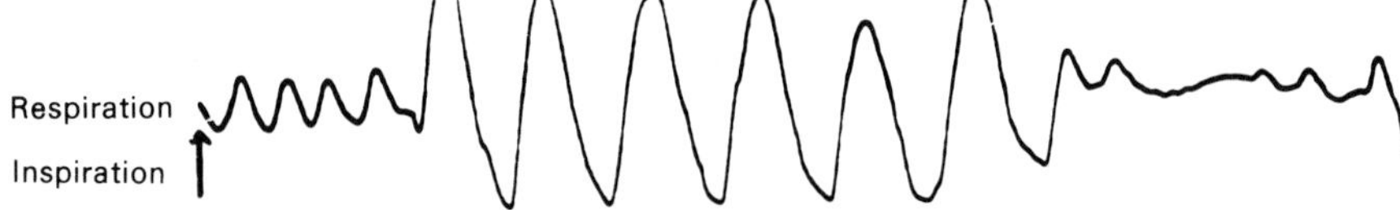

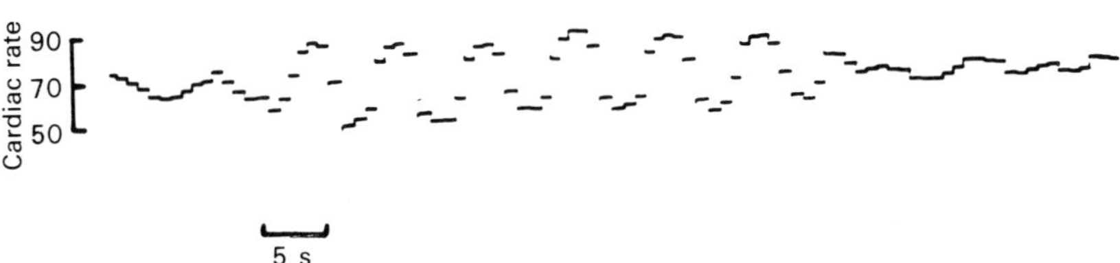

Fig. 16.3. Sinus arrhythmia in normal subject. Respiratory record (upper trace).

SITE OF THE LESION ON THE REFLEX ARC

The tests are listed in Table 16.3 as though they were purely for efferent pathways, but most involve reflex arcs and hence have central and afferent connections as well. The next stage, if postural hypotension and an abnormal Valsalva manoeuvre are demonstrated, is to try to show whether the lesion is afferent or efferent or both (Table 16.4). If the vasoconstrictor response to stress is entirely preserved, the efferent limb must be intact and the lesion is afferent or central. If the sweating response to generalized body heating is preserved, it can be argued, by analogy, that the lesion is probably afferent since sweat glands are innervated by sympathetic (cholinergic) fibres. The loss of sweating and piloerection after intradermal acetylcholine injections has been taken as evidence of a postganglionic lesion but these tests are not easy to

Table 16.4. Principles of localization of lesions in autonomic failure with postural hypotension

Observation	*Conclusion*
1. Vasoconstrictor response to stress preserved	Afferent lesion
2. Defective thermal sweating	Efferent lesion
3. Normal piloerection and sweating to intradermal acetylcholine	Preganglionic lesion
4. Defective piloerection and sweating to intradermal acetylcholine	Postganglionic lesion

interpret (Bárány and Cooper 1956; Macmillan and Spalding 1969). There are of course no single lesions in autonomic failure; lesions occur at more than one site, are progressive, and may be partial rather than complete. Moreover, most tests give information about only one part of an effector mechanism; for example the preservation of the pressor response in one forearm does not mean that it is spared in the remainder of that limb or in the circulation as a whole. It is not usually possible in the presence of an efferent lesion to diagnose with certainty the presence of another lesion of the afferent side of the reflex arc (see Chapter 37). This can sometimes be achieved by comparing two reflexes with the same efferent path but different afferent or central paths and so proving selective involvement of the efferent path (Bannister *et al.* 1967; Aminoff and Wilcox 1971). For example, the lack of change of heart rate after pharmacologically induced hypertension or hypotension in the presence of normal vagally mediated responses to atropine would be strong evidence for an afferent lesion. We have not encountered this in AF.

More precise identification of which fibres are defective is difficult and involves techniques which are not easy to apply in the routine study of patients. The lower-body suction technique has been used to simulate the effects of standing (Bannister *et al.* 1967). The patient remains in the recumbent position with an arterial catheter in place, and forearm blood flow is measured by plethysmography. Suction mimics the shift of blood which occurs on standing. Figure 16.4 shows that if negative pressure is applied in a normal subject to the level of the iliac crest, there is a five-fold increase in the resistance in the forearm muscle blood vessels. Figure 16.4 also shows a patient with autonomic failure in whom forearm bloodflow hardly changes in response to negative pressure applied to the lower half of the body. There is a slight fall, but this is a reflection of the drop in perfusion pressure. At least as important as the total change in resistance or volume of a limb is the rate at which the change occurs in autonomic failure. The volume of the calf increases during suction more quickly in a patient with autonomic failure (Fig. 16.5). Sometimes the effects of suction or postural changes may also be aggravated by active vasodilatation (Abboud and Eckstein 1966;

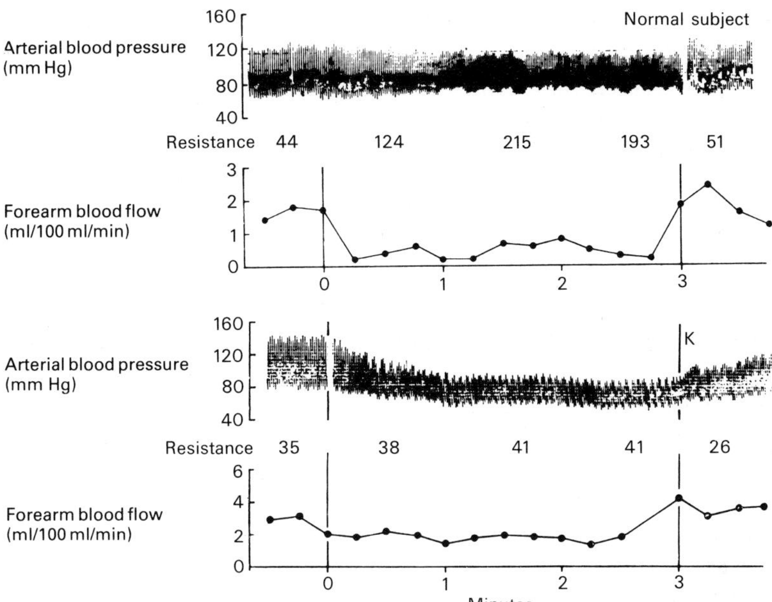

Fig. 16.4. The effect of suction on arterial blood pressure, forearm resistance, and forearm blood flow in a normal subject (upper part), and in a patient with autonomic failure (lower part). (Taken with permission from Bannister *et al.* (1967).)

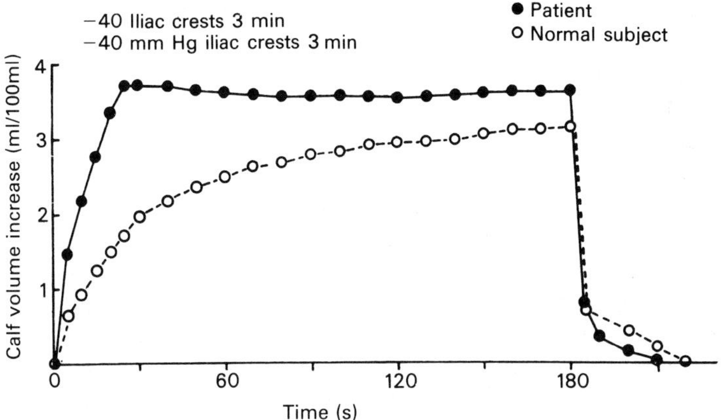

Fig. 16.5. The increase in leg volume during suction in a normal subject and a patient with autonomic failure. Calf volume increase (ml/100 ml) plotted against time in seconds. (Taken with permission from Bannister *et al.* (1967).)

Bannister *et al.* 1967). More complex studies of circulatory control have combined the use of lower-body negative pressure (Abboud *et al.* 1979; Mark 1980; Bennett *et al.* 1980) with neck suction to 'unload' the carotid baroreceptors (Eckberg 1980) (see Chapter 8). These studies have shown that cardiopulmonary 'low-pressure' receptors in general modulate resistance vessels in skeletal muscle but aortic and carotid sinus 'high-pressure' baroreceptors control heart rate and splanchnic resistance. Selective tests of this type have not yet been applied to AF. The direct intraneural recording from sympathetic fibres has provided striking confirmation of the selectivity of the sympathetic vascular control to muscle and skin vessels and is reviewed by Wallin (see Chapter 11).

From such physiological studies in cases of pure autonomic failure or autonomic failure with multiple system atrophy or Parkinson's disease there is good evidence of an efferent sympathetic lesion. The sympathetic efferent lesion affects both resistance and capacity vessels and the heart, and is usually more severe than the vagal central or efferent lesion. This makes an interesting and important contrast to diabetic autonomic neuropathy, in which the vagal efferent lesion is usually more severe than the sympathetic efferent lesion (see Chapters 36 and 37). On the basis of physiological investigation it is difficult to establish the precise site of the lesion distally but recent studies of digital skin temperature and laser doppler blood flow appear to have shown a greater degree of peripheral vasodilatation in patients with PAF by comparison with patients with MSA in whom digital blood flow is similar to that in normal subjects.

BIOCHEMICAL AND PHARMACOLOGICAL TESTS

A variety of pharmacological approaches can now be used to help determine the site of the lesion and determine the status of receptors which are responsible for specific actions.

Pressor responsiveness to noradrenalin and tyramine

There continues to be a major difficulty as to whether the sympathetic efferent lesion is pre- or postganglionic, or both. This is of theoretical and practical importance, as it relates to the degree of denervation supersensitivity (Cannon and Rosenblueth 1949), and determines the response to pressor agents used in therapy. Following complete experimental postganglionic sympathetic denervation, there is supersensitivity of blood vessels to the major neurotransmitter, noradrenalin, together with a loss of response to tyramine, which acts by releasing noradrenalin from the cytoplasmic pool but not from the granular pool, which is accessible only to nerve impulses. Patients with autonomic failure show supersensitivity to intravenously administered noradrenalin (see Fig. 16.6). This response is greater in patients with pure autonomic failure (PAF) as compared to those with MSA (Kontos *et al.* 1975;

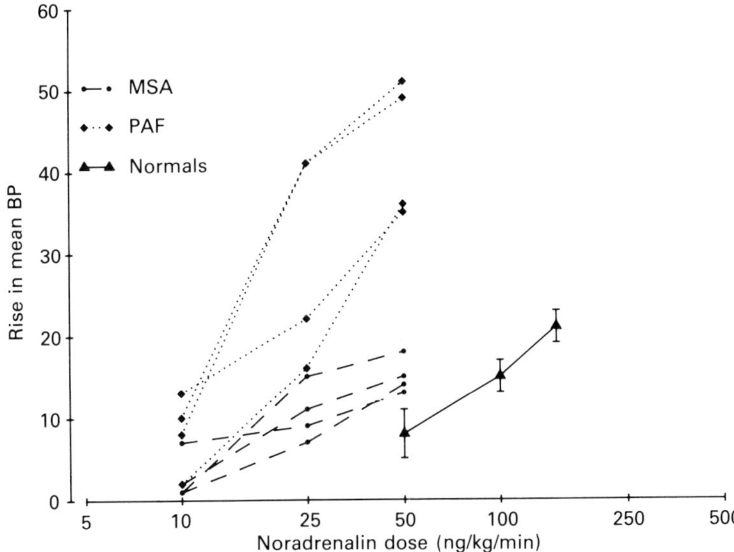

Fig. 16.6. Rise in mean blood pressure (BP) in four patients with pure autonomic failure (PAF) and four patients with multiple system atrophy (MSA); a response in normal subjects is indicated. Both groups of patients with autonomic failure had increased sensitivity to infused noradrenalin. In the PAF patients there appears to be a considerably greater response.

Bannister *et al.* 1979). Because of the exquisite sensitivity in some patients with PAF we first infuse extremely low doses of noradrenalin, with close monitoring of blood pressure, heart rate, and the ECG.

Bradycardia does occur in some patients and, occasionally, this may be a particular problem, as described in a patient who had severe sympathetic failure with an intact, and probably hyperactive vagus (Bannister *et al.* 1986). The upper limit of blood pressure which can be safely reached has to be decided by the clinical investigator in individual patients. Supine hypertension often limits the ability to construct dose-response curves to noradrenalin. It is important that resuscitation facilities, including the ready availability of α-adrenergic blockers, such as phentolamine, are present in case blood pressure needs to be lowered rapidly. Placing patients in the head-up position, however, may often suffice.

The mechanisms responsible for the increased pressor response are probably multiple. There is evidence of an increase in α-receptor number on platelets (Davies *et al.* 1982) (see Chapter 19) and a parallel increase in blood vessels may contribute to the responses. Patients with pure autonomic failure tend to have lower basal plasma levels of noradrenalin than those with multiple system atrophy, which may account for a greater degree of 'up-regulation' in PAF and hence an even greater response to a similar infusion of noradrenalin compared with MSA. Other factors may also clearly contribute; both groups of patients have impairment of the baroreceptor reflex and the inability, therefore, to compensate in different vascular beds would be either impaired or lost. Furthermore, the clearance of noradrenalin is likely to be affected depending upon both the site and the degree of sympathetic efferent impairment.

Studies with intravenous tyramine indicate a small pressor response in patients with autonomic failure, with a lack of rise in plasma noradrenalin levels (Bannister *et al.* 1979); however, the minimal amounts of noradrenalin released probably result in the small pressor response because of the patients' supersensitivity. In cases of pure autonomic failure there is no forearm vasoconstrictor response to tyramine given intra-arterially, which is indicative of the postganglionic lesion (Kontos *et al.* 1975). The nerve terminal and receptor defects, however, probably vary in patients with pure autonomic failure, although they may show similar degrees of severity of postural hypotension. For example, in two patients there was a rise of plasma noradrenalin after tyramine infusion (Bannister *et al.* 1979). In one, however, recumbent and tilt values of noradrenalin were extremely low and there may have been a defect of its release by nerve impulses but not necessarily by tyramine. The second patient probably had a different and less severe defect, so that the resting plasma noradrenalin levels were more nearly normal and the noradrenalin and the nerve ending was accessible to tyramine. The duration of the pressor response to noradrenalin, however, was increased fourfold, suggesting a defect of transmitter re-uptake or metabolism (see Chapter 31).

Chronotropic response to isoprenaline

There is evidence that β-adrenoceptor numbers on lymphocytes are increased in patients with autonomic failure, suggesting that similar changes may occur in relation to β-receptors within the heart and probably blood vessels too (Bannister *et al.* 1981). β_1-adrenoceptors are responsible for mediating chronotropic cardiac changes, while β_2-receptors are present in blood vessels and contribute to vasodilatation. We have used the chronotropic response to isoprenaline, infused in incremental doses, as a means of determining the β-receptor sensitivity. Isoprenaline has both β_1- and β_2-adrenoceptor agonist effects. Initial studies were performed with bolus intravenous injections, but this usually resulted in a depressor response in autonomic failure and the rise in heart rate was probably a combination of its direct effects and those dependent upon cardiac acceleration secondary to vagal withdrawal in response to the fall in pressure. This can make interpretation of this response more difficult, as the degree of baroreceptor impairment can vary between patients. A similar effect occurred in a tetraplegic patient shown in comparison with a paraplegic patient in Fig. 16.7. With infusion of isoprenaline, a fall in systolic and diastolic blood pressure can occur (see Fig. 16.8) but this is often less than that during bolus injections. Figure 16.9 shows the rise in heart rate in patients with autonomic failure after infusions of isoprenaline.

Our studies indicate that in the majority of patients with autonomic failure there is no chronotropic supersensitivity to isoprenaline. Enhanced vasodilatation and a fall in pressure occurs in the majority, suggesting vasodilatation not compensated for by sympathetic nerve activity. The patients with autonomic failure, therefore, may not necessarily be more susceptible to cardiac dysrhythmias when β-receptor agonists are used.

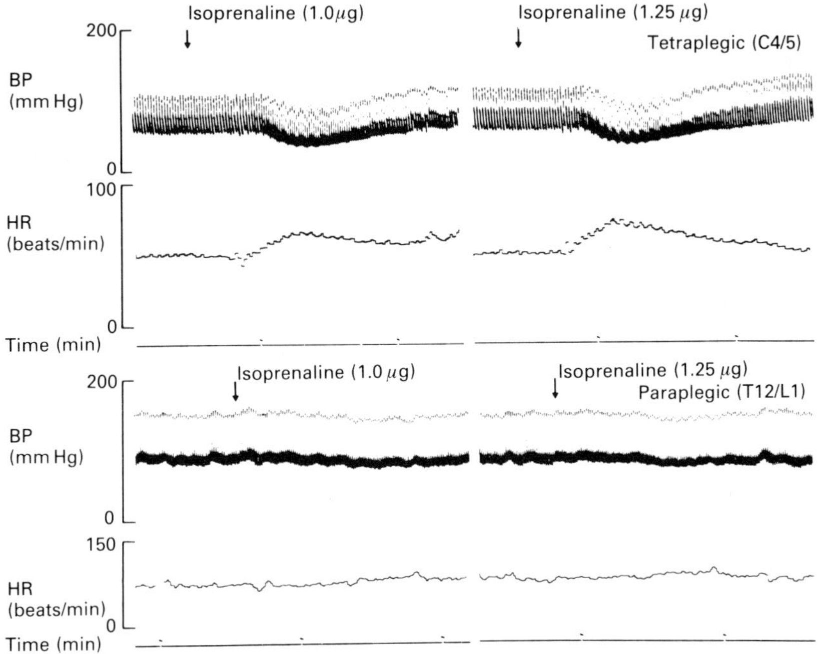

Fig. 16.7. Blood pressure (BP) and heart rate (HR) in a tetraplegic patient (upper panel) and a paraplegic patient (lower panel) (with an almost intact sympathetic nervous system) in response to bolus injections of isoprenaline. In the tetraplegic there is a clear fall in blood pressure after isoprenaline. This probably results from β_2-adrenoceptor mediated vasodilatation. There is a rise in heart rate before the blood pressure falls and this is likely to be a β_1-adrenoceptor mediated effect which is then enhanced by the effects of withdrawal of vagal tonus which is likely to occur in response to the fall in blood pressure. In the paraplegic patient there are considerably smaller changes. (Taken with permission from Mathias and Frankel (1986).)

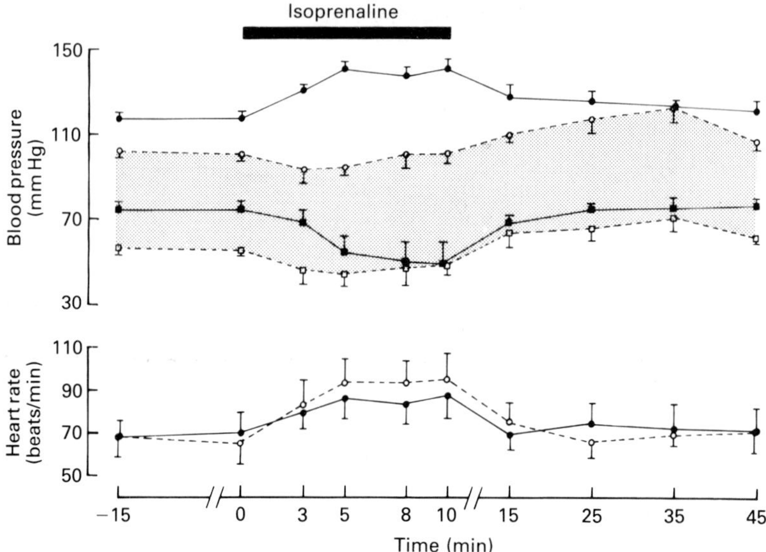

Fig. 16.8. Blood pressure and heart rate in five tetraplegic patients (open circles and squares and broken line) and five control subjects (full circles and squares and continuous line) before, during and after intravenous infusion of isoprenaline (0.01 μg/min/kg). The shaded area indicates blood pressure in the tetraplegic patients; bars indicate ±SEM. In the tetraplegics there is a fall in both systolic and diastolic blood pressure. (Taken with permission from Mathias *et al.* (1981).)

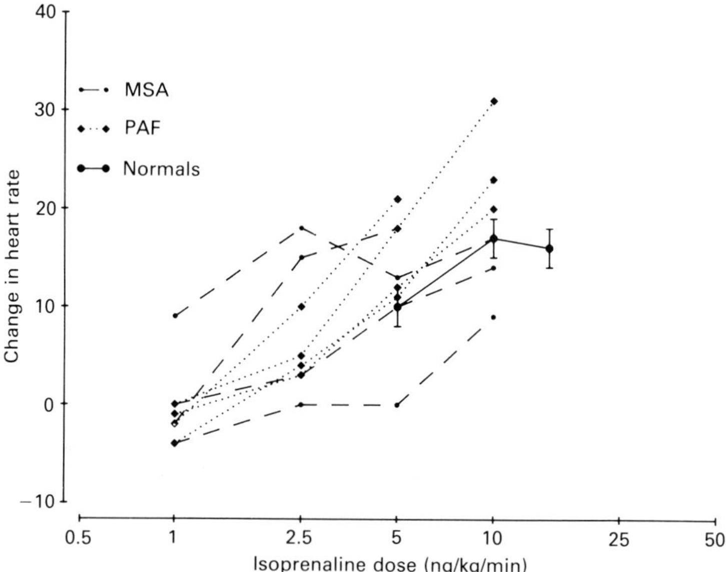

Fig. 16.9. Change in heart rate in response to incremental infusion of isoprenaline in four patients with pure autonomic failure (PAF) and four patients with multiple system atrophy (MSA). The response in normal subjects is indicated. Despite a fall in blood pressure in the majority of patients with autonomic failure only a few had a greater increase in sensitivity. Chronotropic β-adrenergic supersensitivity does not therefore appear to be as marked as pressor supersensitivity in autonomic failure patients.

Atropine

Atropine is a potent muscarinic blocker and has been used to determine the degree of vagal involvement in our patients. Doses of 5 μg/kg are given at 2-min intervals and a dose-response heart-rate curve constructed (Fig. 16.10). The total dose should not exceed 1800 μg. This enables at least four points on the dose-response curve to be plotted in most individuals. The administration is stopped if the heart rate rises above 110 beats/min or, clearly, if there are abnormal beats or rhythms. The drug in these doses causes few symptoms; dilatation of the pupil and blurring of vision may occur because of its cycloplegic effects. In some patients there may be impairment of detrusor-muscle activity and it is therefore best that patients with impaired bladder function empty the urinary bladder before the test. Dryness of mouth lasts for usually no more than an hour.

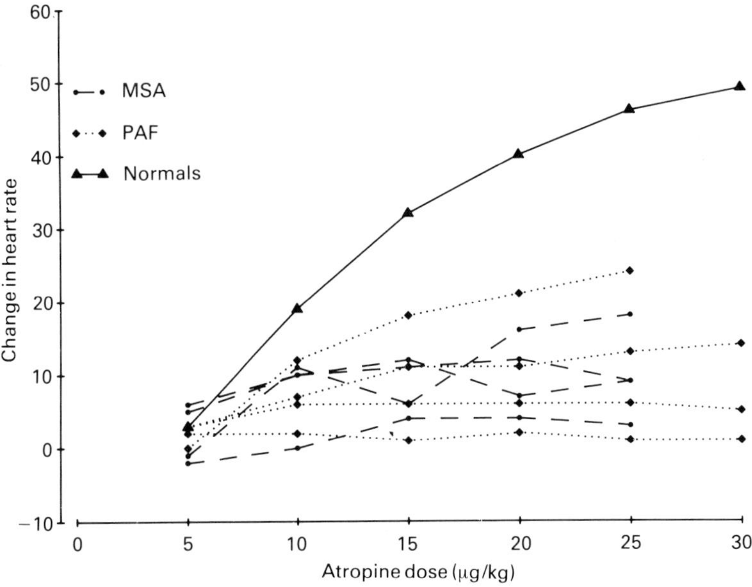

Fig. 16.10. Change in heart rate in four patients with pure autonomic failure and four patients with multiple system atrophy (MSA) in response to atropine. In the majority of patients there is minimal change in heart rate unlike the change expected in normal subjects. Cardiac vagal impairment seems to occur equally in both groups of patients.

The majority of our patients with autonomic failure, either pure or as part of MSA, have vagal impairment as determined by atropine testing. This is consistent with the pathological observations in the brainstem of involvement of the dorsal vagal nuclei.

Clonidine

Clonidine is an α_2-adrenoceptor agonist which lowers blood pressure by its central effects in reducing sympathetic nerve activity. In normal subjects this is accompanied by a reduction in peripheral levels of plasma noradrenalin. It also stimulates the release of growth hormone, and this appears to be dependent on an intact central adrenergic system (Checkley 1980). The growth hormone response to clonidine has been proposed as a test for determining the degree of central sympathetic degeneration in patients with autonomic failure, as the responses based on cardiovascular and peripheral noradrenalin measurements may not distinguish between those with brainstem, spinal, or postganglionic involvement of the sympathetic nervous system.

When intravenous clonidine (1.5 μg/kg) is administered to normal subjects, there is a prompt rise in levels of growth hormone but no change occurs in patients with autonomic failure (Fig. 16.11). There appear to be no differences between those who clearly have pure autonomic failure as compared to those who have autonomic failure with

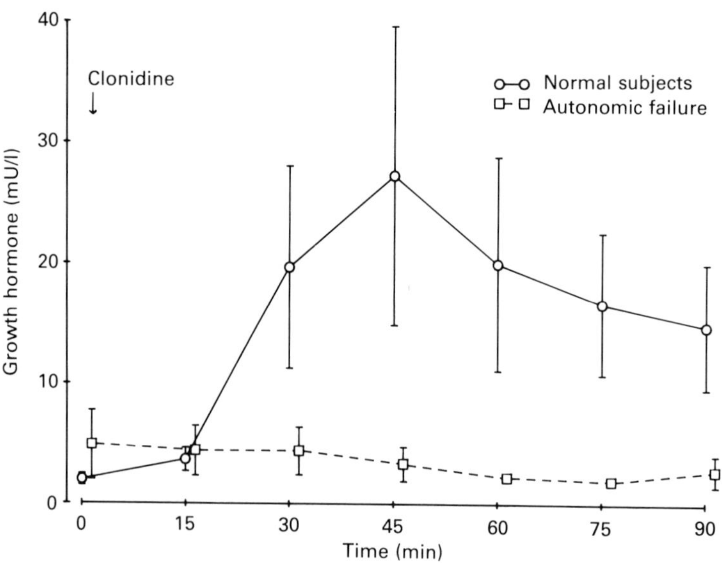

Fig. 16.11. Plasma levels of human growth hormone in normal subjects (open circles, continuous line) and patients with autonomic failure (full squares, dotted lines) in response to 1.5 μg/kg of i.v. clonidine. In the normal subjects there is a significant rise within 30 min which reaches its maximum at 45 min. In the autonomic failure patients the basal levels are not different from the normal subjects but there is no change following clonidine administration. Vertical bars indicate ±SEM. (Taken from da Costa *et al.* (1984).)

MSA, suggesting that the degree of central sympathetic degeneration is similar in both groups, although there is additional peripheral involvement in the former group. The growth hormone release induced by clonidine is therefore a useful neuroendocrine marker for assessing integrity of the central α-adrenergic system in man (da Costa *et al.* 1984).

Plasma vasopressin

The measurement of plasma vasopressin in response to tilt has been used as a test of the afferent part of the baroreflex pathways. Plasma vasopressin levels rise in normal subjects and in patients with a purely efferent autonomic lesion when hypotension on tilt is induced by a saline infusion or hypovolaemia. The lack of a response in a patient with autonomic failure with intact sympathetic efferent function suggests an afferent or central lesion (see Chapter 21).

MISCELLANEOUS TESTS

Recent observations indicate that the blood pressure response to posture can be markedly influenced by two factors—the food intake of patients and the effects of recumbency. These two aspects are now routinely tested in our patients, protocols to obtain the maximum therapeutically valuable information being used.

Effects of food and recumbency

A simple means of determining the response to food ingestion is to use a liquid meal containing glucose alone (1 g/kg body weight) as the hypotensive response to a meal appears to be largely dependent upon carbohydrate intake. Studies with liquid meals containing different food components are in progress. The patient should be tilted prior to administration, then given the glucose so that measurements can be made in a supine position for about an hour, and then the tilt repeated. In the majority of patients there is a fall in blood pressure while supine and an accentuation of postural hypotension. There are occasionally patients in whom the supine blood pressure is lowered modestly but the effects are unmasked by repeated tilt later. Recumbency induces both a diuresis and a natriuresis in patients with autonomic failure (Bannister *et al.* 1979). Studies incorporating salt and water homeostasis together with observations on blood pressure while supine and sitting or standing are necessary to determine the degree of nocturnal polyuria and natriuresis and therefore the appropriateness of therapy with agents such as desmopressin (DDAVP) (Mathias *et al.* 1986). Our routine requires 12-hourly collections of urine between 9 a.m. and 9 p.m. and 9 p.m. and

9 a.m., together with measurements of sodium and potassium excretion together with osmolality, measurements of weight at 9 a.m. and 9 p.m. (to provide the degree of weight loss which occurs overnight), and both supine and sitting and standing blood pressures at intervals through the day prior to meal administration. This provides the major information needed for such evaluation. This also helps decisions on whether the use of agents such as fludrocortisone and salt supplements are needed.

REFERENCES

Abboud, F. M., Eckberg, D. L., Johannsen, U. J., and Mark, A. L. (1979). Carotid and cardiopulmonary baroreceptor control of splanchnic and forearm vascular resistance during venous pooling in man. *J. Physiol., London* **286**, 173–84.

Abboud, F. M. and Eckstein, J. W. (1966). Active reflex vasodilatation in man. *Fed. Proc. Fed. Am. Soc. exp. Biol.* **25**, 1611–17.

Aminoff, M. J. and Wilcox, C. S. (1971). Assessment of autonomic function in patients with a Parkinsonian syndrome. *Br. med. J.* **iv**, 80–4.

Bannister, R. (1979). Chronic autonomic failure with postural hypotension. *Lancet* **ii**, 404–6.

Bannister, R., Ardill, L., and Fentem, P. (1967). Defective autonomic control of blood vessels in idiopathic orthostatic hypotension. *Brain* **90**, 725–46.

Bannister, R., Boylston, A. W., Davies, I. B., Mathias, C. J., Sever, P. S., and Sudera, D. (1981). Beta receptor numbers and thermodynamics in denervation supersensitivity. *J. Physiol. London* **319**, 369–77.

Bannister, R., da Costa, D. F., Hendry, C. H., Jacobs, J., and Mathias, C. J. (1986). Atrial demand pacing to protect against vagal overactivity in sympathetic autonomic neuropathy. *Brain* **109**, 345–56.

Bannister, R., Davies, I. B., Holly, E., Rosenthal, T., and Sever, P. (1979). Defective cardiovascular reflexes and supersensitivity to sympathomimetic drugs in autonomic failure. *Brain* **102**, 163–76.

Bannister, R., Sever, P., and Gross, M. (1977). Cardiovascular reflexes and biochemical responses in progressive autonomic failure. *Brain* **100**, 327–44.

Bárány, F. R. and Cooper, E. H. (1956). Pilomotor and sudomotor innervation in diabetes. *Clin. Sci.* **15**, 533–40.

Bennett, T. (1984). Diabetic autonomic neuropathy and iritis. *Br. med. J.* **289**, 1231.

Bennett, T., Hosking, D. J., and Hampton, J. R. (1980). Cardiovascular responses to graded reductions of central blood volume in normal subjects and patients with diabetes mellitus. *Clin. Sci. mol. Med.* **58**, 193–200.

Cannon, W. B. and Rosenblueth, A. (1949). *The supersensitivity of denervated structures: a law of denervation.* Macmillan, New York.

Checkley, S. A. (1980). Neuroendocrine studies of monoamine function in man. *Psychol. Med.* **10**, 35–53.

Collins, K. J., Exton-Smith, A. N., James, M. H., and Oliver, D. J. (1980). Functional changes in autonomic nervous responses with ageing. *Age Ageing* **9**, 17–24.

da Costa, D. F., Bannister, R., Landon, J., and Mathias, C. J. (1984). Growth hormone response to clonidine is impaired in patients with central sympathetic degeneration. *Clin. exp. Hypertension* **6**, 1843–6.

Davies, I. B., Sudera, D., Sagnella, G., Marchesi-Saviotti, E., Mathias, C., Bannister, R., and Sever, P. (1982). Increased numbers of alpha-receptors in sympathetic denervation supersensitivity in man. *J. clin. Invest.* **69**, 779–84.

Eckberg, D. L. (1980). Carotid baroreceptor stimulus–sinus node relationship in man. In *Arterial baroreceptors and hypertension* (ed. P. Sleight), pp. 476–83. Oxford University Press, Oxford.

Kontos, H. A., Richardson, D. W., and Norvell, J. E. (1975). Norepinephrine depletion in idiopathic orthostatic hypotension. *Ann. intern. Med.* **82**, 336–41.

Low, P. A., Walsh, J. C., Huang, C. Y., and McLeod, J. G. (1975). The sympathetic nervous system in diabetic neuropathy. *Brain* **98**, 341–56.

Macmillan, A. L. and Spalding, J. M. K. (1969). Human sweating response to electrophoresed acetylcholine: a test of postganglionic sympathetic function. *J. Neurol. Neurosurg. Psychiat.* **32**, 155–60.

Mark, A. L. (1980). Reflex control of vascular resistance in borderline hypertension. In *Arterial baroreceptors and hypertension* (ed. P. Sleight), pp. 109–15. Oxford University Press, Oxford.

Marshall, R. J., Schirger, A., and Shepherd, J. T. (1961). Blood pressure during supine exercise in idiopathic orthostatic hypotension. *Circulation* **24**, 76–81.

Mathias, C. J., Fosbraey, P., da Costa, D. F., Thornley, A., and Bannister, R. (1986). Desmopressin reduces nocturnal polyuria, reverses overnight weight loss, and improves morning postural hypotension in autonomic failure. *Br. med. J.* **293**, 353–4.

Mathias, C. J. and Frankel, H. L. (1986). The neurological and hormonal control of blood vessels and heart in spinal man. *J. auton. nerv. Syst.* (Suppl.), 457–64.

Mathias, C. J. and Frankel, H. L. (1988). Cardiovascular control in spinal man. *Ann. Rev. Physiol.* **50**, 577–92.

Mathias, C. J., Frankel, H. L., Davies, I. B., James, V. H. T., and Peart, W. S. (1981). Renin and aldosterone release during sympathetic stimulation in tetraplegia. *Clin. Sci.* **60**, 399–404.

Ungerstedt, U. (1971). Sterotaxic mapping of the monoamine pathways in the rat brain. *Acta physiol. scand.* Suppl. **367**, 1–48.

Wheeler, T. and Watkins, P. J. (1973). Cardiac denervation in diabetes. *Br. med. J.* **iv**, 584–6.

17. Standing, orthostatic stress, and autonomic function

Wouter Wieling

INTRODUCTION

This review is concerned with the short-term circulatory adjustment to orthostatic stress. The first section will deal with basic mechanisms of the heart-rate and blood-pressure responses induced by a change of posture in healthy subjects. We will emphasize that it is important to distinguish between the initial reaction (first 30 s) and the early steady-state response (after 1–2 min upright). We will also discuss that active (standing up) and passive (tilt-table) changes of posture induce distinctly different responses initially. The second section will focus on the application of orthostatic stress as a test procedure in the assessment of neural circulatory control. It will be shown that simple monitoring of the beat-to-beat heart-rate changes induced by standing up and the conventional measurement of blood pressure provide important clinical information about the integrity of cardiovascular adaptation to orthostatic stress, but that an abnormal response can only be fully appreciated by continuous monitoring of both heart rate and blood pressure. We suggest that standing may be superior to head-up tilt as a test for assessing the integrity of heart-rate control. In the third and final section we shall outline the spectrum of normal and abnormal orthostatic responses. We will illustrate how simple non-invasive clinical tests can be used to classify subjects with complaints of orthostatic dizziness.

SHORT-TERM CIRCULATORY RESPONSE TO ORTHOSTATIC STRESS IN HEALTHY SUBJECTS

Initial heart-rate response on standing (first 30 s)

Standing up in healthy subjects induces characteristic changes in heart rate (Fig. 17.1). The heart rate increases abruptly towards a primary peak at around 3 s, increases further to a maximum at about 12 s,

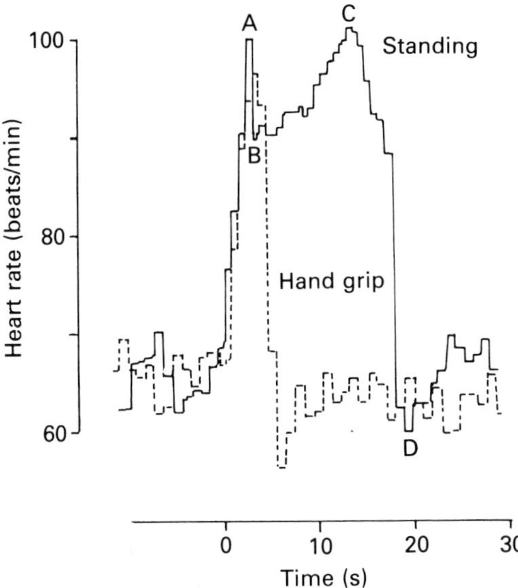

Fig. 17.1. Example of heart-rate changes in a healthy young subject evoked by standing in 2–3 s (solid line). A and C denote primary and secondary peak, respectively. B and D denote primary and secondary valley, respectively. An example of the heart-rate response to handgrip during 3 s has been superimposed (broken line). Handgrip was performed supine at maximal voluntary force. Note the striking resemblance in time course of both responses in the first 4 s. (From Borst *et al.* (1982), with permission.)

declines to a relative minimum at about 20 s, and then gradually rises again (Drischel *et al.* 1963; Borst *et al.* 1982).

The immediate heart-rate increase (A in Fig. 17.1) is the result of abrupt inhibition of cardiac vagal tone and is attributed to the exercise reflex which operates as soon as voluntary (static) muscle contractions are performed (Borst *et al.* 1982). For example, handgrip during 3 s at maximal force causes an acceleration of heart rate very similar to the primary heart-rate peak on standing up (Fig. 17.1). The brief relative heart-rate decrease at about 5 s after the start of standing up (B in Fig. 17.1) is not always present; if not, a distinct transition from a rapid heart-rate increase to a gradual further rise is usually observed (Borst *et al.* 1982, 1984).

The more gradual secondary heart-rate rise, starting around 5 s after the onset of standing up towards the secondary peak (C in Figs 17.1 and 17.2 (a)) is mainly due to further reflex inhibition of cardiac vagal tone and can be attributed to diminished activation of arterial baroreceptors by a temporary fall of arterial pressure. The subsequent decrease in heart rate (D in Figs 17.1 and 17.2 (a)) is associated with the recovery of arterial pressure and is again mediated through the arterial baroreflex

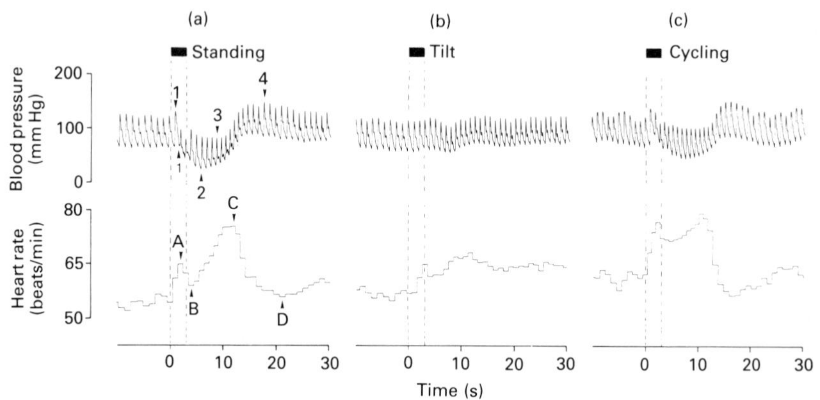

Fig. 17.2. Original tracings of circulatory transients in a healthy 38-year-old male subject evoked by (a) standing, (b) 70° head-up tilt, and (c) cycling. The arrows indicate the timing of various response extremes of interest. Note the striking resemblance of the circulatory transients following standing up and cycling and the more gradual changes following a 70° head-up tilt. The interventions were performed during inspiration. 1, immediate systolic/diastolic pressure increase; 2, diastolic-pressure minimum; 3, systolic-pressure minimum; 4, systolic-pressure maximum. A, primary peak; B, primary valley; C, secondary peak; D, secondary valley.

by rapid vagal inhibition of the sinus node. The relative bradycardia is a vagal reflex, but its occurrence depends on a preceding sympathetically mediated vasoconstriction (see below).

Comparison of initial heart-rate responses upon active and passive changes of posture

The initial heart-rate response upon passive changes of posture differs distinctly from the response on standing. A 70° head-up tilt, which may be considered to induce an identical hydrostatic effect as a 90° head-up tilt (sin 70° = 0.94), results in a less pronounced and a more gradual initial heart-rate rise with little or no overshoot (Fig. 17.2 (a), (b)) (Borst *et al.* 1982, 1984; Wieling *et al.* 1983*a*). These differences have been explained by the active use of muscles during standing up (see below).

Initial blood-pressure response on standing (first 30 s)

The initial blood-pressure response on standing is characterized by an immediate pressure increase, followed by a striking fall, recovery, and sometimes overshoot of arterial pressure (Fig. 17.2 (a)). This is in contrast with the gradual rise in diastolic pressure and little change in systolic pressure after head-up tilt (Fig. 17.2 (b)) (Borst *et al.* 1982, 1984).

The immediate blood-pressure increase (1 in Fig. 17.2 (a)) is probably due to a mechanical increase in total peripheral vascular resistance by the active contracting muscles during standing (Borst *et al.* 1982, 1984).

Two mechanisms have been postulated to account for the temporary fall of systolic and diastolic blood pressure (2 and 3 in Fig. 17.2 (a)). First, the muscular effort at the onset of standing is thought to compress the venous vessels in the contracting muscles of the legs and in the abdomen, resulting in an immediate translocation of blood towards the heart and thereby in an increase in right atrial and ventricular filling pressures (Borst *et al.* 1982, 1984). This mechanism presumably activates the cardiopulmonary receptors. Activation of these receptors results in a reflex release of vasoconstrictor tone (Shepherd and Mancia 1986). Second, activation of the arterial baroreceptor reflex by the immediate arterial-pressure increase at the onset of standing (1 in Fig. 17.2 (a)) may be contributory to the observed reflex release of vasoconstrictor tone (Borst *et al.* 1982, 1984). The recovery and sometimes overshoot of arterial pressure after about 7 s (4 in Fig. 17.2 (a)) is a result of decreased stimulation of the arterial baroreceptor and cardiopulmonary receptors (Borst *et al.* 1982, 1984).

This suggested sequence of events is supported by the results of the responses of heart rate and blood pressure at the onset of bicycle ergometry, where comparable muscle groups come into action (Fig. 17.2 (c)).

Early steady-state circulatory adaptation (after 1–2 min standing)

Characteristic of the adaptation to orthostatic stress in healthy subjects is the rapidity of the counterregulation of the initial disturbance; circulatory readjustment after a change of posture is usually reached within 1 min; in the following minutes only minor changes in heart rate and blood pressure are found. The normal steady-state blood-pressure response to postural change is an increase in diastolic pressure by about 10 per cent, with little or no change in systolic pressure. The steady-state heart-rate increase amounts on average to about 10 beats/min (Blomqvist and Stone 1983).

APPLICATION OF ORTHOSTATIC TESTS

The hallmark of failure of cardiovascular adjustment to orthostatic stress is a significant and persistent reduction in arterial pressure on standing. Orthostatic dizziness and syncope are dramatic expressions of autonomic failure, but may also occur in diverse non-neurogenic clinical disorders. It is not feasible to evaluate all conditions which may cause postural hypotension in each patient. However, a careful evaluation of the patient's history and simple non-invasive clinical tests usually limit the extensive differential diagnosis of orthostatic hypotension to a few possible causes.

Basic to the interpretation of an impaired heart-rate response on standing is the markedly different latency and time constant for the sinus node's response to changes in cardiac vagal and cardiac sympathetic nerve traffic (Shepherd and Mancia 1986). Vagally mediated heart-rate changes have a latency of about 0.5 s and a time constant of a few seconds, whereas these values are on the order of 1–3 and 10 s, respectively, for sympathetically mediated effects (Wieling *et al.* 1985). The initial sympathetically mediated component of the heart-rate response is usually completely obscured by the much larger and faster vagally mediated component. The initial sluggish sympathetic response is unmasked, however, when parasympathetic heart rate control is blocked by atropine (A in Fig. 17.3).

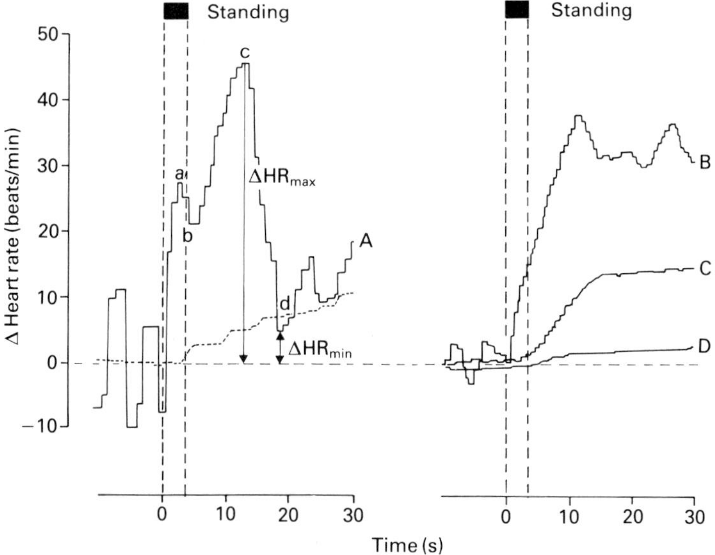

Fig. 17.3. Examples of the heart-rate changes (ΔHR) evoked by standing expressed as deviation from the resting heart rate. A, a 33-year-old male volunteer with a resting heart rate of 55 beats/min. a, Primary peak; b, primary valley; c, secondary peak (ΔHR_{max}); d, secondary valley (ΔHR_{min}). Pharmacological blockade with atropine (– – –) abolished the large transient heart-rate changes (resting heart rate after atropine 105 beats/min). B, a 37-year-old patient with a hyperadrenergic orthostatic response (resting heart rate 90 beats/min). C, a 33-year-old patient with diabetes and orthostatic hypotension with impaired parasympathetic and intact sympathetic heart rate control (resting heart rate 86 beats/min). D, a 36-year-old diabetic patient with severe long-term complications and almost total cardiac denervation (resting heart rate 72 beats/min). (Taken with permission from Wieling *et al.* (1985).)

Below, we shall illustrate how simple monitoring of the beat-to-beat heart-rate changes induced by standing up and the conventional measurement of blood pressure make it possible to distinguish normal from abnormal orthostatic responses. We shall discuss the test procedure first.

Test procedure

The subject is asked to lie down for 5–10 min, while blood pressure is measured with a sphygmomanometer and heart rate is monitored with an electrocardiograph, or more conveniently with a cardiotachometer connected to a pen-recorder. Resting heart rate is taken as the average over a 10-s period prior to standing. However, when marked sinus arrhythmia is present, a 30-s control period should be used. The subject is then asked to stand, while heart rate is monitored continuously for 30 s and again after 1 and 2 min standing. Blood pressure is measured after 1 min in the upright position. If an abnormal response is obtained (see below) and a longer period of standing is tolerated, heart rate and blood pressure are also measured after 2 and 5 min. The following parameters are analysed (A in Fig. 17.3).

Primary heart-rate peak

The primary heart-rate peak (a in Fig. 17.3) is an example of a response that is almost completely vagally mediated. It is therefore an important measure of the integrity of cardiac vagal inhibition; an immediate rise (latency <1 s) and a large primary heart-rate increase exclude the presence of cardiac vagal neuropathy (Wieling *et al.* 1983*a*, 1985). In order to be able to observe vagal withdrawal, some vagal tone should be present. This test, therefore, cannot be interpreted when the resting heart rate is high (>100 beats/min). This general principle applies to all tests aiming to assess withdrawal of cardiac vagal control.

Secondary heart-rate peak and subsequent relative bradycardia

The secondary heart-rate peak (c in Fig. 17.3) is mainly, but not exclusively vagally mediated. Enhanced sympathetic outflow to the sinus node also contributes to the response, in particular when the concomitant initial fall in blood pressure (2 and 3 in Fig. 17.2 (a)) is considerable. The highest heart rate in the first 15 s from the onset of standing is used as a measure for the secondary heart-rate peak (ΔHR_{max}) in Fig. 17.3) (Wieling *et al.* 1982). This approach allows a quantification of the response also in patients with a more gradual heart rate increase, but without a relative bradycardia and consequently without a clear secondary peak (C and D in Fig. 17.3).

As mentioned earlier, the relative bradycardia (d in Fig. 17.3) is the result of a vagal reflex, which depends on a preceding sympathetic mediated vasoconstriction (4 in Fig. 17.2 (a)). Ewing expressed the relative bradycardia originally as the ratio between the thirtieth and fifteenth R–R interval after the onset of standing. Indeed, on average, the maximal heart-rate increase is reached at around the fifteenth beat and the relative bradycardia at around beat 30. However, since there are considerable interindividual differences, measurement of the 30/15 ratio at exactly beats 15 and 30 underestimates the true $R\text{–}R_{max}/R\text{–}R_{min}$ ratio, (Wieling *et al.* 1982). It is now generally recommended to use the $R\text{–}R_{max}/R\text{–}R_{min}$ ratio (A in Fig. 17.3) to quantify the relative bradycardia. Indeed Ewing now recommends measuring the 30/15 ratio by taking the longest and shortest R–R intervals around rather than exactly at beats 15 and 30, making this ratio identical to the $R\text{–}R_{max}/R\text{–}R_{min}$ ratio that we use.

Early steady-state heart-rate response (after 1–2 min standing)

As discussed above, the initial heart-rate transient is mainly vagally mediated. In contrast, the steady-state heart-rate adjustment in the upright position depends predominantly on increased activity of the sympathetic system (Marin Neto *et al.* 1980). An excessive heart-rate increase after being in the upright position for 1–2 min offers therefore useful clinical information: it indicates a strong adrenergic drive to the sinus node (Blomqvist and Stone 1983).

Factors involved in the magnitude of the heart-rate response on standing

An important determinant is age, since in the elderly both the initial and steady-state heart-rate changes on standing are smaller (Fig. 17.4; Table 17.1). Thus, in assessing the heart-rate responses on standing, it is essential to compare responses in patients with those of control subjects of comparable age (Wieling *et al.* 1982; Dambrink and Wieling 1987).

A second important factor in interpreting the magnitude of the initial heart-rate response on standing is the duration of the preceding period of supine rest; the magnitude of the initial heart rate maximum after 20 min rest exceeds the maximum after 1 min rest by about 30 per cent (Borst *et al.* 1982, 1984; Wieling *et al.* 1985).

Early steady-state blood-pressure response (after 1–2 min standing)

Conventional sphygmomanometry is accurate enough for a clinical assessment of the blood-pressure adjustment to standing. A fall in arterial pressure in the upright position can either involve both systolic and diastolic pressure or is restricted to the systolic pressure only. A fall of the systolic pressure only is most likely caused by a non-neurogenic disturbance such as a decrease in blood volume. Orthostatic hypotension due to autonomic failure involves both systolic and diastolic pressure. No agreement exists regarding the normal range of postural changes in

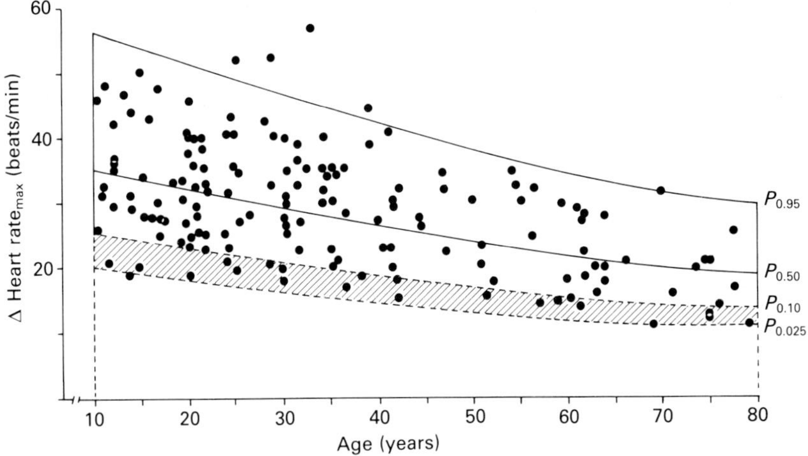

Fig. 17.4. Magnitude of the secondary heart-rate peak (ΔHR_{max}) on standing up in relation to age. The regression line ($P_{0.50}$) and confidence limits were calculated from log-transformed values. Scores below $P_{0.025}$ are considered abnormally small. (Taken with permission from Wieling *et al.* (1982) and Dambrink and Wieling (1987).)

Table 17.1. Assessment of initial heart-rate response following 5–10 min resting period and assessment of early steady-state heart-rate response

	Initial heart-rate response		*Early steady-state*
Age (years)	ΔHR_{max}* *(beats/min)*	HR_{max}/HR_{min}†	$\Delta HR_{2\ minutes}$‡ *(beats/min)*
10–14	< 20	< 1.20	> 30
15–19	19	1.18	29
20–24	19	1.17	28
25–29	18	1.15	28
30–34	17	1.13	27
35–39	16	1.11	26
40–44	16	1.09	25
45–49	15	1.08	25
50–54	14	1.06	24
55–59	13	1.04	23
60–64	13	1.02	22
65–69	12	1.01	21
70–74	12	1.00	21
75–80	11	—	20

* Abnormally low scores for ΔHR_{max} are defined as scores below $P_{0.025}$ in Fig. 17.4

† Abnormally low values for relative bradycardia are numerically expressed as HR_{max}/HR_{min} ratio.

‡ Heart-rate increases above $P_{0.975}$ of early steady-state values (after 2 min standing) are defined as excessive increase in heart rate.

blood pressure despite many studies. There is, however, good evidence that a persistent fall in systolic pressure larger than 20 mm Hg and/or 5 mm Hg in diastolic pressure after a change from the supine to the erect position should be considered abnormal (Wieling *et al.* 1983*b*). Even in elderly subjects an orthostatic fall in systolic pressure of more than 20 mm Hg after 1 min standing appears to be rare, provided supine blood pressure is normal (Dambrink and Wieling 1987).

Limitations of test procedure

An obvious limitation of the above-described simple test procedure is the fact that blood pressure is not monitored on a beat-to-beat base. When a normal initial heart-rate response on standing is observed, it seems reasonable to infer that the underlying blood-pressure response is normal as well (see discussion in previous section). An abnormal initial heart-rate response on standing, however, can only be interpreted in a more general way. Sufficient information for a classification of normal and abnormal orthostatic responses and a selection of patients in need of further investigations can be obtained when the heart-rate response on standing is combined with the conventionally measured steady-state blood-pressure response. The simple test procedure is, however, not sufficient for a full physiological interpretation in case of an abnormal test result.

It has been suggested that a diminished relative bradycardia in patients with a normal secondary heart-rate peak should be considered as an early sign of cardiac vagal neuropathy (see Chapter 38). The importance of these findings remains to be established, since such an abnormal heart-rate response cannot be fully evaluated without monitoring the concomitant blood-pressure response. This fundamental concept applies to the interpretation of all abnormal heart-rate responses which are known to be baroreflex-mediated (Eckberg 1980; Wieling *et al.* 1985).

Head-up tilt and the assessment of autonomic circulatory control

Passive changes of posture have been used for many years to assess orthostatic tolerance. Compared to standing up this procedure induces a hydrostatic redistribution of blood due to pooling in the dependent parts of the body without much counteracting muscular activity, but it is questionable whether this is desirable for routine clinical evaluation of patients.

The heart-rate response induced by head-up tilt does not differentiate between patients with mild vagal impairment and those whose heart-rate control is normal; this in contrast to the response induced by standing up (Wieling *et al.* 1983*a*, 1985). Therefore, it is questioned whether the assessment of the initial heart-rate response induced by head-up tilt should be included in the battery of tests used to assess impaired autonomic control (see Chapter 38).

CLASSIFICATION OF NORMAL AND ABNORMAL ORTHOSTATIC RESPONSES

Five main types of responses are clinically important in the evaluation of complaints of orthostatic dizziness (Table 17.2). The first three are common and transient and are found in subjects with intact circulatory reflexes. The last two are rare and characterized by a significant and persistent fall in blood pressure in the upright position due to autonomic failure.

Table 17.2.

Response	*Early steady-state blood pressure*		*Initial heart-rate response*	*Early steady-state heart-rate response*
Normal	Systolic	=	Biphasic	↑
	Diastolic	↑		
Hyperadrenergic	Systolic	↓	Large ΔHR_{max};	↑↑
	Diastolic	↑↑	little or no relative bradycardia	
Vasovagal	Systolic	↓	Normal or hyperadrenergic	↓
	Diastolic	↓		
Hypoadrenergic (vagus intact)	Systolic	↓	Large ΔHR_{max}; no relative bradycardia	↑↑
	Diastolic	↓		
Hypoadrenergic (with cardiac denervation)	Systolic	↓	Absent	=
	Diastolic	↓		

Orthostatic dizziness on standing in healthy subjects

A normal initial heart-rate response consisting of an immediate heart-rate increase, a large secondary heart-rate peak, and a marked subsequent bradycardia (A in Fig. 17.3) is an important clinical finding. It indicates, for reasons explained above, that intact afferent, central, and efferent cardiac vagal and efferent sympathetic vasomotor control is present.

Nevertheless, it should be realized that subjects with intact autonomic control can still have complaints of dizziness shortly after standing up; in fact most people have experience with a brief feeling of dizziness 5 to 10 s after the onset of standing up rapidly, especially after prolonged supine rest. Such common 'functional' spells of dizziness are characterized by their time of onset and short duration.

Hyperadrenergic orthostatic response

An excessive heart-rate increment after 1–2 min of standing can be considered as a compensatory response to a variety of conditions; an abnormal degree of central hypovolaemia and a strong adrenergic drive in the upright posture are common to these conditions (Blomqvist and Stone 1983). Classically, such a response consists of an immediate heart-rate increase and a large secondary peak with little or no subsequent relative bradycardia resulting in an excessive increase in heart rate in the upright position (B in Fig 17.3), together with a fall in systolic pressure and a marked increase in diastolic pressure. The combination of an excessive increase in heart rate and in diastolic pressure are important clinical findings, indicating functionally intact baroreflex pathways.

Vasovagal orthostatic response

Typical for a vasovagal response is a temporary phase of tachycardia in the upright position, which changes into a decrease in heart rate and a fall in blood pressure due to reflex vagal facilitation and adrenergic inhibition, respectively. The initial circulatory response is normal or hyperadrenergic, indicating integrity of baroreceptor pathways (Blomqvist and Stone 1983).

Hypoadrenergic orthostatic response with intact vagal cardiac control

In patients with sympathetic vasomotor lesions but intact vagal heart-rate control, an immediate large heart-rate increase without a relative bradycardia and consequently a persistent and marked heart-rate rise in the upright position are observed. This response can be attributed to failure of the arterial blood pressure to recover due to the defect of vasoconstrictor mechanisms (compare Fig. 17.2 (a) with Fig. 17.5).

Hypoadrenergic orthostatic hypotension, combined with a marked postural tachycardia can be found in some patients with dysautonomia, in tetraplegic patients, and after extensive sympathectomies. This rare combination may be interpreted as the mirror image of the common pattern of autonomic circulatory denervation, as observed for instance in diabetic autonomic neuropathy, where impaired vagal heart-rate control precedes manifest sympathetic lesions (Wieling *et al.* 1983*b*; van Lieshout *et al.* 1986).

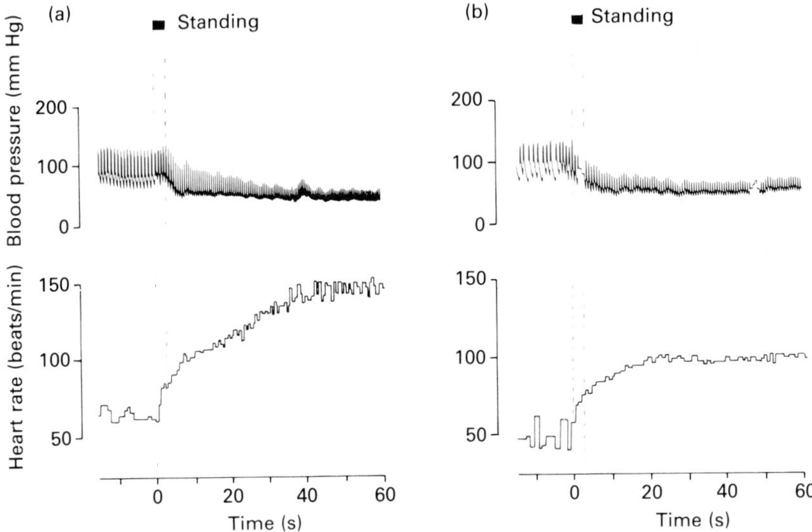

Fig. 17.5. Blood-pressure and heart-rate responses on standing in two patients with isolated sympathetic vasomotor lesions. Note instantaneous large heart-rate increase indicating intact vagal cardiac control, resulting in a marked heart-rate increase in upright position. A relative bradycardia is not observed due to a lack of recovery of arterial pressure. Patient (a), a 22-year-old female, suffered from acute dysautonomia. (Taken with permission from van Lieshout *et al.* (1986).) Patient (b), a 38-year-old female, suffered from orthostatic hypotension after extensive sympathectomies.

Hypoadrenergic orthostatic response with impairment of vagal and sympathetic innervation of the heart

In subjects with a normal resting heart rate, a delayed and sluggish primary heart-rate response indicates that vagal heart rate control is completely lost (compare A and C in Fig. 17.3). The remaining heart-rate increase in these patients is the unmasked sympathetic response mentioned before. Thus, a delayed onset of cardioacceleration and a substantial heart-rate increase afterwards suggest cardiac vagal denervation with intact sympathetic heart-rate control. A small heart-rate increase after prolonged standing in patients with orthostatic hypotension should be interpreted as a sign of impaired sympathetic heart rate control (Wieling *et al.* 1983*a*, 1985). Likewise, almost no heart-rate increase upon standing at all (D in Fig. 17.3) implies complete denervation of the heart.

REFERENCES

Blomqvist, C. G. and Stone, H. L. (1983). Cardiovascular adjustment to gravitational stress. In *Handbook of physiology* (ed. J. T. Shepherd and F. M. Abboud)

Sect. 2, The cardiovascular system, Vol. III (Peripheral circulation and organ blood flow), pp. 1025–63. American Physiological Society, Bethesda, Maryland.

Borst, C., van Brederode, J. F. M., Wieling, W., van Montfrans, G. A., and Dunning, A. J. (1984). Mechanisms of initial bloodpressure response to postural change. *Clin. Sci.* **67**, 321–7.

Borst, C., Wieling, W., van Brederode, J. F. M., Hond, A., de Rijk, L. G., and Dunning, A. J. (1982). Mechanisms of initial heart rate response to postural change. *Am. J. Physiol.* **243**, H676–81.

Dambrink, J. H. A. and Wieling, W. (1987). Circulatory response to postural change in healthy male subjects in relation to age. *Clin. Sci.* **72**, 335–41.

Drischel, H., Fanter, H., Gürtler, H., Labitzke, H., and Priegnitz, F. (1963). Das Verhalten der Herzfrequenz gesunder Menschen beim Übergang vom Liegen zum Stehen. *Arch. F. Kreislauff.* **40**, 135–67.

Eckberg, D. L. (1980). Parasympathetic cardiovascular control: a critical review of methods and results. *Am. J. Physiol.* **239**, H581–93.

Marin Neto, J. A., Gallo Jr, L., Manco, J. C., Rassi, A., and Amorim, D. S. (1980). Mechanisms of tachycardia on standing: studies in normal individuals and in chronic Chagas' heart patients. *Cardiovasc. Res.* **14**, 541–50.

Shepherd, J. T. and Mancia, G. (1986). Reflex control of the human cardiovascular system. *Rev. Physiol. Pharmacol.* **105**, 1–99.

van Lieshout, J. J., Wieling, W., van Montfrans, G. A., Settels, J. J., Speelman, J. D., Endert, E., and Karemaker, J. M. (1986). Acute dysautonomia associated with Hodgkin's disease. *J. Neurol. Neurosurg. Psychiat.* **49**, 830–2.

Wieling, W., Borst, C., van Brederode, J. F. M., van Dongen Torman, M. A., van Montfrans, G. A., and Dunning, A. J. (1983*a*). Testing for autonomic neuropathy: heart rate changes after orthostatic manoeuvres and static muscle contractions. *Clin. Sci.* **64**, 581–6.

Wieling, W., Borst, C., van Dongen Torman, M. A. van der Hofstede, J. W., van Brederode, J. F. M., Endert, E., and Dunning, A. J. (1983*b*). Relationship between impaired parasympathetic and sympathetic cardiovascular control in diabetes mellitus. *Diabetologia* **24**, 422–7.

Wieling, W., Borst, C., van Lieshout, J. J., Sprangers, R. L. H., Karemaker, J. M., van Brederode, J. F. M., van Montfrans, G. A., and Dunning, A. J. (1985). Assessment of methods to estimate impairment of vagal and sympathetic innervation of the heart in diabetic autonomic neuropathy. *Neth. J. Med.* **28**, 383–92.

Wieling, W., van Brederode, J. F. M., de Rijk, L. G., Borst, C., and Dunning, A. J. (1982). Reflex control of heart rate in normal subjects in relation to age: a data base for cardiac vagal neuropathy. *Diabetologia* **22**, 163–6.

18. Neurotransmitter and neuropeptide function in autonomic failure

Ronald J. Polinsky

INTRODUCTION

Autonomic control of vital functions is accomplished through the extensive innervation of many organs by the sympathetic and parasympathetic divisions of the autonomic nervous system. Precise management of circulatory and metabolic parameters results from the successful integration of multiple neurohumoral and hormonal responses. Adjustments are rapidly made according to the changing demands imposed by environmental factors, activity, emotional status, and other stimuli. Although internal variables such as blood pressure or glucose are generally maintained within a 'normal range', they may be altered in various situations as required to achieve functional homeostasis.

Consistent with its primitive but critical role, the autonomic nervous system resembles the most simple nervous system—a reflex arc. In fact, it is really comprised of a series of reflex arcs which permit processing at various levels within the nervous system as well as control and influence exerted by higher brain centres. This organization forms the basis for predictable physiological responses to standardized stimuli and makes the autonomic nervous system ideally suited for clinical and research testing.

Physiologists have examined various aspects of autonomic function for more than a century. However, it is only within the last few decades that biochemical and pharmacological investigation has been possible. Progress in understanding sympathetic neuronal function has been facilitated by the development of sensitive, specific assays for neurotransmitters and their metabolites. Noradrenalin is present in sympathetic nerves and released by nerve stimulation; adrenalin excretion is related to adrenal medullary activity. Biochemical indices of parasympathetic function, however, are extremely limited. Thus, pharmacological responses to drugs with known mechanisms of action have proved in some instances to be a more successful approach towards assessing autonomic function.

Many symptoms of autonomic dysfunction reflect the lack of control due to lesions which interrupt specific reflex mechanisms. The afferent (sensory) limb, central integration pathways, and/or efferent (motor) pathway may be affected at one or several points in the system. Much clinical research in this area has focused on blood-pressure control because orthostatic hypotension is often the most disabling symptom of autonomic failure. Autonomic function may be affected in a number of other neurological and systemic disorders; two distinct syndromes of chronic autonomic failure have been studied in depth. Isolated autonomic failure is also referred to as pure autonomic failure (PAF). Although not all patients with multiple system atrophy (MSA) have autonomic dysfunction, the term MSA will be used in this chapter to distinguish from PAF those patients with autonomic failure attended by central neurological signs. A more thorough discussion of clinical classification is found in Chapters 1 and 15.

Biochemical and neuropharmacological assessment of autonomic function provides a means for localizing the lesion and a rational foundation for pharmacotherapy. The first section of this chapter deals with various aspects of peripheral and central neurotransmitter metabolism and function. The second section describes abnormal hormonal and peptide responses observed in patients with autonomic failure. Some of these results are useful in understanding the different consequences of peripheral and central lesions of the autonomic nervous system. Investigation of patients with autonomic dysfunction has also helped to more clearly define the mechanisms and characteristics of normal neurotransmitter and neuropeptide function and metabolism.

Quantitative release of neurotransmitter substances in response to neuronal action potentials serves as the chemical communication link to bridge the gap between neurons and other post-synaptic tissues. Investigation of peripheral neurotransmitter function is easier because there is access to the biological compartments through which at least a portion of the removal mechanism directly occurs. Assessment of central nervous system metabolism requires the development and validation of indirect strategies.

PERIPHERAL-NERVOUS-SYSTEM NEUROTRANSMITTER FUNCTION AND METABOLISM

Blood pressure is controlled by the sympathetic nervous system through changes in vascular tone and heart rate modulated by activity from sympathetic nerves that release noradrenalin (for review see Polinsky 1984*a*). The type and location of noradrenalin receptors determine the effect of the neurotransmitter. Two different receptors have been postulated to explain the excitatory and inhibitory effects of various sympathomimetic amines. The current classification of α- and β-receptors is based on the relative potencies of noradrenalin, adrenalin, and isoproterenol. Stimulation of vascular α-adrenergic receptors generally causes vasoconstriction in contrast to cardiac receptors and those mediating vasodilation which are of the β-type. Since noradrenalin plays a key role in the maintenance of blood pressure, it is important to understand the relationship between plasma noradrenalin and blood pressure, factors which affect its disposition and metabolism, and characteristics of the interaction between noradrenergic receptors and the end-organ responses.

Noradrenalin

The characteristics of the peripheral noradrenergic neuron illustrated in Fig. 18.1 provide a theoretical framework upon which several approaches have been developed for studying sympathetic neuronal function in man (for review and detailed references see Polinsky 1984*a*). The cell bodies of these neurons are located primarily in sympathetic ganglia. Newly synthesized noradrenalin is stored in vesicles and is released into the synaptic cleft upon stimulation. Released noradrenalin activates both pre- and postsynaptic receptors, the former serving as a negative feed-back control to inhibit further noradrenalin release. The effects of post-synaptic receptor stimulation depend on a number of factors including

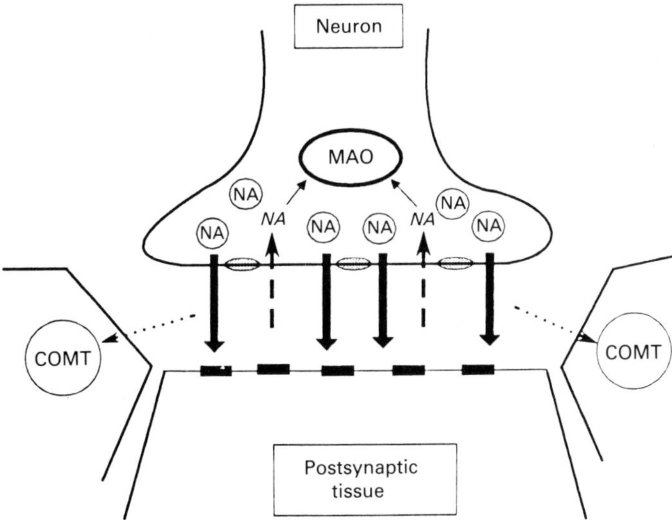

Fig. 18.1. Schematic diagram of a peripheral noradrenergic neuron. NA, nor-adrenalin; MAO, monoamine oxidase; COMT, catechol ortho-methyltransferase.

the type of receptor, but generally, in the case of vascular neuroeffector junctions, the result is vasoconstriction.

Neuronal uptake is the primary mechanism for terminating the actions of released noradrenalin, although local characteristics such as innervation density and synaptic cleft width determine the relative importance of this process. However, a small amount of the released noradrenalin escapes into the circulation and this makes it possible to correlate plasma noradrenalin levels with nerve activity. The plasma concentration is determined by the balance between the rate of noradrenalin entry into the circulation after release by sympathetic nerve endings and its subsequent removal from the plasma. Thus, measurement of plasma noradrenalin and its kinetic disposition yields indices of sympathetic functional integrity. Noradrenalin metabolism will be reviewed in relation to studies of urinary metabolites in autonomic failure. The characteristics of postsynaptic stimulation provide a means for distinguishing differences in pressor responsivity according to the site(s) of the lesion in autonomic failure. Although these various approaches for investigating autonomic dysfunction are complementary, they will be separately discussed to facilitate understanding.

Plasma level and kinetic disposition

Noradrenalin levels in the blood change very rapidly and are affected by a variety of stimuli (e.g. posture, emotion, blood volume, and hypoglycaemia). The site of sampling also affects the plasma level: arterial values are lower than mixed venous samples. In addition, there is a significant rise of plasma noradrenalin with age of the subject. The conditions for taking blood samples must be standardized. In order to obtain a reproducible basal value, sufficient accommodation time must be allowed prior to withdrawing samples from an indwelling catheter since venipuncture increases plasma noradrenalin. Care must also be taken during sample collection, storage, and processing because noradrenalin is relatively unstable in plasma. All of these factors contribute to errors in measurement and complicate comparisons among studies. Despite these limitations, plasma noradrenalin levels correlate with electrophysiologic measurements of sympathetic nerve activity and their use as an index of sympathetic activity in man has been justified under rigorously controlled, standardized conditions for obtaining and analysing samples.

Several investigators have measured plasma noradrenalin levels in groups of PAF and MSA patients (Table 18.1). MSA patients generally have normal or slightly elevated plasma noradrenalin levels. The only exceptions are the studies by Bannister *et al.* (1977) and by Sasaki *et al.* (1983). The former study had very high control values. Values less than 100 pg/ml in plasma from MSA patients are certainly the exception

Table 18.1. Basal plasma noradrenalin levels (pg/ml) in autonomic failure. Numbers in parentheses indicate number of subjects

Basal plasma noradrenalin levels (pg/ml)			
MSA	*PAF*	*Controls*	*References*
310 (6)	95 (4)	315 (10)	Ziegler *et al.* (1977)
76 (10)	—	550 (4)	Bannister *et al.* (1977)
214 (8)	30; 240* (2)	303; 450* (2)	Bannister *et al.* (1979)
—	195 (4)	240 (10)	Esler *et al.* (1980)
318 (7)	62 (6)	233 (11)	Polinsky *et al.* (1981*a*)
255 (7)	91 (5)	—	Polinsky *et al.* (1981*c*)
—	34 (4)	368 (8)	Robertson *et al.* (1983)
88 (4)	—	136 (5)	Sasaki *et al.* (1983)

* Individual values listed since only two subjects were studied.

rather than the rule. However, the question is not resolved as to whether some patients with MSA might have peripheral nerve involvement with a reduced plasma noradrenalin level as observed in neuropathic conditions (e.g. diabetes). Although denervation changes were mentioned in the description by Shy and Drager (1960), findings suggestive of peripheral involvement have been infrequently reported.

Noradrenalin levels in PAF are lower than normal with the exception of those reported by Esler *et al.* (1980) and one patient studied by Bannister *et al.* (1979). Decreased clearance of noradrenalin in PAF was demonstrated by Esler *et al.* (1980). As discussed later in this section, reduced clearance in PAF could certainly elevate the plasma noradrenalin level into the normal range.

The increment in plasma noradrenalin following a standardized stimulus such as postural change is more justified for comparison among studies since each subject serves as their own control. Ziegler *et al.* (1977) found no significant elevation in plasma noradrenalin concentration after 5 or 10 minutes of standing in patients with either PAF or MSA. Bannister *et al.* (1979) also did not observe a significant postural increment in MSA patients although they used a tilt-table with foot support maintained at 60° for 10 minutes. The implication of these observations is that both groups have lesion(s) in the baroreflex arc which prevent an adequate sympathetic nervous system response to a change in posture. The low basal supine noradrenalin levels in PAF suggest a more peripheral localization of the lesion whereas the normal or slightly elevated values observed in MSA are consistent with the failure to activate relatively intact postganglionic sympathetic neurons.

Despite the statistical differences observed between groups of MSA and PAF patients, the clinical utility of plasma noradrenalin as a diagnostic tool in individual cases has not been demonstrated. A larger, unpublished series by the author confirms the distinction between PAF and MSA. The mean (±SEM) supine plasma noradrenalin levels in control subjects ($n = 20$) and patients with PAF ($n = 20$) or MSA ($n = 37$) are respectively 224 (±18), 76 (±18), and 265 (±21) pg/ml. Of greater importance is the fact that, although 20 per cent of PAF patients had plasma noradrenalin levels greater than 100 pg/ml, only 5 per cent of the MSA group had values lower than 100 pg/ml. Thus, while normal basal values are more suggestive of MSA, a low value has much greater significance in establishing the diagnosis of PAF particularly if found early in the course of the disease. The overlap between MSA and PAF highlights the need to use this data in conjunction with other clinical and neuropharmacological investigations. In addition, neuronal re-uptake should be examined as this might be affected out of proportion to the synthesis and release of noradrenalin.

The level of noradrenalin in plasma is determined by the various processes that affect release, re-uptake, or metabolism, and subsequent removal of noradrenalin from plasma. Intravenous administration at a constant rate of a tracer amount of radiolabelled noradrenalin can be used to assess clearance and secretion. When steady-state conditions have been achieved (usually between 3 and 5 half-lives for the compound of interest) the kinetic processes which determine the plasma concentration of noradrenalin are at equilibrium, i.e. the rate of radio-labelled noradrenalin infusion equals the sum of the rates by which noradrenalin leaves the circulation. Thus, it is possible to derive equations for calculating the endogenous secretion rate into plasma and clearance of noradrenalin.

Despite the importance of understanding these aspects of sympathetic neuronal function, there have been only two investigations of noradrenalin kinetics in orthostatic hypotension patients (Esler *et al.* 1980; Polinsky *et al.* 1985*b*). Both studies have shown reduced clearance of noradrenalin only in patients with PAF. However, the patients studied by Esler *et al.* (1980) had normal basal plasma noradrenalin levels presumably from delayed removal of the catecholamine from plasma. The normal noradrenalin clearance in MSA patients is consistent with the view that postganglionic sympathetic neurons are functionally intact (Fig. 18.2).

Isoproterenol is only cleared through extraneuronal mechanisms and hence its disappearance from plasma following a steady-state infusion is normally much slower compared to noradrenalin. The defect in neuronal uptake observed in PAF is striking as shown by the similarity in disappearance rates for noradrenalin and isoproterenol in PAF (Polinsky *et al.* 1985*b*). Very low plasma levels and reduced clearance of noradrenalin in PAF as observed by Polinsky *et al.* (1985*b*) is likely a

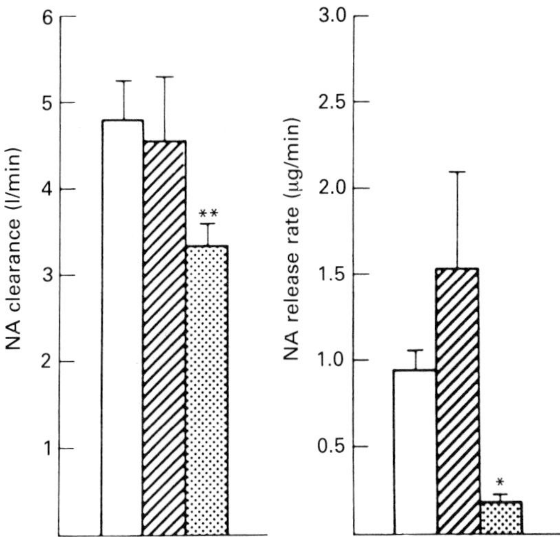

Fig. 18.2. Noradrenalin (NA) clearance and release rate in control subjects (open) and patients with MSA (hatched) and PAF (shaded).

reflection of more severe disease, possibly of longer duration. A lack of correlation between the plasma level and clearance suggests that low plasma levels in these PAF patients are primarily the result of diminished noradrenalin release. Defective neuronal uptake with consequently delayed removal of noradrenalin from plasma in PAF has therapeutic implications. This is a likely explanation for the prolonged pressor effect of exogenously administered noradrenalin observed in some PAF patients (Bannister *et al.* 1979). Extraneuronal uptake and metabolism may take on increasing importance as peripheral sympathetic neurons are affected.

Urinary metabolites

One of the earliest biochemical investigations of patients with postural hypotension showed a reduction in the urinary excretion of catecholamines (Luft and von Euler 1953). Unfortunately, overall estimates of catecholamine excretion provide little insight into the mechanism involved in disorders associated with sympathetic dysfunction. Technical advances over the last 30 years have allowed more precise measurement of specific noradrenalin metabolites. It is necessary to consider some additional aspects of sympathetic neuronal function in order to interpret the findings obtained as these methods have been applied to study autonomic failure.

Released noradrenalin that is taken up into sympathetic neurons is initially deaminated by monoamine oxidase (Fig. 18.3). Subsequent metabolism results in the formation of vanillylmandelic acid (VMA) and 3-methoxy,4-hydroxyphenylglycol (MHPG). Normetanephrine is

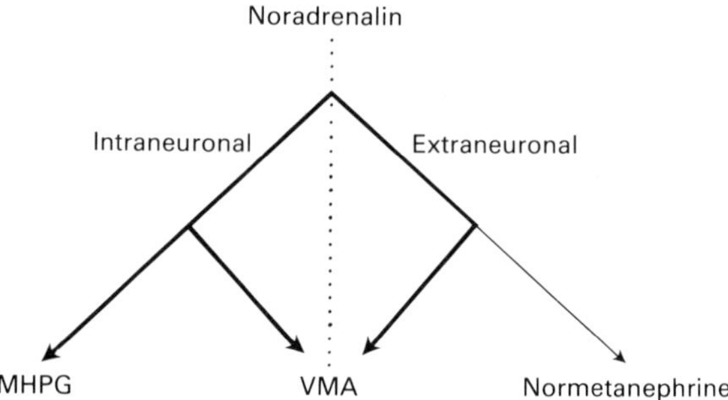

Fig. 18.3. Intra- and extraneuronal peripheral noradrenalin metabolism. See text for detailed explanation.

formed from released noradrenalin that is not taken up by sympathetic nerve endings. Although most of the normetanephrine is later deaminated, a small amount is excreted as conjugated normetanephrine and may reflect the activity of sympathetic neurons. Thus, the urinary excretion and apportionment of metabolites may be used to investigate sympathetic neuronal function (Kopin *et al.* 1983*b*).

All urinary noradrenalin metabolites are low in PAF consistent with a reduction in the number of sympathetic noradrenergic neurons. In MSA the amount of normetanephrine is selectively reduced out of proportion to VMA and MHPG. The slight reduction in overall noradrenalin synthesis and relative decrease in normetanephrine excretion in MSA reflect the failure to appropriately activate the intact peripheral sympathetic nervous system. These results further support the biochemical distinction in pathophysiology between MSA and PAF previously discussed.

Pressor responsivity

Although descriptions of supersensitivity to drugs appeared in the literature more than a century ago, the problem is still not completely understood but sufficient knowledge in this area provides a rational basis for exploring the pharmacological distinction between PAF and MSA. Chronic postganglionic denervation enhances the response to noradrenalin but reduces the effects of indirectly acting sympathomimetics. In contrast, the increased pressor response observed following decentralization is modest compared to denervation and is not accompanied by a loss of peripheral noradrenalin stores; the response to tyramine, an indirect sympathomimetic, is unchanged. Since denervation also interrupts the pathway from the central nervous system to the end-organ the exaggerated blood-pressure responses result from local effects of the lesion as well as impaired reflex modulation. Changes in sensitivity to drugs can result from abnormalities in drug absorption, elimination, and access to the target organ in addition to defective compensatory reflex mechanisms and localized changes at the cellular site of action (e.g. receptor and metabolic derangements). More than one of these mechanisms may be operative in an individual case. Thus, increased sensitivity to sympathomimetic drugs would be expected in patients with autonomic dysfunction but the characteristics of the pressor responses would vary according to the site of the lesion(s). Lesions of postganglionic sympathetic nerves might produce exaggerated responses to noradrenalin, diminished peripheral stores of noradrenalin, decreased neuronal uptake, and poor modulation of pressor responses by the baroreflex. A more central (preganglionic) lesion would also cause an increased pressor response to noradrenalin resulting primarily from interruption of the baroreceptor reflex arc. It is necessary to appreciate the concepts related to interpreting dose–response curves in order to pharmacologically distinguish these different forms of increased pressor responsivity.

When appropriately plotted on a semilogarithmic scale dose–response curves have a sigmoidal shape although the region of interest is really within the linear portion. Normal curves can be perturbed in a variety of ways which can be explained on the basis of four characteristics which may be changed individually or in combination. Two of these features, i.e. threshold and gain, are crucial in differentiating the effects of denervation and decentralization (Fig. 18.4). Gain is the slope of the dose–response curve; a change in gain does not alter the threshold but may be associated with an increase in the maximal response. With respect to blood-pressure control, alterations in baroreflex modulation may change the gain of the blood pressure–log dose of drug curve. Horizontal displacement of the curve changes the threshold of the response; it is this type of change which is a manifestation of true receptor supersensitivity.

Blood-pressure responses to various pharmacological agents have been used to examine adrenoceptor function and localize the lesion(s) in patients with orthostatic hypotension. One of the earliest studies was that of Kontos *et al.* (1976) who measured forearm blood flow during intra-arterial administration of noradrenalin and tyramine. Patients with PAF manifested decreased forearm blood flow in response to noradrenalin but not to tyramine. Normal reductions in forearm blood flow occurred in response to both drugs in MSA patients. Efferent sympathetic dysfunction in PAF was previously suggested by the absence of fluorescent staining of catecholamines in vessel walls of skeletal muscle (Kontos *et al.* 1975). However, loss of catecholamine histofluorescence in sympathetic perivascular nerve endings has also been reported in even mildly affected patients with MSA (Bannister *et al.* 1981*b*). Caution must be used in interpreting histofluorescence studies because this approach has at times given variable results even within the

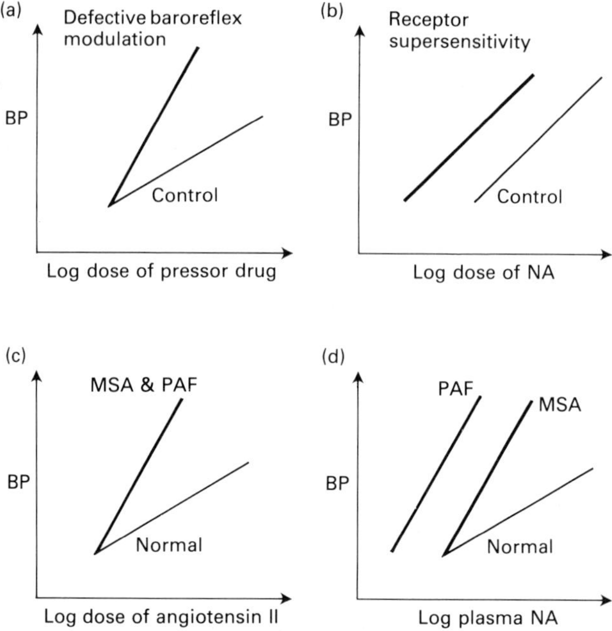

Fig. 18.4. Blood pressure (BP) dose–response curves to pressor drugs: (a) lesion of the baroreceptor reflex; (b) denervation; (c) non-specific gain increase in MSA and PAF; and (d) shift to the left in PAF only in response to noradrenalin (NA).

same laboratory. The absence of a finding should be viewed with reservation, particularly since the results of the pharmacological studies clearly suggest a difference in pathophysiology between PAF and MSA.

Another early study (Wilcox and Aminoff 1976) reported a greater than normal pressor response to noradrenalin and dopamine in five MSA patients. Lack of sweating after intradermal injection of acetylcholine was the basis for the authors to suggest that a postganglionic lesion with reduced noradrenalin clearance caused the exaggerated pressor response. This non-specific increase in pressor responsivity is analgous to the results of decentralization in experimental animals.

More recently, pressor responses to sympathomimetic drugs have been investigated in two larger series of patients with autonomic failure. Eight MSA and two PAF patients studied by Bannister *et al.* (1979) manifested a greater than normal blood-pressure response to noradrenalin. The magnitude of the pressor response appeared to correlate with the degree of baroreflex impairment. One PAF patient had the greatest sensitivity to noradrenalin as well as a prolonged pressor effect following a bolus injection. The prolonged pressor effect and normal basal plasma noradrenalin level suggest delayed clearance of the drugs as demonstrated in other patients with PAF (Esler *et al.* 1980; Polinsky *et al.*

1985*b*). These results were confirmed and extended by Polinsky *et al.* (1981*a*) who examined blood-pressure responses and plasma catecholamine levels before and during infusion of noradrenalin, angiotensin, and tyramine (bolus injections) in eight patients with PAF and nine with MSA (Fig. 18.4). Angiotensin was used as a non-adrenergic pressor agent. Both MSA and PAF patients had an increased gain of their blood pressure–dose response curves to noradrenalin and angiotensin, consistent with a lesion in the baroreflex arc resulting in defective modulation of blood pressure. However, only PAF patients had a shift to the left of their dose–response curve to noradrenalin, a manifestation of true adrenergic receptor supersensitivity. These results further support the distinction between primarily peripheral involvement of the sympathetic nervous system in PAF (denervation) and the central nervous system lesion(s) in MSA (decentralization).

An indirect means for assessing peripheral neuronal uptake and stores of noradrenalin involves measuring the increment in plasma noradrenalin after intravenous administration of tyramine (Polinsky *et al.* 1981*a*). PAF patients had a significantly reduced increment in plasma noradrenalin compared to either MSA patients or control subjects. The normal increment in MSA provides additional evidence for the functional integrity of postganglionic noradrenergic neurons. Impaired sympathetic neuronal uptake in PAF has been confirmed through kinetic studies of noradrenalin disposition as previously discussed. These results with tyramine are consistent with the earlier work by Kontos *et al.* (1976). However, Bannister *et al.* (1979) failed to detect significant elevations of plasma noradrenalin in MSA patients. This might be related to lower plasma tyramine levels achieved with smaller doses and constant rate infusion used to reach the desired blood pressure increase.

Other drugs have been used to examine cardiovascular responses in autonomic failure: methoxamine, isoproterenol, and antidiuretic hormone. Hyperresponsivity to methoxamine in orthostatic hypotension has been observed (Parks *et al.* 1961). Increased chronotropic and vasodepressor responses to isoproterenol have been reported in MSA (Mathias *et al.* 1977); Bannister *et al.* 1981*b*) and PAF (Robertson *et al.* 1984). An enhanced pressor response to antidiuretic hormone was demonstrated in PAF (Mohring *et al.* 1980). This may have therapeutic value since analogues with long duration of action have been developed for intranasal administration. Patients with orthostatic hypotension also appear to have an exaggerated pressor response to somatostatin and its analogues (Hoeldtke *et al.* 1986).

A complementary approach to pharmacological assessment of adrenergic receptors is the measurement of binding to platelets by dihydroergocryptine. Bannister *et al.* (1980) found an increased affinity and number of α-receptors in MSA. These findings have been confirmed and extended to PAF (Kafka *et al.* 1984). The implications are not entirely clear because the relationship between platelet α-receptors and the neuroeffector junction at vascular sympathetic nerve endings is not known.

In summary, it is apparent that the pressor responses are increased in both PAF and MSA. However, the underlying mechanisms causing these changes differ in the two disorders. These pharmacological results provide further support for the clinical and biochemcal distinction between PAF and MSA discussed earlier. The low plasma noradrenalin level, diminished neuronal uptake, shift of the dose–response curve to noradrenalin, and reduced increment in plasma noradrenalin following tyramine provide clear evidence for postganglionic noradrenergic dysfunction in PAF. The normal findings in MSA with a non-specific increase in responsivity to pressor agents are consistent with a more central involvement of the sympathetic nervous system. Neuropathologic findings in MSA support this notion; unfortunately, the pathology of PAF has not been clearly established.

Adrenalin

The adrenal medulla functions as a specialized postganglionic neuron by releasing adrenalin along with a small amount of noradrenalin in response to a variety of stressful stimuli. Although adrenalin certainly plays an important compensatory role in circulatory shock and vascular collapse, the adrenal medullary response is more closely involved with metabolic homeostatis. Catecholamines can affect intermediary metabolism through various mechanisms including an increase of hepatic glucose output, activation of lipolysis, inhibition of insulin secretion, and reduction in glucose utilization. Insulin-induced hypoglycaemia has long been known as a potent stimulus for adrenalin secretion. The primary role of the adrenal medulla in protecting against severe hypoglycaemia is highlighted by the fact that the rise in plasma adrenalin precedes increases in noradrenalin, glucagon, growth hormone, and cortisol.

Luft and von Euler (1953) demonstrated a lack of catecholamine excretion to insulin-induced hypoglycaemia in two patients with postural hypotension. There have been few additional studies of the sympathetic nervous system responses to hypoglycaemia in autonomic failure. Polinsky *et al.* (1980) investigated the catecholamine responses during insulin-induced hypoglycaemia in eight MSA and eight PAF patients as well as normal control subjects. This study will be discussed in depth because it is an excellent example in which the investigation of a disease state helps to elucidate the normal responses.

In normal subjects, the glucose recovery curve following the nadir of hypoglycaemia is biphasic with an initial rapid rise followed by a slower rate of return towards euglycaemia (Figure 18.5). The initial rapid phase of glucose recovery is not present in patients with severe adrenergic insufficiency. This difference in glucose recovery suggests that the rapid phase is due to adrenalin. A precipitous rise in plasma adrenalin and to a lesser extent noradrenalin occurs in normal subjects; the peak in plasma levels is attained within minutes following the nadir of hypoglycaemia. Most patients with either MSA or PAF have deficient catecholamine responses to hypoglycaemia. In a small group of patients (three MSA, one PAF) there was essentially no detectable rise in adrenalin or noradrenalin.

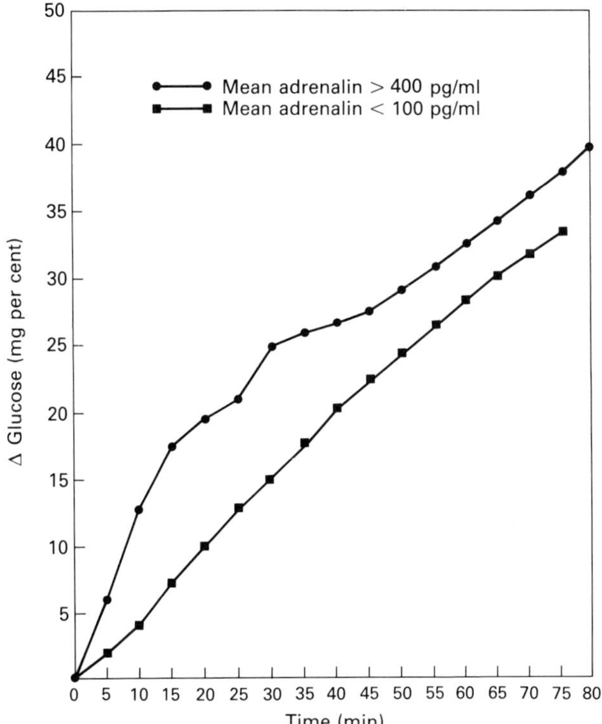

Fig. 18.5. Glucose recovery curves following the nadir of hypoglycaemia in control subjects and patients with adrenergic insufficiency.

Patients with either MSA or PAF manifest deficient catecholamine responses because a lesion located at any point in the pathway from glucose receptors in the hypothalamus or brainstem to the adrenal medulla would block the reflex. Diminished or absent adrenalin responses have also been reported in sympathectomized, splanchnectomized, or adrenalectomized patients. An afferent baroreflex lesion, as presumably occurs in familial dysautonomia, could cause orthostatic hypotension without altering the adrenal medullary response to hypoglycaemia. Hence, although it is important to assess the adequacy of this protective stress response, it is not possible to use this information alone to localize the lesion in patients with autonomic failure. These results also demonstrate that adrenalin rapidly elevates glucose but is not essential for restoring euglycaemia. Thus, hypoglycaemic episodes are fortunately not a feature of autonomic dysfunction.

CENTRAL-NERVOUS-SYSTEM NEUROTRANSMITTER METABOLISM AND FUNCTION

Investigation of central-nervous-system neurotransmitter metabolism and function in man is inherently more difficult because of the limited access to appropriate biological materials. Most of the progress in this area has been achieved through the study of post-mortem brain specimens (see Chapter 25). Two approaches for probing brain neurotransmitter metabolism are currently possible:

1. measurement of neurotransmitter and metabolite levels in cerebrospinal fluid (CSF); and
2. administration of appropriately labelled ligands or precursors coupled with positron emission tomography.

The latter technique is presently in an early stage; only very preliminary studies with low-resolution scans have been obtained and quantitation is limited. This section will describe the results obtained by measuring CSF levels of monoamine metabolites in patients with autonomic failure.

Noradrenalin

In addition to its importance as a neurotransmitter in the peripheral sympathetic nervous system, noradrenalin is also present in the central nervous system (for review see Polinsky 1984). The hypothalamus is innervated by noradrenergic neurons whose cell bodies are located in the locus ceruleus; other fibres project to the cerebellum, hippocampus, cerebral cortex, and hypothalamus. Another ascending pathway has a more diffuse brainstem origin with projections to hypothalamus, limbic system, and other brainstem nuclei. There is also a descending bulbospinal noradrenergic pathway which innervates preganglionic sympathetic neurons and anterior horn cells.

MHPG is the major brain metabolite of noradrenalin (Kopin *et al.* 1983*a*). Although CSF levels of MHPG have been used as an index of central noradrenalin metabolism, it is necessary to correct these values for the contribution from free plasma MHPG which readily crosses the blood–brain barrier. By measuring the relationship between CSF and plasma MHPG in normal subjects and patients with pheochromocytoma, Kopin *et al.* (1983*a*) derived a formula for correcting total CSF MHPG for the contribution from plasma. Since the tumour produces a peripheral source of MHPG which is not under nervous-system control, the elevation of CSF MHPG in these patients results from diffusion of free MHPG from plasma into CSF. The slope of the line relating CSF to plasma MHPG in these subjects gives the proportion of plasma MHPG which must be subtracted from the total CSF level to obtain the amount due to central nervous system noradrenalin metabolism.

Patients with MSA and PAF have decreased total CSF MHPG levels (Polinsky *et al.* 1984). Consistent with their low plasma noradrenalin, only PAF patients have reduced levels of plasma MHPG. Thus, the corrected CSF MHPG level is lower than normal only in the MSA patients, demonstrating that central-nervous-system noradrenalin metabolism is diminished. The low total CSF MHPG in patients with PAF results from the small contribution from peripheral noradrenalin metabolism; the component reflecting central metabolism is normal. These results are consistent with pathologic studies in MSA that demonstrate involvement in those brain areas innervated by noradrenergic pathways. In addition, there is a reduction in the noradrenalin content of locus ceruleus, hypothalamus, and septal nuclei in the brains of MSA patients (Spokes *et al.* 1979). Thus, it seems evident that the low central-nervous-system MHPG production in MSA is the result of lesions caused by the degenerative process.

Dopamine and serotonin

The clinical syndrome of parkinsonism and pathological involvement of extrapyramidal structures in MSA suggest that dopamine deficiency plays a causative role in the non-autonomic neurological aspects of the disease. Concentrations of serotonergic neurons found in the brainstem along with projections to the spinal cord make this system another likely neurochemical target of the degenerative process. Homovanillic acid (HVA) and 5-hydroxyindoleacetic acid (5-HIAA) are the primary metabolites in man of dopamine and serotonin respectively. These acid monoamine metabolites are discussed together because their removal from the CSF occurs through the same active process.

Moskowitz and Wurtman (1975) reported low CSF levels of HVA in a number of neurological disorders including MSA. Using a more sensitive method of analysis (gas chromatography–mass spectrometry), Williams *et al.* (1979) found reduced HVA and 5-HIAA in the CSF of eight MSA patients. In addition, they also showed that CSF HVA but not 5-HIAA was lowered by bromocryptine suggesting that dopaminergic receptors were still functional in MSA. More recently, Polinsky *et al.* (1985*a*) measured CSF levels of HVA and 5-HIAA in 24 control subjects, 14 patients with PAF, and 33 MSA patients. Both metabolites were significantly reduced in MSA to about 50 per cent of the control values. Patients with PAF had normal CSF HVA and 5-HIAA concentrations. Probenecid equally elevated both metabolites in MSA, but less than normal, confirming that the reduced basal levels reflect decreased turnover rather than a deficit in transport. There was also a significant correlation between the HVA and 5-HIAA levels in MSA suggesting that the dopaminergic and serotonin systems are affected in parallel (Fig. 18.6). Reductions in dopamine content have been found in the striatum, nucleus accumbens, substantia nigra, septal nuclei, hypothalamus, and locus ceruleus (see Chapter 25B). Thus, central-nervous-system noradrenalin, dopamine, and serotonin systems appear to be affected in MSA although the serotonin system has not been adequately confirmed through post-mortem studies.

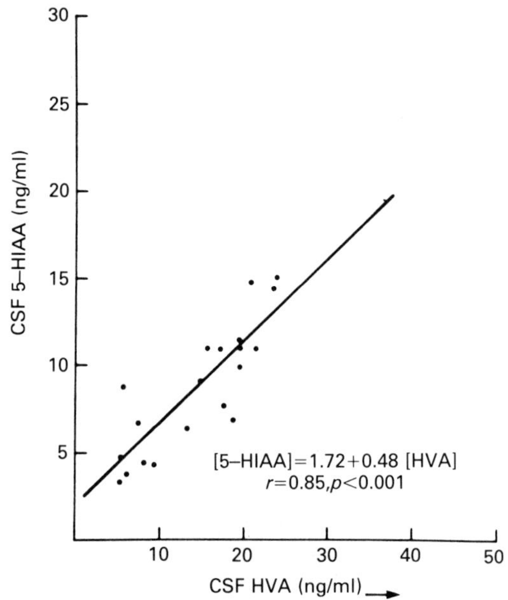

Fig. 18.6. Relationship between CSF levels of 5-HIAA and HVA in MSA patients.

HORMONAL AND PEPTIDE RESPONSES

The extensive ramifications of the autonomic nervous system influence a number of hormonal and peptide systems throughout the body. Most of these substances are involved in a wide variety of activities such as metabolism, digestion, and stress responses. For others, a specific function has yet to be determined in man. The many systems controlled through autonomic function partially accounts for the wide spectrum of symptoms observed in autonomic failure.

With the exception of melatonin, all of the hormonal and peptide responses described in this section have been measured during insulin-induced hypoglycaemia. Although this is not a common physiological situation, hypoglycaemia does evoke numerous hormonal and gastro-enterological responses. Insulin administration provides a standardized method for simultaneously measuring these changes. However, to facilitate discussion, this section is divided into hypoglycaemic counter-regulatory hormones, gut peptides, and central-nervous-system mediated responses.

Hypoglycaemic counterregulatory hormones

Restoration of euglycaemia following insulin administration does not depend on the secretion of adrenalin. Other protective metabolic mechanisms are clearly operational in patients with adrenergic insufficiency to prevent prolonged, dangerously low levels of blood glucose. Examination of the hypoglycaemic counterregulatory hormones in the absence of catecholamine responses provides an opportunity to examine the relationship between the sympathetic nervous system and release of other hormones and peptides.

Glucagon

Pancreatic glucagon is synthesized by α-cells and released in response to various stimuli. Although glucagon appears to function as an acute hyperglycaemic hormone, catecholamine responses precede the glucagon response during insulin-induced hypoglycaemia. The baseline plasma glucagon, maximum levels, and those observed at the nadir of hypoglycaemia were normal in patients with either MSA or PAF who had essentially absent catecholamine responses (Polinsky *et al.* 1981*b*). It is not possible to directly compare these results with the subnormal glucagon responses reported in some patients with autonomic failure and the essentially absent glucagon responses in the four MSA patients reported by Sasaki *et al.* (1983). The low basal noradrenalin levels in the latter investigation suggest that these patients might have peripheral sympathetic involvement. Diminished glucagon responses were also found in another study of MSA patients (Long *et al.* 1979), but the catecholamine levels were not reported. Sympathectomy or adrenalectomy does not affect the glucagon response. Thus, patients with MSA and PAF might have intact glucagon responses to hypoglycaemia despite the lack of significant catecholamine responses.

Growth hormone

Acidophil cells of the anterior pituitary produce growth hormone which is released by stimulation of the hypothalamopituitary axis by many of the same stimuli that also cause catecholamine responses. Sasaki *et al.* (1983) found absent growth-hormone responses to insulin hypoglycaemia in four patients with MSA; these patients also had deficient or absent catecholamine, glucagon, prolactin, and cortisol responses. Although it is certainly plausible that the central nervous system (CNS) lesions of MSA might affect the hypothalamus and its pituitary connections, the normal growth hormone and cortisol responses in the MSA patient studied by Polinsky *et al.* (1981*b*) suggest that this does not invariably occur or that another mechanism may be involved in the abolition of these responses. Three PAF patients with adrenergic insufficiency (Polinsky *et al.* 1981*b*) also had normal growth hormone responses during hypoglycaemia. A lesion at any point beyond the hypothalamus in the sympathetic nervous system would result in disruption of catecholamine release without affecting the other centrally mediated hypothalamopituitary hormonal responses.

Cortisol

Cortisol is released from the adrenal cortex during stressful situations; these responses are superimposed, however, upon the well-established diurnal rhythm. Basal cortisol levels are significantly higher than normal in patients with autonomic failure attended by adrenergic insufficiency (Polinsky *et al.* 1981*b*), probably due to the severe stress of postural hypotension while off medication. The levels do return to the normal range during adequate treatment for the hypotension (Polinsky, unpublished observations). The maximum increment in plasma cortisol during insulin hypoglycaemia is normal in MSA (Wilcox *et al.* 1975) and in orthostatic hypotension patients with adrenergic insufficiency (Polinsky *et al.* 1981*b*). As mentioned above, these findings contrast with the results in four MSA patients studied by Sasaki *et al.* (1983); their patients did not have elevated basal cortisol levels. Similarly to the other counterregulatory hormones it does not appear that a detectable increase in plasma catecholamine levels is required for cortisol release. Furthermore, there is no change in the sequence, magnitude, and temporal profile of these responses in the absence of significant catecholamine increments.

Gut peptides

Many types of peptide-secreting cells have been identified throughout the gastrointestinal tract. They are not, however, always clustered into discrete organs but may be dispersed within the mucosa of structures where their effects are maximal. Unlike circulating hormones, these substances are released locally through nerve stimulation and produce changes in the function of nearby structures including blood vessels. Pancreatic polypeptide and gastrin are two gastrointestinal peptides which have been studied in autonomic failure.

Pancreatic polypeptide

Most of the neurochemical research on autonomic failure has focused on the sympathetic nervous system because of the availability of biological markers for sympathetic activity. The insulin-induced increase in plasma pancreatic polypeptide is blocked by muscarinic anticholinergic drugs and truncal vagotomy but is not affected by splanchnic nerve section. Thus, release of pancreatic polypeptide appears to be under vagally-mediated, cholinergic control (see Polinsky *et al.* 1982 for references). Although pancreatic polypeptide has a variety of effects whose physiological significance remains obscure, measurement of the plasma level provides a biochemical index of vagal function. During insulin-induced hypoglycaemia, the catecholamine and pancreatic polypeptide levels can be measured to simultaneously assess sympathetic and parasympathetic nervous system responses as well as adrenal medullary responses.

Normal subjects manifest a precipitous rise in plasma levels of pancreatic polypeptide during hypoglycaemia. This response is essentially absent in PAF patients and also in most patients with MSA (Polinsky *et al.* 1982). Long *et al.* (1979) previously reported diminished pancreatic polypeptide responses in MSA patients. As anticipated there is no correlation between the catecholamine and pancreatic polypeptide responses (Polinsky *et al.* 1982). In fact, normal catecholamine responses were observed in some patients who lacked pancreatic polypeptide responses (Fig. 18.7) and vice versa. Although the deficiency in pancreatic polypeptide responses was not related to age or duration of illness, the one MSA patient with a normal response was the youngest MSA patient and also had the shortest duration of illness. Parasympathetic involvement in MSA clearly occurs and may respond to cholinergic treatment (Khurana *et al.* 1980). Deficient or absent pancreatic polypeptide and catecholamine responses provide biochemical evidence of pandysautonomia in both patients with PAF and MSA.

Gastrin

Antral motility and stomach acid output are both increased by gastrin and play a major role in the process of digestion. The factors affecting gastrin release are complex. Vagus-nerve stimulation increases gastrin release. However, the basal level of gastrin is increased following vagotomy, presumably because of the resulting gastric distention and increased stomach pH. Local cholinergic reflexes, increased sympathetic

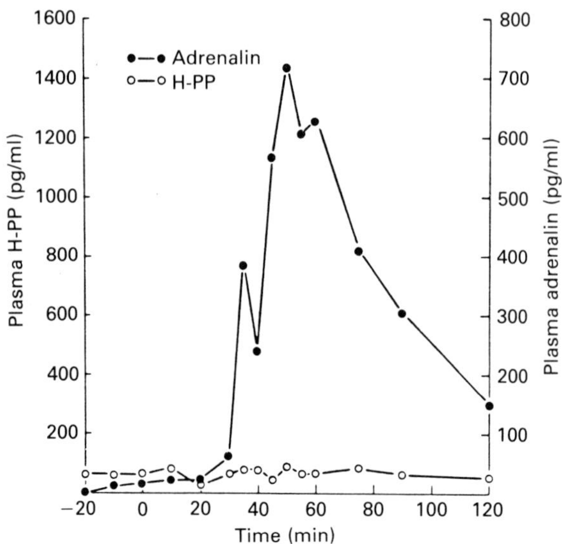

Fig. 18.7. Absent pancreatic polypeptide response in a patient with adequate adrenal medullary response. H-PP, pancreatic polypeptide.

nervous activity, and release of gastrin by adrenalin have been proposed to explain the persistent gastrin response following even highly selective vagotomy. Gastrin can also be released through β-adrenergic stimulation as shown by infusion studies with adrenalin; there is also a correlation between the gastrin increment and plasma adrenalin response during hypoglycaemia. There has only been one study of plasma gastrin in patients with autonomic failure despite the high incidence of symptoms that affect gastrointestinal function. Polinsky *et al.* (1987*b*) found abnormal basal and stimulated gastrin levels in patients with autonomic failure and the pattern differed between PAF and MSA. High basal gastrin levels occurred only in PAF consistent with peripheral vagal involvement. During hypoglycaemia PAF and MSA patients had significantly greater and less than normal increments in gastrin respectively. Since the gastrin response during hypoglycaemia may be controlled through an adrenergic mechanism, the increase observed in PAF might result from adrenergic supersensitivity, whereas the diminished response in MSA is due to reduced catecholamine levels with normal receptor sensitivity. Further investigation will be required to substantiate this explanation. Abnormal gastrin responses may play a role in the development of symptoms such as postprandial fullness.

CNS-mediated responses

Most of the responses discussed up to this point require the functional integrity and activity of the descending sympathetic outflow system. One approach that has been used to determine the anatomic localization of the lesion(s) in autonomic failure patients is the investigation of various systems with divergent efferent pathways that exit at different levels of the nervous system. The centrally mediated responses of the pituitary and pineal glands are two examples studied in patients with PAF and MSA.

Beta-endorphin and adrenocorticotrophic hormone (ACTH)

Hypoglycaemia evokes a number of peripheral hormonal responses as well as the release of pituitary peptides including β-endorphin and ACTH. Both peptides are derived from a common precursor and have hyperglycaemic effects exerted through different mechanisms (for detailed references see Polinsky *et al.* 1987*a*). The effects of ACTH are mediated through cortisol, whereas the hyperglycaemic actions of β-endorphin may involve glucagon secretion and inhibition of somatostatin release. The effects of insulin on β-endorphin release require the development of hypoglycaemia. Of particular relevance are the pharmacological studies with arecoline and atropine which respectively stimulate and block the release of β-endorphin. A central cholinergic pathway appears to mediate its release.

Polinsky *et al.* (1987*a*) found that patients with MSA but not PAF had essentially absent β-endorphin and ACTH responses to insulin-induced hypoglycaemia. The high correlation between β-endorphin and ACTH levels supports the common origin of these peptides from the pituitary. The normal β-endorphin and ACTH responses in PAF patients with markedly reduced or absent catecholamine responses suggests that peripheral catecholamine release is not required for the release of those peptides during hypoglycaemia.

These results provide further confirmation of the distinction between the autonomic involvement in PAF which is limited to peripheral lesions and the more central disturbance in MSA which probably includes the hypothalamus. Furthermore, the defect in β-endorphin release suggests that at least one central cholinergic pathway is affected in MSA. The widespread neuropathological involvement includes several areas with dense, cholinergic innervation. Reduced amounts of choline acetyltransferase activity have been found in the brains of MSA patients (see Chapter 25B).

Melatonin

Synthesis and release of melatonin by the pineal gland occurs in a rhythmic diurnal pattern that appears to be governed by an endogenous circadian oscillator located in the suprachiasmatic nucleus. Environmental light plays a key role in producing the diurnal cycle and its effects are mediated through retinohypothalamic projections. A projection from the suprachiasmatic nucleus terminates in the hypothalamus. Efferent pineal innervation arises from the medial forebrain bundle and midbrain reticular formation which send fibres to the intermediolateral column. The superior cervical ganglion, innervated by preganglionic neurons of the intermediolateral column, provides postganglionic innervation to the pineal through ascending cervical sympathetic-nerve fibres. These postganglionic fibres release increased amounts of noradrenalin at night; stimulation of β-adrenergic pineal receptors causes enhanced synthesis and release of melatonin. Melatonin is rapidly metabolized to 6-hydroxymelatonin which is conjugated and excreted in the urine. Hence, measurement of urinary 6-hydroxymelatonin conjugates provides an index of pineal function and the sympathetic nervous system pathways which innervate this organ.

Tetsuo *et al.* (1981) measured the diurnal pattern of urinary 6-hydroxymelatonin excretion in normal controls and patients with PAF and MSA. Normal subjects excrete most 6-hydroxymelatonin in the urine between midnight and 06.00 h and the least between noon and 18.00 h (Fig. 18.8). The total urinary excretion of 6-hydroxymelatonin was significantly reduced in patients with PAF. However, in those PAF patients with reliably measurable 6-hydroxymelatonin, there was preservation of the normal diurnal pattern with most at night-time and relatively little in the afternoon. Half of the MSA patients had low overall excretion rates but the pattern was altered. Most MSA patients excreted as much and in some cases more urinary 6-hydroxymelatonin during the daytime than between midnight and 06.00 h. These data can also be explained on the basis of the difference in pathophysiology between PAF and MSA. The preserved cyclic pattern with overall reduction in the amount of melatonin released in PAF reflects the

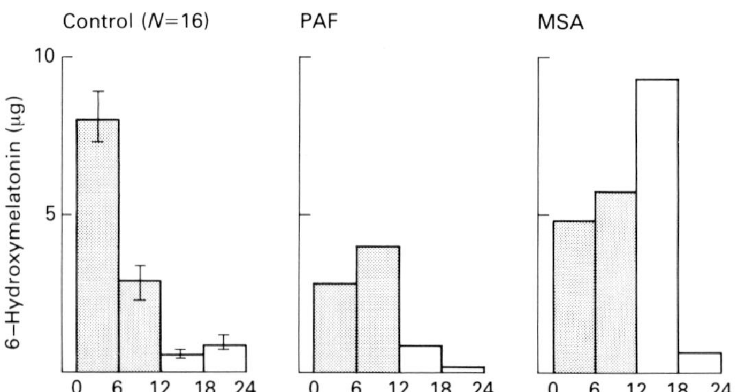

Fig. 18.8. Urinary excretion of 6-hydroxymelatonin in control subjects and an MSA and PAF patient.

decrease in night-time stimulation of the pineal resulting from diminished pineal innervation by postganglionic sympathetic fibres, the primary site of the lesion in PAF. In contrast, alteration of the diurnal pattern in MSA is more consistent with disruption of a central pathway involved in the regulation of pineal function. Plasma melatonin rhythm was found to be attenuated in one MSA patient (Vaughan *et al.* 1979). Further support for a decentralization of the pineal in MSA is found in the study of patients with cord transection; complete cervical but not a lumbar lesion results in a disturbed day–night pattern of melatonin excretion (Kneisley *et al.* 1978). Although the function of the pineal gland is not known in man, investigation of melatonin excretion has demonstrated an abnormality of the β-adrenergic sympathetic nervous system in patients with autonomic failure.

SUMMARY

The overall objective in studying the biochemical and pharmacological consequences of autonomic failure on circulatory and metabolic homeostasis is to enhance our understanding of the pathophysiology so that treatment can be improved. Much of the work presented in this chapter can be applied towards the development of rational therapeutic endeavours. Other aspects of the material included in this review are at a more preliminary stage and require further exploration, confirmation, and integration before they can be exploited for the benefit of patients. The approaches used to study autonomic failure have often yielded valuable insight into normal physiological function and metabolism. Our search in elucidating pathophysiology has forced us to review currently available methods and challenged us to modify and develop strategies that can be applied, albeit in a limited way, to investigate human diseases for which no adequate animal model exists. Table 18.2 is a summary of the current knowledge regarding neurotransmitter and neuropeptide function in autonomic failure.

Substantial progress has been achieved in the management of postural hypotension although this is unfortunately only one aspect of autonomic dysfunction. It is also possible to provide some symptomatic benefit for the other symptoms such as constipation and neurogenic bladder. Unfortunately, the outlook for treating patients with MSA is less optimistic and the overall prognosis is bleak relative to PAF. The extrapyramidal symptoms in MSA do respond to antiparkinsonian medications but this response wanes as the illness progresses. At this time there is no medication for treating the cerebellar symptoms in MSA.

In conclusion, much progress has been made towards understanding the differences between PAF and MSA. However, the similarities have been more useful in a practical sense since there has not yet been

Table 18.2. Biochemical and pharmacological distinction between PAF and MSA

	PAF	*MSA*
Biochemical		
Supine plasma NA	Low	Normal
Urinary NA metabolites		
Total	Decreased	Normal
NM/Total	Normal	Decreased
Responses to hypoglycaemia		
β-endorphin/ACTH	Normal	Decreased
Gastrin	Increased	Decreased
CNS neurotransmitter metabolism		
NA	Normal	Decreased
DA	Normal	Decreased
5-HT	Normal	Decreased
Pharmacological		
Pressor responses		
NA	Markedly increased	Increased
Angiotensin	Increased	Increased
NA release by tyramine	Low	Normal
NA receptor sensitivity	Increased	Normal
NA clearance	Decreased	Normal

NA, noradrenalin; DA, dopamine; NM, normetanephrine.

reported a medication which specifically improves autonomic function in only one of these syndromes. We know even less about the underlying degenerative process in MSA. There remains much work to be done before we can more fully alleviate (or perhaps abolish) the burden of these incapacitating neurological disorders.

REFERENCES

Bannister, R., Boylston, A. W., Davies, I. B., Mathias, C. J., Sever, P. S., and Sudera, D. (1981*a*). Beta-receptor numbers and thermodynamics in denervation supersensitivity. *J. Physiol., London* **319**, 369–77.

Bannister, R., Crowe, R., Eames, R., and Burnstock, G. (1981*b*). Defective catecholamine fluorescence in the sympathetic perivascular nerve plexuses in autonomic failure. *Neurology, Minneapolis* **31**, 1501–6.

Bannister, R., Crowe, R., Eames, R., Rosenthal, T., and Sever, P. (1979). Defective cardiovascular reflexes and supersensitivity to sympathomimetic drugs in autonomic failure. *Brain* **102**, 163–76.

Bannister, R., Crowe, R., Holly, E., Lethbridge, K., Mathias, C. J., Sever, P. S., and Sudera, D. (1980). Different alpha receptor properties and baroreflex loss in alpha-adrenergic denervation supersensitivity in man. *J. Physiol., London* **308**, 44–5P.

Bannister, R., Sever, P., and Gross, M. (1977). Cardiovascular reflexes and biochemical responses in progressive autonomic failure. *Brain* **100**, 327–44.

Barnes, A. J. (1983). Pancreatic endocrine function in autonomic failure. In *Autonomic failure*, 1st edn. (ed. R. Bannister), pp. 249–66. Oxford University Press, Oxford.

Esler, M., Jackman, G., Kelleher, D., Skews, H., Jennings, G., Bobik, A., and Korner, P. (1980). Norepinephrine kinetics in patients with idiopathic autonomic insufficiency. *Circulation Res.* **46** (Suppl. 1), 47–8.

Hoeldtke, R. D., O'Dorisio, T. M., and Boden, G. (1986). Treatment of autonomic neuropathy with a somatostatin analogue SMS-201-995. *Lancet* **ii**, 602–5.

Kafka, M. S., Polinsky, R. J., Williams, A., Kopin, I. J., Lake, C. R., Ebert, M. H., and Tokola, N. S. (1984). Alpha-adrenergic receptors in orthostatic hypotension syndromes. *Neurology, Minneapolis* **34**, 1121–5.

Khurana, R. K., Nelson, E., Azzarelli, B., and Garcia, J. H. (1980). Shy–Drager syndrome: diagnosis and treatment of cholinergic dysfunction. *Neurology, Minneapolis* **30**, 805–9.

Kneisley, L. W., Moskowitz, M. A., and Lynch, H. J. (1978). Cervical spinal cord lesions disrupt the rhythm in human melatonin secretion. *J. neural Transm.* **13** (Suppl.), 311–23.

Kontos, H. A., Richardson, D. W., and Norvell, J. E. (1975). Norepinephrine depletion in idiopathic orthostatic hypotension. *Ann. intern. Med.* **82**, 336–41.

Kontos, H. A., Richardson, D. W., and Norvell, J. E. (1976). Mechanisms of circulatory dysfunction in orthostatic hypotension. *Trans. Am. clin. climatol. Ass.* **87**, 26–33.

Kopin, I. J., Gordon, E. K., Jimerson, D. C., and Polinsky, R. J. (1983*a*). Relation between plasma and cerebrospinal fluid levels of 3-methoxy-4-hydroxyphenylglycol. *Science* **219**, 73–5.

Kopin, I. J., Polinsky, R. J., Oliver, J. A., Oddershede, I. R., and Ebert, M. H. (1983*b*). Urinary catecholamine metabolites distinguish different types of sympathetic neuronal dysfunction in patients with orthostatic hypotension. *J. clin. Endocr. Metab.* **57**, 632–7.

Long, R. G., Barnes, A. J., Albuquerque, R. H., Prata, A., Bannister, R., Adrian, T. E., and Bloom, S. R. (1979). Pancreatic hormone release in Chagas' disease and the Shy–Drager syndrome. *Gut* **20**, A921.

Luft, F. and von Euler, V. (1953). Two cases of postural hypotension showing a deficiency in release of norepinephrine and epinephrine. *J. clin. Invest.* **32**, 1065–9.

Mathias, C. J., Matthews, W. B., and Spalding, J. M. K. (1977). Postural changes in plasma renin activity and responses to vasoactive drugs in a case of Shy–Drager syndrome. *J. Neurol. Neurosurg. Psychiat.* **40**, 138–43.

Mohring, J., Glanzer, K., Maciel, J. A., Dusing, R., Kramer, H. J., Arbogast, R., and Koch-Weser, J. (1980). Greatly enhanced pressor response to antidiuretic hormone in patients with impaired cardiovascular reflexes due to idiopathic orthostatic hypotension. *J. cardiovasc. Pharmacol.* **2**, 367–76.

Moskowitz, M. A. and Wurtman, R. J. (1975). Catecholamines and neurologic diseases. *New Engl. J. Med.* **293**, 274–80, 332–8.

Parks, V. J., Sandison, A. G., Skinner, S. L., and Whelan, R. J. (1961). Sympathomimetic drugs in orthostatic hypotension. *Lancet* **i**, 1133–6.

Polinsky, R. J. (1984). Central nervous system control of blood pressure. In *Mild hypertension—current controversies and new approaches* (ed. M. Weber and C. Mathias), pp. 11–22. Steinkopff-Verlag, Darmstadt.

Polinsky, R. J., Brown, R. T., Burns, R. S., and Kopin, I. J. (1985*a*). Cerebrospinal fluid monoamine metabolites in patients with progressive autonomic failure. *J. Neurol.* **232** (Suppl.), 71.

Polinsky, R. J., Brown, R. T., Lee, G. K., Timmers, K., Culman, J., Foldes, O., Kopin, I. J., and Recant, L. (1987*a*). Beta-endorphin, ACTH, and catecholamine responses in chronic autonomic failure. *Ann. Neurol.* **21**, 573–7.

Polinsky, R. J., Goldstein, D. S., Brown, R. T., Keiser, H. R., and Kopin, I. J. (1985*b*). Decreased sympathetic neuronal uptake in idiopathic orthostatic hypotension. *Ann. Neurol.* **18**, 48–53.

Polinsky, R. J., Jimerson, D. C., and Kopin, I. J. (1984). Chronic autonomic failure: CSF and plasma 3-methoxy-4-hydroxyphenylglycol. *Neurology* **34**, 979–83.

Polinsky, R. J., Kopin, I. J., Ebert, M. H., and Weise, V. (1980). The adrenal medullary response to hypoglycemia in patients with orthostatic hypotension. *J. clin. Endocrinol. Metab.* **51**, 1401–6.

Polinsky, R. J., Kopin, I. J., Ebert, M. H., and Weise, V. (1981*a*). Pharmacologic distinction of different orthostatic hypotension syndromes. *Neurology, Minneapolis* **31**, 1–7.

Polinsky, R. J., Kopin, I. J., Ebert, M. H., Weise, V., and Recant, L. (1981*b*). Hormonal responses to hypoglycemia in orthostatic hypotension patients with adrenergic insufficiency. *Life Sci.* **29**, 417–25.

Polinsky, R. J., Kopin, I. J., Gullner, H. G., and Petersen, L. (1981*c*). Effect of indomethacin inhibition of prostaglandin synthesis on blood pressure and plasma norepinephrine levels in patients with orthostatic hypotension. *Neurology, Minneapolis* **31**, 63.

Polinsky, R. J., Taylor, I. L., Chew, P., Weise, V., and Kopin, I. J. (1982). Pancreatic polypeptide responses to hypoglycemia in chronic autonomic failure. *J. clin. Endocrinol. Metab.* **54**, 48–52.

Polinsky, R. J., Taylor, I. L., Weise, V., and Kopin, I. J. (1987*b*). Gastrin responses in patients with adrenergic insufficiency. *J. Neurol. Neurosurg. Psychiat.* (in press).

Robertson, D., Goldberg, M. R., Hollister, A. S., Wade, D., and Robertson, R. M. (1983). Clonidine raises blood pressure in idiopathic orthostatic hypotension. *Am. J. Med.* **74**, 193–200.

Robertson, D., Hollister, A. S., Carey, E. L., Tung, C.-S., Goldberg, M. R., and Robertson, R. M. (1984). Increased vascular beta 2-adrenoceptor responsiveness in autonomic dysfunction. *J. Am. Coll. Cardiol.* **3**, 850–6.

Sasaki, K., Matsuhashi, A., Murabayashi, S., Aoyagi, K., Baba, T., Matsunaga, M., and Takebe, K. (1983). Hormonal response to insulin-induced hypoglycemia in patients with Shy–Drager syndrome. *Metabolism* **32**, 977–81.

Shy, G. M. and Drager, G. A. (1960). A neurological syndrome associated with orthostatic hypotension: a clinical-pathologic study. *Arch. Neurol., Chicago* **2**, 511–27.

Spokes, E. G. S. (1983). Neurochemistry of autonomic failure. In *Autonomic failure*, 1st edn. (ed. R. Bannister), pp. 284–309. Oxford University Press, Oxford.

Spokes, E. G. S., Bannister, R., and Oppenheimer, D. R. (1979). Multiple system atrophy with autonomic failure: clinical, histological, and neurochemical observations on four cases. *J. neurol. Sci.* **43**, 59–82.

Tetsuo, M., Polinsky, R. J., Markey, S. P., and Kopin, I. J. (1981). Urinary 6-hydroxy-melatonin excretion in patients with orthostatic hypotension. *J. clin. Endocrinol. Metab.* **53**, 607–10.

Vaughan, G. M., McDonald, S. D., Jordan, R. M., Allen, J. P., Bell, R., and Stevens, E. A. (1979). Melatonin, pituitary function, and stress in humans. *Psychoneuroendocrinology* **4**, 351–62.

Wilcox, C. S. and Aminoff, M. J. (1976). Blood pressure responses to noradrenaline and dopamine infusions in Parkinson's disease and the Shy–Drager syndrome. *Br. J. clin. Pharmacol.* **3**, 207–14.

Wilcox, C. S., Aminoff, M. J., Millar, J. G. B., Keenan, J., and Kremer, M. (1975). Circulating levels of corticotrophin and cortisol after infusions of L-DOPA, dopamine, and noradrenaline in man. *Clin. Endocrinol.* **4**, 191–8.

Williams, A. C., Nutt, J., Lake, C. R., Pfeiffer, R., Teychenne, P. E., Ebert, M., and Calne, D. B. (1979). In *Dopaminergic ergots and motor control* (ed. K. Fuxe and D. B. Calne), pp. 271–83. Pergamon Press, New York.

Ziegler, M. G., Lake, C. R., and Kopin, I. J. (1977). The sympathetic-nervous-system defect in primary orthostatic hypotension. *New Engl. J. Med.* **296**, 293–7.

19. Adrenoceptor function

I. Bleddyn Davies and Peter S. Sever

A. Adrenoceptor function in autonomic failure

DENERVATION SUPERSENSITIVITY IN AUTONOMIC FAILURE

Autonomic nervous system failure is associated with changes in the biological effects of adrenoceptor stimulation; the nature and degree of change depends upon the cause of the autonomic failure which may result from a variety of diseases, drugs, or from apparently normal ageing. Impairment of autonomic function in the elderly seems to result in an overall decrease in adrenoceptor-mediated responses and ageing does not seem to be associated with destruction of autonomic neurons although age-associated degenerative changes occur in autonomic ganglia and neurons (Chapter 19B). In contrast, certain diseases lead to destruction of autonomic nerves and, with regard to the sympathetic nervous system, the overriding change produced is one of increased adrenoceptor responses to sympathomimetic drugs. Treatment with adrenoceptor antagonists or drugs which inhibit neuronal catecholamine uptake may also lead to increased responses when the appropriate agonist drug is given.

These increased adrenoceptor responses represent denervation supersensitivity as described by Cannon and Rosenbleuth (1949) for tissues to which the nerve supply has been destroyed and, as noted for 'functional' denervation, where tissue receptors cannot be stimulated because of depletion of the neurotransmitter in their supplying nerves or because of blockade of the receptor by an antagonist drug (Fleming *et al.* 1978). Part A of this chapter summarizes available information about adrenoceptor responses in autonmic failure associated with sympathetic denervation and discusses the changes in adrenoceptors seen in autonomic failure and the mechanisms responsible for denervation supersensitivity. As a background a basic understanding of adrenergic neurotransmission is required as summarized in Part B of this chapter.

ADRENOCEPTOR RESPONSES IN AUTONOMIC FAILURE

In man, increased cardiovascular responses to α- and β-adrenoceptor agonist drugs have been described in autonomic failure associated with a number of diverse conditions including typhoid fever, withdrawal of β-adrenoceptor antagonists, tetraplegia, breast carcinoma, or progressive idiopathic autonomic degeneration occurring alone, with Parkinson's disease or as part of multiple system atrophy (Shy–Drager syndrome) (Bannister *et al.* 1979). The tardive dyskinesia associated with chronic phenothiazine treatment or metoclopramide and other dopamine antagonists may represent supersensitivity of dopamine receptors in response to 'pharmacological' autonomic denervation by chronic receptor blockade. Increased arrhythmias in human cardiac transplants may also reflect supersensitivity of cardiac β-adenoceptors to circulating catecholamines as is the case for experimentally denervated animal hearts.

Postsynaptic α-adrenoceptor changes in autonomic failure

Increased systolic blood pressure caused by intravenous noradrenalin can be used as a measure of *in vivo* α-adrenoceptor responses. Patients with autonomic failure and multiple system atrophy (MSA) show marked left shift of the blood pressure–noradrenalin dose-response curve and have increases in systolic pressure at doses of noradrenalin which do not cause a pressor response in normal subjects (Davies *et al.* 1982*a*). The increased pressor response may be associated with increased α-adrenoceptor numbers. Radioligand binding studies have shown an approximately sevenfold increase in α-adrenoceptor number on blood platelets relative to normal controls using ^{3}H-dihydroergocryptine, an α-adrenoceptor antagonist, to identify the α-adrenoceptors (Davies *et al.* 1982*a*). The affinity of the platelet α-adrenoceptors was unchanged as measured by equilibrium dissociation constants (K_d) for ^{3}H-dihydroergocryptine binding (Nahorski and Barnett 1982). ^{3}H-dihydroergocryptine binds to both α_1- and α_2-adrenoceptors and there are a number of technical problems in its use (Nahorski and Barnett 1982), but the increase in platelet α_2-adrenoceptors in MSA subjects has been confirmed using ^{3}H–yohimbine binding to platelets; yohimbine binds selectively to α_2-adrenoceptors (Fig. 19.1). If platelet α-adrenoceptors reflect the status of vascular α-adrenoceptors then an increase in α-adrenoceptor number could contribute to noradrenalin pressor supersensitivity in patients with autonomic failure and MSA. In animals, too, sympathetic denervation using 6-hydroxydopamine or depletion of neuronal noradrenalin with reserpine cause an increase in α-adrenoceptor number without change in affinity (U'Prichard and

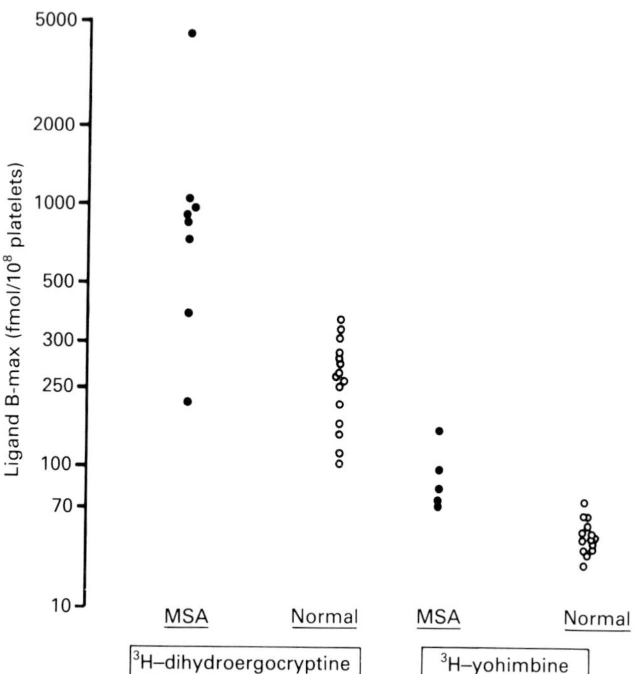

Fig. 19.1. α-Adrenoceptor number (proportional to ligand B-max as ordinate) in platelets isolated from normal subjects (○) and patients with autonomic failure and multiple system atrophy (MSA) (●). α-Adrenoceptors were determined for each subject using ^{3}H-dihydroergocryptine and, separately, ^{3}H-yohimbine. Separate subjects were used in the two studies. (Bannister, Mattin, and Sever, unpublished observations.)

Snyder 1978; U'Prichard *et al.* 1979). The increase in adrenoceptor number may seem puzzling because MSA and autonomic failure in humans and the experimental use of 6-hydroxydopamine in animals are both associated with degeneration and loss of sympathetic nerves. The explanation for the increased α-adrenoceptor numbers is linked to the decreased exposure to noradrenalin which occurs in tissues which have been denervated—the decreased exposure to neurotransmitter leads to a compensatory increase in receptor number. Teleologically, this can be viewed as an adaptive response to maximize the effect of any noradrenalin released from remaining sympathetic nerves (Davies *et al.* 1984). It has been shown that many patients with MSA and autonomic failure have low concentrations of endogenous noradrenalin in blood reflecting the sympathetic nervous degeneration; the range of values obtained in our own series is shown in Fig. 19.2. The situation in MSA patients contrasts with its antithesis, the vast overproduction of catecholamines in phaeochromocytoma; in phaeochromocytoma patients' plasma

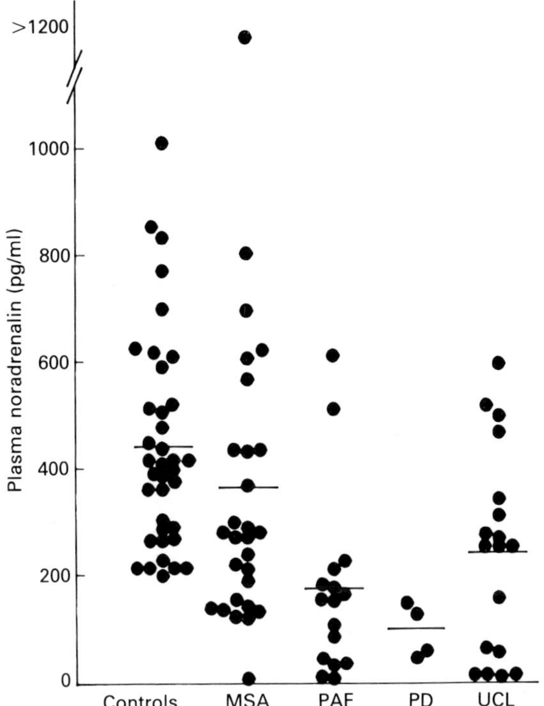

Fig. 19.2. Individual values for recumbent plasma noradrenalin in patients with multiple system atrophy (MSA), pure autonomic failure (PAF), Parkinson's disease and orthostatic hypotension (PD), and a series of unclassified patients with orthostatic hypotension (UCL) who fulfil the biochemical criteria of autonomic failure, namely a failure of plasma noradrenalin to rise with upright posture. Shown also are comparable values for an age-matched healthy control population (40–65 years). Bars indicate mean value for each group.

noradrenalin is markedly increased and platelet α-adrenoceptors decreased below normal (Davies 1982). Platelets have no nuclei and incubation of platelets with catecholamines does not alter the number of α-adrenoceptors on platelet membranes (Davies 1982). However, the bone marrow has a rich autonomic nerve supply in normal subjects and it is likely that α-adrenoceptor status in platelets reflects that at the megakaryocyte stage in the bone marrow (Davies 1982).

In patients with chronic tetraplegia there are increased pressor responses to intravenous noradrenalin (see Part B of this chapter and Davies 1982). Platelet α-adrenoceptors in chronic tetraplegics do not, however, differ from normal control subjects in terms of receptor number and affinity as measured by ^{3}H-dihydroergocryptine binding (Davies *et al.* 1982*a*). This situation may initially seem contradictory to the findings in MSA patients, but it is not. In chronic tetraplegia with lesions of the cervical spinal cord, the spinal cord is isolated from cerebral sympathetic centres and so the sympathetic component of the baroreflex arc is absent but connections with the ninth and tenth cranial nerves are intact. At rest there is little or no sympathetic activity explaining the low plasma noradrenalin concentrations observed in several studies. However, sympathetic reflexes are integrated at a spinal level and stimulation of sympathetic nerve activity, e.g. by percussing the abdominal wall over the urinary bladder, leads to an outpouring of noradrenalin from peripheral nerves with a marked rise in plasma noradrenalin. Therefore, in contrast to MSA where there is continual low exposure of α-receptors to noradrenalin, in chronic tetraplegics, during periods of spinal reflex activity, α-receptors are exposed to large amounts of catecholamines; this may account for the normal numbers of α-receptors observed in chronic tetraplegics: normal agonist concentrations are associated with normal adrenoceptor numbers (see Davies *et al.* 1984). In chronic tetraplegics it is likely that the cause of the supersensitivity to noradrenalin is purely defective baroreflexes, the remaining reflex compensation for a rise in blood pressure being only a vagus-mediated bradycardia which does not seem sufficient to prevent an abnormally brisk response to noradrenalin.

Postsynaptic β-adrenoceptor changes in autonomic failure

In patients with pure autonomic failure and with autonomic failure plus MSA, there is denervation supersensitivity of β-adrenoceptors shown by the greater chronotropic effect on the heart and steeper dose-response curve for isoprenaline (Bannister *et al.* 1981). Patients in studies of adrenoceptor function and autonomic failure tend to be old, but this fact highlights further the effect of the autonomic failure because older people tend to have decreased β-receptor responses and probably decreased α-receptor responses too (see Chapter 19B). In patients with autonomic failure and MSA who were supersensitive to intravenous isoprenaline, ^{3}H-dihydroalprenolol (DHA) binding showed increased numbers of β-adrenoceptors on circulating lymphocytes (Bannister *et al.* 1981; Davies 1982). However, the affinity of the β-adrenoceptors, as measured by equilibrium association constants for DHA binding, was not different in MSA lymphocytes compared with normal. In spite of the difficulty of extrapolating from cardiac β_1-receptors, which mediate the *in vivo* chronotropic isoprenaline response, to *in vitro* lymphocyte β_2-receptors, the increase in β-receptors observed on lymphocytes from MSA subjects suggests that increased β-receptor numbers are likely to be important in the *in vivo* denervation supersensitivity to isoprenaline. Patients with pure autonomic failure and autonomic failure with MSA often have lower concentrations of endogenous catecholamines than normal so that the increased number of β-receptors seen in these patients may (as for platelet α-receptors mentioned above) reflect agonist regulation of adrenoceptor numbers (see Davies *et al.* 1984). The use of DHA to identify β-receptors can be associated with problems (see Nahorski and Barnett 1982). However, the increase of lymphocyte β-adrenoceptors in patients with autonomic failure was confirmed in a subsequent study using [^{125}I]-iodocyanopindolol as the β-receptor binding ligand (Kilfeather *et al.* 1985). Kilfeather *et al.* (1985) also confirmed that β-adrenoceptor affinity was no different from normal in MSA and autonomic failure.

β-Adrenoceptors appear to mediate their effects via stimulation of the adenylate cyclase enzyme complex to which they are linked. The responsiveness of tissue β-adrenoceptors has been tested by measuring the amount of cAMP the tissue can generate in response to isoprenaline (this is not always valid for maximal isoprenaline doses activate only a fraction of the adenyl cyclase present in the tissue). In one study of lymphocytes from patients with MSA, isoprenaline-stimulated cAMP generation was three- to fivefold greater than for normal lymphocytes (Jennings *et al.* 1981). However, this increased cAMP response was not confirmed by Kilfeather *et al.* (1985) who found no difference in isoprenaline-mediated cAMP production between normal and MSA lymphocytes. Increased lymphocyte β-receptors and supersensitivity to intravenous isoprenaline has been described in one case of autonomic failure associated with disseminated breast carcinoma (Hui and Connolly 1981).

Teleologically, β-adrenoceptor antagonist treatment can be viewed as partial pharmacological autonomic failure for endogenous catecholamines are denied access to tissue β-receptors. Sudden β-antagonist withdrawal has been reported to cause tachydysrhythmias, angina, and even myocardial infarction in patients treated chronically with these drugs. This β-blocker withdrawal syndrome may be associated with β-adrenoceptor supersensitivity for some studies have shown increased responses to intravenous catecholamines and increased lymphocyte β-adrenoceptors in patients after β-antagonist withdrawal (Aarons *et al.* 1980).

Mechanisms of denervation supersensitivity in autonomic failure

The increased responses of adrenoceptor-containing denervated tissues when stimulated by sympathomimetic drugs do not in the whole organism depend solely upon local changes in the tissues themselves. In intact man several factors contribute to the overall supersensitivity and these may involve derangement of complex reflexes concerned with interaction between organs in addition to changes at the level of postjunctional adrenoceptors in the effector tissues concerned. Factors known to contribute to denervation supersensitivity in man are summarized in Fig. 19.3.

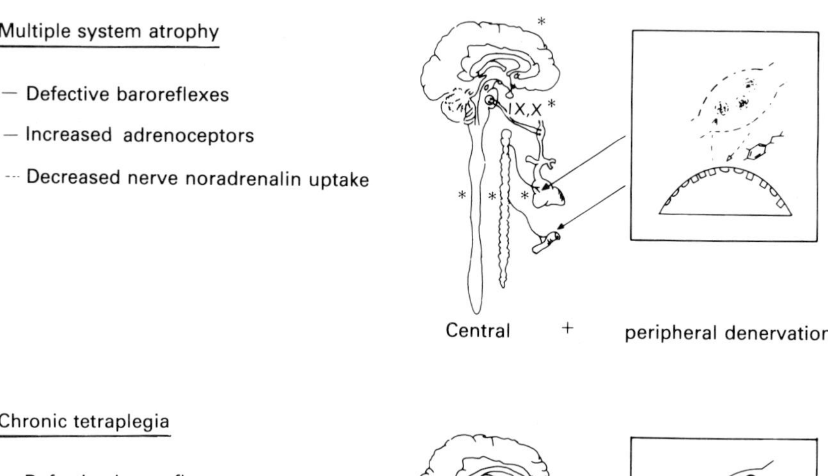

Chronic tetraplegia

— Defective baroreflexes

IX,X

Decentralization

Intact nerve endings

Fig. 19.3. Major mechanisms contributing to denervation supersensitivity in intact humans with autonomic failure due to sympathetic degeneration in multiple system atrophy or decentralization in chronic tetraplegia.

Postsynaptic adrenoceptor changes and receptor–effector coupling

The demonstration of increased platelet α- and lymphocyte β-adrenoceptor numbers in patients supersensitive to, respectively, noradrenalin and isoprenaline, suggests that increased α-adrenoceptor number may be important in the generation of these increased responses. However, increased adrenoceptor number is not necessarily related to increased biological responses. It has become clear for β-adrenoceptors that they may change their coupling to effector mechanisms independently of any change in total receptor number and in some tissues there are more α- and β-adrenoceptors than are required for a maximal tissue response ('spare' receptors). Data on coupling of adrenoceptors with effector mechanisms is scanty in denervation supersensitivity and autonomic failure. Jennings *et al.* (1981) found increased cAMP production in response to isoprenaline in lymphocytes from patients with autonomic failure: this could have been compatible with increased β-receptor numbers leading to increased adenylate cyclase activation, or with increased efficiency of adrenoceptor–adenylate cyclase coupling. Kilfeather *et al.* (1985), however, found no change in cAMP production in response to isoprenaline in lymphocyte membranes from patients with autonomic failure so that increased cAMP generation may not be necessary for causing increased effector tissue responses. The recent elucidation of the roles of inositol phosphates in affecting calcium fluxes in excitable tissues in response to neurotransmitter stimulation needs investigation in autonomic failure, for alteration in the concentrations of metabolic interconversions of inositol phosphate 'second messengers' may explain increased denervated cell responses in the presence of cAMP generation which is only equivalent to that of normal cells (Michel 1986). Increased inositol phosphate turnover has been shown to be coupled with α-adrenoceptor supersensitivity in denervated iris muscle (Abdel-Latif 1986).

ADRENOCEPTOR INTERACTIONS WITH OTHER HUMORAL SYSTEMS

Patients with autonomic failure and MSA show changes in systems other than the sympathetic nervous system; urinary excretion of prostaglandin E and of the renal metabolite of prostaglandin $F_2\alpha$ is increased (Zwada and Kirschenbaum 1979; Davies *et al.* 1980) and there is increased sensitivity to the pressor effects of angiotensin II. Prostaglandins and angiotensin II interact with presynaptic receptors on sympathetic nerve endings and presynaptic receptors provide a means by which complex interactions may occur between remaining adrenergic nerve and other humoral systems in influencing adrenoceptor function in autonomic failure.

Prostaglandins have complex and differing actions, some vasodilator, some constrictor, and some renal prostaglandins are involved in sodium excretion by the kidney. Overactivity of renal prostaglandins, lack of sympathetic-nerve activity to conserve sodium with consequent lack of antagonism of the natriuretic effects of renal dopaminergic nerves could contribute to the salt wasting seen in some patients with autonomic failure and in denervated kidneys. Angiotensin may increase the release of noradrenalin via stimulation of presynaptic angiotensin receptors and can cause release of adrenal catecholamines; an increase in angiotensin responses could be a compensatory mechanism to maximize the release of remaining endogenous catecholamines. However, angiotensin pressor supersensitivity in autonomic failure patients could also be an artefact of the lack of baroreflexes and/or the non-specific increase in reactivity shown by denervated vascular tissue. There is no information upon the role of opioid mechanisms, endothelial relaxing factor of Furchgott, or prostacyclin in control of vascular adrenoceptor responses and vascular reactivity in autonomic failure, but such information would be important.

DEFECTIVE NEUROTRANSMITTER CLEARANCE

Uptake of noradrenalin into sympathetic nerve endings (Uptake$_1$, see Fig. 19.4) is not only important for clearing noradrenalin from the local nerve varicosity, but is also of importance for clearing catecholamines from the blood (Whitby *et al.* 1961). In patients with autonomic failure and in normal ageing people, clearance of noradrenalin is decreased relative to normal or younger controls respectively. Decreased noradrenalin clearance may be another mechanism involved in increased adrenoceptor responses by allowing increased contact of noradrenalin with adrenoceptors.

IMPAIRED PHYSIOLOGICAL DAMPING MECHANISMS

In whole experimental animals or in man, noradrenalin pressor responses are partly compensated by baroreflexes which are defective in autonomic failure and MSA (Bannister *et al.* 1979). Lack of baroreflex activity summates with the other mechanisms causing supersensitivity of adrenoceptor responses in patients with autonomic failure. In chronic tetraplegia, lack of baroreflexes would seem to be the only factor known to cause pressor supersensitivity to noradrenalin because of tetraplegics peripheral sympathetic-nerve endings remain intact and adrenoceptor numbers are normal (see above, 'Postsynaptic adrenoceptor changes in autonomic failure').

B. Adrenoceptor function and ageing

Responses to sympathetic nerve stimulation, adrenoceptor agonist and antagonist drugs change with ageing. The altered responses may be due to true effects of ageing upon adrenergic receptors and effectors, or to the deterioration with age of regulatory systems which modulate adrenoceptor-mediated responses or to disease processes which are often multiple in elderly individuals. There is a paucity of information about the effects of ageing as a continuous process: most studies have compared circumscribed age groups, 'young' and 'old', rather than assessed variation in adrenoceptor function in subjects from the whole age spectrum. Few studies on ageing have controlled for factors that affect sympathetic activity such as time of day, exercise training, fasting, and drugs.

Part B of this chapter summarizes factors affecting adrenoceptor reactivity in relation to ageing, the information available about adrenoceptor responses in ageing humans and experimental animals and in isolated tissues and cells; in the second half of Part B an attempt is made to discuss the mechanism of the effects of ageing on adrenoceptor-mediated processes.

FACTORS REGULATING ADRENOCEPTOR FUNCTION

Processes operating at the whole organism and cellular levels may affect the response to adrenoceptor stimulation by naturally-released noradrenalin or by an exogenous adrenoceptor agonist (Fig. 19.4) (Davies *et al.* 1984). The components regulating adrenoceptor function after

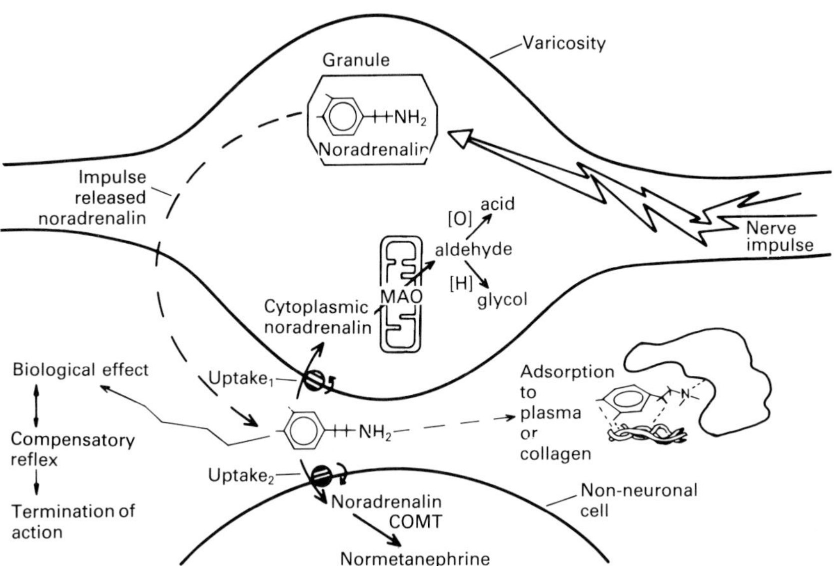

Fig. 19.4. Factors affecting the response of sympathetically innervated tissues. The processes shown lead to the termination of noradrenergic impulse transmission and also govern the degree of exposure of the postjunctional effector cell membrane to noradrenalin. (Taken from Davies (1982).)

agonist has come into contact with adrenoceptors are diagrammed in Fig. 19.5. Nerve impulses trigger exocytotic release of catecholamines from vesicle stores in sympathetic nerves. The catecholamines (or agonist drugs) stimulate membrane receptors. The way in which the adrenoceptor response is mediated is better known for β-adrenoceptors (Rodbell 1980); there is relatively little information about the subcellular mediation of α-adrenoceptor responses. Catecholamine binding to the β-adrenoceptor–adenyl cyclase complex causes the production of cyclic AMP (cAMP) which activates protein kinases. The resulting phosphorylation of proteins may stimulate cell contraction or subcellular calcium fluxes or entry of calcium into the cell; these events are likely to be affected by changes in membrane fluidity and, it would now seem, by inositol phosphates and changes in the microtubular network within cells (Fig. 19.5). The number of adrenoceptors available at the cell surface may increase or decrease, respectively, after abnormally small or large degrees of exposure to agonist drugs or the natural neurotransmitter (Davies *et al.* 1984). The biological effects of catecholamines are rapidly stopped by clearance of catecholamines from the receptors by uptake into sympathetic nerves or other sites such as vascular smooth muscle (Fig. 19.4). The ways in which these processes and adrenoceptor function may be affected by ageing are summarized in Table 19.1.

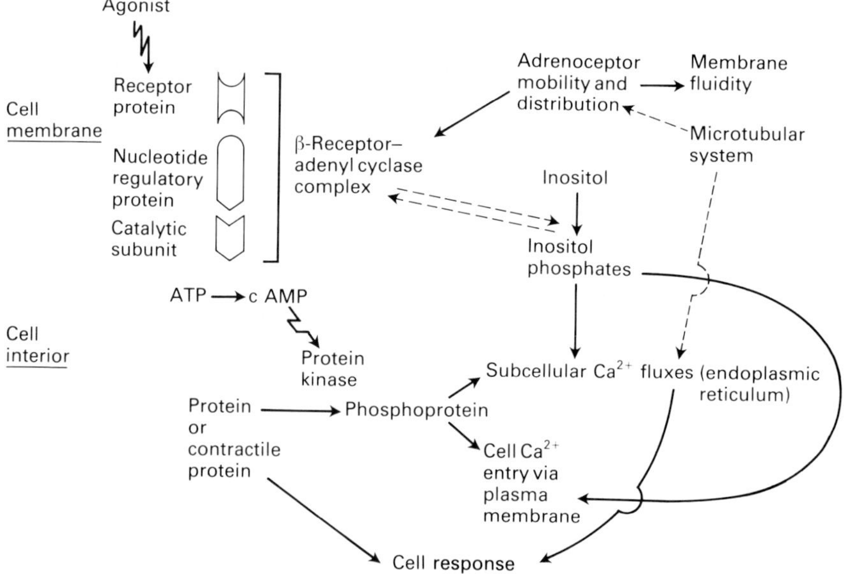

Fig. 19.5. Schematic representation of events in the β-adrenoceptor stimulation–response process. Hypothesized events are indicated by broken line. Inositol phosphate metabolism seems linked to α-adrenoceptors but may not be linked to β-adrenoceptors.

Table 19.1. Effects of age on adrenoceptor responses

Effects at the whole-organism level
Pharmacokinetic and metabolic changes
Defective reflexes modulating sympathetic responses
Deconditioning with less physical exercise
Changes in interacting systems: prostanoids, kinins, opioids, renin–angiotensin
Effects at the cellular level
Altered adrenoceptors
Adrenoceptor stimulation–effector response coupling
Second messengers: changes in phosphoinositides
Altered receptor environment—cell membrane changes

AGEING AND ADRENOCEPTOR-MEDIATED RESPONSES

Ageing clearly decreases the responses of β_1-adrenoceptors, but more information is required for functions of β_2- and α_2-adrenoceptors.

Adrenoceptor responses in elderly humans

At rest and during exercise, the β-blocking effect of propranolol is less in elderly than young subjects. Consistent with this is the right shift of the dose-response curve for isoprenaline-induced increase in heart rate in ageing. Hence, it is presumed that β_1-adrenoceptors are less important in influencing heart rate in elderly people (Kelly and O'Malley 1984). There is no information upon the responsiveness of respiratory β_2-adrenoceptors in ageing in spite of its importance for reversible airways obstruction.

Ageing effects on α_1-adrenoceptor responses are controversial. The pressor effect of phenylephrine may decrease with age (Elliott *et al.* 1982), but adrenalin boluses did not change the blood pressure of younger subjects but increased that of older subjects (Korkushko 1980, p. 288). α-Adrenoceptor antagonists, phentolamine and prazosin, do not seem to have any different effects in old and young subjects (Elliott *et al.* 1982). Interestingly the adrenergically-mediated dark-adapted pupillary responses are decreased in older humans (Halter and Pfeifer 1982).

Adrenoceptor responses in ageing experimental animals

Cardiovascular responses to sympathetic-nerve stimulation or to infusion of adrenalin, noradrenalin, or isoprenaline seem to decrease in older animals. However, at lower doses of agonist, ageing results in increased sensitivity to adrenoceptor agonists (Frolkis 1985). The lower threshold of response in older animals has been attributed to 'denervation' supersensitivity since myocardial catecholamine content decreases with age.

β_2-adrenoceptor function may also decrease with age because adrenalin causes a smaller increase in blood free fatty acids in older animals.

Adrenoceptor responses isolated tissues and cells of humans and experimental animals

In general, evidence from animal and human tissue experiments has suggested decreased functional efficiency of adrenoceptor responses with ageing. Sympathetic ganglia in aged animals show degenerative changes and are more sensitive to ganglion blockers than in young animals. Smooth-muscle cells of mesenteric arterioles and aortic strips isolated from older animals show less potency and efficacy in relaxation (presumably β_2-adrenoceptor) response to catecholamines (Kelly and O'Malley 1984; Frolkis 1985). However, isolated human arteries and veins from elderly subjects have shown no change in contractile (presumably α_1-adrenoceptor) response to noradrenalin relative to young controls. The discrepancies between human and experimental animal studies could result from species differences in vascular adrenoceptors or to the use of tissues from different vascular beds which vary: in ageing rats the threshold for sympathetic nerve-induced or intravenous noradrenalin-induced vasoconstriction varied between hindlimb, small intestinal, and renal vessels (Frolkis 1985). β_2-receptor mediated lipolytic responses and isoprenaline-stimulated cAMP release for adipocytes and polymorphs or lymphocytes (these cells have surface β_2-receptors) isolated from older subjects are also decreased. Respiratory muscle β_2-adrenoceptor function also seems to decrease with age in terms of decreased potency of isoprenaline-induced relaxation in trachea and bronchi isolated from old animals. Data for myocardial β_1-adrenoceptors parallels that for vascular β_2-adrenoceptors. Narayanan and Derby (1982) found impaired guanine nucleotide responses and decreased adenyl cyclase responses in old rats. Data on α_2-adrenoceptor responses is lacking but must be of importance.

MECHANISMS OF AGE-INDUCED CHANGES IN ADRENOCEPTOR FUNCTION

Ageing is associated with changes in factors affecting access of nerve-released and exogenous catecholamines to adrenoceptors, altered neural and endocrine systems that interact with and modulate the biological effects of adrenoceptors. In addition, subcellular effects of ageing seem to be linked with the alterations catalogued by the experimental observations described in Table 19.1. The ultimate effect of ageing upon adrenoceptor function is likely to be the complex summation of all these interacting factors, the relative importance of each factor varying between individuals and, probably, between regional sympathetic beds and animal species.

Ageing, noradrenalin pharmacokinetics and metabolism, and adrenoceptor function

There is evidence that sympathetic-nerve activity increases with age as reflected by increasing plasma catecholamine concentrations in old people and increased impulse traffic in recordings from cutaneous and muscle sympathetic nerves. Controversy surrounds the details, but it seems that the clearance of catecholamines from the circulation is altered and the neural secretion rate of endogenous catecholamines is increased in the elderly (Christensen 1982). Increased sympathetic-nerve activity with ageing is often interpreted as a compensatory phenomenon for failing physiological systems, e.g. increased sympathetic drive to a less efficient, ageing myocardium. However, the increased exposure of post-junctional adrenoceptors to catecholamines could produce changes in adrenoceptor function, for increased exposure to agonist may cause a decrease in adrenoceptor number and/or coupling of adrenoceptor stimulation–effector responses (Davies *et al.* 1984). Causes of increased circulating catecholamines may be decreased removal by uptake into sympathetic nerves or smooth/cardiac muscle or altered metabolism. Some studies have shown decreased synaptosomal uptake of noradrenalin with ageing; thus, the uptake mechanisms for terminating catecholamine action (Fig. 19.4) could be less efficient with age. Alternatively, there may be fewer sympathetic-nerve endings as a result of a subclinical autonomic degeneration in old people. Metabolism does not seem to be important in influencing adrenergic functional changes during ageing, although human brain and serum monoamine oxidase activity may increase with age. The other enzyme important in catecholamine inactivation, catecholamine-O-methyl transferase, does not change with age as reflected by activity in red cells from elderly subjects.

Other age-related factors operative at the whole-organism level

Baroreflex sensitivity decreases with age and impairs the control of cardiovascular adrenoceptor responses. Decreased exercise may also be important because less physically active subjects produce more catecholamines during sympathetic stimulation. Locally-released or circulating humoral factors like prostaglandins, kinins, angiotensin, ions, and nucleotides released from purinergic nerves can all influence effector responses to adrenoceptor stimulation or can alter nerve release of noradrenalin via effects on prejunctional adrenoceptors (Vanhoutte *et al.* 1981). Effects of ageing on prostanoids and kinins are unknown. Renin and aldosterone secretion decreases with age, but sensitivity to angiotensin is increased and angiotensin may have important effects upon adrenoceptor function. Endogenous opioid systems have important connections with central sympathetic pathways, and age-related changes in opioid systems (Rogers and Bloom 1985) could influence adrenoceptor function but such effects have not so far been demonstrated.

Adrenoceptor number and affinity and ageing

Adrenoceptors on cells and membrane fragments isolated from humans and experimental animals can be studied directly by using radiolabelled adrenoceptor antagonists which bind to the receptors (Nahorski and Barnett 1982). These techniques have shown no differences in β-adrenoceptor numbers and affinity for receptors on polymorphs and lymphocytes taken from ageing humans (Kelly and O'Malley 1984). Initially, it was thought that β-receptor numbers decreased with age (reviewed in Kelly and O'Malley 1984), but the study suggesting this may have given artefactual results due to the use of large amounts of radioactive ligand binding to a specific but non-adrenoceptor site (a common problem in radioligand binding studies) (Nahorski and Barnett 1982). No study of human tissues has shown any alteration in β-receptor affinity with ageing. In experimental animals some studies have shown no change in β-receptor numbers with age in myocardium, but some studies have described a decrease in receptor numbers without altered affinity in adipocytes and cerebellum from old rats. However, two studies showed a decreased affinity for agonists at myocardial and lung β_1- and β_2-adrenoceptors, respectively (Zitnik and Roth 1981; Scarpace and Abrass 1983). These findings are important because most studies in ageing tissues (as for most adrenoceptor binding work) have used antagonists but agonist–adrenoceptor interactions are more physiologically relevant and are different from interactions with antagonists.

In summary, there seems to be no decrease in β-receptor number or affinity with ageing so that changes in β-receptors *per se* do not explain the decreased β-receptor responsiveness with age. If the scant data with agonists are to be trusted, decreased β-adrenoceptor affinity may play some role in decreased adrenoceptor responsiveness with ageing.

The situation is more controversial for α-adrenoceptors, studies with human platelet α_2-adrenoceptors variously showing no changes or decreased number of α-receptors with ageing (Kelly and O'Malley 1984). The problems with the human studies are that none of them controlled for endogenous catecholamine concentrations in the subjects studied. Mature platelet α-adrenoceptors do not seem to change in number but they reflect instead the number present at the megakaryocyte stage in the bone marrow which has a very rich autonomic innervation; therefore, different degrees of exposure to endogenous catecholamines, independent of ageing, may alter platelet α-receptor numbers which do change in response to certain conditions (Davies *et al.* 1984). Experimental animal data also concern mainly central α_2-adrenoceptors and do not suggest any difference with ageing.

Adrenoceptor stimulation–effector response coupling in ageing

Measurement of biological responses to correlate with adrenoceptor radioligand binding studies has been made possible by the use of: (1) measurement of cAMP production via β-receptor stimulation by isoprenaline; (2) sodium fluoride stimulation of the guanine nucleotide protein which has a regulatory function in the adenyl cyclase complex (Fig. 19.5); (3) dibutyryl cAMP to bypass the adenyl cyclase mechanism and to stimulate protein kinase directly; (4) forskolin to stimulate directly the catalytic subunit of the adenyl cyclase complex (Fig. 19.5); (5) more recently the R_p diastereomer of adenosine cyclic-3′,5′-phosphorothioate, an antagonist of cAMP.

Evidence from techniques (4) and (5) is as yet lacking in studies of ageing and adrenoceptor function, but data from techniques (1) and (2) have suggested that β-adrenoceptor responses are impaired in ageing mammals because of impaired effector responses rather than because of any change in adrenoceptors (data reviewed in Kelly and O'Malley 1984; Lakatta 1985). In isolated lymphocytes from old people, cAMP production was decreased in response to isoprenaline or to sodium fluoride. However, there was no difference in cAMP production in digitonin-solubilized adenyl cyclase from lymphocytes of old or young people. This strongly suggests an impairment of adenyl cyclase response to β-receptor stimulation in the elderly and implies that this impairment is dependent upon the adenyl cyclase complex being intact and *in situ* in the cell membrane; a similar conclusion was suggested by work with rat myocardium (Lakatta 1985). The function of the catalytic unit of adenyl cyclase remains to be tested in ageing although this should be amenable to experiments with forskolin.

There is no information available about effects of ageing on the coupling of α-adrenoceptor stimulation and response generation; presumably this reflects the paucity of basic information about subcellular events in α-adrenoceptor mediated responses.

Cell membrane, cytoskeletal changes, and adrenoceptor function

Receptor function can be profoundly influenced by changes in the membranes in which they are embedded; for adrenoceptors, increased mobility within the cell membrane may account for adrenoceptor up- and down-regulation (Davies *et al.* 1984). Increased receptor mobility may be achieved by increasing membrane fluidity as a result of decreasing cholesterol content or increasing membrane phosphatidylcholine content. In membranes from older animals, fluidity is decreased in general (Naeim and Walford 1985): this could impair adrenoceptor mobility within the cell membrane, or impair conformational changes so decreasing agonist affinity, or impairing interactions with other proteins involved in generating the adrenoceptor-mediated response (Fig. 19.5). Impaired interaction with other proteins could explain why the age-related impairment of cAMP response to β-adrenoceptor stimulation can only be demonstrated in intact cell membranes and not in solubilized preparations of adenyl cyclase (see above).

Recently, more information has become available for the cytoskeleton, a ubiquitous network of microtubules found in all cells. The microtubules consist of various species of proteins (tubulins) and seem to be important in regulating distribution of membrane receptors and in information relay between subcellular compartments. Microtubules may be rapidly assembled and disassembled from tubulin monomers. Age-related changes in microtubular dynamics deserve attention in relation to adrenoceptor function for cytoskeletal changes may be involved in some receptor-mediated processes (Naeim and Walford 1985).

Adrenoceptor responses and inositol phosphates

One of the most exciting recent discoveries relevant to adrenergically mediated processes involving calcium fluxes was that of the role of receptor-mediated hydrolysis of inositol phosphates as a common mechanism for conveying information across cell membranes following stimulation of specific membrane receptors (Michel 1986). Unfortunately, nothing is known of the effects of ageing on the metabolism of inositol phosphates or of the interaction between adrenoceptors and inositol phosphates in ageing tissues; however, it is likely that information about these processes will be of fundamental importance to the physiology of ageing and design of new drugs for modulation of calcium fluxes in excitable tissues.

REFERENCES

Aarons, R. D., Nies, A. S., Gal, J., Hegstrand, L. R., and Molinoff, P. B. (1980). Elevation of beta-adrenergic receptor density in human lymphocytes after propanolol administration. *J. clin. Invest.* **65**, 949–57.

Abdel-Latif, A. A. (1986). Calcium mobilizing receptors, polyphosphoinositides and the generation of second messengers. *Pharmacol. Rev.* **38**, 228–72.

Bannister, R., Boylston, A. W., Davies, I. B., Mathias, C. J., Sever, P. S., and Sudera, D. (1981). Beta receptor numbers and thermodynamics in denervation supersensitivity. *J. Physiol., London* **319**, 369–77.

Bannister, R., Davies, I. B., Holly, E., Rosenthal, T., and Sever, P. S. (1979). Defective cardiovascular reflexes and supersensitivity to sympathomimetic drugs in autonomic failure. *Brain* **102**, 163–76.

Cannon, W. B. and Rosenblueth, A. (1949). *The supersensitivity of denervated structures. A law of denervation.* Macmillan, New York.

Christensen, N. J. (1982). Sympathetic nervous activity and age. *Eur. J. clin. Res.* **12**, 91–2.

Davies, I. B. (1982). Denervation supersensitivity in man. PhD thesis, University of London.

Davies, I. B., Hensby, C., and Sever, P. S. (1980). The pressor actions of noradrenalin and angiotensin II in chronic autonomic failure treated with indomethacin. *Br. J. clin. Pharmacol.* **10**, 223–9.

Davies, I. B., Mathias, C. J., Sudera, D., and Sever, P. S. (1982*a*). Agonist regulation of alpha-adrenergic receptor responses in man. *J. cardiovasc. Pharmacol.* **4**, 5139–44.

Davies, I. B., Sudera, D., Sagnella, G., Marchesi-Saviotti, E., Mathias, C., Bannister, R., and Sever, P. S. (1982*b*). Increased numbers of alpha-receptors in sympathetic denervation supersensitivity in man. *J. clin. Invest.* **69**, 779–84.

Davies, B., Sudera, D., and Sever, P. S. (1984). Regulation of adrenoceptors in man during different adrenergic states. In *Alpha and beta adrenoceptors and the cardiovascular system* (ed. W. Kobinger and R. P. Ahlquist), pp. 215–44. Excerpta Medica, Princeton, New Jersey.

Elliott, H. E., Summer, D. J., McLean, K., and Reid, J. L. (1982). Effect of age on the responsiveess of vascular adrenoceptors in man. *J. cardiovasc. Pharmacol.* **4**, 388–92.

Fleming, W. W., McPhillips, J. J., and Westfall, D. P. (1978). Post-junctional supersensitivity and subsensitivity of excitable tissues to drugs. *Ergebn. Physiol.* **68**, 55–119.

Frolkis, V. V. (1985). Neurohumoral regulation of cardiovascular function in ageing. In *Geriatric heart disease* (ed. E. Coodley), pp. 53–65. P.S.G. Publ. Co, Littleton, Massachusetts.

Halter, J. B. and Pfeifer, M. A. (1982). Ageing and autonomic nervous system function in man. In *Biological markers of ageing* (ed. M. E. Reff and E. L. Schneider), pp. 168–76. NIH Publ. No. 82-2221, Washington, DC.

Hui, K. K. P. and Connolly, M. E. (1981). Increased numbers of beta-receptors in orthostatic hypotension due to autonomic dysfunction. *New Engl. J. Med.* **304**, 1473–6.

Jennings, G., Bobik, A., and Esler, M. (1981). Beta-receptors in orthostatic hypotension. *New Engl. J. Med.* **305**, 1019.

Kelly, J. and O'Malley, K. (1984). Adrenoceptor function and ageing. *Clin. Sci.* **66**, 509–15.

Kilfeather, S. A., Gorgolewska, G., Davies, I. B., and Turner, P. (1985). Elevated lymphocyte beta-adrenoceptor density in multiple system atrophy with associated sympathetic degeneration. *Br. J. clin. Pharmacol.* **19**, 128–129P.

Korkushko, O. V. (1980). *Clinical cardiology and geriatrics.* Meditsina, Moscow.

Lakatta, E. G. (1985). Heart and Circulation. In *Handbook of the biology of ageing*, 2nd edn. (ed. C. E. Finch and E. L. Schneider), pp. 377–413. Van Nostrand Reinhold, New York.

Michel, R. (1986). Cellular signalling: A second message function for inositol tetrakisphosphate. *Nature* **324**, 613.

Naeim, F. and Walford, R. L. (1985). Ageing and cell membrane complexes: the lipid bilayer, integral proteins and cytoskeleton. In *Handbook of the biology of ageing*, 2nd edn. (ed. C. E. Finch and E. L. Schneider), pp. 272–89. Van Norstrand Reinhold, New York.

Nahorski, S. R. and Barnett, D. B. (1982). Biochemical assessment of adrenoceptor function and regulation: new directions and clinical relevance. *Clin. Sci.* **63**, 97–105.

Narayanan, N. and Derby, J. A. (1982). Alterations in the properties of β-adrenergic receptors of myocardial membranes in ageing: impairments in agonist–receptor interactions and guanine nucleotide regulation accompanying diminished catecholamine responsiveness of adenylate cyclase. *Mechanisms Ageing Develop.* **19**, 127–39.

Rodbell, M. (1980). The role of hormone receptors and GTP-regulatory proteins in membrane transduction. *Nature* **284**, 17–22.

Rogers, J. and Bloom, F. E. (1985). Neurotransmitter metabolism and function in the ageing central nervous system. In *Handbook of the biology of ageing*, 2nd edn. (ed. C. E. Finch and E. L. Schneider), pp. 645–91. Van Nostrand, New York.

Scarpace, P. J. and Abrass, I. B. (1983). Decreased β-adrenergic agonist affinity and adenylate cyclase activity in senescent rat lung. *J. Gerontol.* **38**, 143–7.

U'Pritchard, D. C., Bechtel, W. D., Roust, B. M., and Snyder, S. H. (1979). Multiple apparent alpha-noradrenergic binding sites in rat brain: effect of 6-hydroxy-dopamine. *Mol. Pharmacol.* **16**, 47–60.

U'Pritchard, D. C. and Snyder, S. H. (1978). Increase in alpha-receptor number in reserpine sensitivity in rats. *Eur. J. Pharamacol.* **51**, 145–55.

Vanhoutte, P. M., Verbeuren, T. J., and Webb, R. C. (1981). Local modulation of adrenergic neuroeffector interaction in the blood vessel wall. *Physiol. Rev.* **61**, 151–247.

Whitby, L. G., Axelrod, J., and Weil-Malherbe, H. (1961). The fate of H^3-norepinephrine in animals. *J. Pharmacol. Ther.* **26**, 181–6.

Zitnik, G. and Roth, R. S. (1981). Effects of thyroid hormones on cardiac hypertrophy and β-adrenergic receptors during ageing. *Mechanisms Ageing Develop.* **15**, 19–28.

Zwada, E. T. and Kirschenbaum, M. A. (1979). Evidence for excess renal prostaglandin synthesis in idiopathic orthostatic hypotension. *Clin. Res.* **27**, 65A.

20. Postcibal hypotension in autonomic disorders

Christopher Mathias, David da Costa, and Roger Bannister

INTRODUCTION

In normal subjects food ingestion results in a number of hormonal, neural, and regional haemodynamic changes. A variety of pancreatic and gastrointestinal peptides, some of which have effects on the cardiovascular system either directly or indirectly through modulation of autonomic nervous activity, are released. Although there is a marked increase in intestinal blood flow (Qamar and Read 1986), systemic blood pressure remains virtually unchanged in normal subjects, probably because activation of the sympathetic nervous system, together with release of vasoactive hormones, results in appropriate readjustment. Heart rate rises together with cardiac output and stroke volume; there is a fall in forearm blood flow with a rise in forearm vascular resistance and an elevation in both plasma noradrenalin and plasma renin activity levels (Mathias *et al.* 1986, 1987*b*) (Fig. 20.1). No changes are seen in the cutaneous circulation. There is an overall fall in peripheral vascular resistance. The nervous and endocrine systems therefore exert multiple adjustments which result in maintenance of blood pressure.

In patients with impaired autonomic function, ingestion of food can sometimes substantially lower blood pressure. This was observed in hypertensive patients given ganglionic blockers (Smirk 1953). Postcibal hypotension as a clinical problem was first reported by Seyer-Hansen (1977) in a 65-year-old man with autonomic failure and parkinsonism in whom severe dizziness and visual disturbances occurred during almost every meal and in whom hypotension could be provoked by oral glucose. A series of patients with autonomic dysfunction was studied by Robertson *et al.* (1981) who confirmed a profound fall in both systolic and diastolic blood pressure after food ingestion. In these studies the patients were seated and it was unclear to what degree the upright posture contributed to the hypotensive responses. In one of the first

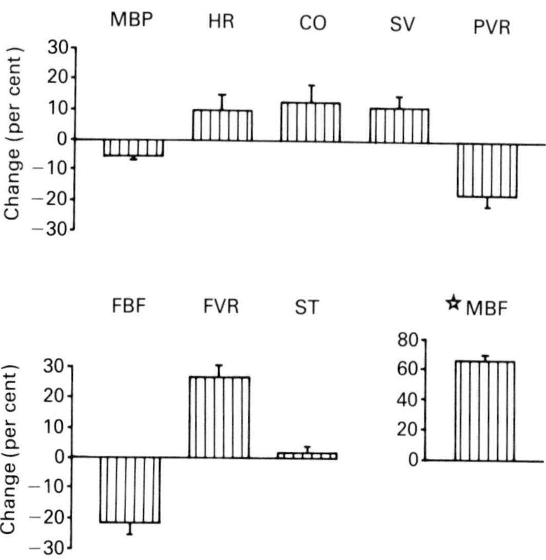

Fig. 20.1. Maximum percentage change in mean blood pressure (MBP), heart rate (HR), cardiac output (CO), stroke volume (SV), calculated peripheral vascular resistance (PVR), forearm muscle blood flow (FBF), calculated forearm vascular resistance (FVR), and skin temperature to the index finger (ST) in six normal subjects in the first hour after food ingestion. Maximum percentage change in mesenteric blood flow (MBF) from the data of Qamar and Read (1986) is included beneath the star. Vertical bars indicate ± SEM.

patients studied, the blood pressure rapidly fell to 80/50 mm Hg after food ingestion and remained low even in the supine position for up to three hours. From our own observations and other studies it was clear that postcibal hypotension could be a major clinical problem in some of our patients with autonomic failure. It was evident that in order to embark on rational approaches of intervention it was necessary to determine the pathophysiological basis for the response, with an emphasis on the haemodynamic and biochemical basis of postprandial hypotension and the determination of which components of the meal were responsible. In this chapter we therefore describe observations on the mechanisms responsible for postcibal hypotension in autonomic failure. Brief descriptions are also provided of responses in other groups of patients with autonomic dysfunction.

HAEMODYNAMIC CHANGES

Food ingestion in patients with autonomic failure, even in the supine position, causes a substantial fall in blood pressure. This may occur within 10 to 15 minutes of ingestion, and reaches its nadir within about 60 minutes (Fig. 20.2) (Bannister *et al.* 1984; Mathias *et al.* 1986). The

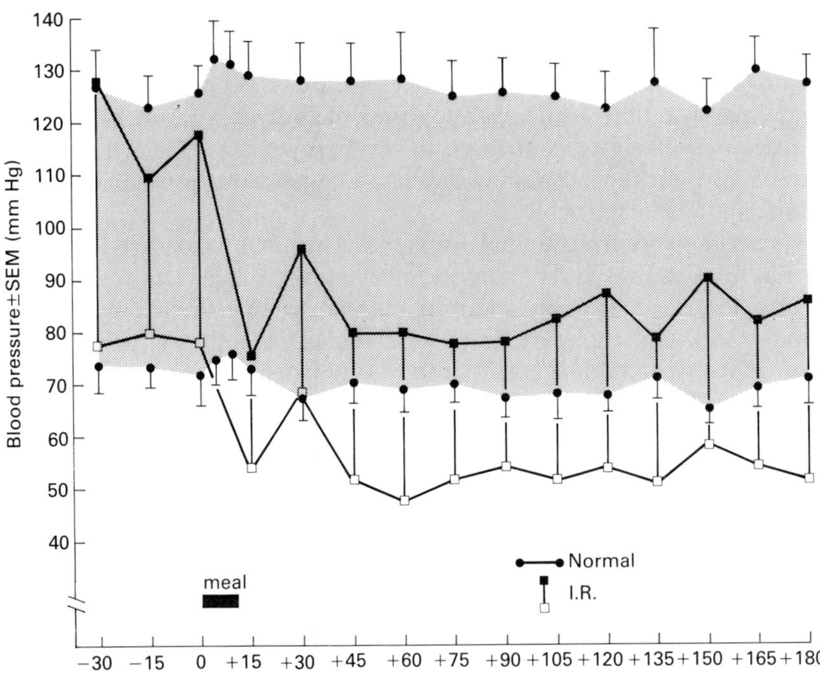

Fig. 20.2. Supine systolic and diastolic blood pressure before and after a standard meal in a group of normal subjects (stippled area with ± SEM) and in a patient with pure autonomic failure (I.R., continuous lines). Blood pressure does not change in the normal subjects. In the patient there is a rapid fall in blood pressure to levels as low as 80/50 mm Hg which remain low even in the supine position over the 3-hour observation period.

fall in blood pressure is not accompanied by changes in blood flow in the forearm and skin, indicating that appropriate haemodynamic adjustments do not occur despite the profound fall in blood pressure. Postural change after food ingestion can therefore markedly enhance symptoms of impaired cerebral perfusion.

BIOCHEMICAL AND HORMONAL CHANGES

In patients with autonomic failure (AF), the fall in blood pressure after food is not accompanied by changes in levels of either plasma noradrenalin or adrenalin, confirming a lack of compensatory sympathetic nervous or sympathoadrenal activity (da Costa *et al.* 1985). In normal subjects there is a small but definite rise in plasma noradrenalin levels. Plasma renin activity levels rise to a similar degree in both groups. In normal subjects the stimuli to release renin include β-receptor stimulation, which would be expected to be diminished or absent in AF patients. It may therefore be argued that the renin rise in the AF patients is impaired, considering the fall in blood pressure. There are no changes in plasma electrolytes or osmolality in either group, suggesting that fluid loss, especially into the gut as a result of osmotic changes, is unlikely to contribute to the hypotension. The haematocrit also remains unchanged, suggesting that a contraction in plasma volume is unlikely to be responsible.

A variety of gastrointestinal hormones have been measured both in normal subjects and in AF patients following fluid ingestion. Changes in plasma levels of gastrin, motilin, vasoactive intestinal polypeptide, somatostatin, and cholecystokinin were similar in both groups (Mathias *et al.* 1986). Enteroglucagon, pancreatic polypeptide, and neurotensin levels rose (Fig. 20.3) to a greater extent in the AF patients. Two of these, enteroglucagon and pancreatic polypeptide, do not have vasodilatatory or negative cardiac inotropic effects and are unlikely to have contributed to the hypotension. Neurotensin, however, has vasodilatatory effects, which may have been increased in AF patients who have exaggerated responses to vasodepressor agents.

The role of gut peptides in the hypotensive responses, may, therefore, be of importance. Although circulating levels of potent vasodilator peptides, such as vasoactive intestinal polypeptide, did not change, this does not exclude significant local or regional effects caused by this peptide. These include splanchnic vasodilatation, which may be an important factor in the causation of hypotension.

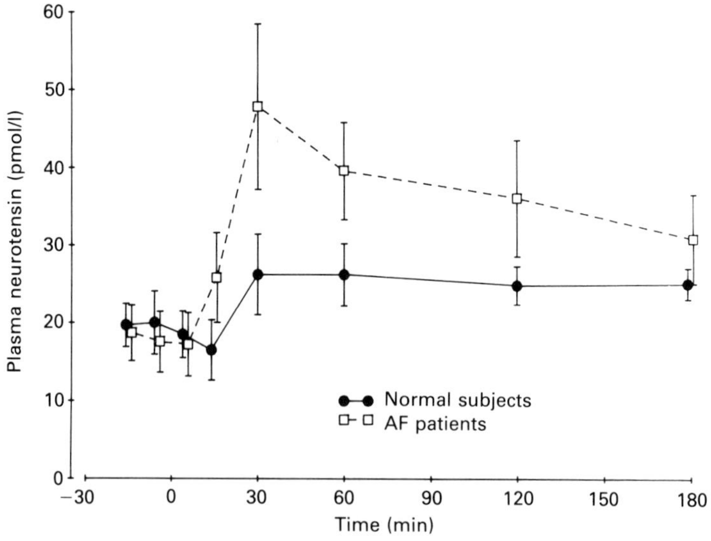

Fig. 20.3. Plasma levels of neurotensin in normal subjects (continuous line) and AF patients (broken line) before and after a standard meal ingested at 0. There is a significantly greater response in the AF patients.

Other peptides released during food ingestion such as insulin, may also play an important role. Evidence from both our laboratory and others indicate that insulin can lower blood pressure substantially in AF patients, even in the absence of changes in blood glucose (Fig. 20.4) (Brown *et al.* 1986; Bannister *et al.* 1987*b*; Mathias *et al.* 1987*a*). Bolus intravenous insulin (0.15 units/kg) causes hypotension without dilatation in forearm muscle or cutaneous vascular beds. Insulin administration in studies using an euglycaemic clamp confirmed that this change occurs independently of changes in blood glucose. In these studies neither cardiac output nor muscle and cutaneous blood flow changed, favouring splanchnic vasodilatation as the cause of the hypotension. Levels of insulin in AF patients are higher in the basal state and after a meal, but

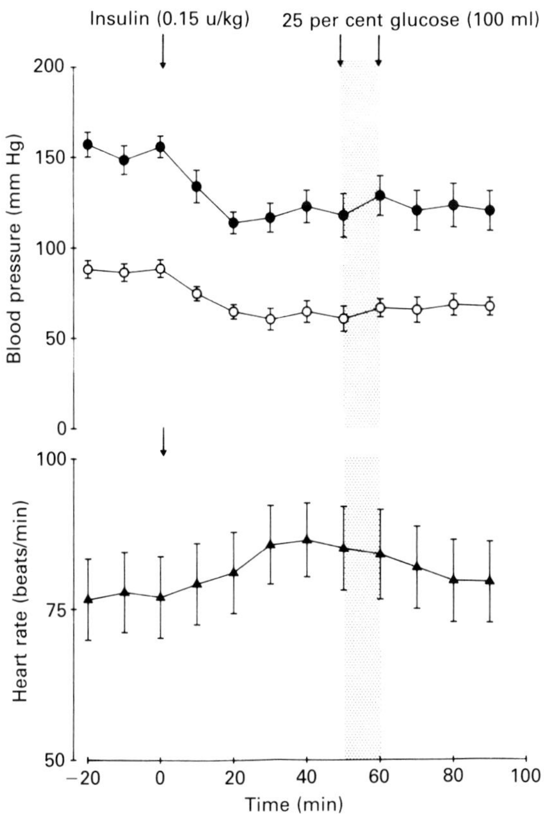

Fig. 20.4. Changes in systolic (filled circles) and diastolic (open circles) blood pressure and in heart rate in five patients with autonomic failure before and after an intravenous bolus of insulin. There is fall in both systolic and diastolic blood pressure within 10 minutes. Hypoglycaemia occurred at around 30 minutes and did not result in a further fall in blood pressure. Reversal of hypoglycaemia with 25 per cent of glucose infused over 10 min did not change blood pressure. (Taken with permission from Mathias *et al.* (1987*b*).)

this probably reflects their greater age rather than a major effect on autonomic control of insulin secretion (Mathias *et al.* 1986). Insulin probably has a role in the hypotension induced by food as carbohydrate is a potent inducer of hypotension; studies in diabetics with autonomic impairment given insulin (Page and Watkins 1976) would favour this.

FOOD COMPONENTS

Studies have been completed in our laboratory comparing food ingestion against isocaloric, isovolumic, and, wherever possible, isotonic solution of different food components (Fig. 20.5). The fall in blood pressure after glucose mimics the changes occurring after food (da Costa *et al.* 1985). Lipid has slower, smaller, and less sustained hypotensive effects, with minimal change caused by protein alone (Bannister *et al.* 1987*a*). The hypotensive effect of glucose is not the result of its osmolality as an isocaloric, isosmotic, and isovolumic solution of xylose caused only minimal changes in blood pressure (Fig. 20.6).

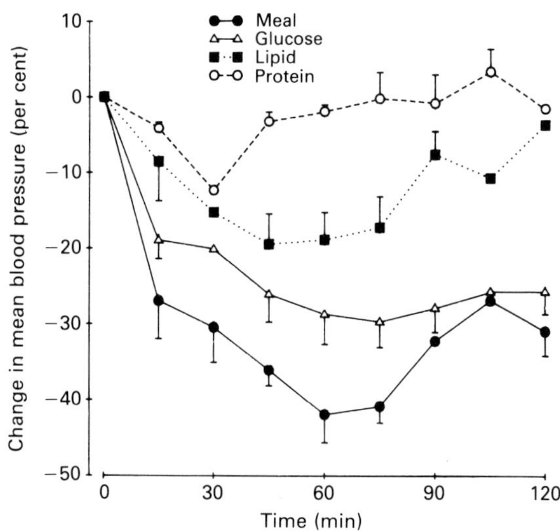

Fig. 20.5. Percentage change in mean blood pressure in six patients with autonomic failure given either a standard meal or an isocaloric and isovolumic solution of carbohydrate (glucose, 1 g/kg body weight), lipid (prosperol 0.95 ml/kg) or protein (maxipro 1 g/kg) alone. Vertical bars indicate ± SEM. (Taken with permission from Mathias *et al.* (1987*a*).)

GASTROINTESTINAL MOTILITY

Patients with autonomic failure often have impairment of motility of the large bowel and diarrhoea may occasionally occur. There is, however,

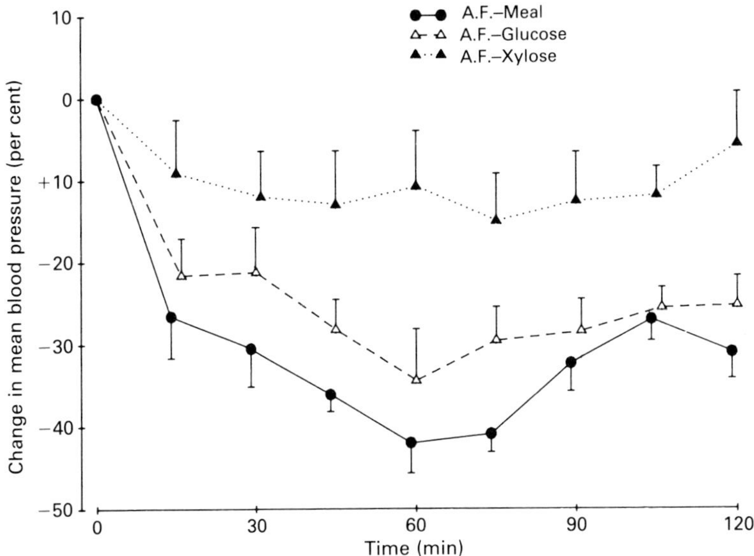

Fig. 20.6. Percentage change in mean blood pressure in patients with autonomic failure after a standard breakfast, oral glucose, or oral xylose. The bars indicate ±SEM. Either standard breakfast or oral glucose cause substantial and prolonged fall in blood pressure. Smaller changes were caused by xylose. In normal subjects (not indicated) neither food nor glucose changed blood pressure. (Taken with permission from da Costa *et al.* (1985).)

little information on motility of the stomach and small bowel and the possibility of 'dumping' was considered. In the classical 'dumping syndrome', which often occurs after gastric drainage procedures, there is rapid entry of a hyperosmotic solution into the jejunum, thus causing fluid absorption within the gut, a reduction in effective plasma volume, and a rise in the haematocrit (Roberts *et al.* 1954; Le Quesne *et al.* 1960). Weakness, sweating, palpitations, and occasionally a modest fall in blood pressure may occur, suggesting an increase in autonomic nervous activity. Studies have been performed using a technetium-labelled bran meal in the sitting position with gamma scintillation scanning to determine the rate of gastric emptying (Mathias *et al.* 1986). In the majority of AF patients increased gastric emptying occurred along with postprandial hypotension (Fig. 20.7). In some patients, however, the rate of emptying was normal and, furthermore, two patients (with amyloidosis) in whom gastric emptying was delayed had marked postprandial hypotension. The precise relationship between the increase in gastric emptying and postprandial hypotension therefore remains unclear.

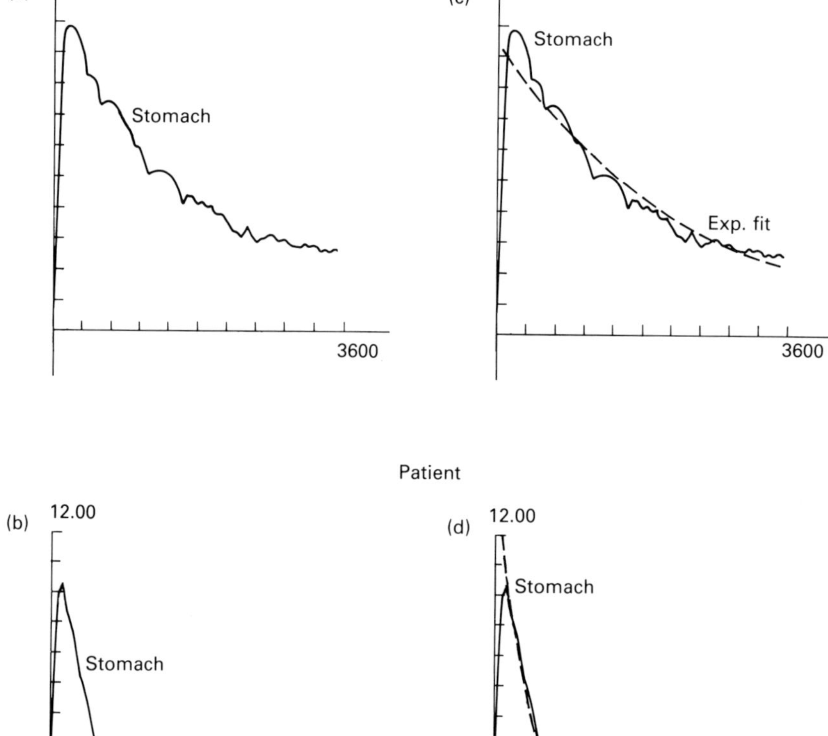

Fig. 20.7. Gastric emptying curves in (a) a normal subject and (b) in a patient with autonomic failure. Integrated counts are indicated on the vertical axis and time in seconds on the horizontal axis. A computer exponential (Exp) fit is indicated. In the autonomic failure patient there is rapid emptying initially (Exp. fit I) with a later slower phase (Exp. fit II).

MANAGEMENT

With a better understanding of the pathophysiological mechanisms responsible there are increasing therapeutic approaches which can be assessed in preventing postcibal hypotension. Advice regarding the quality, quantity, and frequency of meals may help. Carbohydrate can enhance vulnerability to postural hypotension and small meals should be taken at regular intervals. The vasodilatatory effects of alcohol are likely to enhance hypotension.

A variety of drugs have been used in postcibal hypotension. In the initial studies of Robertson *et al.* (1981) propranolol, diphenhydramine, cimetidine, and indomethacin were evaluated in single doses. Propranolol (40 mg orally) had no beneficial effect and may have worsened postcibal hypotension. The h1 antihistaminic (diphenhydramine) and the h2 blocker (cimetidine) had no effect, making it unlikely that histamine played a role in the responses. The hypotensive response to food was attenuated by indomethacin (50 mg orally) suggesting that prostaglandins or arachnidonic acid metabolites, which were vasodilatatory, might be responsible. No long-term studies with indomethacin have been reported in relation to food-induced hypotension.

Alternative approaches have more recently emerged. Caffeine normally raises blood pressure by stimulating sympathetic nervous activity or activating the renin–angiotensin system. It is effective in preventing postprandial hypotension in autonomic failure (Onrot *et al.* 1985) (Fig. 20.8). This occurs independently of sympathetic nervous activation or renin–angiotensin stimulation and may be the result of its ability to block vasodilatatory adenosine receptors. It continues to be effective when administered in a dose of 250 mg daily over a 7-day period and it has been suggested that two cups of coffee (which contain the equivalent of 250 mg of caffeine) may be effective in long-term management.

A further approach, which was initially assessed in patients with postprandial hypotension complicating autonomic failure due to alcoholism and diabetes was the use of the somatostatin analogue, SMS 201-995 (Hoeldtke *et al.* 1986) (Fig. 20.9). This drug appears to block the release of a variety of peptides, presumably including those which may cause dilatation and contribute to hypotension during food ingestion. Our own studies confirm the beneficial effects of SMS 201-995 in patients with chronic autonomic failure.

EFFECTS OF FOOD IN OTHER GROUPS OF PATIENTS WITH AUTONOMIC DYSFUNCTION

Patients on ganglionic blockers or with splanchnic denervation

The hypotensive effect of food was first recorded in hypertensive patients who had been given ganglionic blockers (Smirk 1953). Observations on the fall in blood pressure after insulin were recorded in patients who had undergone splanchnic denervation (T7–L3 inclusive), for the

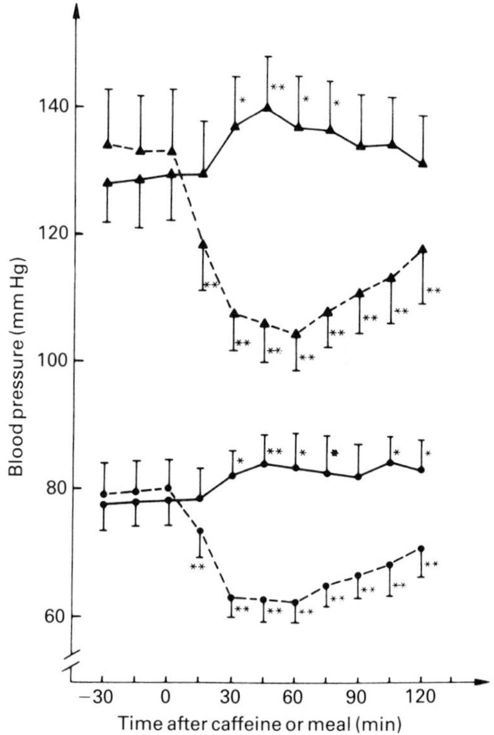

Fig. 20.8. Mean systolic (triangles) and diastolic (circles) blood pressure. Five patients with autonomic failure given either placebo (continuous lines) or 250 mg caffeine (interrupted lines) 30 minutes before a meal. Patients had been on 250 mg per day of caffeine for 7 days. Postprandial blood pressures remained significantly higher after caffeine than after placebo. (Taken with permission from Onrot *et al.* (1985).)

relief of severe hypertension (French and Kilpatrick 1955). Similar changes occurred in normal subjects given ganglionic blockers (di Salvo *et al.* 1956). It was likely that in both groups of patients splanchnic vasodilatation, unaccompanied by appropriate compensatatory sympathetic nervous activity, was responsible for the fall in blood pressure.

Diabetes mellitus

Insulin lowers blood pressure in diabetics with baroreceptor abnormalities and can provoke postural hypotension (Miles and Hayter 1968; Page and Watkins 1976). In these studies the effect of food was not assessed, unlike the study of Hoeldtke *et al.* (1986). In their study it was difficult to separate the effects of insulin from that induced by food itself. The latter is likely to have hypotensive effects in addition to those induced by insulin as in the four patients with diabetes studied by Hoeldtke *et al.*

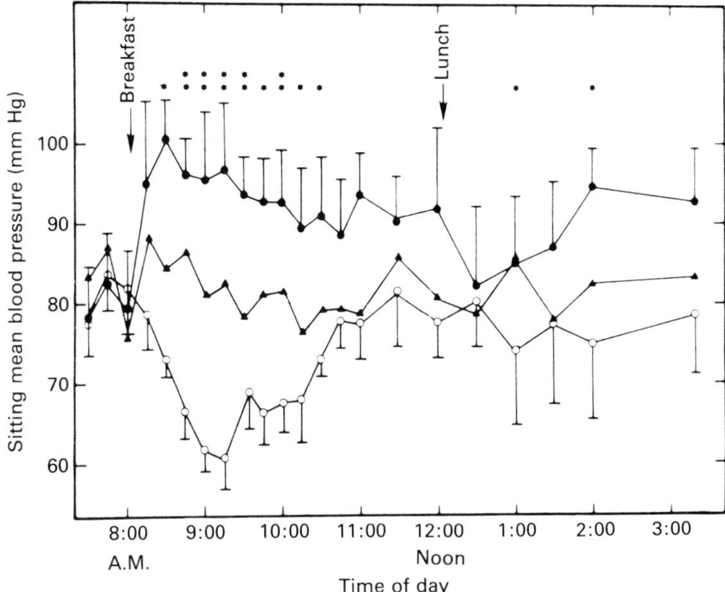

Fig. 20.9. Sitting mean blood pressure after breakfast and lunch in six patients with autonomic failure of different aetiology with given placebo (open circles) or two different doses of the somatostatin analogue SMS-201-995 (filled circles 0.4 μg/kg and filled triangles 0.2 μg/kg). For comparisons of drug and placebo single asterisks signify $p<0.05$ and double asterisks $p<0.001$. SEM for low doses of drug are omitted for clarity. (Taken with permission from Hoeldtke *et al.* (1986).)

(1986) the somatostatin analogue SMS 201-995 prevented the fall in blood pressure and this is unlikely to have been the result of antagonism of the vascular effects of exogenously administered insulin.

The elderly

Autonomic dysfunction of varying degree can occur in elderly patients. Studies of these patients indicate that a large number develop postprandial hypotension (Lipschitz *et al.* 1983) (Fig. 20.10). These studies were in patients over the age of 80 years and a fall in systolic blood pressure mainly was reported after food in patients maintained in the sitting position. This fall in pressure, together with the often increased sensitivity in such patients to drugs which impair autonomic nervous function, may make elderly patients particularly susceptible to hypotension and attendant cerebral ischaemia.

Patients with tabes dorsalis and afferent lesions

We have studied one patient with tabes dorsalis who had, on exhaustive

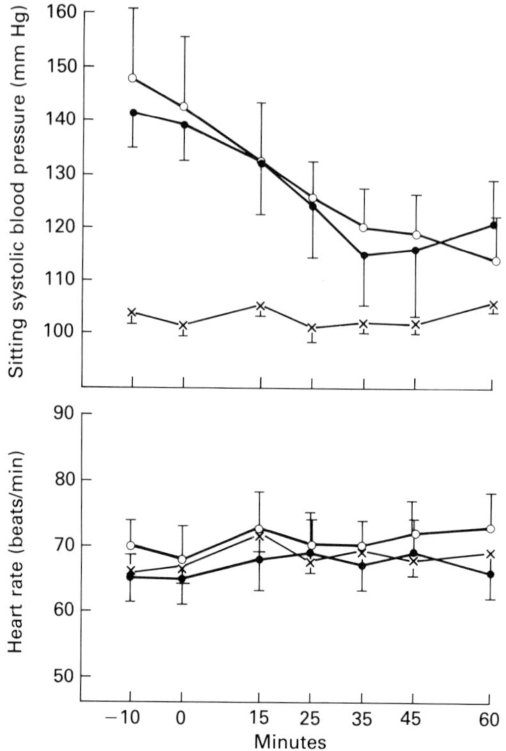

Fig. 20.10. Sitting systolic BP and heart rate before and after food ingestion. The upper panel shows mean systolic blood pressure (±SEM) at intervals before and after the start of the meal (zero time) in elderly subjects with syncope (filled circles) and 10 elderly subjects without syncope (open circles). Data from 11 young normal subjects (X) is included. The lower panel shows a mean heart rate taken at the same time. (Taken with permission from Lipschitz *et al.* (1983).)

autonomic testing, evidence of an afferent baroreceptor lesion, with no impairment of central and peripheral sympathetic pathways. The patient had pronounced hypotension after food, suggesting that afferent lesions, some of which may have involved afferents from the gut, may block the normal corrective reflexes and so contribute to the fall in blood pressure after food.

Tetraplegics

Patients with complete cervical spinal-cord transection cannot activate sympathetic activity in response to a fall in blood pressure (see Mathias and Frankel 1986). They share with AF patients in enhanced depressor response to agents with vasodilatatory properties. In these patients, using a similar protocol, ingestion of either food or glucose did not change either systolic or diastolic blood pressure in the supine position. The reason for this lack of change is unclear.

Acknowledgement

We thank Professor S. R. Bloom of the Hammersmith Hospital, London and the Department of Clinical Physics of St. Mary's Hospital, London, for his help with these studies.

REFERENCES

Bannister, R., Christensen, N. J., da Costa, D. F., Mathias, C. J., Wright, H., and Ukachii-lois, J. (1984). Mechanisms of post-prandial hypotension in autonomic failure. *J. Physiol., London* **349**, 67P.

Bannister, R., da Costa, D. F., Forster, S., Fosbraey, P., and Mathias, C. J. (1987*a*). Cardiovascular effects of lipid and protein meals in autonomic failure. *J. Physiol., London* **377**, 62P.

Bannister, R., da Costa, D. F., Kooner, J. S., MacDonald, I. A., and Mathias, C. J. (1987*b*). Insulin-induced hypotension in autonomic failure in euglycaemia in man. *J. Physiol., London* **382**, 36P.

Brown, R. T., Polinsky, R. J., Lee, G. K., and Deeter, J. A. (1986). Insulin-induced hypotension and neurogenic orthostatic hypotension. *Neurology* **36**, 1402–6.

da Costa, D. F., McIntosh, C., Bannister, R., Christensen, N. J., and Mathias, C. J. (1985). Unmasking of the cardiovascular effects of carbohydrate in subjects with sympathetic denervation. *J. Hypertens.* **3** (Suppl. 3), S447–S448.

di Salvo, R. J., Bloom, W. L., Brust, A. A., Ferguson, R. W., and Ferris, E. B. (1956). A comparison of the metabolic and circulatory effects of epinephrine, norepinephrine and insulin hypoglycaemia with observations on the influence of autonomic blocking agents. *J. clin. Invest.* **35**, 568–77.

French, E. B. and Kilpatrick, R. (1955). The role of adrenalin in hypoglycemic reactions in man. *Clin. Sci.* **14**, 639–51.

Hoeldtke, R. D., O-Dorisio, T. M. and Boden, G. (1986). Treatment of autonomic neuropathy with a somatostatin analogue SMS-201-995. *Lancet* **ii**, 602–5.

Le Quesne, L. P., Hopsley, M., and Hand, B. A. (1960). The dumping syndrome. *Br. med. J.* **1**, 141–51.

Lipschitz, L. A., Nyquist, R. H., Wei, J. Y., and Rowe, J. W., (1983). Postprandial reduction in blood pressure in the elderly. *New Engl. J. Med.* **309**, 81–3.

Mathias, C. J., da Costa, D. F., Fosbraey, P., Bannister, R., and Christensen, N. J. (1986). Post-cibal hypotension in autonomic failure. In *The sympatho-adrenal system*, Alfred Benzon Symposium, No. 23 (eds. N. J. Christensen, O. Henriksen, and N. A. Lassen), pp. 402–13. Munksgaard, Copenhagen,

Mathias, C. J., da Costa, D. F., Fosbraey, P., Christensen, N. J., and Bannister, R. (1987*a*). Hypotensive and sedative effects of insulin in autonomic failure. *Br. med. J.* **295**, 161–3.

Mathias, C. J., da Costa, D. F., Fosbraey, P., McIntosh, C. and Bannister, R. (1987*b*). Factors contributing to food induced hypotension in patients with autonomic dysfunction. In *Proceedings of the 4th International Symposium on Vasodilatation* (ed. P. M. Van Houtte). Raven Press, New York. (In press).

Mathias, C. J. and Frankel, H. L. (1986). The neurological and hormonal control of blood vessels and heart in spinal man. *J. auton. nerv. Syst.* (Suppl.), 457–64.

Miles, D. W. and Hayter, C. J. (1968). The effects of intravenous insulin on the circulatory responses to tilting in normal and diabetic subjects with special reference to baroreceptor reflex block and atypical hypoglycemic reactions. *Clin. Sci.* **34**, 419–30.

Onrot, J., Goldberg, M. R., Biaggioni, I., Hollister, A. S., Kincaid, D., and Robertson, D. (1985). Haemodynamic and humoral effects of caffeine in autonomic failure. Therapeutic implications for post-prandial hypotension. *N. Engl. J. Med.* **313**, 549–54.

Page, M. N. and Watkins, P. J. (1976). Provocation of postural hypotension by insulin in diabetic autonomic neuropathy. *Diabetes* **25**, 90–5.

Qamar, M. I. and Read, A. E. (1986). The effect of feeding and sham feeding on the superior mesenteric blood flow in man. *J. Physiol. London.* **377**, 59P.

Roberts, R. E., Randall, H. T., and Farr, H. W. (1954). Cardiovascular and blood volume alterations resulting from intra-jejunal administration of hypotonic solutions to gastrectomised patients. The relationship of these changes to the dumping syndrome. *Ann. Surg.* **140**, 631–40.

Robertson, D., Wade, D., and Robertson, R. M. (1981). Post-prandial alterations in cardiovascular haemodynamics in autonomic dysfunctional states. *Am. J. Cardiol.* **48**, 1048–52.

Seyer-Hansen, K. (1977). Post-prandial hypotension. *Br. med. J.* **2**, 1262.

Smirk, F. M. (1953). Action of a new methonium compound (M&B 2050A) in arterial hypertension. *Lancet* **i**, 457.

21. Hypothalamic function in autonomic failure

Stafford L. Lightman and T. D. M. Williams

INTRODUCTION

Post-mortem studies of brain tissue from patients with multiple system atrophy (MSA) reveal marked reductions in hypothalamic noradrenalin, dopamine, and tyrosine hydroxylase (Spokes *et al.* 1979). Although the cell bodies of the tuberoinfundibular dopamine system are located within the mediobasal hypothalamus, there are no noradrenalin or adrenalin cell bodies in spite of the high concentration of these amines. The rich network of noradrenalin and adrenalin terminals in the hypothalamus is derived from cell bodies in the pons and medulla, and it is therefore not surprising that the decreased hypothalamic noradrenalin and adrenalin in MSA is also associated with a decrease in brainstem catecholamines, notably in the locus ceruleus (Spokes *et al.* 1979). The catecholamine brainstem nuclei play an important role in the communication of visceral information from the ninth and tenth nerves to the hypothalamus. These nerves synapse in the nucleus of the tractus solitarius (NTS) in the dorsomedial medulla (Fig. 21.1) whence catecholamine pathways radiate to the hypothalamus and forebrain structures. It would therefore be expected that derangements of these ascending catecholamine pathways and of the local dopaminergic tubero-infundibular system would result in changes in neuroendocrine control. Before we consider our clinical studies in patients with autonomic failure, it is important to summarize our current understanding of the role of catecholamines in hypothalamic function (Fig. 21.2 (a), (b)).

DOPAMINE

The dopaminergic neurons in the hypothalamic arcuate nucleus have long been of major interest to neuroendocrinologists. They are the source of dopamine in the external layer of the median eminence (Everitt and Hökfelt 1986) and thus of dopamine in the hypothalamo–

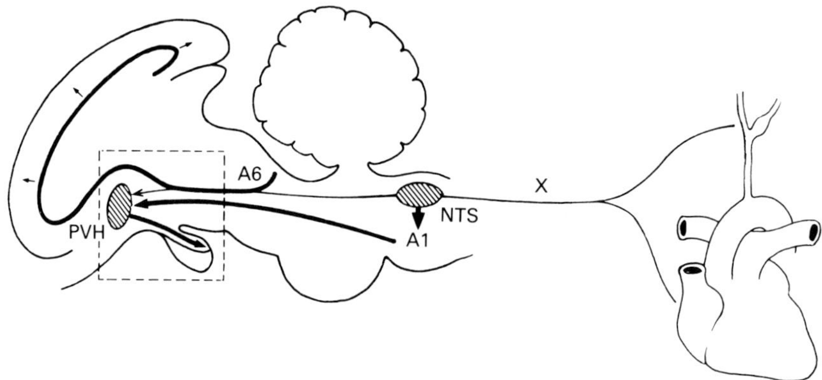

Fig. 21.1. Schematic representation of the catecholamine projections from the brainstem to the paraventricular nucleus of the hypothalamus (PVH) and of neurosecretory fibres from the hypothalamus to the pituitary neural lobe. The dorsal noradrenergic bundle runs between A6 (the locus ceruleus) and the hypothalamus, the ventral noradrenergic bundle between A1 and the hypothalamus. NTS, nucleus of the tractus solitarius.

hypophyseal portal blood. This dopamine is recognized to be the major prolactin inhibitory factor, and dopamine antagonists cause hyperprolactinaemia in man and experimental animals while dopaminergic agonists suppress prolactin release. These are direct actions on the pituitary lactotroph cells.

In the hypothalamus there is immunocytochemical evidence for an association between dopamine and luteinizing hormone releasing hormone (LHRH) neurons, and the demonstration that many of the arcuate nucleus dopaminergic neurons accumulate the sex steroid oestradiol (Heritage *et al.* 1975) suggests that these cells may have an important role in the feedback regulation of LHRH secretion. *In vivo* studies indeed suggest that dopamine inhibits LHRH secretion, but, unfortunately, *in vitro* studies contradict this. In man dopamine usually reduces luteinizing hormone (LH) secretion and in females this effect depends upon the oestrogen status or time of the menstrual cycle.

Dopamine inhibits thyroid stimulating hormone (TSH) secretion *in vitro* with the same specificity and sensitivity as it does prolactin (Foord *et al.* 1968) and dopamine antagonists increase TSH secretion by an action on pituitary thyrotrophs. In man inhibitory effects of dopamine on TSH secretion can be demonstrated, but the effect is small and the physiological significance uncertain.

Dopamine has both stimulatory and inhibitory effects on growth hormone secretion, with stimulation of growth hormone release *in vivo* and an inhibitory effect both at the hypothalamus and directly at the level of the pituitary (Quabbe 1986). Dopamine has recently been

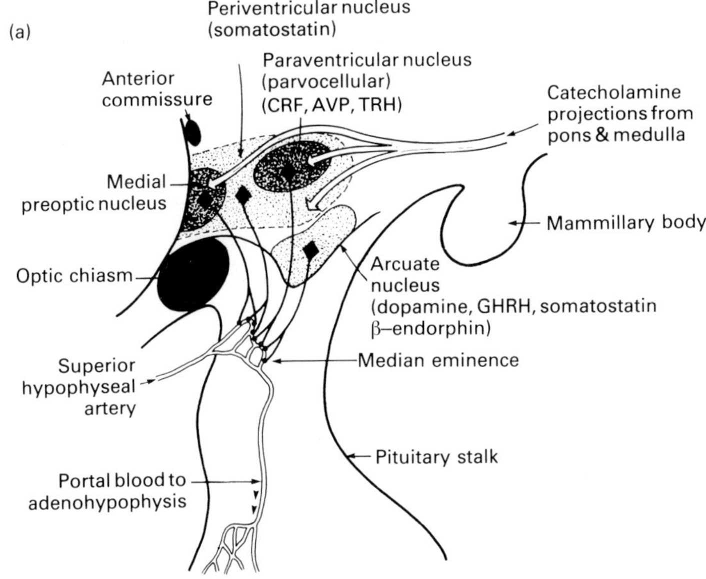

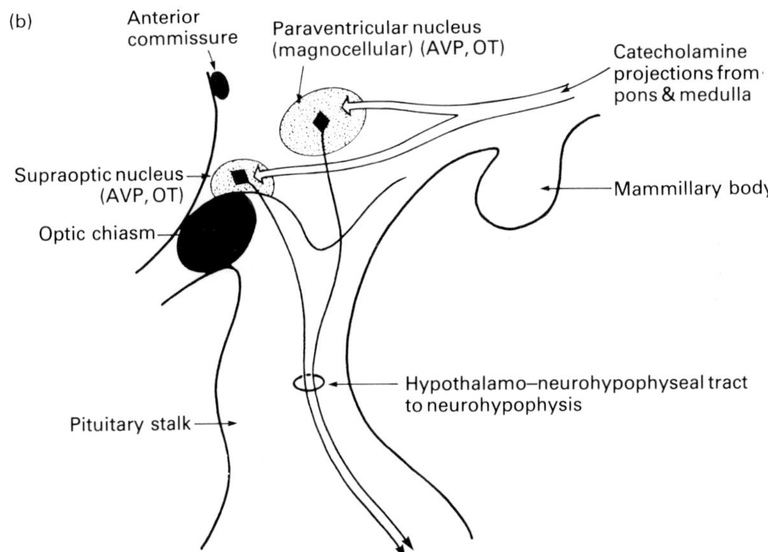

Fig. 21.2. (a) Schematic representation of the hypothalamic nuclei which project to the external layer of the median eminence where hypophysiotrophic factors are secreted into the portal circulation. CRF, corticotrophin releasing factor; AVP, arginine vasopressin; TRH, thyrotrophin releasing hormone; GHRH, growth hormone releasing hormone. (b) Schematic representation of the hypothalamic nuclei which send axons to the neurohypophysis where vasopressin and oxytocin are neurosecreted directly into the circulation. AVP, arginine vasopressin; OT, oxytocin.

demonstrated to coexist with growth hormone releasing hormone (GHRH) in arcuate neurons and this suggests that a significant interaction may occur between these agents. In man administration of dopamine results in increased basal growth hormone but a reduced growth hormone response to hypoglycaemia, while in acromegaly dopamine usually reduces growth hormone secretion.

Dopamine does not seem to be an important component of the control of basal or stress-induced adrenocorticotrophic hormone (ACTH) secretion in the rat. In man dopamine can result in ACTH release but it is unclear whether this is a direct effect of the amine or an indirect effect via other neurotransmitters in the hypothalamus.

Dopamine also plays a role in the control of neurohypophyseal secretion. Dopamine inhibits electrical activity in vasopressinergic neurons and has direct effects on the neural lobe, inhibiting the release of vasopressin (see Carter and Lightman 1985). In man there is also evidence that L-dopa diminishes arginine vasopressin (AVP) secretion by a direct effect at the level of the neural lobe.

NORADRENALIN AND ADRENALIN

There is little evidence that adrenalin or noradrenalin are involved in the physiological control of prolactin secretion either in man or experimental animals. There is, however, a close relationship between noradrenalin turnover and LHRH secretion in the rat suggesting that medullary catecholamine nuclei modulate hypothalamic LHRH secretion. Since these medullary nuclei accumulate oestradiol, the phenomenon of oestrogen positive feedback may even occur at this level. Hypothalamic adrenalin also correlates with plasma LH and this amine may also influence pre-ovulatory and oestrogen-induced LH release. Studies are difficult in man since catecholamines do not cross the blood–brain barrier, but neither α-adrenoceptor agonists or antagonists affect pulsatile LH secretion.

The role of noradrenalin and adrenalin in TSH secretion is unclear (Foord *et al.* 1986). Noradrenalin has been reported to release thyrotrophin releasing hormone (TRH) from hypothalamic slices and depletion of hypothalamic amines by 6-hydroxydopamine abolishes the TSH response to cold exposure. Rat pituitary cells release TSH in response to α_1-adrenoceptor stimulation, and adrenalin and TRH act additively to release TSH. Since hypophyseal blood adrenalin levels are much higher than those in peripheral blood, this may represent an additional mechanism for the control of TSH. In man the α_1-antagonists have been shown to decrease basal TSH and prevent the nocturnal rise found in mildly hypothyroid subjects.

There is considerable evidence for a major role of noradrenalin in the control of growth hormone secretion (Quabbe 1986). Noradrenalin stimulates the release of growth hormone through an α-adrenergic mechanism and inhibits growth hormone via β-receptors. These effects are probably indirect via actions on somatostatin neurons in the periventricular hypothalamus—an area innervated by the locus ceruleus. In man the α_2-agonist clonidine and the β-blocker propranolol stimulate growth hormone secretion while the α_1-antagonist phentolamine reduces and clonidine increases the growth hormone responses to hypoglycaemia.

Noradrenalin inhibits hypothalamic corticotrophin releasing factor (CRF) release both *in vivo* and *in vitro*. This action has been demonstrated in isolated hypothalami and after i.c.v. injections. Clonidine crosses the blood–brain barrier and inhibits CRF release when administered either i.v. or i.c.v. suggesting an action on postsynaptic α-receptors. Stress, however, increases brain noradrenalin turnover so the picture is far from clear. In man α-agonists and β-blockers have little effect on ACTH secretion, but β-blockers enhance the cortisol response to hypoglycaemia or to amphetamines. This suggests that α-receptors may be stimulatory and β-receptors inhibitory to ACTH secretion at the hypothalamic level.

The role of brainstem catecholamine pathways has been much more clearly defined in the control of neurohypophyseal activity. The cell bodies which secrete vasopressin and oxytocin are easy to locate and can be recorded electrophysiologically. Although there has been some dispute about the effects of amines on these cells it is now generally agreed that noradrenalin facilitates the firing of vasopressinergic cells and the release of vasopressin (Day *et al.* 1984). The adrenergic and noradrenergic pathways which relay the hypothalamic response to changes in NTS activity have now been mapped and it is clear that two major tracts are involved: the ventral noradrenergic bundle in the ventral brainstem and the dorsal noradrenergic bundle in the dorsal midbrain. Selective lesions with the neurotoxin 6-hydroxydopamine have demonstrated that the dorsal noradrenergic bundle (which includes fibres from the locus ceruleus) plays an important role in the vasopressin response to cardiovascular stimuli (Lightman *et al.* 1984*a*). These results confirm the facilitatory nature of noradrenalin on vasopressin release. It is difficult to obtain any data in man since not only do adrenalin and noradrenalin fail to cross the blood–brain barrier, but they also have major cardiovascular effects which result in secondary changes in vasopressin secretion. Thus, although infusions of noradrenalin and adrenalin have been shown to increase water clearance with negligible effects on renal plasma flow and glomerular filtration rate, these results are difficult to interpret.

STUDIES IN AUTONOMIC FAILURE

It is with a background of the great difficulties encountered in the study of the role of amines in the control of hypothalamic function in normal man that we must consider our patients with autonomic failure. Patients with MSA have a major loss of ascending catecholamine pathways with an associated decrease in hypothalamic amines. There is also a marked decrease in intrinsic hypothalamic dopamine. Although these subjects present us with a complex pathology, they also provide us with the unique situation of human subjects with abnormal hypothalamic catecholamines, and it is clearly very interesting to assess whether this is associated with any changes in the control of their hypothalamopituitary function. Since the experimental animal data is clearest for neurohypophyseal function, we shall consider this first.

Posterior pituitary function

Vasopressin is secreted in response to both osmotic and cardiovascular stimuli, as well as to oropharyngeal and non-specific stimuli such as nausea and hypoglycaemia (Lightman and Everitt 1986). Since the osmoreceptors are located within the hypothalamus, probably in the area anterior and ventral to the third ventricle, they have relatively direct neuronal access to the vasopressin-containing cells of the magnocellular supraoptic and paraventricular nuclei. Cardiovascular information, however, travels from the thorax in the ninth and tenth nerves to synapse in the NTS in the dorsomedial medulla. Two major pathways—the dorsal and ventral noradrenergic bundles—have been described in the rat (Sawchenko and Swanson 1982), and we have demonstrated (Lightman *et al.* 1984*a*) that lesions of the dorsal bundle very markedly reduce the vasopressin response to haemorrhage. Interestingly, the lesion is specific for the cardiovascular stimulus to vasopressin release since the responses to osmotic and nicotine stimuli are unaffected (Lightman *et al.* 1984*a,b*). Thus, we have evidence in rats that the integrity of the brainstem noradrenergic pathways is important for the relay of cardiovascular information from the dorsomedial medulla to the vasopressin cells of the hypothalamus.

The loss of brainstem catecholamine pathways in MSA is probably the closest we shall be able to get in man to our model of 6-hydroxydopamine lesioned brainstem pathways in the rat. Any studies on these subjects, however, are complicated by the associated degeneration of their sympathetic nervous system which presents major problems for the assessment of any cardiovascular stimulus to vasopressin secretion. In order to get over this problem we have now studied three groups of subjects: normal subjects; subjects with MSA; and patients with midcervical spinal-cord transections. This last group of subjects has no sympathetic output and can act as a control for the sympathetic nervous system loss in the patients with MSA.

The integrity of the vasopressin response to hypertonic saline is good evidence for normal function of the hypothalamo–neurohypophyseal system itself. We tested the vasopressin response to an osmotic stimulus in all three groups of subjects (Williams *et al.* 1985; Poole *et al.* 1987). Hypertonic (0.85 M) saline was infused i.v. at a rate of 0.05 ml/kg/min over a period of 2 hours, and blood samples were taken every 30 min for assessment of plasma osmolality and vasopressin concentrations. There was a similar change in plasma osmolality in all three groups, and the changes in plasma vasopressin can be seen in Fig. 21.3. Although the increase in the subjects with spinal-cord transection is greater than for the other two groups, the difference was not significant.

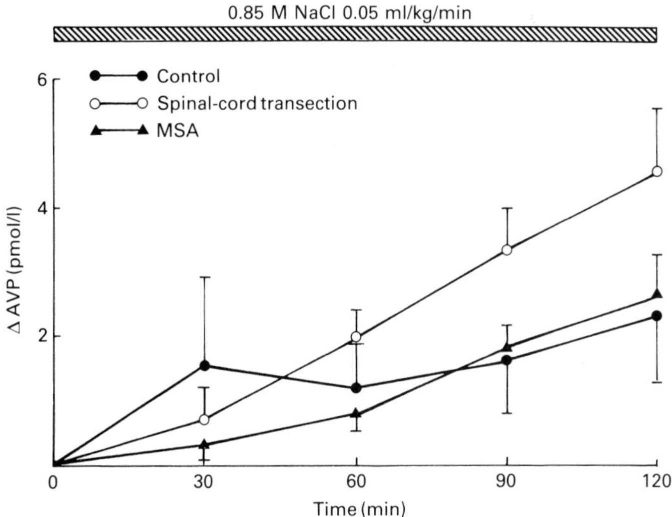

Fig. 21.3. Changes in plasma vasopressin (ΔAVP) during intravenous infusion of 0.85 mol saline, 0.05 ml/kg/min over 2 hours in control subjects, patients with MSA, and patients with spinal-cord transection.

In the knowledge that all three groups of subjects have a normal vasopressin response to an osmotic stimulus, any differences in the vasopressin response to a cardiovascular stimulus must result from abnormalities proximal to the hypothalamo–neurohypophyseal unit itself. In order to assess the functioning of the vasopressin response to changes in blood pressure and plasma volume we tested the response of all three groups to head-up tilt (Fig. 21.4) (Puritz *et al.* 1983; Poole *et al.* 1987). Normal subjects show a significant rise in plasma vasopressin following tilt, while the additional stimulus of postural hypotension in the subjects with spinal-cord transection resulted in a markedly

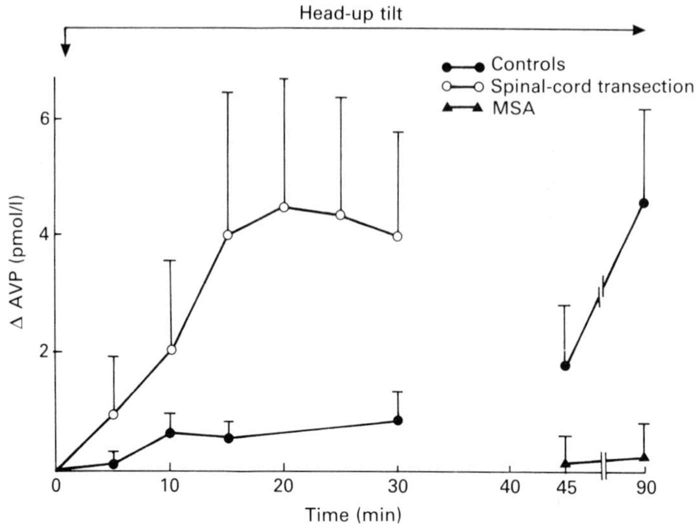

Fig. 21.4. Changes in plasma vasopressin (ΔAVP) during head-up tilt in control subjects, patients with MSA, and patients with spinal-cord transection.

increased release of vasopressin. In marked contrast to this—and in spite of a very similar hypotensive response to tilt—the patients with MSA have a minimal vasopressin response amounting to only 10 per cent of the rise found in their control group.

It is clear from these studies that patients with MSA have abnormalities of vasopressin secretion very similar to those found in our rats with lesions of the dorsal noradrenergic bundle. The response to an osmotic stimulus is intact but there is a severely blunted response to a cardiovascular stimulus. This suggests that in man, as in the rat, ascending catecholamine pathways are important in mediating the vasopressin response to cardiovascular stimuli.

Anterior pituitary function

Anterior pituitary function was studied in five male subjects with MSA (Carmichael, Williams, Bannister, and Lightman, unpublished data). Three investigations were performed on separate occasions. (1) TRH (200 μg) plus LHRH (100 μg) were given i.v. and LH, follicle-stimulating hormone (FSH), TSH, and prolactin measured every 30 min for 2 hours; (2) Metoclopramide (10 mg) was given i.v. and prolactin and TSH measured every 30 min for 2 hours; (3) A control infusion of saline was administered between 09.00 and 13.00 hours followed by an infusion of naloxone (10 mg) between 13.00 and 17.00 hours. LH, FSH, prolactin, cortisol, and growth hormone were measured at half-hourly intervals.

TRH/LHRH test (see Fig. 21.5)

There was a normal response of TSH and prolactin to TRH. There was a reversal of the normal LH:FSH ratio (basal LH 5.8 ± 0.8 U/l, FSH 9.3 ± 5.1 U/l), due to an increased FSH in these elderly subjects. There was a brisk LH response to LHRH with a relatively poor stimulation of FSH.

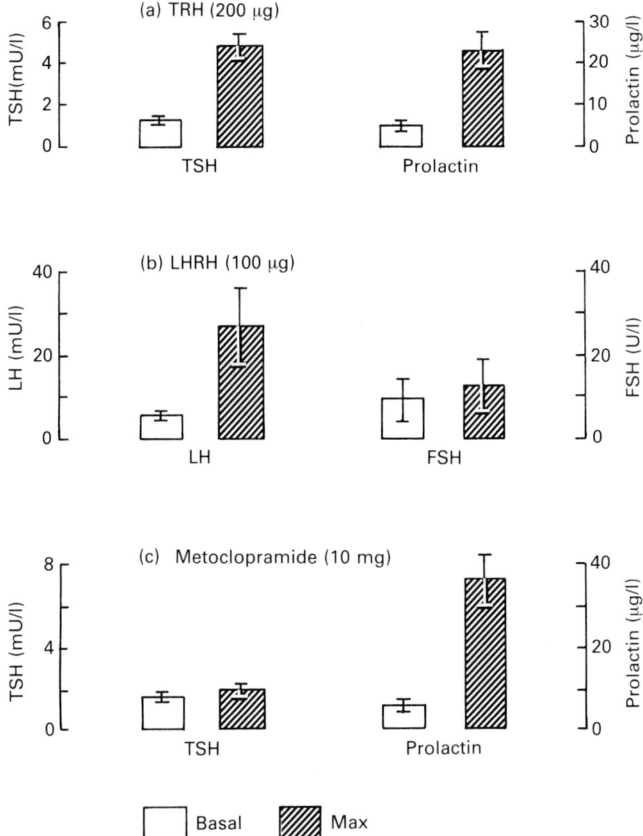

Fig. 21.5. Basal hormone concentrations and maximal responses following intravenous administration of TRH (200 μg), LHRH (100 μg), and metoclopramide (10 mg), in five subjects with MSA.

Metoclopramide test (see Fig. 21.5)

There was a good prolactin response to metoclopramide and no significant change in TSH.

Naloxone infusion

Naloxone had no effect on mean prolactin levels (control 5.9 ± 1.3 μg/l, naloxone 6.0 ± 1.6 μg/l). Mean plasma cortisol concentrations were the same during the placebo (388 ± 38 nmol/l) and naloxone infusion (385 ± 61 nmol/l) infusion periods—not showing the expected fall in cortisol due to its diurnal rhythm. This loss of diurnal fall in cortisol has been previously reported during naloxone infusion in normal subjects (Lightman 1981).

Naloxone did not increase LH (control 5.1 ± 1.0 U/l, naloxone 5.9 ± 1.4 U/l) or FSH (control 6.7 ± 3.3 U/l, naloxone 7.2 ± 3.7 U/l) unlike the response found in normal subjects (Lightman 1981), nor did it alter the frequency of LH pulses during the infusion. LH pulse frequency was in fact markedly depressed in these subjects. There was an overall pulse frequency of 0.125 pulses/hour which is half the rate recently found in elderly monks with a mean age of 73 years (Deslypere *et al.* 1987). Indeed, three of our subjects showed no LH pulses during the 8 hours of testing and the other two had only a total of 5 pulses between them.

Growth hormone levels are markedly lower than those recently reported in men of comparable age (Ho *et al.* 1987). These levels increased during naloxone infusion from 1.7 ± 0.7 mU/l to 3.9 ± 1.0 mU/l ($p < 0.01$ by paired *t*-test) as did the overall number of neurosecretory pulses from 1 to 6.

Conclusions

Although there is a reported decrease in hypothalamic dopamine content in MSA, we do not find evidence for a lack of hypothalamo–hypophyseal portal dopamine, as evidenced by a normal prolactin response to the dopamine antagonist metoclopramide. TSH and prolactin responses to TRH are also normal. The reason for the reversal of the usual LH:FSH ratio is uncertain, but more studies need to be performed on age-matched controls. The relatively high FSH and the brisk LH response to LHRH may be due to poor functioning of the ageing testis with decreased secretion of inhibin and testosterone. The loss of cortisol rhythm during naloxone infusion is quite normal but the marked decrease in LH secretory episodes and the lack of LH and FSH response to naloxone was unexpected. As described earlier in this chapter, data in experimental animals suggests that gonadotrophin secretion is influenced by ascending catecholamine pathways and the abnormality we have now found in MSA should be amenable to further investigation. The growth hormone secretion was not fully tested in these studies but the low mean plasma concentrations of growth hormone, a report by Mathias of a defect in the growth hormone response to clonidine, and the marked response to naloxone suggest a significant abnormality. There is good experimental data for an important role of catecholamines in the control of growth hormone secretion and the present studies suggest that similar mechanisms may occur in man.

SUMMARY

Patients with MSA provide a unique opportunity to study the neuroendocrine effects of a condition associated with abnormal hypothalamic amines. The clearest abnormalities are found in the control of posterior pituitary secretion of vasopressin where there are very similar abnormalities to those found in rats with lesions of their dorsal noradrenergic bundles. Abnormalities of anterior pituitary function are less clear, but there is evidence for altered regulation of LH and growth hormone secretion. It seems likely that these abnormalities are related to the degeneration of ascending noradrenergic and adrenergic pathways. Although hypothalamic dopamine concentrations are decreased, dopaminergic neuroendocrine control appears intact as evidenced by the normality of prolactin responses.

REFERENCES

Carter, D. A. and Lightman, S. L. (1985). Neuroendocrine control of vasopressin secretion. In *The posterior pituitary* (ed. P. H. Baylis and P. L. Padfield), pp. 53–118. Marcel Dekker, New York.

Day, T. A., Ferguson, A. V., and Renaud, L. P. (1984). Facilitatory influence of noradrenergic afferents on the excitability of rat paraventricular nucleus neurosecretory cells. *J. Physiol.* **355**, 237–49.

Deslypere, J. P., Kaufman, J. M., Vermeulen, T., Vogelaers, D., Vandalem, J. L., and Vermeulen, A. (1987). Influence of age on pulsatile luteinizing hormone release and responsiveness of the gonadotrophs to sex hormone feedback in men. *J. clin. Endocrinol. Metab.* **64**, 68–73.

Everitt, B. J. and Hökfelt, T. (1986). Neuroendocrine anatomy of the hypothalamus. In *Neuroendocrinology* (ed. S. L. Lightman and B. J. Everitt), pp. 5–31. Blackwell Scientific Publications, Oxford.

Foord, S. M., Peters, J. R., Dieguez, C., Lewis, M. D., Lewis, B. M., Hall, R., and Scanlon, M. F. (1986). Thyroid stimulating hormone. In *Neuroendocrinology* (ed. S. L. Lightman and B. J. Everitt), pp. 450–71. Blackwell Scientific Publications, Oxford.

Heritage, A. S., Grant, L. D., and Stumpf, W. E. (1975). Oestradiol in catecholamine neurons of the rat brainstem: combined localisations by autoradiography and formaldehyde-induced fluorescence. *J. comp. Neurol.* **176**, 607–30.

Ho, K. Y., Evans, W. S., Blizzard, R. M., Veldhuis, J. D., Merriam, G. R., Samojlik, E., Furlanetto, R., Rogol, A. D., Kaiser, D. L., and Thorner, M. O. (1987). Effects of sex and age on the 24-hour profile of growth hormone secretion in man: importance of endogenous oestradiol concentrations. *J. clin. Endocrinol. Metab.* **64**, 51–8.

Lightman, S. L. (1981). Studies on the responses of plasma renin activity and aldosterone and cortisol levels to dopaminergic and opiate stimuli in man. *Clin. Endocrinol.* **15**, 45–52.

Lightman, S. L. and Everitt, B. J. (1986). Water excretion. In *Neuroendocrinology* (ed. S. L. Lightman and B. J. Everitt), pp. 197–206. Blackwell Scientific Publications, Oxford.

Lightman, S. L., Everitt, B. J., and Todd, K. (1984*a*). Ascending noradrenergic projections from the brainstem; evidence for a major role in the regulation of blood pressure and vasopressin secretion. *Exp. Brain Res.* **55**, 145–51.

Lightman, S. L., Jacobs, H. S., Maguire, A. K., McGarrick, G., and Jeffcoate, S. L. (1981). Constancy of opioid control of luteinising hormone in different pathophysiological states. *J. clin. Endocrinol. Metab.* **52**, 1260–3.

Lightman, S. L., Todd, K., and Everitt, B. J. (1984*b*). Role for lateral tegmental noradrenergic neurons in the vasopressin response to hypertonic saline. *Neurosci. Lett.* **42**, 55–9.

Poole, C. J. M., Williams, T. D. M., Lightman, S. L., and Frankel, H. L. (1987). Neuroendocrine control of vasopressin secretion and its effect on blood pressure in subjects with spinal cord transection. *Brain* **110**, 727–35.

Puritz, R., Lightman, S. L., Wilcox, C. S., Forsling, M., and Bannister, R. (1983). Blood pressure and vasopressin in progressive autonomic failure. *Brain* **106**, 503–11.

Quabbe, H. J. (1986). Growth hormone. In *Neuroendocrinology* (ed. S. L. Lightman and B. J. Everitt), pp. 409–49. Blackwell Scientific Publications, Oxford.

Sawchenko, P. E. and Swanson, L. W. (1982). The organisation of noradrenergic pathways from the brainstem to the paraventricular and supraoptic nuclei in the rat. *Brain Res. Rev.* **4**, 275–325.

Spokes, E. G., Bannister, R., and Oppenheimer, D. R. (1979). Multiple system atrophy with autonomic failure: Clinical, histological and neurochemical observations on four cases. *J. neurol. Sci.* **43**, 59–82.

Williams, T. D. M., Lightman, S. L., and Bannister, R. (1985). Vasopressin secretion in progressive autonomic failure: evidence for defective afferent cardiovascular pathways. *J. Neurol. Neurosurg. Psychiat.* **48**, 225–8.

22. Pupillary function in autonomic failure

Shirley A. Smith

INTRODUCTION

This chapter describes how pupillary function is affected by autonomic failure confined to the eye and as part of more widespread neuropathies, particularly that associated with diabetes mellitus. First, the anatomy and physiology which underlies normal pupillary function is described.

PUPILLARY CONSTRICTION

Contraction of the circular smooth-muscle fibres of the sphincter pupillae constricts the pupil during the reflex responses to light and near vision. Both reflexes involve activation of parasympathetic preganglionic neurons whose cell bodies lie in the Edinger–Westphal nuclei, a pair of slim columns of small cells situated dorsorostrally to the main mass of the oculomotor nuclear complex in the anterior midbrain. These preganglionic neurons pass uncrossed with the third cranial nerve to synapse in the ciliary ganglion which lies about 10 mm in front of the superior orbital fissure in the loose fatty tissue at the orbital apex. This ganglion contains cell bodies of the postganglionic parasympathetic fibres whose axons travel forward to the ciliary muscle and iris sphincter via the short ciliary nerves which penetrate the eyeball at its posterior pole. Fibres subserving pupillary constriction comprise only 3 per cent of the parasympathetic outflow from the ciliary ganglion; the majority subserve accommodation.

The course of the light reflex pathway from the retina to the sphincter is illustrated in Fig. 22.1. Afferent impulses for visual perception and pupillary constriction diverge in the posterior (central) third of the optic tracts. The visual fibres relay in the lateral geniculate bodies, whereas the pupillary fibres leave the optical tract and synapse in the pretectal nuclei in the midbrain. Fibres from these nuclei carry the pupillomotor impulses to Edinger–Westphal nuclei of both sides. In man this crossing,

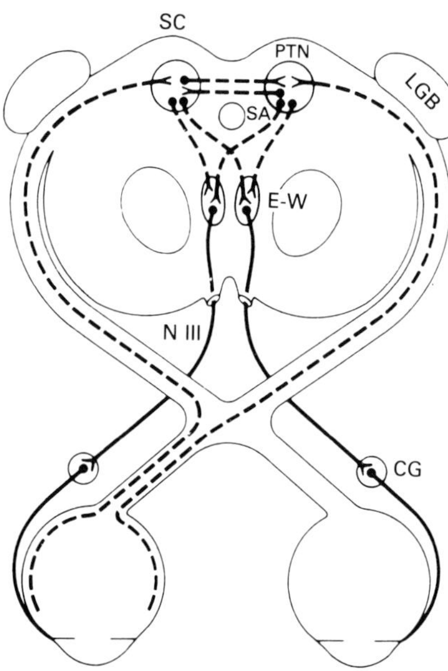

Fig. 22.1. The light reflex pathway from the retina to the iris sphincter. SC, superior colliculus; PTN, pretectal nucleus; LGB, lateral geniculate body; SA, Sylvian aqueduct; E–W, Edinger–Westphal nucleus; N III, oculomotor (third) nerve; CG, ciliary ganglion. (Taken with permission from Alexandridis (1985).)

together with the preceding one at the optic chiasm, is essentially symmetrical. Thus, illumination of only one eye produces reflex constriction of both pupils of approximately equal magnitude.

During near vision, the pupil constricts in association with accommodation produced by ciliary muscle contraction and convergence elicited by contraction of the medial rectus muscles. The light and near pupillary reflexes share a common neuronal path only from the Edinger–Westphal nucleus onward. Prior to that, the near reflex pathway descends from the cortex bypassing the pretectal nucleus on its way to the Edinger–Westphal nucleus. As the fibres approach the nucleus, they are probably situated more ventrally than the light reflex fibres because they are often spared in patients in whom pineal or collicular tumours have abolished the light reflex by pressure from the dorsal side (Lowenstein and Loewenfeld 1969).

The postganglionic nerves release acetylcholine which activates muscarinic receptors to contract the circular smooth muscle fibres of the sphincter pupillae. There is evidence that muscarinic receptors are present on the dilator, which relax the radial smooth muscle fibres during the pupil constriction. However, the physiological significance of these in man remains uncertain.

PUPILLARY DILATATION

Dilatation of the pupil in darkness and during arousal is elicited by two mechanisms: central inhibiton of the Edinger–Westphal nucleus and activation of the peripheral sympathetic innervation of the radial smooth muscle fibres of the dilator pupillae. The central inhibition is said to be via sympathetic fibres from the posterior hypothalamus to the oculomotor nucleus (Lowenstein and Loewenfeld 1950).

The peripheral sympathetic pathway comprises three parts (Fig. 22.2). The first neuron arises in the hypothalamus where connections from higher centres, including the cortex, influence sympathetic control of the pupil. From the hypothalamus the fibres descend uncrossed through the brainstem to the ciliospinal centre of Budge in the intermediolateral columns at the level of the last cervical and the first two thoracic segments. This centre contains the cell bodies of the preganglionic neurons which form the second stage of the pathway. Their axons leave the cord by the ventral roots of the first two thoracic segments and enter the cervical sympathetic trunk. They traverse the inferior and middle cervical ganglia before reaching the superior cervical ganglion near the bifurcation of the internal and external carotid arteries. Since these preganglionic axons pass close to the apex of the lung, the sympathetic pathway to the pupil may be interrupted by malignancy in this area

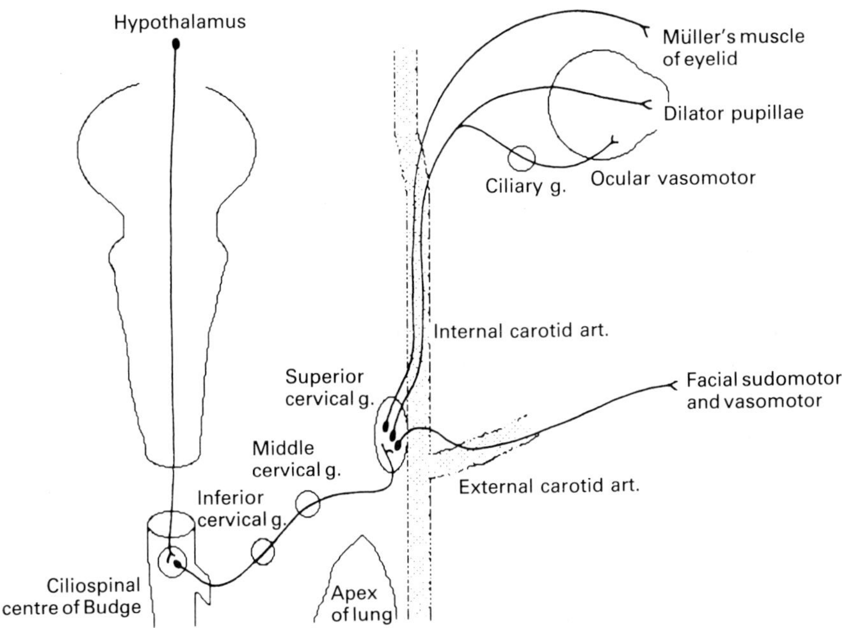

Fig. 22.2. The sympathetic pathway subserving pupillary dilatation.

arising from pulmonary or breast tissue. Within the superior cervical ganglion they synapse with the cell bodies of the postganglionic nerves which form the third stage of the pathway. Fibres subserving pupillary dilatation, movement of the eyelids via Müller's (smooth) muscle, and vasomotor function in and around the eye leave the ganglion and follow the course of the internal carotid arteries into the cranium. The pupillary fibres join the fifth (trigeminal) nerve and approach the orbit in its ophthalmic branch, entering via the superior orbital fissure. They continue in its nasociliary division and enter the eye in the long ciliary nerves. In man, some of the sympathetic fibres to the pupil may cross, but do not synapse in, the ciliary ganglion.

The postganglionic sympathetic nerves release noradrenalin which acts on α-adrenoceptors to contract the radial smooth muscle fibres of the dilator pupillae. There is evidence that β-adrenoceptors on the sphincter relax these circular fibres during pupillary dilatation. As with the cholinergic reciprocal innervation, there is, however, no indication that these are of physiological significance.

AUTONOMIC FAILURE LOCALIZED TO THE EYE

In general, acute parasympathetic dysfunction gives a large pupil with poor reactions to light and near vision, whereas sympathetic dysfunction causes a small pupil which fails to dilate in darkness.

Tumours or vascular accidents which damage the third cranial nerve in its passage from the oculomotor nucleus to the ciliary ganglion will reduce pupillary constriction. Postganglionic parasympathetic neuropathy caused by damage to the ciliary ganglion or the short ciliary nerves results in 'tonic' pupils. These can occur with orbital infections, choroidal tumours, or trauma from retrobulbar injections. They are, however, seen most commonly in Adie's syndrome, a benign condition in which the idiopathic ciliary ganglion pathology is associated with loss of deep tendon reflexes (Adie 1932). Rarely, there is in addition a segmental hypohidrosis, a condition termed Ross syndrome.

Usually, a patient with Adie's syndrome of recent onset presents with accommodative paresis and has one large pupil with poor light reactions. Further examination shows segmental sphincter palsy, diminished or absent tendon reflexes, and enhanced miosis to cholinomimetic eyedrops (such as 0.125 per cent pilocarpine) indicative of denervation supersensitivity.

Many cases of Adie's pupils are investigated in the clinic some time after the initial onset of symptoms when the affected pupil is in fact smaller than the normal one. Adie's pupils only remain larger than the fellow one for about 2–6 months (Thompson 1977). Thereafter, it is said that aberrant regeneration of fibres subserving accommodation (which are far in excess of those subserving pupil constriction) grow to innervate the affected sections of the sphincter pupillae. The neuronal drive associated with ciliary muscle function then constricts the pupil via its aberrent nerves to give a small pupil. This also results in a 'light–near dissocation' with pupillary constriction to near exceeding that to light, though both reflexes are abnormally slow. The initial accommodative difficulties resolve as the ciliary muscle reinnervates. The pupils at this stage may be difficult to distinguish from spastic miotic pupils (Argyll Robertson syndrome, see below) caused by midbrain lesions anterior to the oculomotor nucleus. The differential diagnosis may be made on the presence of segmental sphincter palsy and denervation supersensitivity (as in Adie's pupils) and the nature of the pupillary near reflex response which is slow (tonic) in Adie's but brisk in Argyll Robertson's syndrome.

Adie's syndrome is a progressive condition with loss of the light reaction in further segments of the sphincter, further loss of the deep tendon reflexes, and eventual second-eye involvement. This has lead to the suggestion that a slow virus may be the cause of Adie's syndrome although immunological studies have, as yet, proved inconclusive (Meek and Thompson 1979).

Small pupils due to sympathetic dysfunction (Horner's syndrome) have normal reflex constriction to light and near, are usually accompanied by ptosis, and, in preganglionic lesions, by sweating deficits of the face and neck. There is sometimes an apparent, not a real, enophthalmos due to the narrowing of the palpebral fissure caused by denervation of Müller's smooth muscles of the eyelids. Horner's syndrome results from partial or complete interruption of the sympathetic pathway in any of its three parts. Patients with damage to the first neuron may have had a medullary infarction or may have cervical-cord disease. Second-neuron lesions can occur when a lung or breast malignancy has spread to the thoracic outlet, or when surgery or trauma to the neck has involved the sympathetic nerves. Causes of postganglionic lesions include vascular headache (Raeder's) syndrome, intraoral or retroparotid trauma, internal carotid-artery pathology, and tumours of the middle cranial fossa or the cavernous sinus.

The pupillary behaviour in Horner's syndrome is illustrated in Fig. 22.3. This pupillographic record from a 62-year-old patient with cluster headaches shows a left-sided Horner's pupil. Compared with the normal right pupil, the affected one shows reduced dilatation in the dark, normal constriction to light, and a redilatation lag in the latter part of the recovery phase. Redilatation can be quantified as shown in Fig. 22.4 as the time taken for the pupil to recover to three-quarters of its size at the start of the light reflex, at which time the peripheral sympathetic nerves are active. Measurement of this from Fig. 22.3 shows that the $t_{3/4}$

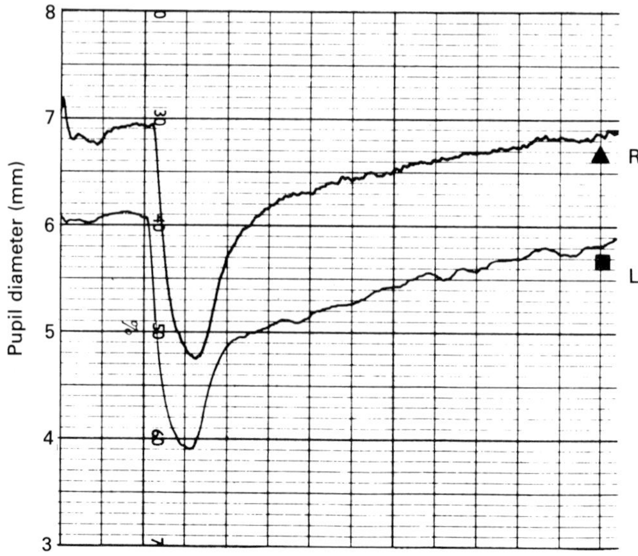

Fig. 22.3. Pupillograph from a patient with a left-sided Horner's syndrome obtained with infra-red television pupillometry. The right (R) and left (L) traces are separated on the time axis (1 vertical bar = 1 second) for convenience.

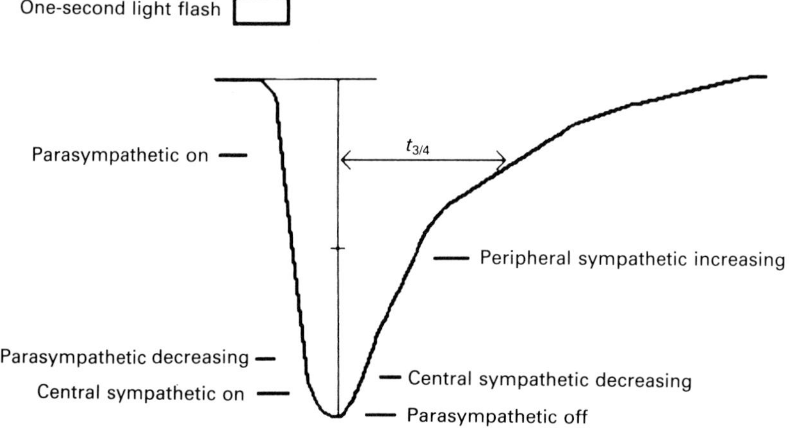

Fig. 22.4. Diagram of a pupillographic tracing of a light reflex to show the $t_{3/4}$ measure of redilatation time. The presumed activity of the autonomic system in shaping the reflex is indicated.

time in the affected pupil was 6.4 seconds, considerably prolonged in comparison with the 3.1 seconds measured in the fellow eye.

Drug tests can be useful in the diagnosis of Horner's syndrome (Maloney *et al.* 1980). Confirmation that the small pupil is indeed due to a sympathetic deficit is provided by either the phenylephrine or cocaine tests. An enhanced mydriasis to 2 per cent phenylephrine, a directly-acting α-adrenoceptor agonist, indicates denervation supersensitivity resulting from partial or complete lesions at any point in the sympathetic pathway. A reduced response to 4 per cent cocaine, which dilates the normally innervated pupil by blocking the inactivation by re-uptake of noradrenalin, also indicates the existence but not the locality of a sympathetic lesion. Pre- and postganglionic damage can be differentiated with a third mydriatic, hydroxyamphetamine 0.5 per cent. This acts indirectly, getting into the sympathetic nerve ending and displacing noradrenalin which leaks from the nerve to activate receptors. It has no effect in postganglionic lesions since there is no noradrenalin for it to release and the agent itself has no agonist activity. If the lesion is in the first or second neuron, hydroxyamphetamine will dilate the pupil, often by more than normal, since decentralized nerves may have increased stores of transmitter (Brown *et al.* 1967).

The response to phenylephrine and hydroxyamphetamine increase with advancing age (Smith and Smith 1983*a*); thus, the sensitivity of these drug tests is increased by reference to their age-related normal range (Table 22.1). The reason for this age effect, which is more marked with phenylephrine than with hydroxyamphetamine, is not understood. The pupils in elderly subjects respond to these drugs in the same way as pupils from younger patients with partial preganglionic sympathetic lesions. The change with advancing age parallels the gradual decrease in darkness of pupil size, called senile miosis in the elderly. Perhaps, decreased central sympathetic drive with age is responsible for the small pupil and the altered mydriatic responses.

Table 22.1. Age-related normal ranges for 2 per cent phenylephrine and 0.5 per cent hydroxyamphetamine drug tests. Values shown are the 2.5, 50, and 97.5 percentiles which define the lower, mean, and upper limits of normal

Age range (year)	*Mean (year)*	*Phenylephrine mydriasis (mm)*			*Hydroxyamphetamine mydriasis (mm)*		
		Lower	*Expected*	*Upper*	*Lower*	*Expected*	*Upper*
15–19	17	—	0.2	1.6	0.25	1.6	2.9
20–24	22	—	0.4	1.8	0.3	1.7	3.0
25–29	27	—	0.6	2.0	0.4	1.7	3.05
30–34	32	—	0.85	2.2	0.5	1.8	3.1
35–39	37	—	1.1	2.4	0.55	1.9	3.2
40–44	42	—	1.3	2.6	0.6	1.9	3.2
45–49	47	0.2	1.5	2.8	0.7	2.0	3.3
50–54	52	0.4	1.7	3.0	0.75	2.05	3.4
55–59	57	0.6	1.9	3.25	0.8	2.1	3.4
60–64	62	0.8	2.1	3.5	0.9	2.2	3.5
65–69	67	1.0	2.4	3.7	0.9	2.25	3.6
70–74	72	1.2	2.6	3.9	1.0	2.3	3.6

PUPIL DYSFUNCTION IN WIDESPREAD AUTONOMIC DISORDERS

Clinical signs of pupillary dysfunction are often complex and variable in these conditions, since both branches of the autonomic may be involved in addition to local iris myopathy. Pupil signs in progressive autonomic failure and familial dysautonomias are included in other chapters. Sarcoidosis, porphyria, leprosy, and alcoholic neuropathy may involve the pupil although few detailed studies with modern pupillographic techniques are available. In contrast to most of the generalized autonomic neuropathies, that associated with diabetes mellitus occurs commonly and much is now understood about pupillary dysfunction in this condition, detailed in the section below.

Pupillary dysfunction does not only result from decreased autonomic drive to the iris, since in some diseases pathology in the central nervous system leads to disinhibition of autonomic nuclei leading to spastically increased tone. Such is the case of Argyll Robertson pupils of neurosyphilis, now a rarity but still of considerable theoretical interest.

In the Argyll Robertson syndrome the pupils are small, light reflexes are reduced or absent, whereas the pupillary constriction to near vision is well preserved. The pupil signs are usually bilateral and may be associated with tabes dorsalis and general paresis although vision is not impaired. The pupillary abnormalities are thought to be due to pathology close to and slightly anterior to the oculomotor nucleus in the midbrain (Lowenstein and Loewenfeld 1969). Such a lesion would destroy the terminal branches of both the crossed and the uncrossed pretectal fibres subserving the light reflex, but would spare the more ventrally situated supranuclear paths for the near-vision reaction. Other inhibitory inputs to the Edinger–Westphal nuclei from higher brain centres would also be interrupted, disinhibiting the parasympathetic motor nuclei to give spastically miotic pupils. The pupils are often irregular and tonic, which is thought to be due to postganglionic parasympathetic function in addition to the central pathology.

Other situations in which there is a small pupil due to central disinhibition are fatigue, sleep, narcotic addiction, and narcolepsy, a condition of chronic hypersomnia for which pupillography can be a valuable diagnostic tool (Yoss *et al.* 1969). Responses to light and near are normal, but measurement in darkness reveals abnormally small pupils which show large spontaneous oscillations in diameter reflecting the sleepiness that characterizes this condition. Treatment with amphetamines, which gives an excellent clinical response, reverses these pupillary abnormalities which represent one end of the spectrum of arousal effects on pupil size. The other end, the large pupils seen in anxiety or fear, result from central inhibition of the parasympathetic together with excitation of the sympathetic iris innervation.

The pupils in diabetic autonomic neuropathy

There is evidence that pupillary function is affected by central, sympathetic, and parasympathetic damage in diabetes. However a mild sympathetic deficit appears to be the earliest sign, and pupils showing a partial Horner's syndrome are common whereas signs resembling an acute Adie's pupil are rare.

Diabetic miosis

It is well recognized that diabetic patients have small pupils (Rundles 1945; Smith *et al.* 1978; Hreidarsson 1982; Pfeifer *et al.* 1984). This can be demonstrated most clearly when pupil size is measured in darkness, which can be done quite simply from a Polaroid photograph of the eye taken at threefold manification (Smith and Dewhirst 1986). Pupils become smaller in healthy subjects with advancing age and therefore it is important to use an age-related normal range for identification of miosis in diabetic patients (Table 22.2). Results from a large screening survey have shown that 21 per cent of diabetic patients had pupils that failed to dilate normally for age in darkness (Fig. 22.5). This is only an estimate of the true prevalence as the population was not demographically complete. There was a highly significant association between miosis and autonomic neuropathy elsewhere, measured in this study as reduced cardiac beat-to-beat variation in response to deep breathing (Smith 1982).

Significant associations between small pupils and a wide range of diabetic complications have been recorded: cardiovascular autonomic

Table 22.2. Age-related normal range for pupil diameter in darkness expressed as the absolute measure and as a percentage of iris diameter (PD%). Values shown are the 2.5, 50, and 97.5 percentiles which define the lower, mean, and upper limits of normal

Age range (year)	*Mean (year)*	*Pupil diameter (mm)*			*PD%*		
		Lower	*Expected*	*Upper*	*Lower*	*Expected*	*Upper*
15–19	17	6.0	7.4	8.8	52.0	63.3	74.6
20–24	22	5.8	7.2	8.6	50.5	61.8	73.1
25–29	27	5.6	7.0	8.4	49.0	60.3	71.5
30–34	32	5.4	6.8	8.2	47.5	58.8	70.0
35–39	37	5.2	6.6	8.0	46.0	57.3	68.5
40–44	42	5.0	6.4	7.8	44.5	55.8	67.0
45–49	47	4.8	6.2	7.6	43.0	54.3	65.5
50–54	52	4.6	6.0	7.4	41.5	52.7	64.0
55–59	57	4.4	5.8	7.2	40.0	51.2	62.5
60–64	62	4.2	5.6	7.0	38.5	49.7	61.0
65–69	67	4.0	5.4	6.8	37.0	48.2	59.5
70–74	72	3.8	5.2	6.6	35.4	46.7	58.0

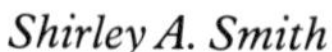

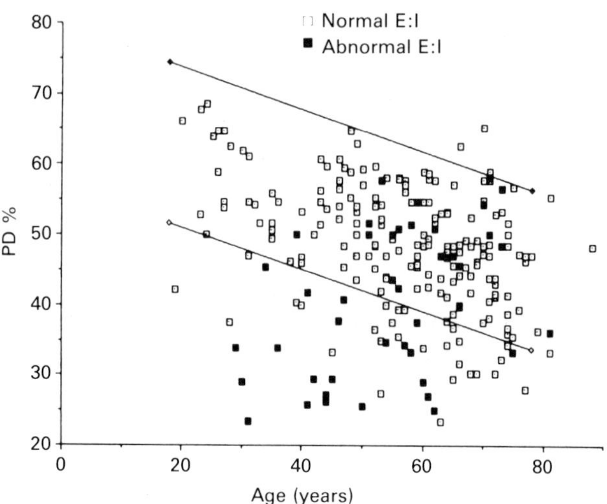

Fig. 22.5. Pupil diameter in darkness in 243 diabetic patients. The PD% (horizontal pupil diameter as a per cent of iris diameter) was abnormally small in 21 per cent of patients and abnormally large in 1 per cent when compared with the age-related normal range described by the lines. The presence (■) or absence (□) of abnormal cardiac beat-to-beat variability, measured as the expiratory:inspiratory ratio (E:I), is indicated. The data was obtained when screening for diabetic complications in London and Oxford. (Oxford data kindly supplied by Dr H. A. W. Neil.)

dysfunction (Smith and Smith 1983*a*); peripheral sensory loss (Smith *et al.* 1978; Hreidarsson 1982); retinopathy (Hayashi and Ishikawa 1979); and nephropathy (Hreidarsson 1982). Patients are more likely to have small pupils if their hyperglycaemia has been of a marked degree and duration (Smith and Smith 1983*a*; Hreidarsson 1982).

The common occurrence of a small pupil with normal light reflexes, in contrast to the rarity of a large pupil with poor light reflexes, suggests that the sympathetic innervation of the iris is more sensitive to damage than the parasympathetic innervation in diabetes. Histological studies of irides from diabetic patients removed during cataract surgery has confirmed that loss of nerve terminals occurs mostly from the dilator pupillae (Ishikawa *et al.* 1985). The reason for the greater sensitivity of the sympathetic pathway to damage is not understood. The sympathetic pathway to the iris is longer than the parasympathetic, which may make it more susceptible to damage. Certainly in the sensory deficits of diabetic neuropathy, it is the longer pathways of the feet that are affected before those of the hands.

The measurement of darkness pupil diameter has provided a simple, accurate method of testing autonomic function in the diabetic patient. Only one pupil need be measured for identification of abnormality since binocular discrepancies in darkness diameter are no different from normal in diabetic autonomic neuropathy (Smith *et al.* 1978). Addition of a pupil test to the conventional battery of cardiovascular tests provides a more comprehensive investigation of autonomic function. The test compares favourably with the cardiovascular tests in terms of repeatability. The coefficient of variation for the Polaroid photographic measure is 3.2 per cent, compared with 15.4 per cent for the Valsalva ratio, for example (Smith 1984). Some groups measure pupil size after treating the eye with a large dose of an anticholinergic mydriatic to block the small parasympathetic input present in darkness (Pfeifer *et al.* 1984). This has the disadvantage for the patient of mydriatic photophobia and accommodative paralysis.

Redilatation lag

Delayed redilatation following light reflex stimulation is one of the characteristic signs in Horner's syndrome (see Fig. 22.3). It is easy to identify in unilateral Horner's syndrome from television pupillometer recordings since there is a normal pupil trace available for comparison. In order to aid identification of redilatation lag in binocular neuropathies, the normal times for redilatation have been defined precisely from studies made in 63 healthy subjects (unpublished observations). The index of redilatation time, the $t_{3/4}$ time (Fig. 22.4), is defined as the time taken for the pupil to recover from its peak constriction during a light reflex to three-quarters of its initial darkness diameter. The length of the $t_{3/4}$ time depends principally on the size of the light reflex, increasing linearly by 0.8 seconds for each mm increase in amplitude. The percentiles of this relationship describe the normal range, from which one can identify whether a pupil is redilating too slowly for the light reflex size.

This index of sympathetic function was found to be abnormal in diabetic patients with other signs of autonomic neuropathy. Figure 22.6 shows redilatation in two healthy non-diabetic subjects and one diabetic with autonomic neuropathy. The diabetic patient has small pupils in darkness which constrict well to light but qualitatively appear to lag in the redilatation phase when compared with the pupils of the healthy subjects. The $t_{3/4}$ times in the diabetic are 6 and 6.5 s in the right and left eyes, respectively. The normal $t_{3/4}$ time for reflexes of this size (1.4 mm) is 1.8 s and the upper limit of normal is 3.3 s. The results in a group of 31 diabetic patients with and without autonomic neuropathy are shown in Fig. 22.7. About half of those with autonomic neuropathy had delayed redilatation whereas all those with normal function tests elsewhere redilated normally. Thus, redilatation lag is often present in diabetic neuropathy of the pupil. It becomes more difficult to identify in the more advanced cases in which parasympathetic dysfunction markedly reduces light reflex amplitude.

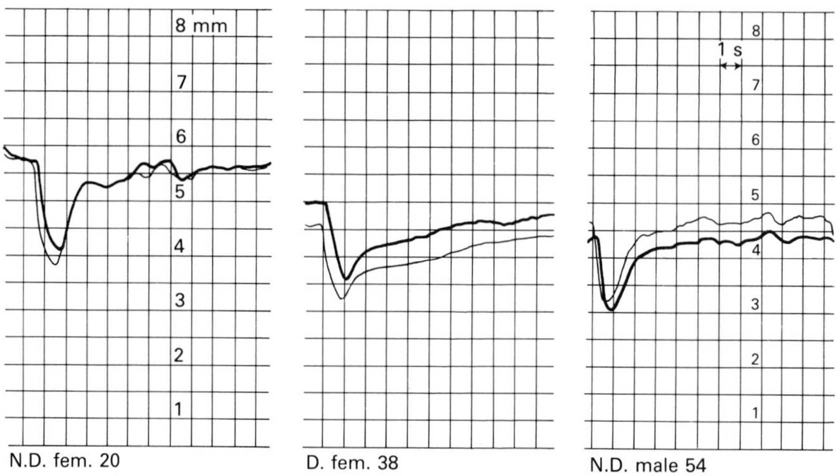

Fig. 22.6. Pupillographs from a non-diabetic (N.D.) 20-year-old female, a diabetic (D.) 38-year-old female with autonomic neuropathy, and a non-diabetic 54-year-old male subject. The bolder line indicates the right pupil, and the responses from the two pupils are separated on the time axis (1 vertical bar=1 second) for convenience. For each subject, measurements were made in darkness interrupted by a single 1-second light flash. The diameter scale in mm is shown on the left graph. Note the bilateral redilatation lag and absent hippus in the diabetic patient.

Sympathetic denervation supersensitivity

The mydriatic response to directly acting sympathomimetic agents is exaggerated in patients with diabetic autonomic neuropathy suggesting that there is denervation supersensitivity as in Horner's syndrome (Hayashi and Ishikawa 1979; Smith and Smith 1983*a*).

Smith and Smith (1983*a*) tested mydriatic responses in 34 diabetic patients divided into four groups according to how well their pupils dilated in darkness. The division was made on the number of standard deviations by which their darkness diameter differed from the normal for age. Group 1 had diameters above or within 1 SD below normal ($n=9$); group 2 between 1 and 2 SD ($n=9$); group 3 between 2 and 3 SD ($n=10$); group 4 between 3 and 4 SD ($n=6$). The groups were balanced for age, but those with small pupils had poorer glycaemic control, longer duration of disease, and poorer neurological function generally. Each patient was tested with the sympathomimetics, phenylephrine (2 per cent) and hydroxyamphetamine (0.5 per cent), and the results are shown in Fig. 22.8. Results are expressed as a difference between the mydriasis observed and that expected for age. The two groups with abnormally small pupils (groups 3 and 4) showed supersensitivity to phenylephrine which confirms that the aetiology is likely to

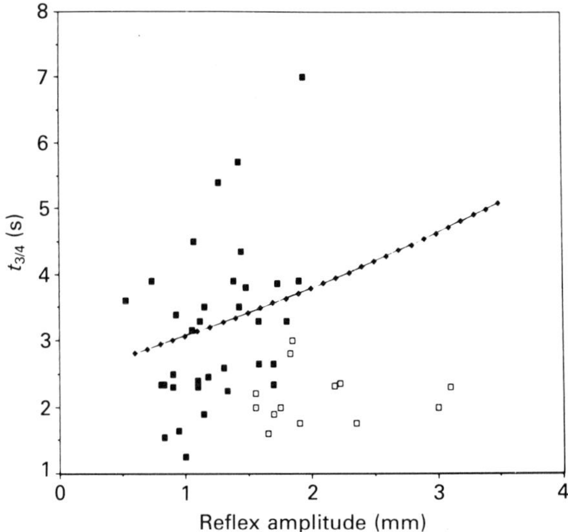

Fig. 22.7. Redilatation time in diabetic patients with or without autonomic dysfunction as indicated by darkness pupil diameter and cardiovascular (CVS) function tests. Fourteen eyes from nine patients (□) with normal autonomic function and 34 eyes from 22 patients (■) with abnormal function were studied. The line defines the upper limit of normal. Abnormally slow redilatation ($t_{3/4}$ time exceeding the upper limit) was found only in the autonomic neuropaths.

be sympathetic dysfunction. The response of all the groups to hydroxyamphetamine did not differ significantly from normal, from which one can conclude that postganglionic nerve function is essentially normal. It would be surprising if a multifactorial disorder such as diabetes caused dysfunction at one specific point in the pathway. More probably, the sympathetic deficit results from a composite of mildly reduced function throughout.

An enhanced response to phenylephrine but a normal response to hydroxyamphetamine argues against a non-specific cause of drug supersensitivity, such as increased penetration through a damaged cornea. Further, the finding that the small diabetic pupils dilated well with drugs shows that damage to the muscle itself is not responsible for the limited movement in darkness. In severe diabetic eye disease, rubeosis iridis and glaucoma might be expected to limit pupillary movements but the evidence available shows that muscle function is remarkably well preserved.

Sympathetic denervation supersensitivity in the diabetic patient with neuropathic and retinopathic complications has been utilized in an effective regimen for mydriasis for fundal inspection (Huber *et al.* 1985).

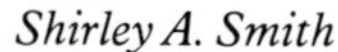

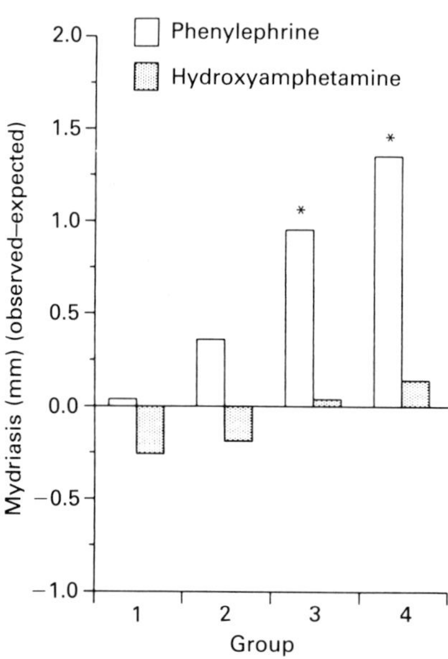

Fig. 22.8. Age-corrected mydriasis in four groups of diabetic patients with normal (Groups 1 and 2) and abnormal (Groups 3 and 4) pupils. The response to phenylephrine was significantly larger than normal in Groups 3 and 4 (*$p < 0.05$), whereas the hydroxyamphetamine responses were normal in all four Groups.

Pupils of such patients are often difficult to dilate with conventional anticholinergic agents because there is inadequate sympathetic drive to activate the dilator. A combination of phenylephrine (10 or 2.5 per cent) with 1 per cent tropicamide is very effective. The supersensitive dilator reacts very well to phenylephrine to give a widely dilated pupil. This permits use of the weaker anticholinergic tropicamide to block the light reflex prior to ophthalmoscopy. Tropicamide has minimal postclinic accommodative paralysis compared with stronger agents such as cyclopentolate.

Ptosis

Another classical sign of Horner's syndrome is ptosis which results from damage to the sympathetic innervation of Müller's muscles, the smooth-muscle component of the eyelid levators. Ptosis is difficult to identify in binocular neuropathies but has been observed in diabetics with autonomic neuropathy (Fig. 22.9). It can be differentiated from ptosis due to third-nerve palsy by its ready reversal with weak concentrations of phenylephrine.

Lack of hippus

When pupils from healthy subjects are stimulated with continuous

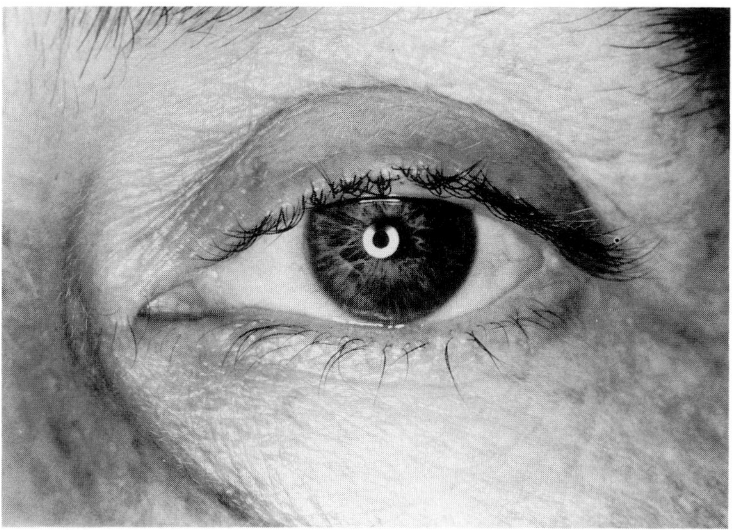

Fig. 22.9. Ptosis in a diabetic patient with autonomic neuropathy.

bright light they constrict initially, then redilate partially as the eye adapts to the stimulus. Pupil size oscillates slowly as the redilatation ensues, a phenomenon known as hippus (Lowenstein and Loewenfeld 1969). This pupillary unrest is always symmetrical in the two eyes and is therefore likely to be central in origin. Diabetics with neuropathy show reduced hippus (Smith *et al.* 1978), which indicates that the central control of the pupillary autonomic innervation may be affected in diabetic autonomic neuropathy. This greater stability of pupil size in diabetic eyes can be seen in the pupillographs of Fig. 22.6.

Reduced light reflex size

The amplitude of the pupillary constriction to light is reduced in diabetic autonomic neuropathy (Smith and Smith 1983*b*; Hreidarsson and Gundersen 1985). This reduction is usually only seen in pupils which are already small from sympathetic dysfunction. Figure 22.10 shows a pupil recording from a patient with severe autonomic neuropathy. Pupil size remained almost the same despite a change in illumination from darkness to bright flash stimulation. Myopathy was not responsible for the limited mobility since drugs were effective in changing pupil size, nor was an afferent defect reducing reflex response since visual perception was intact. Presumably the iris was essentially denervated in both autonomic branches.

Testing for reduction of the parasympathetically-mediated constriction to light is complicated by the presence of other ocular pathology that may limit the effectiveness of the light stimulus. Retinopathy and

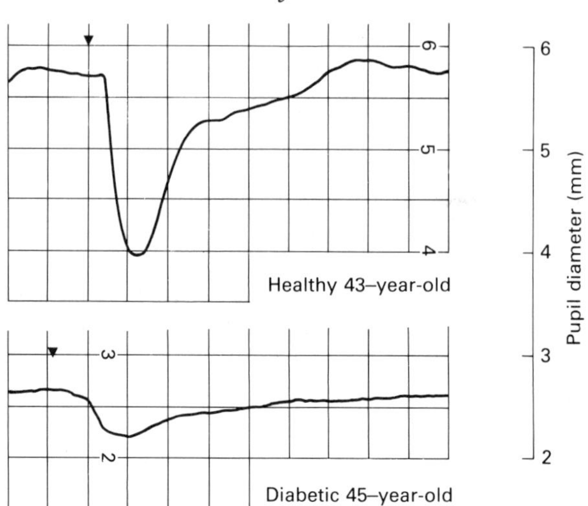

Fig. 22.10. Pupillographic record from a diabetic patient with marked autonomic neuropathy (lower trace). A normal light reflex from an age-matched healthy subject (upper trace) is shown for comparison. The pupil of the diabetic patient failed to dilate in the dark, and constricted poorly to a bright 1-second light flash (▼).

optic-nerve disease will give an afferent pupillary defect and these are inevitably present to some extent in patients under examination for neuropathy. This can be overcome by relating the intensity of the stimulating light to the visual perception threshold measured by a forced choice method (Smith and Smith 1983*b*), enabling the efferent side of the light reflex arc to be tested independently.

A second difficulty in establishing reductions in reflex amplitude is the limited range of movement possible in pupils made small by sympathetic dysfunction. The extent of this mechanical restriction has been investigated (Smith and Smith 1983*b*) by comparing responses in diabetic patients with those in elderly healthy subjects with senile miosis. Twenty-five healthy subjects (mean age 60.5 years) with darkness diameters below 6 mm were studied. Light reflex size was found to decrease by 0.55 mm per mm decrease in darkness diameter. Age did reduce reflex size, but only as a consequence of the progressive reduction of diameter seen with advancing years. The results in 43 diabetic patients (mean age 39.7 years) with similar small resting diameters showed that the reflexes were on average 0.34 mm smaller than in non-diabetics with the same starting diameter.

These findings show that miosis due to old age or diabetes is associated with reduced reflex amplitudes but the reduction is greater in diabetic pupils. It is likely that mechanical restriction is responsible in both groups but the additional reduction in diabetics is due to parasympathetic dysfunction. The enhanced response of the diabetic pupil to cholinomimetic drugs (Hayashi and Ishikawa 1979), indicating denervation supersensitivity, supports this hypothesis.

Delayed pupil cycle time

Another method of testing pupillary parasympathetic function is measurement of the pupil cycle time (Martyn and Ewing 1986). Regular oscillations of the pupil are induced by focusing a narrow beam of light on the pupil margin using a slit lamp. The constricting pupil interrupts the light beam, removing the stimulus and thereby dilating the pupil enabling the light to restimulate the retina ('closed loop stimulation'). The mean time is calculated from 100 cycles with a stop watch. It has been found to increase with increasing age (Clark and Mapstone 1986). The pupil cycle time was lengthened by parasympathetic, but not sympathetic, drug blockade. It was found to be prolonged in diabetics with autonomic neuropathy, presumably due to parasympathetic dysfunction. It does not differentiate between afferent and efferent pupillary defects and pupils in a small proportion of patients cannot be made to cycle.

Light reflex latency and velocity

These indices are affected by diabetic neuropathy, and prolonged latency times have been used to identify abnormality in a pupillary autonomic function test (Pfeifer *et al.* 1984). Diabetic patients with neuropathy have longer latencies and slower maximum velocities of constriction and dilatation compared with normal pupils (Smith *et al.* 1978; Hreidarsson and Gundersen 1985). However, analysis of these dynamic variables in normal pupils has shown that they are strongly related to the size of the reflex. Thus latency times are always longer and maximum velocities of constriction and dilatation slower in low-amplitude reflexes elicited by low-intensity light stimuli in healthy pupils (Fig. 22.11). This relationship is maintained in diabetic pupils indicating that the reflexes are sluggish because they are small. Prolonged latency, slow maximum velocities, and reduced amplitudes are thus all likely to be caused by parasympathetic dysfunction.

The maximum velocity of dilatation occurs in the first half of the recovery phase from a light reflex when the withdrawal of parasympathetic tone is determining pupil size (Fig. 22.4). It differs from the $t_{3/4}$ redilatation time which occurs in the latter phase of the recovery when the peripheral sympathetic nerves are actively dilating the pupil. Thus the $t_{3/4}$ time, but not the maximum dilatation velocity, may be abnormal even if reflex amplitude is of normal size. Such a situation occurs when the sympathetic nerves are affected but the parasympathetic nerves are working normally.

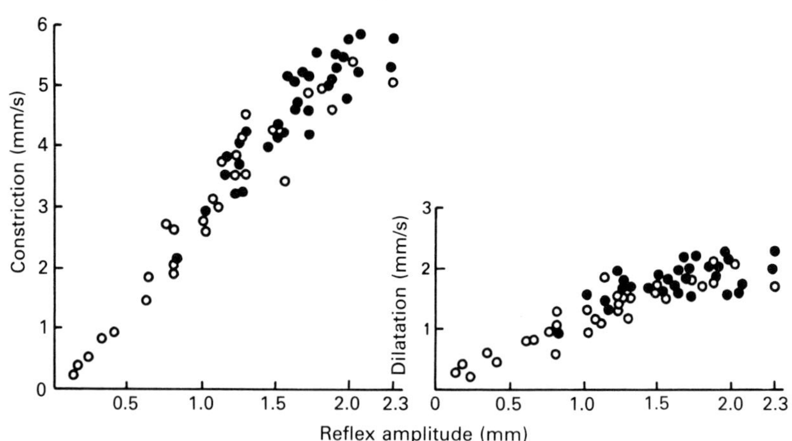

Fig. 22.11. The dependence of maximum velocities of pupillary constriction and dilatation on light reflex amplitude in normal (●) and diabetic (○) subjects. The speed of pupillary movements are slower in diabetic eyes because the size of the reflexes are reduced.

Irreversibility of pupillary signs

The realization that chronic hyperglycaemia is a significant risk factor for the development of neuropathy in diabetes stimulated hope that improved control could reverse nerve dysfunction. Assessment of pupil function is particularly useful in studies relating control to complications because pupil tests are repeatable enough to be able to identify small changes in nerve function. The St Thomas's Diabetic Study Group (1986) reported a prospective trial of a 2-year improvement in glycaemic control in 20 insulin-treated diabetic patients with established autonomic dysfunction. There was no reversal of the neuropathy and, in fact, two pupillary and three cardiovascular tests indicated a significant deterioration which exceeded that explicable by ageing. It may be that in diabetes, nerve function like glomerular function declines beyond some critical threshold after which further deterioration is inevitable. It remains to be seen whether the aldose reductase inhibitor drug treatments for diabetic complications, which are said to reverse the metabolic abnormalities in nerve cells, will reverse the autonomic neuropathy.

CONCLUSIONS

Advanced pupillometric techniques have increased our understanding of the pupillary manifestations of autonomic failure. Experience gained in the common conditions, notably diabetic neuropathy, should be a useful guide for future research in the rarer autonomic neuropathies.

REFERENCES

Adie, W. J. (1932). Complete and incomplete forms of the benign disorder characterized by tonic pupils and absent tendon reflexes. *Br. J. Ophthalmol.* **16**, 449–61.

Alexandridis, E. (1985). *The pupil.* Springer-Verlag, New York.

Brown, G. L., Dearnaley, D. P., and Geffen, L. B. (1967). Noradrenaline storage and release in the decentralized spleen. *Proc. R. Soc.* **B168**, 48–56.

Clark, C. V. and Mapstone, R. (1986). Pupil cycle time in primary closed-angle glaucoma. *Can. J. Ophthalmol.* **21**, 88–91.

Hayashi, M. and Ishikawa, S. (1979). Pharmacology of pupillary responses in diabetics—correlative study of the responses and grade of retinopathy. *Jap. J. Ophthalmol.* **23**, 65–72.

Hreidarsson, A. B. (1982). Pupil size in insulin-dependent diabetes. *Diabetes* **31**, 442–8.

Hreidarsson, A. B. and Gundersen, H. J. G. (1985). The pupillary response to light in Type I (insulin-dependent) diabetes. *Diabetologia* **28**, 815–21.

Huber, M. J. E., Smith, S. A., and Smith, S. E. (1985). Mydriatic drugs for diabetic patients. *Br. J. Ophthalmol.* **69**, 425–7.

Ishikawa, S., Bensaoula, T., Uga, S., and Mukono, K. (1985). Electron microscopic study of iris nerves and muscles in diabetes. *Ophthalmologica* **191**, 172–83.

Lowenstein, O. and Loewenfeld, I. E. (1950). Mutual role of sympathetic and parasympathetic in shaping of the pupillary reflex to light. Pupillographic studies. *Arch. Neurol. Psychiat.* **64**, 341–77.

Lowenstein, O. and Loewenfeld, I. E. (1969). The pupil. In *The eye* (ed. H. Davson), Vol. 3, pp. 255–337. Academic Press, New York.

Maloney, W. F., Younge, B. R., and Moyer, N. J. (1980). Evaluation of the causes and accuracy of pharmacologic localization in Horner's syndrome. *Am. J. Ophthalmol.* **90**, 394–402.

Martyn, C. N. and Ewing, D. J. (1986). Pupil cycle time: a simple way of measuring an autonomic reflex. *J. Neurol. Neurosurg. Psychiat.* **49**, 771–4.

Meek, E. S. and Thompson, H. S. (1979). Serum antibodies in Adie's syndrome. In *Topics in neuro-ophthalmology* (ed. H. S. Thompson, R. Daroff, L. Frisen, J. S. Glaser, and M. D. Sanders), pp. 119–21. Williams and Wilkins, Baltimore.

Pfeifer, M. A., Weinberg, C. R., Cook, D. L., Reenan, A., Halter, J. B., Ensink, J. W., and Porte, D. (1984). Autonomic neural dysfunction in recently diagnosed diabetic subjects. *Diabetes care* **7**, 447–53.

Rundles, R. W. (1945). Diabetic neuropathy. General review with report of 125 cases. *Medicine* **24**, 111–60.

Smith, S. A. (1982). Reduced sinus arrhythmia in diabetic autonomic neuropathy: diagnostic value of an age-related normal range. *Br. med. J.* **285**, 1599–601.

Smith, S. A. (1984). Diagnostic value of the Valsalva ratio reduction in diabetic autonomic neuropathy: use of an age-related normal range. *Diab. Med.* **1**, 295–7.

Smith, S. A. and Dewhirst, R. R. (1986). A simple diagnostic test for pupillary abnormality in diabetic autonomic neuropathy. *Diab. Med.* **3** 38–41.

Smith, S. A. and Smith, S. E. (1983*a*). Evidence for a neuropathic aetiology in the small pupil of diabetes mellitus. *Br. J. Ophthalmol.* **67**, 89–93.

Smith, S. A. and Smith, S. E. (1983*b*). Reduced pupillary light reflexes in diabetic autonomic neuropathy. *Diabetologia* **24**, 330–2.

Smith, S. E., Smith, S. A., Brown, P. M., Fox, C., and Sonksen, P. H. (1978). Pupillary signs in diabetic autonomic neuropathy. *Br. med. J.* **2**, 924–7.

St Thomas's Diabetic Study Group (1986). Failure of improved glycaemic control to reverse diabetic autonomic neuropathy. *Diab. Med.* **3**, 330–4.

Thompson, H. S. (1977). Adie's syndrome: some new observations. *Trans. Am. Ophthalmol. Soc.* **75**, 587–626.

Yoss, R. E., Moyer, N. J., and Ogle, K. N. (1969). The pupillogram and narcolepsy. *Neurology* **19**, 921–8.

23. Bladder and sexual dysfunction in diseases affecting the autonomic nervous system

Roger S. Kirby and Clare J. Fowler

INTRODUCTION

The urinary bladder and genitalia receive a rich innervation from the autonomic nervous system. It is not surprising, therefore, that disturbances of continence, micturition, and sexual function are commonly encountered in patients with autonomic dysfunction. When an individual presents with these symptoms, it may be difficult to decide whether they are the result of disease affecting the autonomic nervous system or simply the result of local abnormalities of the bladder and urethra, together with the changes of ageing. In such circumstances, sophisticated urodynamic, electromyographic, and neurohistochemical testing may be helpful in establishing the diagnosis. Although the management of such patients is usually supportive rather than curative, much may be done to prevent renal impairment and alleviate their symptoms.

METHODS OF INVESTIGATION

An intravenous urogram and measurement of urinary flow rate are good initial screening tests. If the bladder empties completely with a normal flow pattern, a significant abnormality of the innervation of the bladder is unlikely. Urodynamic assessment of the detrusor response to filling and the pressure-flow characteristics of micturition are often helpful; these may usefully be combined with fluoroscopy to study bladder neck competence and urethral configuration during voiding. The striated muscle of the urethra is tonically active and only normally relaxes at the time of micturition. Kinetic studies of the electromyographic (EMG) activity of the sphincter during urodynamics may demonstrate a failure of relaxation resulting in obstruction of urinary flow.

EMG examination of the urethral muscle with a coaxial needle electrode allows individual motor units to be analysed. Abnormalities of their proportions and configuration provide a sensitive index of muscle re-innervation, which occurs after denervation (Fowler *et al.* 1984).

The measurement of sacral reflex latencies and cortical evoked responses has been advocated by some, but these techniques are usually more appropriate for the investigation of lesions affecting the somatic rather than autonomic nervous system.

Histochemical studies of bladder biopsies have revealed marked differences in patients with diseases affecting the autonomic nervous system compared with controls. However, caution should be exercised in the interpretation of such data in individual cases, as the peripheral innervation of the bladder may be profoundly affected by local factors such as outflow obstruction and overdistension and advancing age (Gilpin *et al.* 1986; Gosling *et al.* 1986).

AUTONOMIC FAILURE WITH MULTIPLE SYSTEM ATROPHY

Urinary and sexual dysfunction are prominent features of autonomic failure with multiple system atrophy (MSA) and were described in the original report of Shy and Drager in 1960. Indeed, erectile impotence occurring in middle age is usually the first symptom of the disease in males; later ejaculatory failure occurs. Frequency and urgency of micturition occur, together with a reduced and intermittent stream, and may closely mimic prostatic obstruction. Urinary leakage is associated with an urgent desire to void at first but, as the disease progresses, stress leakage develops; later, incontinence becomes almost constant and is associated with a large residual urinary volume. In spite of this retained urine, dilatation of the ureters and kidneys is unusual in this condition. On examination the bladder is usually impalpable, but the anal sphincter tone is greatly reduced. The most important general sign of autonomic failure is a pronounced fall in blood pressure on standing.

Urodynamic investigation reveals normal urethral and bladder sensation. Bladder filling provokes involuntary bladder contractions which result in leakage that the patient appears powerless to prevent (Fig. 23.1(a), (b)). In more advanced cases the magnitude of these unstable contractions appears diminished, and the bladder becomes 'atonic'. At all stages of bladder filling the proximal urethra is widely incompetent—an important feature best demonstrated by a cystogram with the patient in the erect position (Fig. 23.2).

The ability to develop a voluntary bladder contraction appears to be lost in the early stages of the disease and voiding is intermittent, incomplete, and achieved by abdominal straining. The explanation for

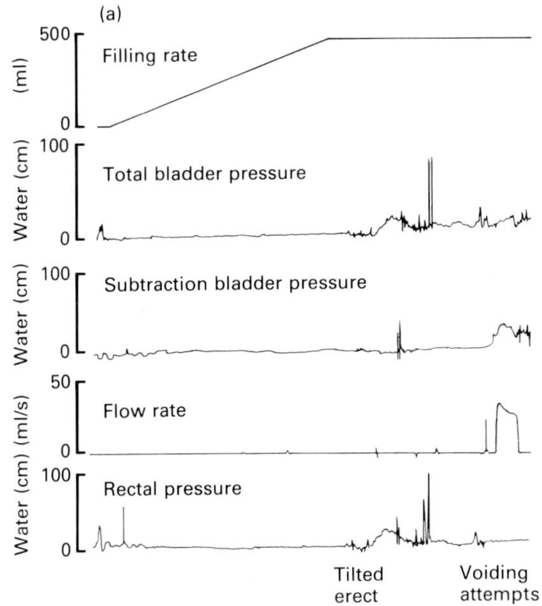

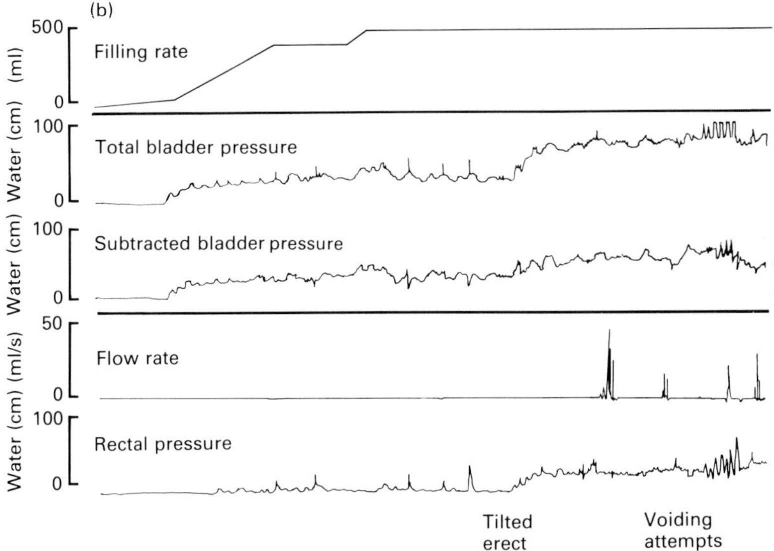

Fig. 23.1. (a) A cystometrogram in a normal subject demonstrating accommodation (i.e. the absence of an intravesicular pressure rise) in response to bladder filling at a rate of 50 ml/min. Normal micturition is achieved at a pressure of 25 cm of water and at a maximum flow of 25 ml/s. (b) A cystometrogram in a patient with autonomic failure and MSA. Note the rise in bladder pressure in response to filling and the absence of a voluntary bladder contraction when the patient is asked to micturate.

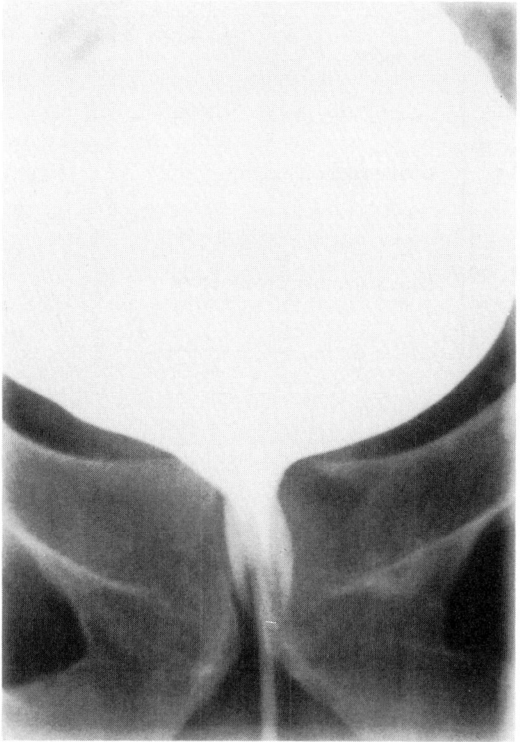

Fig. 23.2. A cystogram showing the open bladder neck which is characteristic of autonomic failure with MSA.

these features lies in the degenerative changes that affect the basal ganglia and midbrain; both the corpus striatum and pontine nuclei have been shown to profoundly influence bladder activity in experimental animals. These more central effects are undoubtedly compounded by progressive cell loss from the preganglionic autonomic neurons of the thoracolumbar and sacral spinal segments, which will eventually result in a decentralized bladder akin to that seen after injury to the cauda equina or pelvic nerves.

Patients who suffer from autonomic failure with MSA show a characteristic inability to contract the distal urinary sphincter adequately to prevent urinary leakage. Urethral sphincter EMG studies have shown that individual motor units, which appear polyphasic and of long duration, are clearly abnormal when compared with controls (Kirby *et al.* 1986) (Fig. 23.3(a)–(d)). Sakuta *et al.* (1978) reported the same phenomenon in the external anal sphincter muscle of patients with this disorder. The presence of these abnormal motor units provides unequivocal evidence of continuing denervation and attempts at re-

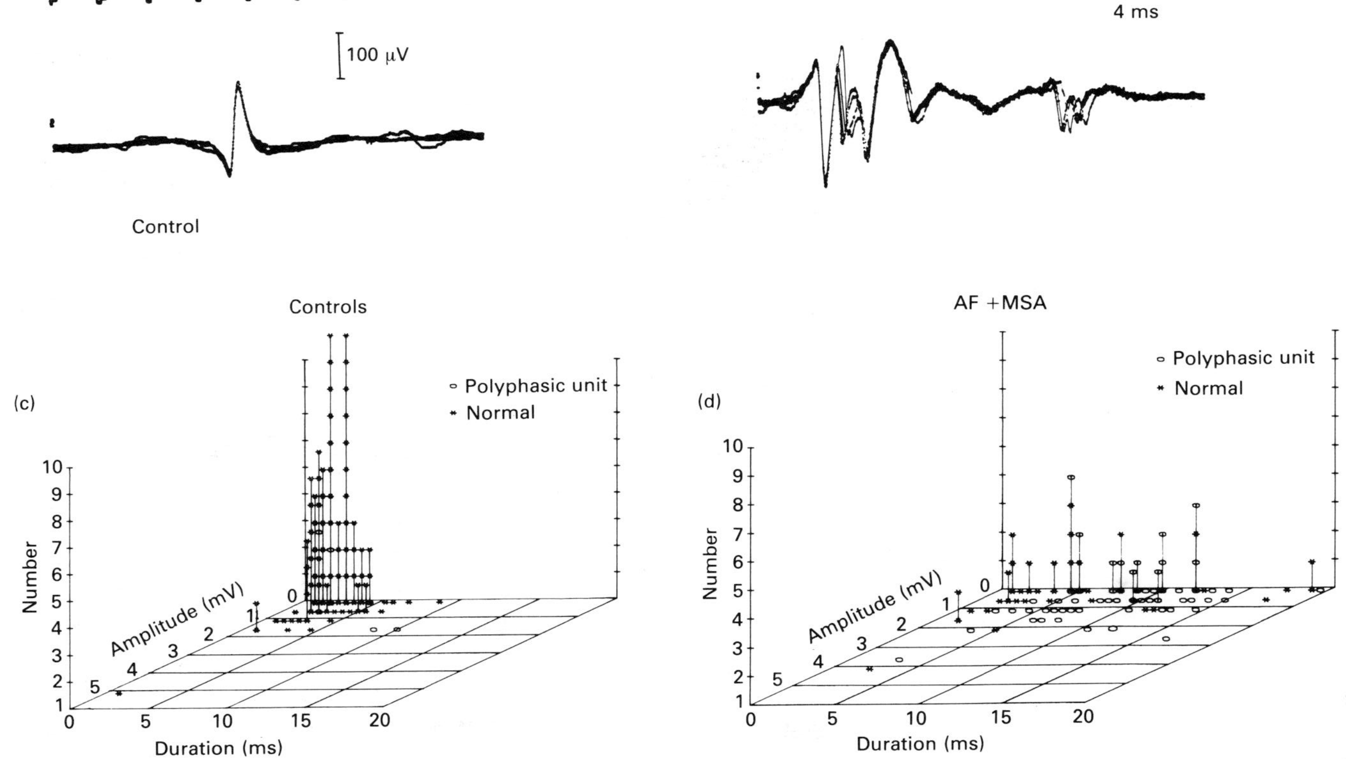

Fig. 23.3. (a) An individual motor unit recorded from the striated muscle of the urethra in a control patient. (b) An individual motor unit from a patient with autonomic failure and MSA. (c) A three-dimensional histogram showing the characteristics of motor units recorded from the urethral sphincter of 20 control subjects. Note how they are clustered and how most units are less than 6 mV in amplitude and shorter than 2 ms in duration. (d) A three-dimensional histogram showing the characteristics of motor units recorded from the urethral sphincter muscle of 16 patients with autonomic failure (AF) with MSA. The majority of units are outside the control parameters for amplitude and duration.

innervation of the striated sphincter muscle. Sung *et al.* (1978) demonstrated that patients with autonomic failure and MSA suffer specific neuronal degeneration of Onuf's nucleus, a particular area within the anterior horn of the sacral cord which has been shown in experimental animals to be responsible for the innervation of the external anal and striated urethral sphincters.

Degeneration of motor neurons at this site would result in denervation of sphincter muscle fibres; and re-innervation could occur from collateral sprouting of surviving motor nerves, as is seen in skeletal muscle in motor neuron disease. It is known that the striated muscle of the urethra plays a part in the rapid adjustments of urethral pressure necessary to prevent urinary leakage when intra-abdominal pressure rises or involuntary bladder contractions occur. Loss of this ability to achieve such adjustments, especially when associated with an unstable detrusor activity and incompetence of the proximal urethra, may account for the severity of the incontinence in patients with autonomic failure and MSA.

While denervation affecting voluntary skeletal muscle occasionally occurs in autonomic failure with MSA, it is never a prominent feature. It is a matter for speculation as to why the motor neurons of the urethral and anal sphincters should be selectively vulnerable in this disease. In other degenerative disorders, such as motor neuron disease, where there is severe generalized anterior horn cell loss, the cells of Onuf's nucleus have been shown to be spared. Clearly, these cells differ in some fundamental way from other motor neurons. The striated muscle of the urethral and anal sphincters differs from other skeletal muscle in exhibiting tonic EMG activity, which persists even in sleep and light general anaesthesia. The only structure that bears close comparison is the larynx, whose posterior cricoarytenoid muscle is constantly active to maintain abductor tone.

Significantly, EMG studies of the cricoarytenoid muscles have revealed evidence of denervation in patients with autonomic failure and MSA (Guindi *et al.* 1981) and histological examination has confirmed changes consistent with denervation atrophy (Bannister *et al.* 1981). It seems that there is some property of these neurons (located in Onuf's nucleus in the case of the urethral and anal sphincters, and the nucleus ambiguus in the case of the larynx), perhaps related to their capacity to fire tonically, that distinguishes them from the neurons of other skeletal muscles and determines their vulnerability in this disease.

Since the degenerative neuronal loss that occurs in autonomic failure and MSA cannot be arrested or reversed, treatments of the bladder disturbances are, at best, supportive. Most important is the recognition of the diagnosis and avoidance of transurethral surgery, which invariably makes incontinence worse. Unfortunately, cholinergic agents do not seem to improve voluntary bladder contractions and, although sympathomimetic drugs may increase urethral resistance, they also carry a risk of hypertension, due to the extreme supersensitivity of agonist agents in this disorder. Eventually, urinary incontinence may need to be treated by external urinary appliances in men or either intermittent or indwelling catheterization in females. The poor prognosis in patients suffering this condition generally precludes treatment by implantation of artificial sphincter devices.

PARKINSON'S DISEASE

Although idiopathic Parkinson's disease is not usually considered as a disease which prominently affects the autonomic nervous system, bladder disturbances are common in this condition. The nature of the vesicourethral dysfunction encountered in the disease differs markedly from that found in autonomic failure with MSA and produces some interesting contrasts. These differences may sometimes be valuable in distinguishing patients with idiopathic Parkinson's disease from those with autonomic failure with parkinsonism.

Patients with idiopathic Parkinson's disease commonly suffer frequency of micturition and urge continence. Occasionally, urinary retention occurs, which necessitates catheterization. Many patients report that their bladder symptoms vary markedly according to the efficiency of therapeutic control of their disease.

Urodynamic studies in these patients have revealed a high incidence of involuntary detrusor contractions which occur in response to bladder filling. Because the basal ganglia, especially the globus pallidus and substantia nigra, have been shown to exert an inhibitory influence on the bladder in animals (Lewin *et al.* 1967), it has been argued that an absence of this inhibition may account for the involuntary bladder contractions seen in humans with Parkinson's disease. If this theory is correct, improvement in the cystometrogram might be expected when the patients' parkinsonism symptoms are adequately controlled by medication.

In a study designed to investigate this, 10 parkinsonian patients with the 'on–off' syndrome were assessed both 'on' and 'off' their antiparkinsonian treatment. Although there were differences in the cystometrograms in the two states, the changes were unpredictable (Fitzmaurice *et al.* 1986). This would seem to indicate that, although the basal ganglia are involved in the neurophysiological control of bladder function, their influence is more complex than simple inhibition of the pontine micturition centre.

Incontinence in Parkinson's disease is much less troublesome than that encountered in autonomic failure with MSA. This may partly be explained by the observation that the innervation and function of the striated muscle of the urethra is unimpaired in idiopathic Parkinson's disease. Individual motor units recorded from the striated muscle of the urethra in parkinsonian patients were indistinguishable from those recorded in a series of age-matched controls (Fig. 23.4).

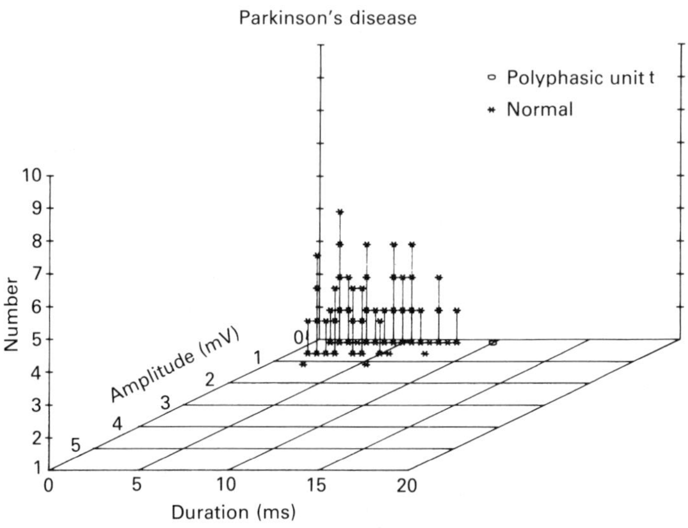

Fig. 23.4. A three-dimensional histogram showing the characteristics of motor units recorded from the urethral sphincter of 10 patients with idiopathic Parkinson's disease. The units are clustered as in normal subjects (Fig. 23.3(c)) and few exceed the control limits of 6 mV and 2 ms. This confirms that peripheral sphincter innervation is preserved in idiopathic Parkinson's disease.

This finding has important implications in the management of the bladder problems of these patients. Because the disease affects mainly elderly people, a proportion of patients will also suffer coexistent prostatic obstruction. When this occurs, there is usually urodynamic evidence of a high voiding pressure and a low flow rate, and also radiological narrowing of the prostatic urethra during voiding. In these circumstances a carefully performed transurethral resection of the prostate carries little risk of subsequent incontinence; however, the patient should be warned that some degree of frequency and urgency or micturition may persist as a result of the involuntary bladder contractions that occur in Parkinson's disease.

DISTAL AUTONOMIC NEUROPATHY

In 1969 Young *et al.* reported a case of autonomic neuropathy of subacute onset, which developed over a period of a few weeks and was followed by a complete recovery. Normal function of central and peripheral somatic nervous systems was preserved. Since this publication 14 other reports of distal autonomic neuropathy, involving both sympathetic and parasympathetic functions, have appeared in the literature and the condition has become known as pandysautonomia. A variant of the disorder which affects only the parasympathetic limb of the autonomic nervous system has also been described; there have been five patients reported with this condition, which has been termed cholinergic dysautonomia.

These conditions appear to affect both sexes, but children seem especially susceptible to the cholinergic type. Painful urinary retention invariably occurs. In addition, there may be an acute or subacute onset of lethargy with symptoms of blurred vision, decreased tear formation, loss of sweating, and abdominal distension. Male patients experience erectile impotence and, in pandysautonomia, also lose their ability to ejaculate. Recovery in either pandysautonomia or cholinergic dysautonomia is often incomplete and occurs over a variable period.

Peripheral nerve conduction studies have been normal in those patients who have no features of a more generalized neuropathy (Guillain–Barré syndrome). Sural nerve biopsy of patients with pandysautonomia has revealed no abnormality of myelinated fibres, but in the case reported by Appenzeller and Kornfield (1973) there was an increase in the density of small unmyelinated (C) fibres which corresponded to recovering function and which might be regarded as consistent with regeneration of autonomic nerve fibres. Detailed study of the bladder dysfunction which occurs in these conditions has been limited to two patients (Kirby *et al.* 1985). Urodynamic investigation revealed normal bladder sensation in both pandysautonomia and cholinergic dysautonomia. However, the conditions differed in their response to bladder filling; in cholinergic dysautonomia the intravesicular pressure remained low, as in the normal individual, while in pandysautonomia there was a steep rise in intravesicular pressure that denotes a loss of bladder compliance. This is probably the result of a loss of normal β-adrenergically mediated inhibition of detrusor smooth-muscle tone in pandysautonomia. In both conditions there is a loss of the ability to achieve a voluntary detrusor contraction with consequent retention of urine.

Bladder muscle biopsies processed to demonstrate tissue acetylcholinesterases revealed a profound loss of enzyme-positive nerves from the muscular layers of the bladder wall in both conditions. By contrast, there was a striking preservation of the subepithelial plexus of acetylcholinesterase-containing nerves (Fig. 23.5). These results lend weight to the view that enzyme-containing nerves in the muscular layer of the

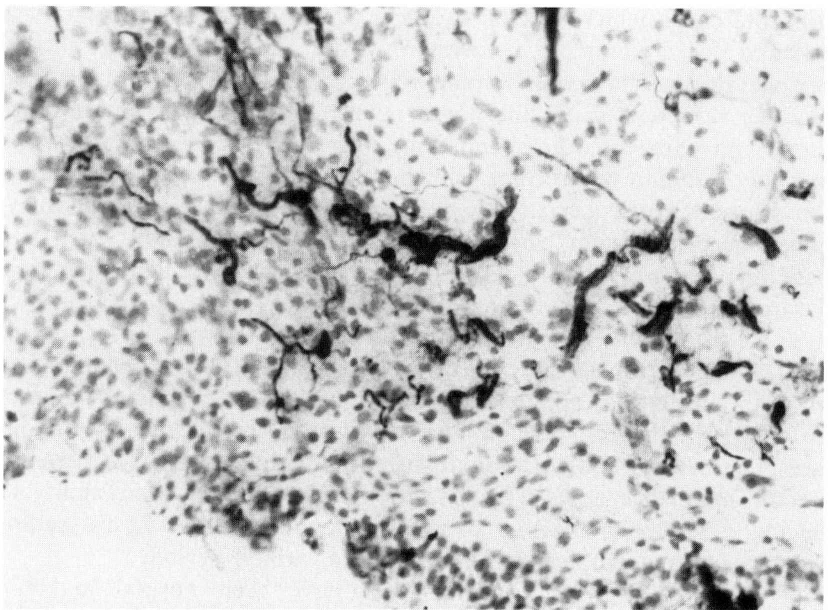

Fig. 23.5. A bladder biopsy from a patient with pure cholinergic dysautonomia showing the preservation of sub-epithelial plexus of acetylcholinesterase-positive nerves.

bladder are motor in function, while those lying beneath the urothelium are sensory nerves.

Urethral sphincter electromyography in both patients with distal dysautonomia revealed normal motor units which were neither significantly greater in duration or amplitude than those encountered in controls, nor were they polyphasic. Although Elbadawi and Schenk (1974) reported that the striated muscle of the canine urethra has a unique triple innervation by sympathetic, parasympathetic, and somatic nerve fibres, the results in patients with distal autonomic neuropathy suggest that this is unlikely to be the case in man. Instead a purely somatic peripheral innervation seems more probable.

A point of contrast in the two variant forms of dysautonomia is the observed difficulty in the state of bladder-neck competence. In pure cholinergic dysautonomia the bladder neck is tightly closed (Fig. 23.6) while in pandysautonomia it is widely incompetent (Fig. 23.7). This observation supports the view that bladder-neck competence is dependent on a reflex arc, involving pelvic afferent fibres and hypogastric efferent (sympathetic) nerves, which is, of course, intact in cholinergic dysautonomia, but interrupted in pandysautonomia.

The management of the bladder dysfunction in either form of dysautonomia is supportive in anticipation of eventual partial recovery

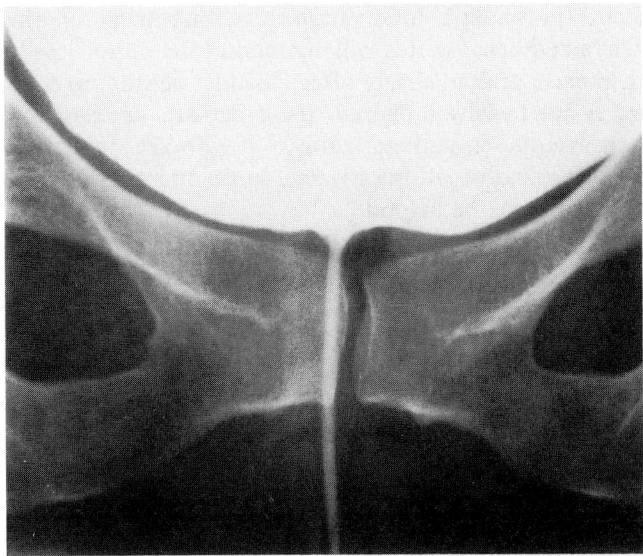

Fig. 23.6. A cystogram in a patient with pure cholinergic dysautonomia showing the preservation of sub-epithelial plexus of acetylcholinesterase-positive nerves.

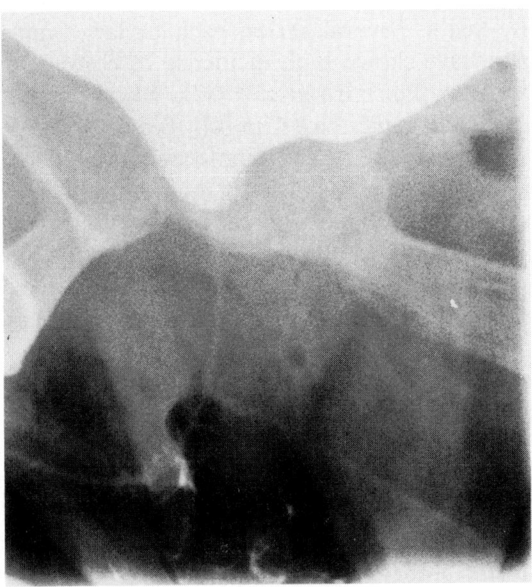

Fig. 23.7. A cystogram in a patient with pandysautonomia showing an open bladder neck.

of peripheral autonomic innervation. Overdistension of the bladder should be avoided because this will compound the motor loss by damage to smooth muscle and adversely affect bladder sensation. Since urinary continence is not usually impaired, these patients are best managed by clean intermittent self-catheterization. If urinary infections become troublesome, a low dose of prophylactic antibiotic such as trimethoprim or nitrofurantoin may be helpful.

DIABETES MELLITUS

Many different types of neuropathy may complicate diabetes, some of which include damage to unmyelinated fibres. The unmyelinated fibre component of peripheral nerve comprises autonomic efferent and afferent fibres conveying sensations of warmth and pain. Although in some unusual cases of diabetic neuropathy the neuropathic process appears initially to be selective for either the large myelinated fibres or thin unmyelinated fibres, the commonest presentation is of an insidious and gradually progressive neuropathy affecting the entire range of fibres.

Sexual dysfunction

An association between erectile impotence and diabetes has been recognized for many years. Several series, each of large numbers of male diabetic patients, have shown high incidence of between 39 and 59 per cent for this problem (Fairburn *et al.* 1982). Whether the complaint has an organic or psychogenic bases in all these cases is not known. Measurements of nocturnal penile tumescence reveal that, in a proportion of diabetics, the problem is non-organic (Hosking *et al.* 1979). Also, a rather brief but much quoted study claims that the incidence of impotence in diabetes is no higher than that of an age-matched control population (Lester *et al.* 1980). Despite these papers, the clinical impression that erectile impotence is a common complaint in diabetes persists.

The explanation for the high incidence of impotence in diabetics is not known. An incomplete knowledge of the mechanism of normal erection has made pathophysiological studies difficult, but over the years various hypotheses have been proposed. Current research suggests that penile erection results from a neurovascular reflex, mediated by the release of the powerful vasodilatory peptide VIP into cavernosal vessels from parasympathetic fibres. Either vascular insufficiency or autonomic neuropathy can reasonably be implicated in the pathogenesis of diabetic erectile impotence. Hormonal imbalance and an androgen deficiency have now been eliminated from the list of possible causes (Kolodny *et al.* 1974).

The production and maintenance of an erection requires a marked increase in penile blood flow. In impotent diabetics vascular lesions have been reported in both large vessels within the pelvis and small penile vessels. These arterial changes worsen with age, and, when diabetics were compared with non-diabetic men, the penile microangiopathy showed accelerated progression in diabetics (Rubarsky and Michel 1977).

It seems likely that the neuropathy which affects unmyelinated nerve fibres is important in the pathogenesis of erectile impotence. The difficulty with proving this hypothesis is a lack of appropriate investigations. Several studies have shown that the latency of the bulbocavernosus response may be abnormal in a proportion of men with diabetic impotence, but other diabetic men, who are also impotent, may have entirely normal reflex responses (Ertekin and Reel 1976). This is not surprising since such tests examine the conduction velocity of the largest myelinated nerve fibres innervating the pudenda, which are probably of no importance in erection. Tests for autonomic neuropathy are based largely on examining cardiovascular responses to deep breathing, the Valsalva manoeuvre, or sustained handgrip. These reflexes have been shown to be abnormal in diabetics with symptoms of autonomic neuropathy such as postural hypotension or nocturnal diarrhoea and impotence, but in men with impotence alone, no abnormality may be found (Ewing *et al.* 1974). This does not exclude the possibility that erectile failure is the earliest manifestation of autonomic neuropathy becoming a problem before abnormalities of the cardiovascular reflexes develop. However, the claim of preserved potency by men with demonstrably abnormal cardiovascular reflexes argues against the hypothesis.

More light may be shed on this problem by the advent of methods for accurately measuring cutaneous thresholds for warming, a sensation conveyed in the unmyelinated fibres. A preliminary study (Fowler *et al.* 1987) has shown that, of 15 diabetics attending a clinic for the treatment of impotence and who were considered neuropathic on grounds of history and response to corporeal injections of papaverine, 14 had lost the ability to perceive warming on the feet. Four diabetics and 12 other non-diabetic men also attending the clinic, who were not thought to have neurogenic impotence, had thresholds within the normal range. This finding argues strongly that an unmyelinated fibre neuropathy is an important cause of impotence in diabetics.

Characteristically, the impotence of diabetes has a gradual onset, with diminishing firmness of erections, ending in complete failure. Sexual interest is maintained at a normal level and ejaculation and orgasm are preserved. By contrast, psychogenic impotence has an abrupt onset, and failure of erection is most marked with attempts at sexual intercourse, but present in other circumstances.

Ejaculatory failure in diabetes is much less common than erectile impotence. When it does occur it may be the result of impairment of sympathetic innervation of the bladder neck. This structure normally closes tightly at the time of ejaculation, directing semen down the urethra. If the bladder neck is incompetent, retrograde ejaculation of semen into the bladder will occur.

Investigations should be directed towards distinguishing between psychogenic and organic impotence. A normal male experiences three to five erections, each lasting 25–35 minutes, during a nights' sleep. This ability may be assessed by nocturnal tumescence testing in which two strain gauges are placed around the penis and connected to a strip recorder. The investigation is usually performed over two or three consecutive nights. Complete absence of nocturnal erections is highly suggestive of an organic cause for the impotence. Recently, intra-corporeal injections of papaverine (30–60 mg) have been used as a means of diagnosing impotence. This substance, which may be combined with the α-adrenergic blocking agent, phentolamine, normally produces an erection which lasts from 2 to 6 hours. This effect is the combined result of vasodilatation of the arteries supplying the corpora and simultaneous reduction of venous outflow. An absent or reduced response to these agents is suggestive of organic impotence, but there is still controversy as to whether this test is useful in distinguishing between neurogenic and vasculogenic lesions.

The blood supply to the corpora may be assessed by penile plethysmography or by Doppler probes. Pudendal arteriography may be employed to diagnose large-vessel disease, which may improve with percutaneous angioplasty or vascular bypass procedures. Infusion cavernosography, usually combined with intracorporeal papaverine, is used to diagnose 'venous leaks' which may be the cause of one form of organic impotence. These may be successfully corrected by ligation of the abnormal venous communications.

There is no treatment to restore potency once it has been lost as a result of autonomic neuropathy in diabetes. The problem should be discussed with the patient and his partner, and many, particularly older patients, will opt for a sexual relationship which is not based on coitus. Younger patients may choose to undergo operation for insertion of penile prostheses. It must be explained to the patient that, although the prosthesis will provide the means of vaginal penetration, the sensory aspects of sexual relations may be lacking.

The choice of penile prostheses rests between the malleable and inflatable varieties. The former are extremely reliable, but concealment is sometimes a problem, since the penis remains semi-rigid at all times. Inflatable prostheses are more natural, in being rigid only at the time of intercourse, but are considerably more expensive. Brantley–Scott prostheses provide the best cosmetic results but are prone to mechanical failure. The newer *Flexiflate* and *Hydroflex* prostheses have incorporated the pump mechanism and reservoir and are therefore simpler to implant and less susceptible to malfunction.

Retrograde ejaculation due to autonomic neuropathy is not usually a serious problem, unless the patient wishes to impregnate his partner. In these circumstances it may be necessary to retrieve spermatozoa from the urine for insemination. If the failure is of recent onset, or incomplete, it is sometimes possible to restore ejaculation with sympathomimetic agents such as ephedrine or disipramine.

Bladder dysfunction

Considering the frequency with which erectile impotence is encountered in diabetic males, it is surprising that symptomatic disturbances of bladder function are comparatively uncommon. Ellenburg and Weber (1967) argued that this simply reflects the fact that many diabetic patients suffer asymptomatic impairment of lower-urinary-tract function and that this often goes unrecognized. The exact prevalence of neurocystopathy among diabetics remains a matter of debate; the reported incidence varies from 25 (Rundles 1945) to 87 per cent (Faerman *et al.* 1971)—a divergence that probably reflects differences in methods of diagnosis and patient selection.

The onset of diabetic cystopathy is usually insidious with progressive impairment of bladder emptying which may culminate in chronic urinary retention. An intravenous urogram will often reveal a large post-micturition urinary volume (Fig. 23.8), but dilatation of the upper tracts is unusual. Urodynamic assessment shows a hypotonic, large-capacity bladder with reduced sensation and impaired voluntary detrusor contraction.

The bladder and urethra are innervated by efferent and afferent sympathetic, parasympathetic, and somatic nerves, all of which may be affected in diabetic neuropathy. However, the observation that the proximal urethra is competent in most cases of diabetic neurocystopathy suggests that, as in the cardiovascular system, sympathetic denervation of the urinary tract is a relatively late feature of diabetes.

The predominant neural lesion in diabetic neurocystopathy probably affects sensory afferent axons which pass in the pelvic nerves to the posterior horns of the second to fourth sacral segments. Impaired conduction of bladder-wall tension and stretch-receptor information will

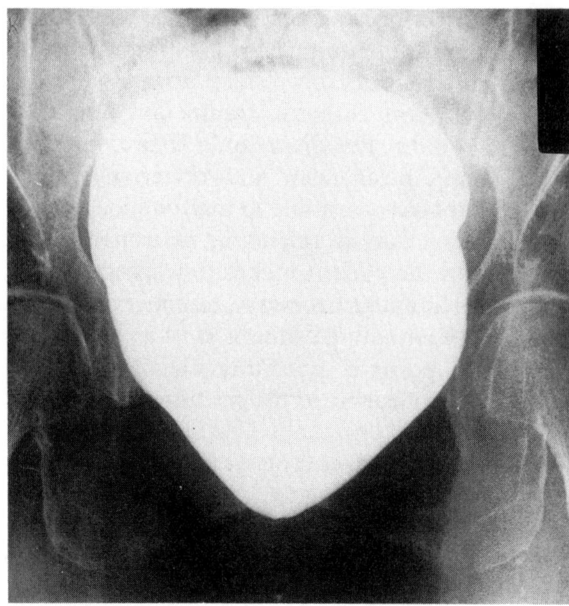

Fig. 23.8. A cystogram in a patient with diabetes showing an enormously distended bladder.

reduce conscious sensation of bladder filling and also impair the facilitation of pontine micturition centre activity that normally occurs during micturition.

The ability of the detrusor muscle to contract may be further impaired by neuropathic involvement of efferent parasympathetic fibres. Faerman and colleagues (1973) studied the axons in the bladder wall of 10 diabetic patients and demonstrated morphological changes consistent with a peripheral autonomic neuropathy. These workers reported that the density of acetylcholinesterase-positive nerve fibres appeared markedly reduced compared with controls, and we have confirmed this observation quantitively. However, the significance of this finding is uncertain because it is not clear to what extent motor efferent nerves to the bladder have to be lost before there is an appreciable decline in detrusor contractility.

The striated muscle of the urethral sphincter is supplied by the perineal branches of the pudendal nerves. The denervation and re-innervation processes which affect all striated muscle in diabetic neuropathy do not spare the striated muscle of the urethral sphincter. The state of sphincter innervation has a bearing on the management of diabetic patients with disturbances of bladder function. The principal aim should be to improve bladder emptying and to reduce the risk of urinary-tract infection. Urodynamic evaluation should be performed in order to distinguish those patients with large bladders due to neurocystopathy from those with bladder outflow obstruction. The patient with a grossly overdistended bladder should undergo an initial period of catheter drainage, which in itself seems to improve bladder sensation and contractility. Thereafter, instructions should be given to void by the clock, rather than waiting for a conscious sensation of bladder distension, which may, of course, be absent. The ability of the bladder to empty more completely should theoretically be enhanced by cholinergic agents, such as carbachol or bethanechol, but in practice these agents are seldom effective. Although bladder-neck incision or resection has been advocated in diabetic patients with the aim of reducing urethral resistance (Emmett *et al.* 1949), such an irrevocable step should be approached with caution. Destruction of the proximal urethral sphincter mechanism will leave the patient dependent on a distal striated sphincter which may be demonstrably neuropathic. An incidence of urinary incontinence following this procedure has even been reported by its advocates (Zinke *et al.* 1974). Ideally, urethral sphincter electromyography should be undertaken to confirm the integrity of the innervation of the striated urethral muscle before transurethral surgery to the proximal urethra is considered. Urethral resistance may be reversibly reduced by the α_1 selective adrenoceptor blocking agent prazosin, which seems to have fewer adverse effects than phenoxybenzamine. However, its efficiency is usually insufficient to achieve satisfactory bladder emptying and most patients are best managed by clean intermittent self-catheterization.

REFERENCES

Appenzeller, O. and Kornfield, M. (1973). Acute pandysautonomia: clinical and morphological study. *Arch. Neurol.* **29**, 334–9.

Bannister, R., Gibson, M., Michaels, L., and Oppenheimer, P. (1981). Laryngeal abductor paralysis in multiple system atrophy. *Brain* **104**, 351–86.

Elbadawi, A. and Schenk, E. (1974). A new theory of the innervation of the vesico-urethral junction and the external urethral sphincter. *J. Urol.* **111**, 613–15.

Ellenberg, M. and Weber, H. (1967). The incipient asymptomatic diabetic bladder. *Diabetes* **16**, 331–5.

Emmett, J. L., Daut, R. V., and Sprague, R. G. (1949). Transurethral resection for neurogenic vesical dysfunction in cases of diabetic neuropathy. *J. Urol.* **61**, 244–56.

Ertekin, C. and Reel, F. (1976). Bulbocavernosus reflex in normal men and patients with neurogenic bladder and/or impotence. *J. neurol. Sci.* **28**, 1–15.

Ewing, D. J., Campbell, I. W., Burt, A. A., and Clarke, B. F. (1974). Sexual dysfunction in diabetic men. *Diabetes* **23**, 306–9.

Faerman, I., Glocer, L., Celener, S., Jadzinsky, M., Fox, D., Maler, M., and Alvanez, E. (1973). Autonomic nervous system and diabetes. Histological and histochemical study of nerve fibres of the urinary bladder in diabetic patients. *Diabetes* **22**, 225–37.

Faerman, I., Maler, M., Jadinsky, M., Arranes, E., Fox, D., Silberrang, J., Cibeira, J. B., and Colinas, R. (1971). Asymptomatic neurogenic bladder in juvenile diabetes. *Diabetologia* **7**, 168–72.

Fairburn, C. G., McCullock, D. W., and Win, F. C. (1982). The effects of diabetes on male sexual function. *Clin. Endocrinol. Metabol.* **11**, 749.

Fitzmaurice, H., Fowler, C. J., Rickards, D., Kirby, R. S., Quinn, N. P., Marsden, C. D., Milroy, E. J. G., and Turner-Warwick, R. T. (1986). Micturition disturbances in Parkinson's disease. *Br. J. Urol.* **57**, 652–6.

Fowler, C. J., Ali, Z., Kirby, R. S., and Pryor, J. P. (1987). The value of testing for unmyelinated fibre sensory neuropathy in diabetic impotence. *Br. J. Urol.* (In press.)

Fowler, C. J., Kirby, R. S., Harrison, M. J. G., Milroy, E. J. G., and Turner-Warwick, R. T. (1984). Individual motor unit analysis in the diagnosis of disorders of urethral sphincter function. *J. Neurol. Neurosurg. Psychiat.* **47**, 637–41.

Gilpin, S. A., Gilpin, C. J., Dixon, J. S., Gosling, J. A., and Kirby, R. S. (1986). The effect of age on the autonomic innervation of the bladder. *Br. J. Urol.* **58**, 378–81.

Gosling, J. A., Gilpin, S. A., Dixon, J. S., and Gilpin, C. J. (1986). Decrease in autonomic innervation of human detrusor muscle in outflow obstruction. *J. Urol.* **136**, 501–4.

Guindi, G. M., Bannister, R., Gibson, W. P. R., and Payne, J. H. (1981). Laryngeal electromyography in multiple system atrophy with autonomic failure. *J. Neurol. Neurosurg. Psychiat.* **44**, 49–53.

Hosking, D. J., Bennet, T., Hampton, J. R., Evans, D. F., Clark, A. J., and Robertson, G. (1979). Diabetic impotence: studies of nocturnal erection during REM sleep. *Br. med. J.* **ii**, 1285–454.

Kirby, R. S., Fowler, C. J., Gosling, J. A., and Bannister, R. (1985). Bladder dysfunction in distal autonomic neuropathy of acute onset. *J. Neurol. Neurosurg. Psychiat.* **48**, 762–7.

Kirby, R. S., Fowler, C. J., Gosling, J., and Bannister, R. (1986). Urethro-vesical dysfunction in progressive autonomic failure with multiple system atrophy. *J. Neurol. Neurosurg. Psychiat.* **49**, 554–62.

Kolodny, R. C., Kahn, C. B., Goldstein, H. H., and Barnett, D. M. (1974). Sexual dysfunction in diabetic men. *Diabetes* **23**, 306–9.

Lester, E., Wordraffe, F. J., and Smith, R. J. (1980). Impotence in diabetic and non-diabetic outpatients. *Br. med. J.* **281**, 354–5.

Lewin, R. J., Dillard, G. V., and Porter, R. W. (1967). Extrapyramidal inhibition of the urinary bladder. *Brain Res.* **4**, 301–7.

Rubarsky, V. and Michel, V. (1977). Morphological changes in the arterial bed of the penis with ageing. Relationship to the pathogenesis of impotence. *Invest. Urol.* **15**, 194.

Rundles, R. W. (1945). Diabetic neuropathy. General review with a report of 125 cases. *Medicine* **24**, 111–52.

Sakuta, M. S., Nakaniski, T., and Toyakuru, M. (1978). Anal muscle electromyograms differ in lateral sclerosis and Shy–Drager syndrome. *Neurology* **28**, 1289–93.

Shy, G. M. and Drager, G. A. (1960). A neurological syndrome associated with orthostatic hypotension. *Arch. Neurol.* **2**, 511–27.

Sung, J. H., Mastri, A. R., and Segal, E. (1978). Pathology of the Shy–Drager syndrome. *J. Neuropathol. exp. Neurol.* **38**, 253–68.

Young, R. R., Ashbury, A. K., Adams, R. D., and Corbett, J. L. (1969). Pure pandysautonomiea with recovery. *Trans. Am. neurol. Ass.* **94**, 355–7.

Zinke, H., Campbell, J. T., Palumbo, P. J., and Furlow, W. L. (1974). Neurogenic vesical dysfunction in diabetes: another look at vesical neck resection. *J. Urol.* **111**, 488–90.

24. Sleep apnoea and respiratory disturbances in multiple system atrophy with autonomic failure

Sudhansu Chokroverty

INTRODUCTION

Since the original description of Shy and Drager (1960) of a neurodegenerative disorder characterized by autonomic failure and multiple system atrophy there have been numerous reports (Bannister *et al.* 1967, 1972, 1981; Chokroverty *et al.* 1969; Chokroverty 1984) of the condition which has generally come to be known as the Shy–Drager syndrome or autonomic failure with multiple system atrophy (Chokroverty 1984). Multiple system atrophy (MSA) presents initially with autonomic failure (AF) and is associated later with progressive somatic neurological manifestations affecting multiple systems, particularly the extrapyramidal and cerebellar pathways. Because of the close proximity of the central autonomic, respiratory, and hypnogenic neurons (Chokroverty 1986), and known degeneration of these structures in the brainstem in MSA it is plausible to expect dysfunction of the respiratory control mechanism in parallel fashion along with the autonomic and somatic deficits. This chapter is concerned with respiratory dysrhythmias during sleep and wakefulness in MSA. A basic familiarity with the control of breathing during wakefulness and sleep and with the interrelationship among the neurons responsible for the control of breathing, sleep–wake states, and autonomic functions is a prerequisite to an understanding of the ventilatory dysrhythmias in MSA.

THE STATES OF SLEEP

Based on the electroencephalographic (EEG), behavioural, and physiological observations, two types of sleep have been recognized (Chokroverty

1986): non-rapid eye movement (non-REM) or slow-wave sleep comprising 75–80 per cent and rapid eye movement (REM) or paradoxical sleep comprising 20–25 per cent of sleep time in adults. EEG criteria establish four stages of non-REM sleep: Stages I–IV. The EEG findings during stage I consist of general disorganization of background rhythm, diminution of the alpha rhythm, and the appearance of a mixture of theta (4–7 Hz) and beta (> 13 Hz) rhythms. Stage II is characterized by sleep spindles of 12–14 Hz and K complexes, and the record contains less than 20 per cent delta (< 4 Hz) activity. EEG during stage III sleep shows 20–50 per cent of delta activity. In stage IV the EEG contains more than 50 per cent of delta waves.

In normal individuals REM sleep begins 60 to 90 minutes after sleep onset and recurs in a cyclical manner every 90 minutes throughout the night. REM sleep is divided into tonic and phasic stages (Chokroverty 1986). Desynchronized EEG, hypotonia of the axial muscles (antigravity, orofacial, and posterior neck muscles), and depression of monosynaptic and polysynaptic reflexes constitute the tonic stage. The phasic stage is discontinuous and superimposed on tonic stage. The phasic events consist of bursts of rapid eye movements, myoclonic twitchings of the facial and limb muscles, irregular heart rate, and respiration with variable blood pressure, spontaneous middle ear muscle activity, and phasic tongue movements (Chokroverty 1986).

Based on the ablation and stimulation experiments, and pathological findings, it is believed that non-REM or synchronized sleep results from a combination of two factors (Chokroverty 1986): reduced activity of the ascending reticular activating system and an increased activity of the two hypnogenic centres (a diencephalic centre in the basal pre-optic region of the hypothalamus and a lower brainstem centre in the region of the nucleus tractus solitarius). REM sleep is dependent upon an interaction between the REM-off cells in the dorsal raphe nuclei and locus ceruleus and the REM-on cells in the gigantocellular tegmental fields located in the brainstem (Hauri 1982). The caudal third of the locus ceruleus is responsible for muscle hypotonia and the middle third triggers the phasic events of REM sleep. The locus ceruleus inhibits the gigantocellular tegmental field during non-REM sleep; during REM sleep this inhibition disappears and the gigantocellular tegmental field triggers the phasic events by generating ponto-geniculate-occipital spikes and desynchronizes the EEG (Hauri 1982; Chokroverty 1986). During REM sleep there is maximum cholinergic hyperactivity and aminergic hypoactivity. The serotonergic neurons located in the midline raphe nuclei of the brainstem are involved in the production of non-REM sleep. The serotonergic neurons initiate and maintain non-REM by inhibiting the cholinergic ascending reticular activating system; they also trigger REM sleep.

CONTROL OF BREATHING DURING WAKEFULNESS AND SLEEP

Two separate and independent controlling systems are responsible for breathing (Chokroverty 1986): a metabolic or automatic system and a voluntary or behavioural system. Both voluntary and metabolic systems operate during wakefulness but respiration during sleep depends upon the inherent rhythmicity of the automatic respiratory control system located in the medulla. These two controlling systems are complemented by a third system, the reticular arousal system exerting a tonic influence on the brainstem respiratory neurons (McNicholas *et al.* 1983). Two fundamental mechanisms are responsible for various changes in breathing during sleep: the reticular inhibition and the loss of wakefulness stimulus on automatic respiration.

Upper brainstem respiratory neurons are located (Cherniack and Longobardo 1986) in the rostral pons (pneumotaxic centre), and in the dorsolateral region of the lower pons (apneustic centre). These two centres influence the automatic respiratory neurons located in the medulla. The medullary respiratory neurons consist of two principal groups (Chokroverty 1986; Cherniack and Longobardo 1986): dorsal respiratory groups located in the nucleus tractus solitarius (NTS) responsible predominantly but not exclusively for inspiration and the ventral respiratory group located in the region of the nucleus ambiguus and retroambigualis responsible for both inspiration and expiration (Fig. 24.1). These respiratory premotor neurons send axons which decussate below the obex and descend in the reticulospinal tracts in the ventro-lateral spinal cord to synapse with spinal respiratory motor neurons innervating the various respiratory muscles. Respiratory rhythmogenesis depends on tonic inputs converging on the medullary neurons. The parasympathetic (vagal) afferents, the carotid and aortic body peripheral chemoreceptors, the central chemoreceptors located on the ventral surface of the medulla, the supramedullary (forebrain, midbrain, and pontine regions), and the reticular activating systems all influence the medullary respiratory neurons to regulate the rhythm, rate, and amplitude of breathing and internal homeostasis (Cherniack and Longobardo 1986; Chokroverty 1986). Figure 24.2 shows schematically the effects of various brainstem and vagal transections on the ventilatory patterns.

The voluntary breathing system originating in the cerebral cortex (forebrain and limbic system) controls respiration during wakefulness (Chokroverty 1986) in addition to participating in non-respiratory functions. This system descends partly to the automatic medullary controlling system but mostly descends with the corticobulbar and corticospinal tracts to the spinal respiratory motor neurons where these

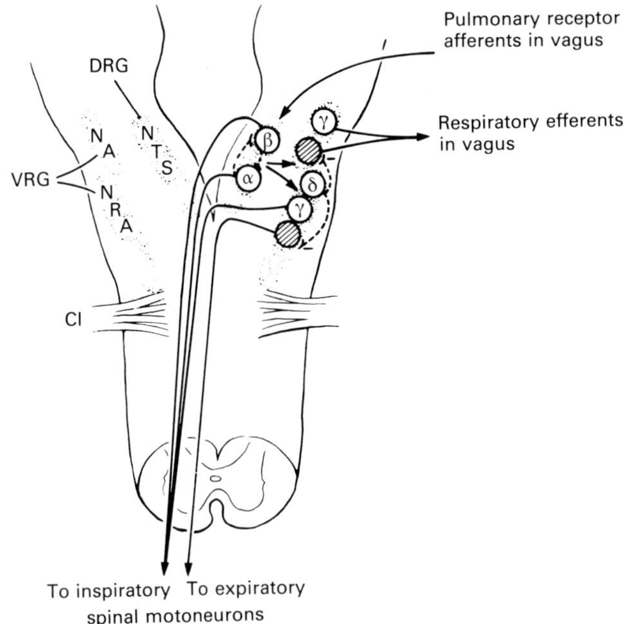

Fig. 24.1. Medullary respiratory neurons, cell types, and interconnections are shown schematically. DRG, Dorsal respiratory group; VRG, ventral respiratory group; NTS, nucleus tractus solitarius; NA, nucleus ambiguus; NRA, nucleus retro-ambigualis; CI, first cervical dorsal root; subscripts α, β, γ, δ, inspiratory cell subtype designations. The DRG located in the ventrolateral NTS is the site where vagal sensory information is first incorporated into a respiratory motor response. The DRG drives the VRG and some spinal inspiratory motoneurons. The VRG is composed of NA and NRA. Vagal respiratory motoneurons arise from NA. Axons from NRA project to some spinal inspiratory and probably all spinal expiratory motoneurons. Inspiratory cells are indicated by open circles, and expiratory by hatched circles. Dashed lines indicate some of the hypothesized intramedullary neural interconnections. (Taken with permission from Berger *et al.* (1977).)

fibres integrate with the reticulospinal fibres originating from the automatic medullary respiratory neurons.

There is a close interrelationship between the respiratory, central autonomic, and lower brainstem hypnogenic neurons in the pontomedullary region. Direct projections from the caudal portion of the NTS to the hypothalamic nuclei and hypothalamic fibres to the NTS and some to the nucleus ambiguus have been demonstrated (Brodal 1981). This reciprocal interrelationship suggests a delicate balance between the autonomic nervous system and the neurons controlling respiration and sleep–wake stages.

The control of respiration during non-REM sleep in normal individuals is entirely dependent upon the automatic control system

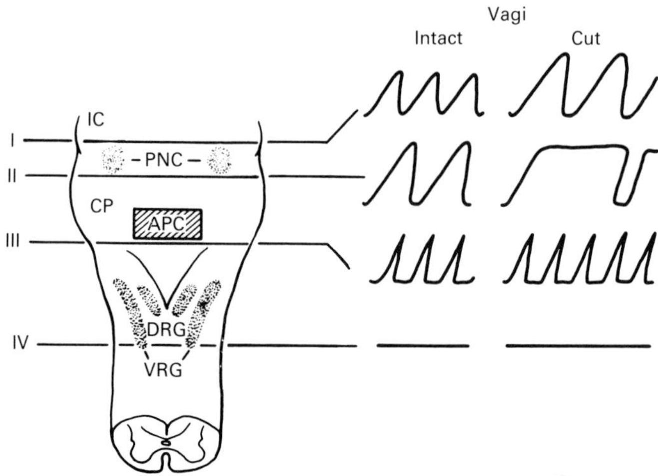

Fig. 24.2. Schematic representation of effects of various brainstem and vagal transections on the ventilatory pattern of the anaesthetized animal. IC, Inferior colliculus; PNC, pneumotaxic centre; CP, cerebellar peduncle; APC, apneustic centre; DRG, dorsal respiratory group; VRG, ventral respiratory group. On the left is a representation of the dorsal surface of the lower brainstem, and on the right, a representation of tidal volume with inspiration upwards. Transection I, just rostral to the PNC, does not affect normal breathing, but in combination with vagotomy, slow deep breathing results. Transection II, isolating the PNC from the lower brainstem, causes slow deep breathing with the vagi intact, and either apneusis (sustained inspiration) or apneustic breathing (rhythmic respiration with marked increase in inspiratory time) when the vagi are cut. Transection III, isolating structures rostral to the medulla, results in most cases in a regular gasping breathing that is generally not affected by vagotomy. Transection IV, at the medullospinal junction, results in respiratory arrest. (Taken with permission from Berger *et al.* (1977).)

(Phillipson and Bowes 1986). As a result of hyposensitivity of the respiratory neurons to CO_2, the inhibition of the reticular activating system, and alteration of the metabolic control of the respiratory neurons during sleep, the ventilation, tidal volume, and respiratory rate decrease in non-REM sleep. Ventilatory responses to hypercapnoea and hypoxia are attenuated during non-REM sleep in normal individuals (Phillipson and Bowes 1986). In REM sleep respiration is rapid and erratic; tonic and phasic activities in the intercostal and upper airway muscles decrease while activity is maintained in the diaphragm (Chokroverty 1986; Phillipson and Bowes 1986). There is uncertainty about the ventilatory responses to CO_2 and hypoxia during REM sleep (Phillipson and Bowes 1986). The REM-related respiratory control system is at least in part independent of the non-REM related system. The voluntary respiratory control system may be active during some part of REM sleep. Thus, in normal individuals, respiration is vulnerable during sleep; mild respiratory irregularities and pauses may occur in normals but in disease states these may assume a pathological significance.

THE SPECTRUM OF VENTILATORY DISTURBANCES IN MSA

Respiratory disturbances usually appear in the second and third stages (Chokroverty 1984) of the disease affecting men and women equally. Initially the patients present with autonomic failure comprising dysfunction of both the sympathetic and parasympathetic systems. They may present with two or more of the autonomic tetrad, namely, symptoms related to orthostatic hypotension (e.g. postural dizziness and faintness or even frank loss of consciousness), urinary sphincter dysfunction (e.g. frequency, urgency, hesitancy, dribbling or overflow incontinence), hypo- or anhidrosis, and impotence in men. After 2 to 6 years the second stage ensues with varying combinations of pyramidal, extrapyramidal, upper-motor-neuron, and lower-motor-neuron dysfunction including bulbar deficits. Most commonly the patients manifest a parkinsonian–cerebellar syndrome. In some patients, atypical parkinsonian features (e.g. bradykinesia, rigidity, postural instability) predominate while in others pancerebellar dysfunction predominates. At this stage of the illness a variety of respiratory disturbances, both in wakefulness and sleep, add to the progressive disability. Occasionally, respiratory dysfunction, particularly dysrhythmic breathing in wakefulness becoming worse in sleep manifests in the initial stage of the illness. In the third stage there is progressive autonomic and somatic dysfunction compounded by respiratory failure. The ventilatory disturbances may be present both in wakefulness and sleep. Because of the physiological vulnerability of the brainstem respiratory neurons in sleep (Chokroverty 1986) the waking abnormalities are worse in sleep.

The clinical manifestations resulting from the respiratory dysfunction may consist of: breathlessness; daytime hypersomnolence; early morning headache; daytime fatigue; disturbed nocturnal sleep; and intellectual deterioration. Examination may reveal respiratory irregularity in rate, rhythm, and depth with asynchrony in wakefulness and sleep. Breathlessness is usually present in patients with affections of the respiratory motor neurons or the respiratory muscles. But breathlessness is not an important symptom in patients with dysfunction of the medullary respiratory control system. It is important to recognize alveolar hypoventilation during sleep since patients may die from fatal sleep apnoea. Furthermore, because of episodic or prolonged hypoxaemia, hypercapnoea, and respiratory acidosis in sleep, pulmonary hypertension, cor pulmonale, and congestive cardiac failure may develop.

The spectrum of respiratory dysrhythmias in MSA may be summarized:

1. Central, upper airway obstructive, and mixed apnoeas in non-REM and REM sleep associated with oxygen desaturation.
2. Irregularities in rate, rhythm, and amplitude of respiration with and without oxygen desaturation becoming worse in sleep (dysrhythmic breathing).
3. Transient occlusion of the upper airway or transient uncoupling of the intercostal and diaphragmatic muscle activities.
4. Prolonged periods of central apnoea accompanied by mild oxygen desaturation in relaxed wakefulness.
5. Cheyne–Stokes pattern and Cheyne–Stokes variant pattern of breathing which become worse in sleep.
6. Periodic breathing in the erect posture accompanied by postural fall of blood pressure.
7. Inspiratory gasps and apneustic-like breathing.
8. Transient sudden respiratory arrest.

Figure 24.3 schematically shows the various breathing patterns.

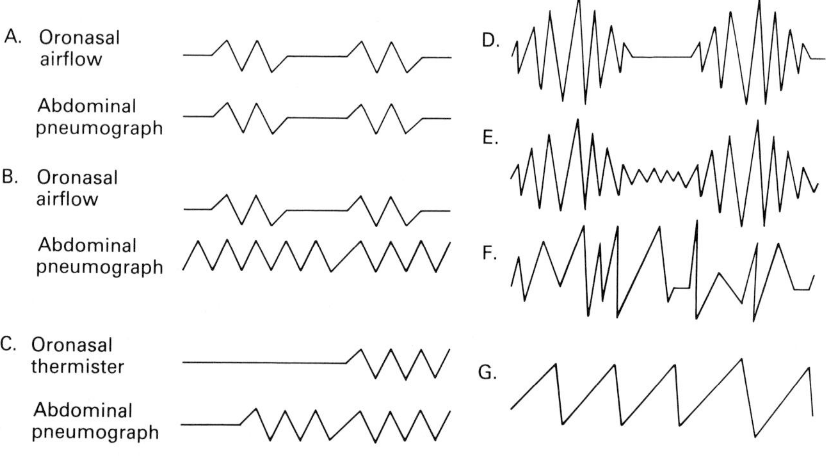

Fig. 24.3. Different respiratory patterns in MSA are shown schematically. A, central apnoea; B, upper airway obstructive apnoea; C, mixed apnoea; D, Cheyne–Stokes breathing; E, Cheyne-Stokes variant pattern; F, dysrhythmic breathing; G, apneustic breathing.

Recurrent episodes of apnoea predominantly during non-REM stages I and II and REM sleep have been noted in patients with MSA (Chokroverty 1986). Sleep-related hypopnoeas should have the same significance as sleep apnoeas. To be significant the apnoea or the hypopnoea should be at least 10 seconds in duration and the patient should have at least 30 periods of apnoea–hypopnoea during 7 hours of all night sleep or an apnoea–hypopnoea index (number of apnoea–hypopnoeas per hour of sleep) of at least 5 (Chokroverty 1986).

Three types of apnoeas may be recognized (Chokroverty and Sharp 1981):

1. Central apnoea, characterized by the suppression of diaphragmatic and intercostal muscle activity and absence of air exchange through the nose or mouth.
2. Upper-airway-obstructive apnoea manifested by an absence of air exchange detected by the oronasal thermistors but persistence of the diaphragmatic and intercostal muscle activities.
3. Mixed apnoea manifested by an initial period of central apnoea followed by a period of upper-airway-obstructive apnoea before resumption of regular breathing.

Cheyne–Stokes breathing is a special type of central apnoea characterized by cyclical changes in breathing with crescendo–decrescendo sequence separated by central apnoeas (Chokroverty 1986; Cherniack and Longobardo 1986). The Cheyne–Stokes variant pattern of breathing is distinguished by the substitution of hypopnoeas for apnoeas (Chokroverty 1986). Dysrhythmic breathing is characterized by a non-rhythmic respiration with irregularity in rate, rhythm, and amplitude during wakefulness and becoming worse in sleep resulting from an abnormality in the automatic respiratory pattern generator in the brainstem (McNicholas *et al.* 1983); Chokroverty 1986). The apneustic breathing is characterized by a short inspiratory but prolonged expiratory time (Cherniack and Longobardo 1986).

Bannister and Oppenheimer (1972) reported periodic inspiratory gasps resembling apneustic breathing in two patients with MSA; however, polysomnographic or respiratory recordings were not obtained.

Lockwood (1976) described a 54-year-old man with MSA who had cluster breathing with periods of apnoea, recorded by a thermistor of up to 20 s duration during wakefulness and up to 40 s during sleep. The patient had a sudden respiratory arrest at night and died. The pathological findings showed widespread diffuse lesions typical of MSA in addition to gliosis in the pontine tegmentum and medulla severely involving the reticular formation. The author suggested that the presence of periodic apnoea without impaired ventilatory response to CO_2 indicated that neurons responsible for respiratory rhythmogenesis functioned independently from the medullary chemoreceptors controlling ventilation.

Castaigne *et al.* (1977) described a 65-year-old man with MSA who had central alveolar hypoventilation, arrhythmic respiration, many episodes of apnoea, and probable apneustic breathing 4 years after the onset of the illness. Necropsy findings included diffuse lesions in the brainstem and the spinal cord consistent with the diagnosis of MSA.

Laryngeal abductor paralysis giving rise to laryngeal stridor and excessive snoring during sleep has been described in cases of MSA by Bannister *et al.* (1967, 1981), Israel and Marino (1977), Guilleminault *et al.* (1977), and Williams *et al.* (1979). The nocturnal stridor can be inspiratory, expiratory, or both. This stridor may give rise to a striking noisiness which may be likened to a 'donkey braying'. Williams *et al.* (1979) noted this abnormality in eight of 12 cases of MSA. The stridor was relieved by tracheostomy. Bannister *et al.* (1981) described the clinical and pathological findings in three cases of MSA with laryngeal stridor requiring tracheostomy. Pathologically, there was a marked atrophy of the posterior cricoarytenoid muscles which are the abductors of the vocal cords. The exact pathogenesis of the muscle atrophy could not be determined but was thought to be due to denervation; however, quantitative cell count in the nucleus ambiguus was normal implying that a biochemical defect may be the basis for denervation of laryngeal muscles in at least some of these cases.

Briskin *et al.* (1978) described three patients with MSA. Polygraphic studies documented that more than 70 per cent of the apnoeic episodes were obstructive in nature and the mean apnoea index was 75–79 in two of these patients. All three had daytime hypersomnolence. One needed resuscitation at night on two occasions because of respiratory arrest and, ultimately, all three died of respiratory arrest at night. Hypercapnoeic ventilatory responses were normal in all three but the hypoxic ventilatory responses were normal in two and severely impaired in another patient. Sleep scoring showed very little non-REM sleep stages III and IV and almost total absence of REM sleep.

Guilleminault *et al.* (1981) described another four patients with MSA who had predominantly upper-airway-obstructive apnoea during sleep. The apnoea–hypopnoea index ranged from 12 to 62. These authors noted a clear dissociation between heart rate and respiratory response, and found no correlation between waking hypercapnoeic and hypoxic response and the degree or presence of sleep apnoea.

McNicholas *et al.* (1983) described two patients with MSA who had overnight polysomnographic studies. Hypoxic ventilatory resposes were impaired in both patients and the hypercapnoeic ventilatory response was impaired in one suggesting a defect in the metabolic control system. During sleep the patients' pattern of breathing was highly irregular. They had a total of 61 to 79 apnoeic episodes during non-REM stages I and II but without oxygen desaturation. The apnoeic periods were mostly central but occasionally they had transient occlusion of the upper airway or transient uncoupling of the intercostal and diaphragmatic muscle activities. The most striking abnormality, however, was an irregular pattern of breathing during sleep. These findings during sleep and wakefulness in their patients suggested a defect in the automatic respiratory rhythm generator in the brainstem.

Chokroverty *et al.* (1978) described four patients with MSA who had periodic central apnoea in the erect position. One of these patients also had Cheyne–Stokes respiration during the late stage of the illness that was worse during sleep. In one patient hypercapnoeic ventilatory response in the supine position was impaired and the necropsy findings in the same patient of neuronal loss and astrocytosis in the pontine tegmentum suggested involvement of the respiratory neurons in the brainstem.

Recently, the author had the opportunity of studying respiratory patterns in collaboration with other investigators in nine patients with MSA showing a variety of respiratory dysrhythmias. The respiratory disturbances consisted of central apnoea including Cheyne–Stokes or Cheyne–Stokes like breathing, upper-airway-obstructive and mixed apnoeas accompanied by oxygen desaturation predominantly during non-REM sleep stages I and II and REM sleep. Seven patients had central, two had upper-airway-obstructive (Fig. 24.4), and two had mixed apnoeas during sleep (Fig. 24.5). The apnoea–hypopnoea index varied from 20 to 80. The duration of apnoeas ranged from 10 to 65 seconds. Heart-rate variation during apnoeic–eupnoeic cycles was not seen in those patients showing evidence of cardiac autonomic denervation. This finding was in contrast to relative bradycardia during apnoea and relative tachycardia on resumption of normal breathing as seen in patients with primary sleep apnoea syndrome (Chokroverty and Sharp 1981). Four patients had several episodes of central apnoeas during relaxed wakefulness as if the respiratory centre 'forgot' to breathe.

These findings suggest impairment of the metabolic respiratory control system. Impaired hypercapnoeic ventilatory response and mouth occlusion pressure response in one patient supported this suggestion. Normal hypercapnoeic and hypoxic ventilatory response in another patient in the presence of an abnormal respiratory pattern supported the suggestion of Lockwood (1976) that the chemoreceptor control and respiratory pattern generator are probably subserved by different population of neurons with selective vulnerability of these neurons in MSA. It should be noted, however, that there may not be any correlation between waking hypercapnoeic response and apnoeic events during sleep (Guilleminault *et al.* 1981). The finding that in eight of nine patients dysrhythmic breathing occurred mostly during sleep and in four patients also during wakefulness implied that this type of respiratory disturbance is very common in MSA. These observations are in agreement with the

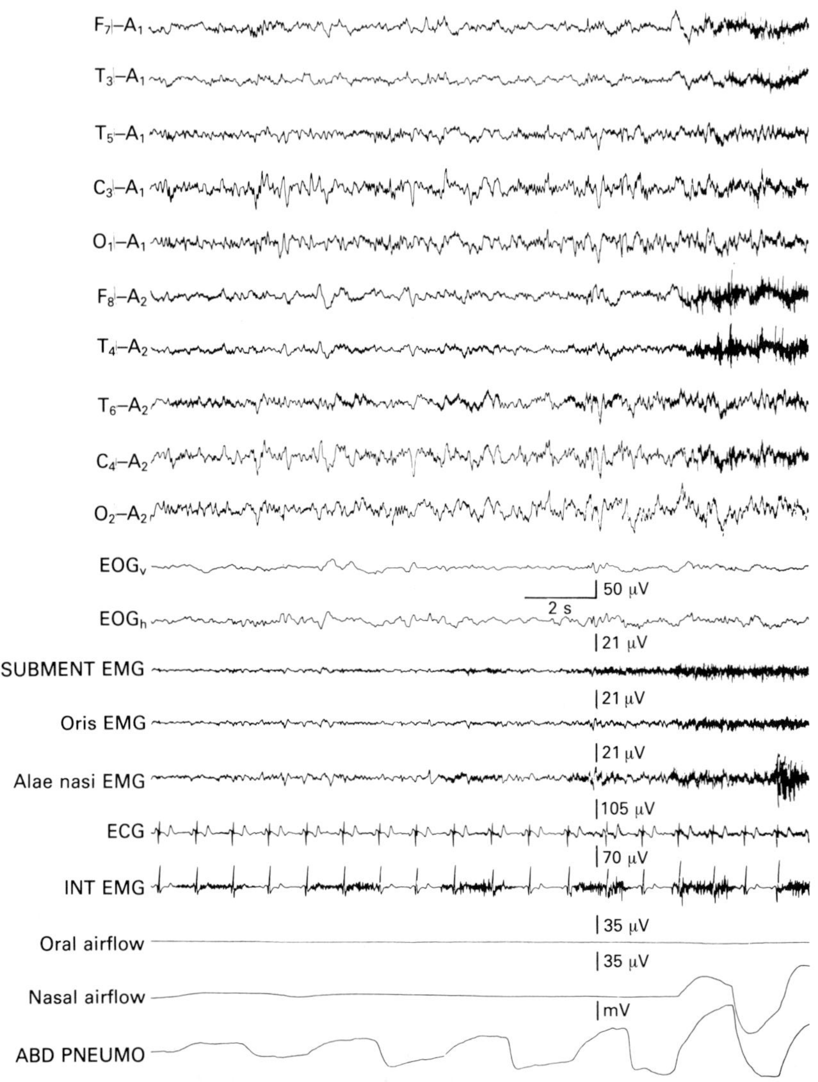

Fig. 24.4. Upper airway obstructive apnoea (only a portion of an episode is shown) during stage II non-REM sleep in a patient with MSA. Polygraphic recording shows EEG (top 10 channels), vertical (EOG_v) and horizontal (EOG_h) electrooculograms, electromyograms (EMG) of submental (SUBMENT), oris, alae nasi, and intercostal (INT) muscles, electrocardiogram (ECG), oral and nasal airflow, and abdominal pneumogram (ABD PNEUMO).

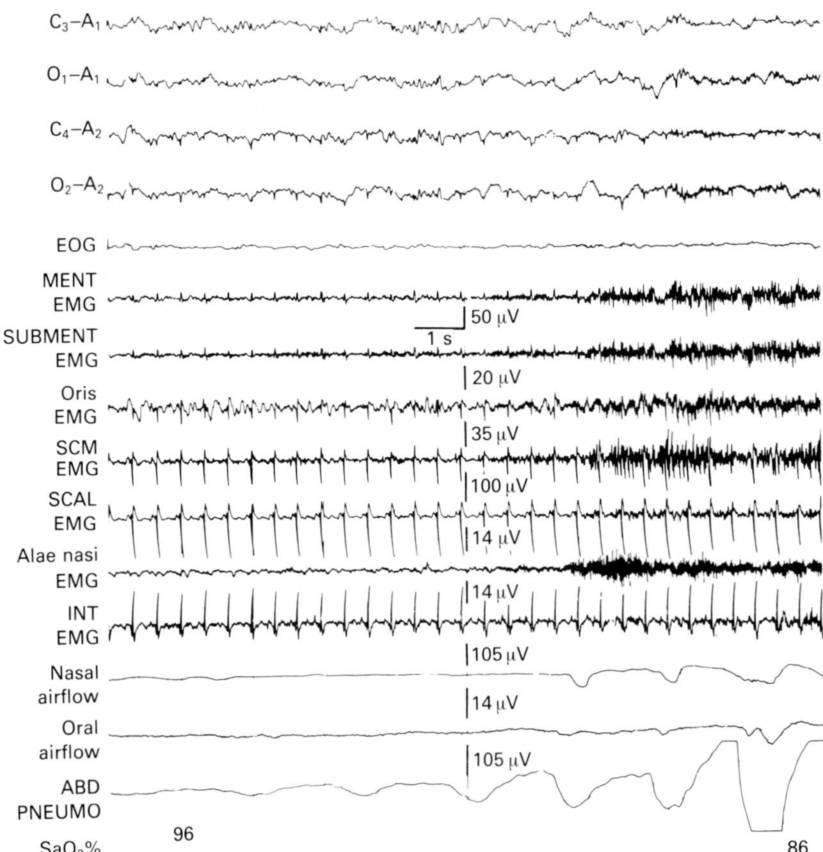

Fig. 24.5. Polygraphic recordings in a patient with MSA showing EEG (top four channels), vertical electrooculogram (EOG), EMG of mentalis (MENT), submental, oris, sternocleidomastoideus (SCM), scalenus anticus (SCAL), alae nasi and intercostal (INT) muscles, nasal and oral airflow, abdominal pneumogram (ABD PNEUMO), and oxygen saturation (SaO_2%). The patient has mixed apnoea (only a portion of the episode is shown) associated with oxygen desaturation during stage II non-REM sleep.

suggestion of McNicholas *et al.* (1983) that such findings imply an impaired respiratory pattern generator in these patients.

Two patients had inspiratory gasps and two required tracheostomy for respiratory dysrhythmia. All-night polysomnographic studies in two patients by the author revealed marked reduction of non-REM sleep stages III and IV and REM sleep, increased awakenings after sleep onset, snoring, excessive body movements, and frequent arousal responses in the EEG accompanied by mild-to-moderate oxygen desaturation.

MECHANISM OF VENTILATORY DYSRHYTHMIA IN MSA

Respiratory abnormalities in sleep and wakefulness in MSA result from both central and peripheral mechanisms secondary to autonomic and somatic denervation. The following are the suggested pathogenetic mechanisms for respiratory dysrhythmia in MSA.

1. Direct involvement of the medullary respiratory neurons affecting the pattern- and rhythm-generating mechanism with or without involvement of the central chemoreceptors may give rise to central sleep apnoea and respiratory dysrhythmia in wakefulness and sleep.
2. Involvement of the arousal system (ascending reticular activating system) and severe compromise of the wakefulness stimulus will raise the arousal threshold thus prolonging the apnoea.
3. Involvement of the respiratory and the non-respiratory motor neurons in the brainstem, e.g. nucleus ambiguus and hypoglossal nucleus causing laryngeal abductor paresis and pharyngeal and genioglossal weakness may cause upper-airway-obstructive apnoea.
4. Involvement of the respiratory motor neurons (anterior horn cells) in the cervical and thoracic spinal cord, thereby reducing impulse traffic along the phrenic and intercostal nerves to the diaphragm and intercostal muscles may cause central apnoea. If there is differential affection between the upper-airway motor neurons and spinal-respiratory motor neurons, there may be obstructive and mixed apnoea.
5. Interference with the supramedullary (forebrain, midbrain, and pontine) inputs to the medullary respiratory neurons may cause dysrhythmic and apneustic breathing.
6. Involvement of the hypothalamic projections directly (Brodal 1981) to the respiratory neurons in the NTS and nucleus ambiguus may promote apnoea and respiratory dysrhythmia.
7. Involvement of the parasympathetic (vagal) afferents from the lower and upper airway receptors may reduce the input to the central respiratory neurons causing respiratory dysrhythmia.
8. Sympathetic denervation of the nasal mucosa causing increased nasal resistance and greater narrowing downstream from the nose (Strohl 1986) may promote upper airway obstructive apnoea.
9. Finally, discrete neurochemical alterations in MSA may interfere with normal regulation of breathing.

These suggested mechanisms are based on evidence of involvement of the anatomical, physiological, and neurochemical pathways in MSA.

There is ample evidence in the literature (Shy and Drager 1960; Chokroverty 1984) of pathological involvement of the pontine tegmentum, the reticular formation, the NTS, nucleus ambiguus, hypoglossal nucleus, and, in some patients, anterior horn cells of the cervical and thoracic spinal cord. Lockwood (1976) and Chokroverty *et al.* (1978) correlated the physiological and clinical features of respiratory dysrhythmias with a direct involvement of the regions containing the respiratory neurons in the brainstem. In addition, studies of respiratory control showed impairment of hypercapnoeic and hypoxic ventilatory and mouth occlusion pressure responses (McNicholas *et al.* 1983; Chokroverty, unpublished data) indirectly suggesting impairment of the metabolic respiratory control system. Vagal and sympathetic denervation in patients with MSA is also well established (Shy and Drager 1960; Chokroverty 1984).

The anatomical proximity of adrenergic and serotonergic neurons to the respiratory related units in the brainstem suggests a role for these monoamines in the regulation of breathing (Dempsey *et al.* 1986). There is experimental evidence that noradrenalin, serotonin, and dopamine play distinct roles in the control of breathing (Dempsey *et al.* 1986). Dopamine has a biphasic action on respiration (Dempsey *et al.* 1986): by its central mechanism it stimulates breathing and by its peripheral mechanism through the carotid body chemoreceptor it inhibits breathing, and, therefore, an imbalance between these two mechanisms may cause respiratory dysrhythmia. Patients with MSA have been found to have low levels of dopamine and noradrenalin in the basal ganglia, the limbic–hypothalamic region including the septal nuclei, and the locus ceruleus (Spokes *et al.* 1979). Furthermore, these patients may also have specific catecholamine enzyme deficits in the brain and sympathetic ganglia (Chokroverty 1986). In summary then, in any one patient a variety of neurophysiological, neuropathological, and neurochemical mechanisms may play a role in the pathogenesis of sleep apnoea and respiratory disturbances in MSA.

LABORATORY DIAGNOSIS OF RESPIRATORY DYSFUNCTION IN MSA

The diagnosis of MSA is based on a combination of clinical manifestations, documentation of autonomic dysfunction, and exclusion of other causes of dysautonomia and somatic neurological diseases. CT brain scan, magnetic resonance imaging, EMG and nerve conduction studies, cerebrospinal fluid examination, and routine EEG in addition to special autonomic function studies may be necessary to establish the diagnosis of MSA. Once the diagnosis of MSA is made, further studies are necessary in patients suspected of respiratory dysrhythmia to diagnose and possibly treat the specific respiratory disturbance. A careful history and physical examination including otolaryngological examination to detect laryngeal and oropharyngeal muscle weakness should precede the special studies described next.

Polysomnographic study

It is important to obtain a complete polysomnographic study to understand and evaluate sleep-releated respiratory dysrhythmia. The initial study may consist of daytime polysomnography which will document the presence of sleep apnoea and other respiratory abnormalities. However, to assess the severity of the respiratory dysfunction and to fully understand the structure of sleep, all-night recordings should be obtained. The study should include simultaneous recordings of multiple channels of EEG, electromyograms (EMG) of orofacial muscles, electrocardiogram, electrooculogram, respiratory recordings, and continuous oxygen saturation by an ear oximeter (Chokroverty and Sharp 1981). Respiration can be monitored by nasal and oral thermistors to detect airflow and by use of an abdominal pneumograph or inductive plethysmograph (respitrace). The inductive plethysmograph has an advantage over the abdominal pneumograph because of its ability to provide quantitative data which can be used to measure tidal volume.

It is important to record multiple channels of EEG to diagnose accurately different sleep stages and their relationship to respiration. EEG may reveal focal and diffuse neurological lesions and seizure disorders that may sometimes complicate sleep apnoea. Recording of the electrooculogram and EMGs of multiple orofacial muscles is necessary to define REM sleep accurately and to document upper-airway muscle hypotonia. The recording should include REM sleep which is usually seen in all-night rather than daytime recordings because the most severe breathing abnormalities are often noted during this sleep stage.

It is important to study the sleep structure because sleep may accentuate respiratory abnormalities and respiratory dysfunction may affect sleep structure adversely (Chokroverty 1986); both these factors may alter the long-term course of the illness. One can also obtain 24-hour ambulatory recording of sleep and breathing to accurately assess sleep and breathing dysfunction throughout the day.

Pulmonary function test

In order to exclude intrinsic bronchopulmonary disease contributing to respiratory dysfunction in MSA, one should obtain measurements of spirometry, lung volumes, pulmonary diffusing capacity, and blood gases (Chokroverty 1986). One should also measure the maximal static inspiratory and expiratory pressures. These are more important than the dynamic measurements in detecting respiratory muscle weakness.

To measure the chemical control of breathing hypercapnoeic or hypoxic ventilatory and mouth occlusion pressure ($P_{0.1}$) responses, with or without load should be studied (Chokroverty 1986; Phillipson and Bowes 1986). Mouth occlusion pressure reflects central respiratory drive and inspiratory muscle strength independent of pulmonary mechanical factors. These measurements may be impaired in patients with dysfunction of the metabolic respiratory control system in MSA.

EMG of respiratory muscles

Electrical activity of the respiratory and upper airway including genioglossus and laryngeal muscles (Guindi *et al.* 1981) may be obtained to assess ventilatory activity and upper airway muscle tone. Measurements may be quantitated with a moving averager. Laryngeal EMG is important in patients suspected of having laryngeal paresis (Guindi *et al.* 1981).

TREATMENT OF RESPIRATORY DYSFUNCTION IN MSA

In the absence of an adequate understanding of the pathogenesis and a lack of a definite aetiological agent causing the disease, treatment remains unsatisfactory and consists of symptomatic measures only. Similarly, the pathogenesis of respiratory dysfunction in MSA is not clearly understood and therefore the treatment remains difficult. One should first diagnose and assess the type of respiratory dysrhythmia. Repeated hypoxaemias during sleep is potentially harmful not only to the immediate health of the patient but also to the long-term course of the illness. It is, therefore, important to be aware of their respiratory problem and to take appropriate measures to ameliorate the disability.

General measures

The patients must avoid alcohol and sedative–hypnotic drugs which may further depress the respiratory centre. The role of alcohol and sedative–hypnotic drugs in increasing the frequency and duration of sleep apnoeas is well established but the mechanism is not known. It has been suggested that these agents may selectively depress genioglossal muscle activity thus promoting upper-airway-obstructive apnoea (Chokroverty 1986).

Pharmacological treatment

Pharmacological treatment should ideally be directed towards a search for agents which will change the respiratory-centre motor output selectively to stimulate the upper-airway muscles to overcome the hypotonia of the genioglossus and other upper-airway muscles and so prevent central and obstructive apnoeas. However, no such selective and ideal agents have been found yet. Protriptyline, a non-sedating tricyclic antidepressant drug has been used with some success in patients with mild-to-moderate obstructive sleep apnoea (Chokroverty 1986). This agent may be tried in patients with MSA showing predominantly obstructive apnoea during sleep. The drug may improve oxygenation, reduce hypersomnolence, and improve sleep structure. Other agents which may be tried are medroxyprogesterone acetate and acetazolamide. Some patients with upper-airway-obstructive apnoea may show some improvement in breathing after medroxyprogesterone treatment (Chokroverty 1986). Acetazolamide has been used to treat central apnoea in MSA. One must, however, be cautious because of the danger of increasing orthostatic hypotension resulting from diuresis and natriuresis. The value of the pharmacological treatment of the respiratory dysfunction in patients with MSA cannot be ascertained definitively because a sufficient number of patients have not yet been carefully treated to understand the short- and long-term effects of these agents.

Neuromechanical measures

Continuous positive-airway pressure (CPAP) delivered through the nose has been shown to cause improvement in many patients with obstructive sleep apnoea (Chokroverty 1986). CPAP may be tried in patients with MSA showing predominantly obstructive sleep apnoea. One should use the lowest pressure which will be effective in decreasing the number and duration of obstructive apnoeic events. If nasal CPAP shows a good response during polysomnographic study, this treatment may be considered in patients with moderate-to-severe obstructive sleep apnoea. The role of nasal CPAP in MSA patients cannot be ascertained without treating a sufficient number of patients with this device. In the author's experience in a limited number of patients with MSA showing respiratory dysfunction, pharmacological treatment and nasal CPAP have not proved very useful.

Tracheostomy

This remains the only effective treatment used as an emergency measure in patients with severe respiratory dysfunction accompanied by marked hypoxaemia and cyanosis, and in patients with sudden respiratory arrest after resuscitation by intubation. Tracheostomy is also the only form of treatment used successfully in patients with severe laryngeal stridor due to laryngeal abductor paralysis. Gradually, one may try to wean a patient from a tracheostomy but the weaning procedure may be difficult in patients with MSA because of the progressive course of the illness.

Despite considerable advances in our understanding of MSA and the respiratory disturbances observed in this illness, an effective therapy for the respiratory dysrhythmias continues to elude us. Future research should be directed towards improving our understanding of the neurotransmitter deficiencies in MSA and pharmacological manipulation to find an effective agent to treat the disease as well as the respiratory dysrhythmia which is potentially life-threatening and is generally responsible for the final demise of the patients.

Acknowledgements

The author wishes to thank Dr Roger C. Duvoisin for reviewing the manuscript and Lena DiMauro for typing it.

REFERENCES

Bannister, R., Ardill, L., and Fentem, P. (1967). Defective autonomic control of blood vessels in idiopathic orthostatic hypotension. *Brain* **90**, 725–46.

Bannister, R., Gibson, W., Michaels, L., and Oppenheimer, D. R. (1981). Laryngeal abductor paralysis in multiple system atrophy. *Brain* **104**, 351–68.

Bannister, R. and Oppenheimer, D. R. (1972). Degenerative disease of the nervous system associated with autonomic failure. *Brain* **95**, 457–74.

Berger, A. J., Mitchell, R. A., and Severinghaus, J. N. (1977). Regulation of respiration. *New Engl. J. Med.* **297**, 138–43.

Briskin, J. G., Lehrman, K. L., and Guillemninault, C. (1978). Shy–Drager syndrome and sleep apnea. In *Sleep apnea syndromes* (ed. C. Guilleminault and W. C. Dement), pp. 316–22. Alan R. Liss, New York.

Brodal, A. (1981). Neurological anatomy, 3rd edn. Oxford University Press, Oxford.

Castaigne, P., Laplane, D., Autrel, A., Bousser, M. G., Gray, F., and Baron, J. C. (1977). Syndrome de Shy et Drager avec troubles du rhythme respiratoire et de la vigilance. *Rev. Neurol., Paris* **133**, 455–6.

Cherniack, N. S. and Longobardo, G. S. (1986). Abnormalities in respiratory rhythm. In *Handbook of physiology*, Section 3: *The respiratory system*, Volume II, Part 2 (ed. A. F. Fishman, N. S. Cherniack, and J. G. Widdicombe), pp. 729–49. American Physiological Society, Bethesda, Maryland.

Chokroverty, S. (1984). Autonomic dysfunction in olivopontocerebellar atrophy. In *The olivopontocerebellar atrophies* (ed. R. C. Duvoisin and A. Plaitakis), pp. 105–41. Raven Press, New York.

Chokroverty, S. (1986). Sleep and breathing in neurological disorders. In *Breathing disorders of sleep* (ed. N. H. Edelman and T. V. Santiago), pp. 225–64. Churchill Livingstone, New York.

Chokroverty, S., Barron, K. D., Katz, F. M., Del Greco, F., and Sharp, J. T. (1969). The syndrome of primary orthostatic hypotension. *Brain* **92**, 743–68.

Chokroverty, S. and Sharp, J. T. (1981). Primary sleep apnoea syndrome. *J. Neurol. Neurosurg. Psychiat.* **44**, 970–82.

Chokroverty, S., Sharp, J. T., and Barron, K. D. (1978). Periodic respiration in erect posture in Shy–Drager syndrome. *J. Neurol. Neurosurg. Psychiat.* **41**, 980–6.

Dempsey, J. A., Olson, E. B., Jr., and Skatrud, J. B. (1986). Hormones and neurochemicals in the regulation of breathing. In *Handbook of physiology*, Section 3: *The respiratory system*, Volume II, Part I (ed. A. F. Fishman, N. S. Cherniack, and J. G. Widdicombe), pp. 181–221. American Physiological Society, Bethesda, Maryland.

Guilleminault, C., Briskin, J. G., Greenfield, M. S., and Silvestri, R. (1981). The impact of autonomic nervous system dysfunction on breathing during sleep. *Sleep* **4**, 263–78.

Guilleminault, C., Tilkian, A., Lehrman, K., Forno, L., and Dement, W. C. (1977). Sleep apnoea syndrome: States of sleep and autonomic dysfunction. *J. Neurol. Neurosurg. Psychiat.* **40**, 718–25.

Guindi, G. M., Bannister, R., Gibson, W., and Payne, J. K. (1981). Laryngeal electromyography in multiple system atrophy with autonomic failure. *J. Neurol. Neurosurg. Psychiat.* **44**, 49–53.

Hauri, P. (1982). *The sleep disorders.* The Upjohn Company, Kalamazoo, Michigan.

Israel, R. H. and Marino, J. M. (1977). Upper airway obstruction in the Shy–Drager syndrome. *Ann. Neurol.* **2**, 83.

Lockwood, A. H. (1976). Shy–Drager syndrome with abnormal respirations and antidiuretic hormone release. *Arch. Neurol.* **33**, 292–5.

McNicholas, W. T., Rutherford, R., Grossman, R., Moldofsky, H., Zamel, N., and Phillipson, E. A. (1983). Abnormal respiratory pattern generation during sleep in patients with autonomic dysfunction. *Am. Rev. resp. Dis.* **128**, 429–33.

Phillipson, E. A. and Bowes, G. (1986). Control of breathing during sleep. In *Handbook of physiology*, Section 3: *The respiratory system*, Volume II, Part 2 (ed. A. F. Fishman, N. S. Cherniack, and J. G. Widdicombe), pp. 649–89. American Physiological Society, Bethesda, Maryland.

Shy, G. M. and Drager, G. A. (1960). A neurological syndrome associated with orthostatic hypotension. *Arch. Neurol., Chicago* **2**, 511–27.

Spokes, E. G., Bannister, R., and Oppenheimer, D. R. (1979). Multiple system atrophy with autonomic failure: clinical, histological and neurochemical observations on 4 cases. *J. neurol. Sci.* **43**, 59–82.

Strohl, K. P. (1986). Control of the upper airway during sleep. In *Breathing disorders of sleep* (ed. N. H. Edelman and T. V. Santiago), pp. 115–37. Churchill Livingstone, New York.

Williams, A., Hanson, D., and Calne, D. B. (1979). Vocal cord paralysis in the Shy–Drager syndrome. *J. Neurol. Neurosurg. Psychiat.* **42**, 151–3.

25. Neuropathology and neurochemistry of autonomic failure

A. Neuropathology of autonomic failure

David Oppenheimer

The first neuropathological description of a case of autonomic failure was that of Shy and Drager (1960), who reported on a man dying at age 56 after an illness lasting 6½ years in which the main features were orthostatic hypotension and disturbances of micturition. There were no significant findings outside the central nervous system, in which the authors observed varying degrees of cell loss and/or gliosis in many sites, including the caudate nuclei, substantia nigra, cerebellar Purkinje cells, inferior olives, dorsal vagal nuclei, and the lateral horns of the thoracic cord. They made no comment on the possible significance of this last observation in accounting for their patient's autonomic disturbances. The second neuropathological report came from Fichefet *et al.* (1965), whose patient was a man dying at age 72 after an illness lasting two years, starting with orthostatic hypotension and later developing parkinsonism. The pathology was typical of Parkinson's disease, with loss of pigmented nerve cells from the subtantia nigra and locus ceruleus, and cytoplasmic inclusions of Lewy type in remaining pigmented cells. In addition, the authors observed some cell loss in the anterior and lateral horns of the spinal cord.

In 1966, Johnson *et al.* described two cases with neuropathological findings. Clinically, the first case was one of 'pure' autonomic failure, with orthostatic hypotension, loss of sweating, and sexual impotence, of 4 years duration. Detectable cell loss was practically confined to the lateral horns of the thoracic cord. Cell counts, carried out at 12 thoracic levels, with controls, indicated that nearly 90 per cent of the preganglionic sympathetic cells in the intermediolateral columns of the thoracic cord had been lost. The other finding was of Lewy-type inclusion bodies in the substantia nigra and locus ceruleus and elsewhere, though there was no detectable loss of pigmented cells. The second case was of a man dying at age 54 after a 4½ year illness in which autonomic failure was combined with motor and cerebellar disturbances. The findings were of olivopontocerebellar atrophy (OPCA), with additional cell loss in the putamen, pigmented nuclei, vestibular nuclei, and intermediolateral columns. Lewy bodies were not present. Cell loss in the lateral horns was estimated at about 75 per cent; and the authors concluded that in their two cases autonomic failure was attributable to loss of preganglionic autonomic neurons.

Three very similar cases were reported in the following year, one by Nick *et al.* (1967) and two by Schwarz (1967). All of these showed cell loss in the putamen, pigmented nuclei, olives, dorsal vagal nuclei, cerebellar cortex, and intermediolateral columns. Cell loss in the pontine nuclei was seen in two of these three cases. No Lewy bodies were observed. In their dicussion, Nick *et al.* (1967) remarked on a possible relationship between their case and those recently described by Adams *et al.* (1961, 1964) under the heading of striatonigral degeneration (SND). Graham and Oppenheimer (1969) described a similar case, in which the lesions of OPCA were combined with those of SND, as they had been in three previously described cases of autonomic failure, and in one of the cases as described by Adams *et al.* (1964). They suggested that SND and OPCA were, in fact, different manifestations of the same basic disease, for which they proposed the term *multiple system atrophy* (MSA)—i.e. a primary degneration of the nervous system, familial or sporadic, with onset in middle life, and affecting a *selection* of the following structures: striatum, pigmented nuclei (substantia nigra and locus ceruleus), pontine nuclei, inferior olives, cerebellar Purkinje cells, and dorsal vagal and vestibular nuclei. Among the structures at risk in this condition are the intermediolateral cell columns; when these are depleted, autonomic failure results. Graham and Oppenheimer also pointed out that cases of autonomic failure appeared, from the pathological evidence, to belong to one of two groups, the first having affinities with Parkinson's disease and the second having the lesions of MSA. This twofold grouping was accepted by Vanderhaeghen *et al.* who in 1970 described a further case of the first type.

As published case-records accumulated, it became apparent that there were clinical as well as histological differences between the two groups. When Bannister and Oppenheimer (1972) gave their findings in four cases of autonomic failure, three with MSA and one with clinical and pathological signs of Parkinson's disease, they were able to point out that in five published cases of the Lewy-body type the mean age of onset was 65 years (mean age at death, 70), whereas in 11 cases with MSA the corresponding means were 49 and 55—a difference of 15–16 years. In the first group, apart from autonomic failure, neurological disturbances were either not present or were confined to parkinsonism. In the second, there were additional neurological complaints, which frequently but not always included parkinsonism. In both groups, clinical parkinsonism was

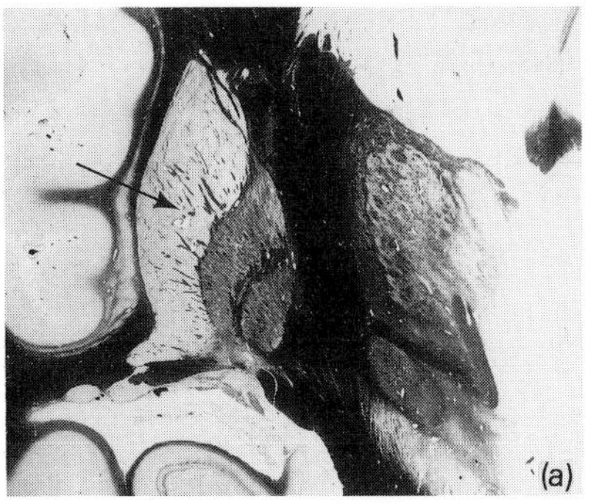

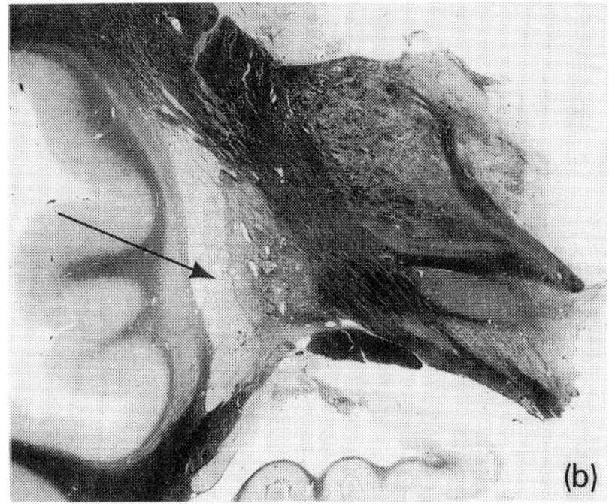

Fig. 25.1. Basal nuclei in coronal section, showing (a) normal-sized putamen (arrow), with well-marked myelinated bundles; (b) shrunken putamen (arrow), with loss of myelinated bundles, from a case of MSA with autonomic failure (Oppenheimer 1980, case 19). Myelin stain.

related to loss of pigmented cells in the substantia nigra. Cell counting showed similar degrees of intermediolateral cell loss in the two groups.

At the time of writing (1987) the European and American literature contains some 56 reports, with reasonably full histological descriptions, on cases of progressive autonomic failure (Table 25.1).* The cases are still clearly divisible into two groups. In the first group, characterized by Lewy bodies (see Chapter 26) in substantia nigra, locus ceruleus, and elsewhere, there are 10 cases, eight in males, two in females. Ages at death range from 66 to 83, with a mean of 72. Five of these cases (Fichefet *et al.* 1965; Bannister and Oppenheimer 1972, case 3; Schober *et al.* 1975, case 2; Rajput and Rozdilsky 1976, case 6; Oppenheimer 1980, case 5) had clinical parkinsonism and pathological evidence of Parkinson's disease. In four non-parkinsonian cases (Johnson *et al.* 1966, case 1; Vanderhaeghen *et al.* 1970, case 2; Oppenheimer 1980, cases 7 and 8) the substantia nigra contained Lewy bodies, but there was no detectable loss of pigmented cells. In three cases (Johnson *et al.* 1966, case 1; Roessmann *et al.* 1971, case 1; Oppenheimer 1980, case 8) autonomic failure was the sole neurological disorder. Loss of intermediolateral column cells was noted in the nine cases in which the spinal cord was examined. Cell loss in the dorsal vagal nuclei was noted in seven of the 10 cases. None of them showed lesions of SND or of OPCA.

The second group (46 cases) consists (with one possible exception) of cases of multiple system atrophy. Thirty cases are in males, 16 in females. Ages at death range from 41 to 79 years, with a mean of 58.6. In 35 cases parkinsonism was recorded, in 11 it was not; but all 46 are reported as showing some degree of nigral cell damage. Shrinkage, cell loss, and gliosis in the putamen are reported in all but nine cases (Fig. 25.1). Where local variations are recorded, it is often observed that the

* I know of 11 autopsied cases in the Japanese literature. These are listed and tabulated by Takahashi (1973). All except one appear to have been cases of MSA.

Table 25.1. Clinical features, sites of cell loss, and occurrence of Lewy inclusion bodies in 56 autopsied cases of primary autonomic failure. Note that only positive findings are recorded here. A gap in the table may mean that the lesion was not looked for, or that it was looked for and not found

No. Reference	*Case number*	*Sex*	*Age at death*	*Duration (y)*	*Parkinsonism (p)*	*Striatum*	*Subst. nigra*	*Locus cerul.*	*Cerebellar cortex*	*Pontine nuclei*	*Inf. olives*	*Dorsal vagal nuc.*	*Anterior horns*	IML *(thoracic)*	IML *(sacral)*	*Onuf's nucleus*	*Symp. ganglia*	*Pyram. tract*	*Lewy bodies*
1. Fichefet *et al.* (1965)		F	72	1½	p		SN	LC				X	AH	Tho			G		LB
2. Johnson *et al.* (1966)	1	M	66	4										Tho					LB
3. Vanderhaeghen (1970)	2	M	75	2								X							LB
4. Roessmann *et al.* (1971)	1	M	69	13			SN	LC			O	X		Tho			G		LB
5. Bannister and Oppenheimer (1972)	3	M	67	4	p							X		Tho					LB
6. Schober *et al.* (1975)	2	M	76	3	p		SN	LC				X		Tho					LB
7. Rajput and Rozdilsky (1976)	6	F	72	14	p		SN	LC				X		Tho			G		LB
8. Oppenheimer (1980)	5	M	66	15	p		SN	LC				X		Tho					LB
9. Oppenheimer (1980)	7	M	83	½				LC						Tho					LB
10. Oppenheimer (1980)	8	M	70	5										Tho					LB
11. Shy and Drager (1960)	2	M	56	6½	p	St	SN	LC			O	X		Tho					
12. Johnson *et al.* (1966)	2	M	54	4½		St	SN	LC	C	P	O			Tho				Pyr	
13. Schwarz (1967)	1	F	41	4½	p	St	SN	LC			O	X		Tho			G		
14. Schwarz (1967)	2	M	57	11	p	St	SN	LC	C	P	O	X		Tho					
15. Nick *et al.* (1967)		F	61	5	p	St	SN	LC		P	O	X	AH	Tho			G		
16. Graham and Oppenheimer (1969)		M	62	4		St	SN		C	P	O	X		Tho				Pyr	
17. Fischer and Petri (1969)		F	62	4½	p		SN		C		O	X	AH	Tho					
18. Mark (1969)		M	45	3½	p		SN		C	P	O								
19. Hughes *et al.* (1970)	1	M	58	7	p	St	SN	LC									G	Pyr	

20. Thapedi *et al.* (1971)		M	58	5	p	St	Sn	LC	C		O		AH	Tho			G		LB
21. Evans *et al.* (1972)		M	48	4	p		SN	LC	C	P	O	X						Pyr	
22. Bannister and Oppenheimer (1972)	1	M	47	10	p	St	SN	LC	C	P	O	X		Tho				Pyr	
23. Bannister and Oppenheimer (1972)	2	M	57	6	p	St	SN					X		Tho					
24. Bannister and Oppenheimer (1972)	4	F	64	6	p	St	SN	LC	C	P	O	X	AH	Tho				Pyr	
25. Takei and Mirra (1973)	4	F	46	3		St	SN	LC		P	O			Tho				Pyr	
26. Rohmer *et al.* (1973)		M	61	5	p		SN	LC				X	AH	Tho					
27. Guard *et al.* (1974)		F	54	6	p	St	SN	LC	C		O	X		Tho					LB
28. Schober *et al.* (1975)	1	F	59	4	p	St	SN	LC	C			X	AH	Tho				Pyr	
29. Vuia (1975)		M	55	2	p	St	SN					X							
30. Rajput and Rozdilsky (1976)	7	M	52	4	p	St	SN	LC	C			X	AH	Tho					
31. de Lean and Deck (1976)		M	60	6	p	St	SN	LC				X	AH	Tho				Pyr	
32. Lockwood (1976)		M	54	5		St	SN			P			AH	Tho					
33. Kluyskens *et al.* (1977)	5	M	60	6	p	St	SN		C	P	O		AH	Tho					
34. Castaigne *et al.* (1977)		M	69	4			SN	LC		P				Tho					
35. Spokes *et al.* (1979)	1	M	70	9	p	St	SN		C	P	O		AH	Tho				Pyr	
36. Spokes *et al.* (1979)	2	M	48	8	p	St	SN		C	P	O		AH	Tho				Pyr	
37. Spokes *et al.* (1979)	3	M	51	4	p	St	SN							Tho					
38. Spokes *et al.* (1979)	4	F	52	5	p	St	SN	LC	C	P	O	X		Tho				Pyr	
39. Sung *et al.* (1979)	1	F	79	5	p	St	SN	LC	C	P	O	X	AH	Tho	Sac	On		Pyr	
40. Sung *et al.* (1979)	2	F	52	4	p	St	SN	LC	C	P	O	X	AH	Tho	Sac	On		Pyr	
41. Sung *et al.* (1979)	3	M	63	3		St	SN	LC	C	P	O	X	AH	Tho	Sac	On		Pyr	
42. Sung *et al.* (1979)	4	M	66	7	p	St	SN	LC	C	P	O	X	AH	Tho	Sac	On		Pyr	
43. Oppenheimer (1980)	17	M	58	5		St	SN	LC	C	P	O			Tho					
44. Oppenheimer (1980)	18	M	67	5		St	SN							Tho					
45. Oppenheimer (1980)	19	F	58	8	p	St	SN	LC	C	P	O			Tho				Pyr	
46. Oppenheimer (1980)	24	F	66	6	p	St	SN	LC	C	P	O	X	AH	Tho				Pyr	
47. Oppenheimer (1980)	26	F	59	3		St	SN	LC	C	P	O			Tho					
48. Oppenheimer (1980)	27	M	68	5	p		SN	LC						Tho					

Table 25.1. (*cont.*)

No.	*Reference*	*Case number*	*Sex*	*Age at death*	*Duration (y)*	*Parkinsonism (p)*	*Striatum*	*Subst. nigra*	*Locus cerul.*	*Cerebellar cortex*	*Pontine nuclei*	*Inf. olives*	*Dorsal vagal nuc.*	*Anterior horns*	*IML (thoracic)*	*IML (sacral)*	*Onuf's nucleus*	*Symp. ganglia*	*Pyram. tract*	*Lewy bodies*
49.	Reznik (1980)		F	76	6	p	St	SN	LC	C	P	O	X	AH	Tho			G	Pyr	
50.	Bannister *et al.* (1981)	2	F	72	3	p	St	SN			P	O	X		Tho					
51.	Bannister *et al.* (1981)	3	M	60	7			SN		C		O			Tho					
52.	Konno *et al.* (1986)	1	M	45	9	p		SN	LC	C	P	O	X	AH	Tho	Sac	On			
53.	Konno *et al.* (1986)	2	M	64	4	p	St	SN	LC	C	P	O	X	AH	Tho	Sac	On			
54.	Konno *et al.* (1986)	3	M	60	8	p	St	SN	LC	C	P	O	X	AH	Tho	Sac	On			
55.	Konno *et al.* (1986)	4	M	62	7	p		SN	LC	C	P	O	X	AH	Tho	Sac	On			
56.	Konno *et al.* (1986)	5	F	58	3	p	St	SN	LC	C	P	O	X	AH	Tho	Sac	On			

IML, intermediolateral column.

lateral parts of the substantia nigra suffer most, whereas in Parkinson's disease the middle third is most affected (Hassler 1938). In the putamen, the lesions tend to be in the lateral and posterior parts, whereas the anterior part, and the caudate nucleus, tend to be spared. This distribution is in accordance with Szabo's (1962, 1967) account of the nigrostriatal projections. In 25 cases (i.e. over half the total) there was olivopontocerebellar atrophy, and in 21 this was combined with striatonigral degeneration. The rest of the cases showed various combinations of lesions (see Table 25.1). Lewy inclusion bodies were seen in two cases (Thapedi *et al.* 1971; Guard *et al.* 1974). In both instances the lesions in the striatum, olives, and cerebellum make it plain that the condition was of MSA rather than of Parkinson's disease.

Taking both groups together, loss of cells from the lateral horns of the thoracic cord (see Chapter 27) has been reported in all but five cases. In two of these, the cord was not examined. In another, it is not clear whether the lateral horns were looked at. In the case of Hughes *et al.* (1970) the authors say 'The intermediomedial and intermediolateral columns were examined in all thoracic segments, and although formal counting was not employed, the numbers of cells did not differ from control sections'. In the case reported by Evans *et al.* (1972) cell counts were carried out on the intermediolateral columns and compared with normal controls. No significant difference was found. In many cases, loss of intermediolateral cells is reported, without evidence of quantitative assessment. Such reports should be treated with reserve. In normal subjects, the distribution of cells within the lateral grey horns is somewhat irregular, and one needs to examine numerous sections before making a qualitative judgement on whether cell loss has occurred.

Apart from the case of Evans *et al.* (1972), formal counts have been carried out by Guard *et al.* (1974, one case), de Lean and Deck (1976, one case), Sung *et al.* (1979, two cases), Oppenheimer (1980, 21 cases, including 11 previously reported cases), and Kennedy and Duchen (1985, two cases). Severe loss of intermediolateral column cells was demonstrated in all 27 cases. Oppenheimer (1980) compared his findings in cases of autonomic failure (a) with 'normal' controls, (b) with cases of Parkinson's disease without autonomic disturbances, and (c) with cases of multiple system atrophy without autonomic disturbances. The findings are shown graphically in Fig. 25.2. Briefly, they show that: (1) there is a very obvious correlation between autonomic failure and loss of lateral horns cells; (2) at all levels, the control counts are higher than in any case of autonomic failure; (3) the counts in three cases of uncomplicated Parkinson's disease do not differ from the controls; (4) the counts in cases of MSA without clinical autonomic failure are about half the control counts, and overlap with recorded cases of autonomic failure.

Other parts of the CNS concerned with autonomic function have been

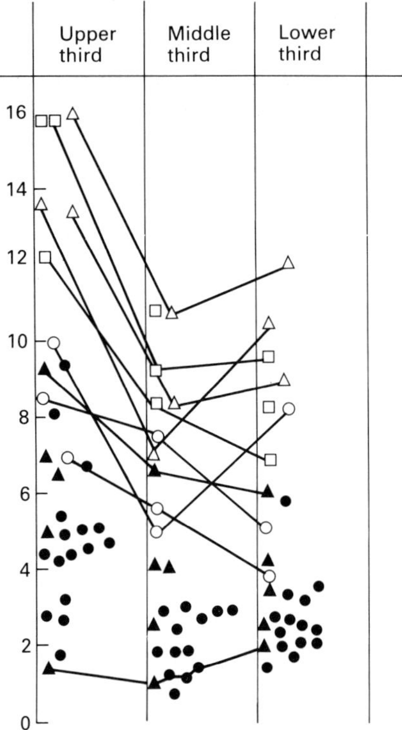

Fig. 25.2. Chart showing results of cell counts on lateral horns in upper, middle and lower thirds of thoracic cord. Figures on left show mean numbers of cells in a single lateral horn in 20-μm sections. □ Control cases. △ Three cases of Parkinson's disease, without autonomic failure. ○ Three cases of MSA without autonomic failure. ▲ Five cases of autonomic failure, showing Lewy bodies in brainstem. ● Sixteen cases of MSA with autonomic failure. (Taken with permission from Oppenheimer (1980).)

less intensively studied. Shy and Drager (1960) reported slight cell loss in the posterior hypothalamus, but most reports in which the hypothalamus is mentioned describe it as normal. I have routinely examined the hypothalamus at 1-mm intervals, and have never encountered a definite lesion there. Regarding the parasympathetic system, Shy and Drager (1960) reported cell loss in the Edinger–Westphal and dorsal vagal nuclei. The former has rarely been mentioned in subsequent reports; but damage to the dorsal vagal nuclei has been reported in 36 out of 56 cases—seven in cases of the Lewy-body type, and 29 in cases of MSA. Regarding the parasympathetic cells of the sacral cord, our information dates from 1977, when Mannen *et al.* reported that in motor neuron disease (amyotrophic lateral sclerosis) a particular cell group, referred to as 'Onuf's nucleus', is spared in spite of severe depletion of large cells of motor type in the anterior horns of the sacral, as in other segments. This group, first noted by Onufrowicz in 1900, is found at the ventral margin of the ventral horn in the lower part of the second sacral segment, extending into the upper part of the third sacral segment. Similar selective sparing was observed by Iwata and Hirano (1978) in three cases of Werdnig–Hoffman disease and two cases of healed poliomyelitis. From the clinical observation that sphincter control is preserved in such cases, these authors concluded that Onuf's nucleus contained the cells innervating the 'voluntary' sphincters of the anus and bladder neck. In 1979 Sung observed that in five cases of Fabry's disease there was lipidotic distension of certain cells in the spinal cord. In the thoracic segments, only the preganglionic sympathetic cells of the intermediolateral columns were affected. In the sacral cord, not only the corresponding parasympathetic cells of the intermediolateral columns were affected, but also the cells of Onuf's nucleus. Sung and his colleagues (1979) reported on four cases of multiple system atrophy (cases 39 to 42 in Table 25.1), in which they found severe loss of cells in the thoracic and sacral intermediolateral columns, and in Onuf's nuclei.

More recently, Konno and colleagues (1986) used cell-counting methods to compare the sacral cords in five multiple system atrophy cases (cases 52–6 in Table 25.1), five cases of motor neuron disease, and four age-matched controls. They found marked loss of cells from the postero-lateral (somatic motor) groups in both multiple system atrophy and motor neuron disease; severe cell loss from the intermediolateral groups and Onuf's nucleus in the multiple system atrophy cases; and less severe loss from these two sites in motor neuron disease. The general conclusions from all these results are: (1) that both autonomic and somatic efferents are at risk, though in different degrees, in both diseases; and (2) that the cells of Onuf's nucleus enjoy a status intermediate between ordinary somatic motor neurons and autonomic efferents, being morphologically indistinguishable from the former, but sharing the risks (in Fabry's disease and in MSA) of the latter. There seems to be no doubt that they innervate the anal and urethral sphincters, and that their loss can be blamed for the common sphincter disturbances in Shy–Drager syndrome. To what extent they are affected in Lewy-body disease is still uncertain.

Other central nervous structures commonly reported as showing damage in cases of autonomic failure, though not known to be implicated in autonomic functions, include the vestibular (particularly the medial vestibular) nuclei, motor cells of the anterior horns, and the corticospinal tracts. In the Lewy-body group, six out of 10 have shown loss of pigmented cells in the locus ceruleus. This is not surprising, in view of the affinities of this group with Parkinson's disease. In the MSA group cell loss from the locus ceruleus has been reported in 28 cases; from the vestibular nuclei in 15 cases; and from the anterior horns in 18 cases. Some degree of pyramidal-tract degeneration has been observed in 19 cases. These figures should probably be regarded as minima, since it is clear, in many reports, that these changes were not specifically looked for. It must also be stressed that lesions in all these sites have been observed in some, but not all, reported cases of MSA without clinical evidence of autonomic failure.

The same is true of lesions in the peripheral nervous system, which are present in some but not all cases of MSA without autonomic disturbances. It appears that the peripheral nerves and ganglia have been examined in only about half the reported cases of autonomic failure. Among these there are about eight reports of changes in sympathetic ganglia—mostly in the form of mild cell loss, with some proliferation of supporting cells. Most of these reports are unconvincing, as they do not give evidence that the material has been compared with control material from middle-aged and elderly subjects. Hyaline eosinophilic inclusion bodies, similar to those described by Jager and Bethlem (1960) in cases of Parkinson's disease, have been observed in four cases, all in the Lewy-body group; but the only convincing account of serious damage in sympathetic ganglia is that of Rajput and Rozdilsky (1976). Their case 6 had Parkinson's disease, with autonomic failure. Apart from the expected intermediolateral cell loss, the sympathetic ganglia from this case showed severe cell loss and cellular degeneration, and numerous eosinophilic inclusion bodies. Lesions in parasympathetic ganglia or visceral nerve plexuses have not, as far as I know, been reported. My own observations on the innervation of gut and bladder, on cardiac and other peripheral ganglia, and on sweat glands in the skin have disclosed no significant changes. Several reports mention the finding of degenerative changes in somatic nerves; but such changes are not uncommon in Parkinson's disease and in MSA without clinical autonomic disturbances. The most severe sensory neuropathy I have encountered was in case 1 of Bannister and Oppenheimer (1972). Here the ninth and tenth cranial nerves were involved, and there was gross loss of fibres in the tractus solitarii.

This account of the pathology of autonomic failure leaves several important questions unanswered, or only partially answered. The first problem concerns the nature of the disease or diseases from which these patients are suffering. All that one can say at present is that both groups of patients—those with Lewy bodies and those with MSA—are suffering from a primary (i.e. totally unexplained) degenerative disease of the nervous system. There are no known provoking factors, metabolic, infectious, or other. In general, the disease is not familial, although

Lewis (1964) described a family in which four members suffered a combination of ataxia, parkinsonism, and orthostatic hypotension. I have myself examined a case of MSA with autonomic failure (Oppenheimer 1980, case 17) with a fairly convincing history of dominant inheritance. One might be tempted to suppose that a sporadically-occurring disease was essentially different from one with dominant inheritance, whatever the clinical and pathological resemblances; but this expectation is probably naive. The same problem is met in Pick's disease (see Corsellis 1976) and in OPCA (see Konigsmark and Weiner 1970).

The second main problem is in identifying the lesion or lesions responsible for autonomic failure. Figure 25.2 leaves no room for doubt that there is an association between autonomic failure and loss of preganglionic autonomic neurons; but the two recorded cases (Hughes *et al.* 1970; Evans *et al.* 1972) of autonomic failure without detectable loss of intermediolateral cells lead one to look for a primary cause elsewhere. For example, it might be that cell loss in the intermediolateral columns is a transsynaptic effect of degeneration in the upper sympathetic pathway, occurring in most but not in all cases of autonomic failure. To test this possibility we should need to know more than we do about the location of the cells of origin of these pathways. If, as could well be the case, these cells are diffusely scattered through the brainstem reticular formation, it will be difficult to decide whether, or how much, their numbers are depleted. In any case, it would be a mistake to assume that the relevant lesion necessarily involves loss of cells. Nerve cells may be in good health but yet be unable to function normally because of a chemical inadequacy—as appears to be the case for the striatal nerve cells in Parkinson's disease. This leads to a further question, relevant to all types of multisystem degeneration. When several neuronal structures degenerate in a selective manner, leaving neighbouring structures intact, to what extent is this due to common physiological or biochemical properties of the cells concerned, and to what extent do the cells undergo transsynaptic, or 'chain' degeneration? Selective atrophy of pigmented cells in various brainstem nuclei in Parkinson's disease suggests the former. Concomitant degeneration of olives and Purkinje cells in OPCA, and of striatum and substantia nigra in SND, suggests the latter. Yet loss of nigral cells does not cause loss of striatal cells in Parkinson's disease, and loss of striatal cells does not entail loss of nigral cells in Huntington's chorea. These problems seem to be no nearer solution now than when they were discussed by Bannister and Oppenheimer in 1972, by Takei and Mirra in 1973, and by Schober *et al.* in 1975.

Finally, there is the broader question of the nosological placing of these cases. Some of them show unmistakable clinical and pathological evidence of Parkinson's disease, with preganglionic cell loss and autonomic failure as additional features. Others, not showing either nigral-cell loss or clinical parkinsonism, nevertheless show Lewy-type inclusions. Should these cases be regarded as *formes frustes*, or pre-clinical stages, of Parkinson's disease? It is known that Lewy bodies are not found exclusively in Parkinson's disease. They have been observed by Lipkin (1959) and Forno (1966) in as many as 5 per cent of 'normal' controls; in two cases of familial ataxia by Sigwald *et al.* (1964); in a case of SND by Jellinger and Danielczyk (1968); in one out of 21 autopsied cases of OPCA by Jellinger and Tarnowska-Dziduszko (1971); in cases of MSA with autonomic failure by Thapedi *et al.* (1971); and by Guard *et al.* (1974), and in a similar case from Japan by Yamamura *et al.* (1973); and in a case of multiple system atrophy, with intermediolateral cell loss but without clinical signs of autonomic failure, by Kaiya (1974).

Cases such as these appear at first to blur the line of distinction between the two groups of cases in which autonomic failure occurs. In view of the fact that cells may be lost in the substantia nigra and in the intermediolateral columns and that Lewy bodies may be found in both groups, one might be tempted to suppose that Parkinson's disease and MSA form parts of a continuous spectrum of degenerative disease: but such a view is not, I think, justified in the present state of ignorance concerning the aetiology of both conditions. Cases with 'borderline' pathological changes, such as those referred to above, are exceedingly rare, whereas Parkinson's disease, without lesions in the striatum or cerebellar system, is common. In contrast, only a small minority of cases of OPCA fail to show lesions in the substantia nigra and/or striatum (Jellinger and Tarnowska-Dziduszko 1971), while five out of seven cases of SND examined by Takei and Mirra (1973) showed lesions in the cerebellar system. It is this extensive overlap which justifies the inclusion of OPCA and SND under the same heading of multiple system atrophy.*

Clinical differences between MSA and Parkinson's disease include the earlier age of onset, and age at death, in the former. For 21 cases of OPCA, Jellinger and Tarnowska-Dziduszko (1971) give a mean age at onset of 18.7 for familial cases and 35.2 for sporadic ones, with mean survivals of 21.8 and 6.3 years respectively. For 15 sporadic cases, the mean age at death was 57.7; and the same figure—57.7—is given by Takei and Mirra (1973) as the mean age at death in 17 recorded cases of SND. These figures contrast with those given by Hoehn and Yahr (1967) for 293 patients dying with idiopathic Parkinson's disease: duration of symptoms 1 to 33 years (mean 9.4 years), and age at death 43 to 91

* A similar view of the unity of OPCA and SND is taken by Takei and Mirra (1973); these authors, however, carry assimilation to much greater lengths by including Pick's disease, Friedreich's ataxia, and Huntington's chorea in the group. They do not include Parkinson's disease.

years, with a mean of 67.0. This difference (67.0 in Parkinson's disease as against 57.7 in MSA) is similar to that recorded in the two groups of cases with autonomic failure (72 as against 58.7).

One of the most noticeable clinical differences between the two groups is that in cases of MSA the parkinsonian features, if present, tend to be little affected by levodopa. This has been attributed to the loss of striatal cells, which are thought to be the point of action of the drug. Other biochemical and physiological differences are discussed in other chapters of this book. A common defect in such studies has been that the investigators have rarely been able to carry out parallel studies, with consistent techniques, on cases of the two groups. An exception is the work of Wilcox and Aminoff (1976). These authors observed cardiovascular responses to infusions of either noradrenalin or dopamine in normal subjects, five patients with Parkinson's disease, and five patients with the Shy–Drager syndrome. In general, the altered responses in patients with Parkinson's disease tended to be in the opposite direction from those in the Shy–Drager patients.

The twofold grouping of the cases of primary autonomic failure has been accepted by several authors. These include Schober *et al.* (1975), who described the clinical and pathological findings in two cases, one of each group. Where they differ from the view put forward here is in using the term 'idiopathic orthostatic hypotension' (IOH) as the name of the disease with two 'subtypes', one characterized by the finding of Lewy bodies, the other having the lesions of MSA. The two 'subtypes' share the common features of autonomic failure and loss of intermediolateral cells. In the view which I am proposing, there is no disease entity to which the term 'IOH' can properly be applied. Rather, there are two disease entities—Parkinson's disease and MSA—in both of which a minority of cases undergo degeneration in certain parts of the autonomic nervous system. The difference between these two views may seem to be largely verbal, having little to do with the practical management of cases; but it should be borne in mind that effective clinical research depends on finding a system of classification of cases which ensures that like is grouped with like. Real differences exist between the two groups of cases in which the autonomic centres degenerate. Confusion can result when cases of both kinds are lumped together for the purpose of clinical trials or biochemical investigations, and the results applied to all cases of autonomic failure.

B. Central neurochemistry of autonomic failure

E. G. S. Spokes

INTRODUCTION

Post-mortem studies on cases of primary autonomic failure have delineated two distinct pathological groups: a smaller group, showing lesions characteristic of Parkinson's disease, and a larger group, showing lesions of multiple system atrophy (MSA—a variable disease entity including olivopontocerebellar atrophy, striatonigral degeneration, and pyramidal degeneration). Patients in the second group display a variety of neurological deficits in addition to autonomic failure, which together constitute the Shy–Drager syndrome (Shy and Drager 1960). Although definite histological differences exist between these groups, they share certain common clinical and pathological features. First, in both, autonomic failure is associated with cell loss from the intermediolateral columns of the spinal cord; second, the clinical state of parkinsonism is related to loss of pigmented cells from the substantia nigra in both Parkinson's disease and the striatonigral form of MSA.

The supraspinal control of the autonomic nervous system is effected through complex loop systems connecting the limbic system, hypothalamus, and brainstem reticular formation which influence impulse traffic in spinal preganglionic neurons of the intermediolateral nuclei through a variety of descending tracts. An up-to-date anatomical summary based on animal studies is shown in Fig. 25.3.

The possible contribution of supraspinal lesions to autonomic failure is unclear and morphometric data on nuclear structures concerned with central control of autonomic outflow are scant. However, Evans *et al.* (1972) reported a case of autonomic failure without significant cell loss from the intermediolateral columns. Thus, it is conceivable that, in some cases at least, the primary lesion may be central with neuronal death in the intermediolateral columns perhaps occurring through transsynaptic degeneration as the disease evolves. The biochemical changes observed in plasma as a consequence of defective autonomic output are discussed in Chapters 18 and 19; those present in the central nervous system are very inadequately documented, due largely to the relative rarity of these conditions, and are based on neurochemical examinations of brain tissue obtained at autopsy and cerebrospinal fluid (CSF).

Spokes *et al.* (1979) performed neurochemical measurements on post-mortem brain tissue from four well-documented patients with autonomic failure, in all of whom there were additional non-autonomic

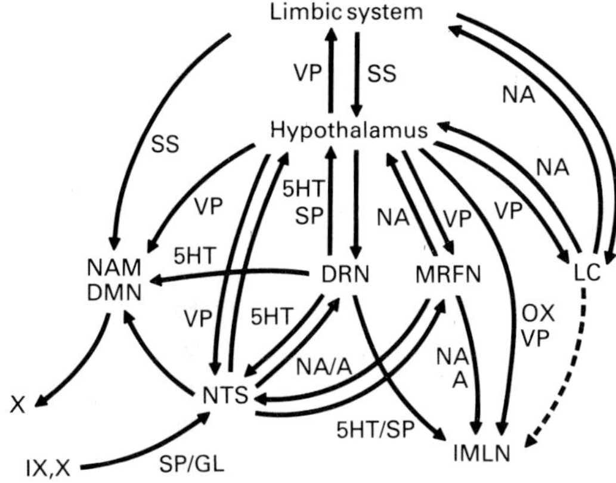

Fig. 25.3. Supraspinal pathways controlling autonomic output. NTS, nucleus of tractus solitarius; NAM, nucleus ambiguus; DMN, dorsal motor nucleus of the vagus; DRN, dorsal raphe nucleus; MRFN, medullary reticular formation nuclei; LC, locus ceruleus; IMLN, intermediolateral nuclei of spinal cord; IX, X, glossopharyngeal and vagus nerves respectively. Neurotransmitters: NA, noradrenalin; A, adrenalin, 5HT, serotonin; SP, substance P; VP, vasopressin; OX, oxytocin; GL, glutamate; SS, somatostatin. References: Saper *et al.* (1976); Ricardo and Koh (1978); Hopkins and Holstege (1978); Moore and Bloom (1979); Loewy (1981); Smith and De Vito (1984); Veening *et al.* (1984).

abnormalities including pyramidal, extrapyramidal, and cerebellar features, i.e. cases of multiple system atrophy. More recently, Kwak (1985) reported the findings in seven such cases.

MONOAMINES

Spokes *et al.* (1979) found low dopamine (DA) values in the corpus striatum, substantia nigra, septal nuclei, hypothalamus, and locus ceruleus (Table 25.2). Similar results were obtained by Kwak (1985). The finding of reduced DA concentrations in the basal ganglia (corpus striatum and substantia nigra) is consistent with the clinical state of parkinsonism resulting from striatonigral degeneration, and is similar to that observed in Parkinson's disease (Spokes and Bannister 1981). Loss of DA from the septal nuclei, nucleus accumbens, and hypothalamus implicates involvement of mesolimbic and intrinsic hypothalamic DA systems, which also occurs in Parkinson's disease. Thus, in both Parkinson's disease and striatonigral degeneration there is evidence for a widespread drop-out of dopaminergic neurons, reflected in low CSF levels of homovanillic acid, the major cerebral metabolite of dopamine (Williams 1981). It is of interest that parkinsonism associated with striatonigral degeneration responds poorly to dopaminergic agents

Table 25.2. Mean alterations in dopamine (DA), noradrenalin (NA), and tyrosine hydroxylase (TOH) values in four cases of MSA

Brain region	*Percentage change from control levels*		
	DA	*NA*	*TOH*
Corpus striatum	↓80	↓65	
Substantia nigra	↓75	↓80	
Nucleus accumbens	↓70	↓70	
Septal nuclei	↓55	↓80	
Hypothalamus	↓50	↓85	↓90
Locus ceruleus	↓60	↓75	

For quantitative data, see Spokes *et al.* (1979).

(Spokes *et al.* 1979), unlike that due to Parkinson's disease. This difference in therapeutic response could relate to a number of factors, one of which may be a reduction in striatal DA-receptor affinity in the former condition (Spokes and Bannister 1981). It is well established that central DA depletion profoundly affects motor function but its possible relevance to autonomic disturbance has yet to be evaluated. It would seem unlikely, however, that the nigrostriatal, mesolimbic, or hypothalamic DA systems are important as autonomic regulators as most cases of Parkinson's disease are not complicated by significant abnormal autonomic features. Whether medullary DA fibres are spared in Parkinson's disease is still unknown.

Noradrenergic fibres are diffusely distributed throughout the brain and spinal cord and arise from two major groups of cell bodies: the locus ceruleus in the central pontine grey matter and scattered nuclei throughout the medullary reticular formation (Moore and Bloom 1979). Ascending fibres from both groups innervate limbic structures and the hypothalamus. A crossed cerulospinal tract innervates the ventral horns (Commissiong 1981) and fibres from the medullary reticular nuclei innervate brainstem regions concerned with autonomic reflexes as well as sympathetic preganglionic neurons via a partly crossed bulbospinal pathway (Glazer and Ross 1980).

Both Spokes *et al.* (1979) and Kwak (1985) found reduced noradrenalin (NA) levels in multiple system atrophy cases (Table 25.2). The most marked depletion was seen in areas normally very rich in this amine—the septal nuclei, hypothalamus, and locus ceruleus. Losses from the basal ganglia were similar to those observed in Parkinson's disease (Spokes and Bannister 1981), but greater than those reported for Parkinson's disease in regions other than the basal ganglia. In accord with these findings, Williams (1981) has found significantly low levels of

NA in CSF from parkinsonian and MSA patients, especially pronounced in the latter group.

It is likely that some central NA fibres have a somatic function and modulate motor activity. At least some L-dopa is converted to NA within the brain and, indeed, NA depletion is less prominent in parkinsonian cases treated with this agent (Spokes and Bannister 1981). Animal experiments indicate that this process may contribute to L-dopa's efficacy as an anti-akinesia drug, perhaps via a facilitatory noradrenergic input from the locus ceruleus to nigral dopaminergic neurons or even through the influence of the cerulospinal pathway on anterior horn cells. Thus impaired ability to synthesize NA may to some extent limit the success of L-dopa therapy for parkinsonism. Certainly, loss of pigmented cells from the locus ceruleus occurs in Parkinson's disease and may also occur in multiple system atrophy. However, in multiple system atrophy (Spokes *et al.* 1979) NA depletion in the locus ceruleus occurred in the absence of prominent cell drop-out, except for one case, suggesting that this biochemical change is not merely a reflection of cell death. Consistent with this finding of NA loss, Black and Petito (1976) reported a tyrosine hydroxylase (TOH) deficit in the locus ceruleus of three patients dying with progressive autonomic failure (two of whom probably had associated Parkinson's disease and one multiple system atrophy).

Reduced NA concentrations in the septal nuclei and hypothalamus, and the gross depletion of hypothalamic TOH activity (Table 25.2), indicates, if comparisons with animal studies are valid, involvement of NA cell groups in the medullary reticular formation in the multiple system atrophy patients. It is probable, therefore, that noradrenergic innervation of brainstem nuclei and the intermediolateral columns of the spinal cord is also deficient, although measurements to substantiate this point are lacking. If such is indeed the case, the control of autonomic outflow could be profoundly affected. A finding possibly relevant to these speculations is that of Lloyd *et al.* (1975) who reported near normal levels of hypothalamic TOH activity in two cases of Parkinson's disease uncomplicated by autonomic failure, suggesting, perhaps, a relative sparing of medullary noradrenergic cell groups in this condition.

Serotonin (5HT)-containing neurons lie in the vicinity of the midline or raphe regions of the brainstem. Rostral groups of cells innervate forebrain areas whereas more caudal groups project to the medulla and spinal cord where they richly innervate sympathetic preganglionic neurons (Loewy and McKellar 1981). Serotonin has been shown to be reduced by 50 per cent in post-mortem striatal tissue from parkinsonian patients (Bernheimer *et al.* 1961) but there are no comparable data for patients with autonomic failure associated either with Parkinson's disease or multiple system atrophy. Sharpe *et al.* (1973) found normal striatal 5HT concentrations in a single case of striatonigral degeneration without autonomic impairment. Measurements of CSF 5-hydroxyindole acetic acid, the 5HT metabolite, have been used as an index of central serotonin turnover (although this is a dubious assumption), and fell within the normal range in parkinsonian cases (Williams 1981). In the same study, multiple system atrophy patients had a tendency to low values, but individuals remained within the normal range. Thus, at present there is no convincing evidence to implicate lesions of central serotonergic fibres in multiple system atrophy.

ACETYLCHOLINE

The integrity of central cholinergic neurons, as measured by regional analyses of choline acetyltransferase (CAT) activity, is shown in Table 25.3. In general, the findings of Spokes *et al.* (1979) and Kwak (1985) were similar for this enzyme. The changes in the basal ganglia parallel those observed in parkinsonian subjects and do not correlate with histopathological findings (Spokes *et al.* 1979; Kwak 1985). Thus reduced CAT activity need not necessarily imply cell death but rather functional underactivity of cholinergic neurons. In any event, the inconsistency of CAT loss from the basal ganglia in multiple system atrophy and its occurrence in Parkinson's disease and Huntington's chorea renders a connection with autonomic failure most unlikely.

On the other hand, low CAT was found in the dentate, red, olivary, and pontine nuclei, structures interconnected by fibre projections, in all

Table 25.3. Choline acetyltransferase (CAT) activities in various regions of post-mortem brain from four MSA cases

Brain region	*CAT levels*
Basal ganglia	N(2) or ↓(2)
Nucleus accumbens	N(2) or ↓(2)
Septal nuclei	N(1) or ↓(3)
Hypothalamus	↓(4)
Dentate nucleus	↓(4)
Red nucleus	↓(4)
Basal pons	↓(4)
Olive	↓(4)
Cerebellar cortex	N(1) or ↓(3)
Hippocampus	N(1) or ↓(3)
Motor cortex	N(3) or ↓(1)

N, normal level; ↓, reduction in CAT level. Number of cases in brackets.

For quantitative data, see Spokes *et al.* (1979).

the multiple system atrophy cases, those with the most marked depletion showing degenerative changes, an observation confirmed by Kwak (1985). Olivopontocerebellar atrophy is a common feature of multiple system atrophy and autonomic failure frequently develops. The CAT loss from the hypothalamus, a consistent finding in the MSA group, might also be relevant to some aspects of autonomic failure.

In three MSA cases reported by Spokes *et al.* (1979) there was deficient CAT activity in the septum and hippocampus which may mirror changes in the cholinergic septohippocampal pathway. It seems improbable that this observation is related to autonomic failure as similar changes are seen in Huntington's chorea and Alzheimer's disease, conditions in which autonomic disturbances are not prominent.

AMINO ACIDS

Glutamic acid decarboxylase (GAD), an enzyme marker for gamma aminobutyric acid (GABA)-containing neurons, shows a global loss in MSA cases (Spokes *et al.* 1979; Kwak 1985). GAD is markedly affected by agonal status, and any cause of a slow death, such as bronchopneumonia, reduces the activity of this enzyme, rendering interpretation of results very difficult. Measurements of GABA concentrations probably provide a more accurate index of the integrity of GABA-containing neurons. Kwak (1985) reported normal levels of GABA in the basal ganglia indicating preservation of GABA-containing striatal interneurons and striatonigral neurons. However, markedly reduced levels were found in the dentate nucleus correlating with Purkinje cell loss from the cerebellar cortex. Kwak (1985) also observed depletion of glutamate and aspartate in the cerebellum correlating with cell loss in the inferior olivary nucleus from which climbing fibres containing these amino acids arise, and loss of glutamate-containing granule cells in cerebellar cortex.

Cerebellar connections may be important in mediating orthostatic circulatory reflexes (Doba and Reis 1974) and loss of these pathways reflected in depleted levels of CAT, GABA, glutamate, and aspartate may contribute to postural hypotension.

SUBSTANCE P

About 30 peptide hormones are known to occur intraneuronally and act as neurotransmitters or neuromodulators. Substance P (SP) is the oldest putative peptide transmitter and the only one to be investigated in autonomic failure. Kwak (1985) measured SP in the basal ganglia in four cases and found markedly reduced levels in the substantia nigra with lesser reductions in the corpus striatum, consistent with Williams's

(1981) finding of a 50 per cent reduction in CSF SP concentrations in MSA patients. A similar pattern of loss occurs in Huntington's chorea and is believed to indicate degeneration of SP-containing striopallidonigral fibres. This latter observation renders a connection with autonomic failure unlikely although loss of the SP-containing striopallidonigral pathway may contribute to the poor response to L-dopa of patients with striatonigral degeneration as SP is believed to facilitate activity in the dopaminergic nigrostriatal tract.

CONCLUSION

An understanding of the biochemical lesions in autonomic failure is fundamental to rational therapy. The detection of such abnormalities in post-mortem brain tissue remains largely unexplored but the potential exists for major progress in this area using methods currently available which are being applied to animal studies. Early results on MSA have revealed changes in dopaminergic, noradrenergic, and cholinergic systems, as well as amino-acid neurotransmitters and substance P. It is unknown to what extent these relate to autonomic dysfunction, and comparative data from patients with MSA uncomplicated by autonomic failure and from parkinsonian subjects with autonomic failure will be needed before any useful deductions can be made.

C. Neuropathological approaches to degenerative disorders

Donald L. Price

INTRODUCTION

During the past decade, investigators have identified at least three degenerative disease syndromes manifested as autonomic failure (AF): patients with AF without other neurological manifestations (PAF); individuals with AF combined with Parkinson's disease (AF–PD); and patients with AF associated with a variety of other neurological abnormalities, i.e. multiple system atrophy (AF–MSA) (see Chapter 25A). In PAF, the number of neurons in the intermediolateral cell column is decreased as is the number of myelinated fibres in the ventral roots. AF–PD is characterized by Lewy bodies in the substantia nigra pars compacta (SNpc), loss of dopaminergic neurons in the SNpc, reductions in the number of nerve cells in the dorsal nucleus of the vagus, and a decrease in neurons in the intermediolateral cell column of the thoracic spinal cord. Individuals with AF–MSA exhibit evidence of involvement of neurons in a variety of regions of brain, including the striatum, SNpc, locus ceruleus, vestibular and pontine nuclei, inferior olives, Purkinje cells, dorsal nucleus of the vagus, pyramidal tracts, intermediolateral cell columns, and motor neurons. Levels of catecholaminergic markers may be decreased in locus ceruleus, septal nuclei, striatum, substantia nigra, and hypothalamus; levels of choline acetyltransferase (CAT) may be decreased in several nuclei of the brainstem and cerebellum (see Chapter 25B).

The challenge for neuropathologists is to use information derived from these studies to define the cellular and molecular abnormalities involved in the pathogeneses of these syndromes. Recently developed approaches (Table 25.4) have proved to be extraordinarily useful in the

Table 25.4. Neurobiological strategies for the study of degenerative disorders

Biological measures	*Techniques*	*Examples*
Clinical evaluation	Neuropsychological tests; assessment of changes in blood pressure	Memory impairments in patients with AD; postural hypotension in individuals with AF
Animal models	Studies of models	Memory impairments in aged monkeys; parkinsonian syndrome in monkeys with MPTP intoxication; motor neuron disease in dogs with HCSMA
Brain metabolism	Dynamic imaging studies	In AD, reduced glucose utilization in neocortex; in PD, alterations in striatal dopamine receptors
Gross and microscopic examination of brain	Inspection; histology; histochemistry; immunocytochemistry	In AD, neurofibrillary tangles in neurons in neocortex and hippocampus, and dopamine β-hydroxylase-immunostained neurites in plaques; in PD, neurofilament antigen sites in Lewy bodies; in ALS, neurofilamentous swellings of proximal motor axons
Quantitation of pathological changes	Morphometric studies	In AD, reduced number of neurons in basal forebrain cholinergic system; in PD, reduced number of neurons in SNpc; in AF, decreased number of neurons in the intermediolateral cell column
Neuron shape and size	Golgi stains	In AD, abnormal dendritic arborizations of pyramidal neurons in hippocampus

Table 25.4. (*cont.*)

Biological measures	*Techniques*	*Examples*
Ultrastructure	Electron microscopy; immunocytochemistry	Neurofilament and tau epitopes associated with paired helical filaments
Transmitters, enzymes, and receptors	Assays of markers; binding assays; *in vitro* autoradiography	In AD, reduced levels of CAT, somatostatin, and CRF in cortex; in PD and MPTP model, decreased dopamine in striatum; in ALS, loss of glycine receptors in ventral horn
Proteins of abnormal organelles	Purification of constituents; analyses of proteins and other components; immunocytochemistry	In AD, actin in Hirano bodies, tubulin in generalized vascular disease, and β-amyloid protein in plaque cores
Proteins and their modifications	Gels/Western blots; immunocytochemistry	In AD, A68 present in neurofibrillary tangles; presumed aberrant processing of β protein to form amyloidogenic fragment
Transport of proteins	In experimental models, radiolabelling and gel fluorography	In HCSMA, axonal swellings associated with impaired transport of neurofilament proteins
mRNAs	Hybridization *in situ* or on gels	β protein mRNA in neurons
Genes	DNA technology	Amyloid gene on chromosome 21; anonymous marker on 21 linked to familial AD

analyses of structural and chemical abnormalities occurring in the brains of individuals with a variety of adult-onset degenerative disorders, including Alzheimer's disease (AD), amyotrophic lateral sclerosis (ALS), and Parkinson's disease (PD) (Price 1986; Price *et al.* 1986; Tandan and Bradley 1985). In each of these diseases, significant progress has been made in demonstrating regional distributions of brain abnormalities, the involvement of specific neuronal systems, and aspects of the cellular and molecular abnormalities occurring in at-risk populations of nerve cells. Because it is likely that some of the approaches used in studies of other disorders will prove helpful in investigations of syndromes associated with autonomic failure (AF), results of these strategies are briefly reviewed using, as illustrations, studies of AD, ALS, and PD as well as animal models sharing features with these human disorders. Moreover, some of the same populations of neurons are affected in these diseases (i.e. motor neurons and SNpc cells) and in AF syndromes.

REGIONAL PATTERNS OF PATHOLOGY: THE NEOCORTEX IN ALZHEIMER'S DISEASE (AD)

AD involves neurons of the locus ceruleus, dorsal raphe, basal forebrain, amygdala, hippocampus, and neocortex (Price 1986). For heuristic purposes, this review focuses on the evidence of involvement of transmitter-specific populations of neocortical neurons in AD (Mountjoy *et al.* 1983). Somatostatinergic neurons develop neurofibrillary tangles and form neurites in plaques; levels of somatostatin-like and neuropeptide Y-like immunoreactivity are reduced in cortex. The number of somatostatin receptors is also decreased. GABAergic markers may be decreased, particularly in the temporal lobe; rare glutamic acid decarboxylase-immunoreactive neurites in plaques have been visualized in aged primates. Radioimmunoassays have detected reductions in levels of corticotrophin-releasing factor (CRF), a 41 amino-acid peptide present in some cortical neurons, and in some brainstem neurons projecting to cortex (DeSouza *et al.* 1986); moreover, CRF-immunoreactive neurites are present in small numbers of plaques. In regions showing low levels of CRF immunoreactivity, numbers of CRF receptors are reciprocally up-regulated. Although a variety of neuropeptides do not appear to be significantly altered in neocortex, these peptidergic systems do contribute neurites to plaques. In entorhinal cortex (Brodmann area 28), layer II and IV neurons develop neurofibrillary tangles (Kemper 1984), and the terminal fields of this system, i.e. the perforant pathway, show a high density of plaques; these observations suggest that individual neurons may develop perikaryal tangles and neuritic abnormalities of distal axons. Some of the neurons at risk are believed to use excitatory amino acids as transmitters; in cortex, glutamate concentrations and the uptake of [^{3}H] aspartate (a marker of glutaminergic terminals) may be mildly decreased.

INVOLVEMENT OF SPECIFIC NEURONAL SYSTEMS: MOTOR SYSTEMS IN AMYOTROPHIC LATERAL SCLEROSIS (ALS) AND THE NIGROSTRIATAL SYSTEM IN PARKINSON'S DISEASE (PD)

In many of these degenerative disorders of the central nervous system, specific populations of neurons are selectively vulnerable, although other cell groups are spared. For the purpose of discussion, we consider the evidence for involvement of motor neurons in ALS and dopaminergic neurons of the SNpc in PD.

Motor systems in ALS

ALS and its variants provide examples of diseases that affect specific neurons, i.e. motor neurons in brainstem and spinal-cord motor and upper motor neurons in neocortex (Hughes 1982; Tandan and Bradley 1985). Involvement of pyramidal neurons in motor cortex leads to secondary degeneration in corticospinal pathways. Ventral horns show: neurofibrillary swellings of proximal axons; reductions in the calibre of myelinated motor axons; decreased numbers of motor neurons; and lower levels of glycinergic, benzodiazepine, and muscarinic cholinergic receptors. Impaired axonal transport of neurofilament proteins (composed of 200-, 160-, and 68-kilodalton (kDa) proteins) may play a role in the pathogenesis of neurofilamentous axonal swellings and atrophy of distal axons. Consistent with this concept are experimental studies of parameters of axonal transport and axon calibre in experimental models of neurofibrillary axonal pathology (see below) (Cork *et al.* 1982; Griffin *et al.* 1978; Troncoso *et al.* 1985).

Nigrostriatal systems in PD

Abnormalities of the dopaminergic nigrostriatal system are a hallmark of PD (Forno 1986). Nerve cells in the SNpc are reduced in number, and some surviving nigral neurons contain Lewy bodies, i.e. concentric, intracytoplasmic inclusions containing neurofilament antigens. Dopaminergic markers are decreased in the striatum (80–95 per cent), and the ratio of striatal dopamine to homovanillic acid (an index of dopamine turnover and release) is decreased (Hornykiewicz 1982). Thus, surviving nigral neurons may increase their activity in response to loss of some of the SNpc cells. Postsynaptic striatal nerve cells may compensate by increasing the number of dopamine receptors.

CELLULAR AND MOLECULAR PATHOLOGIES

As neuronal systems at risk in a disease are defined, cellular and molecular biological strategies (Table 25.4) can be used to analyse structural/chemical abnormalities occurring in affected cells. These approaches are illustrated by studies of the biology of neurofibrillary tangles and amyloid-containing senile plaques occurring in AD.

Neurofibrillary tangles

These inclusions in the cell bodies of neurons represent accumulations of insoluble 10-nm paired helical filaments (Kidd 1963), the protein composition of which has not yet been defined. Immunocytochemical studies have demonstrated that tangles are associated with a variety of antigens, including tau, microtubule-associated protein 2, phosphorylated epitopes of the 200-kDa neurofilament protein, A68 (a 68-kDa protein enriched in the brains of individuals with AD), and, a 4-kDa protein (A4) that appears to share N-terminal amino-acid sequence homology with the β-amyloid protein (Wolozin *et al.* 1986). Ubiquitin, a protein that plays a proteolytic role in degradation of intracellular proteins, is also present in paired helical filaments, suggesting that diseased neurons may be attempting to degrade the insoluble constituents of paired helical filaments.

Senile plaques

Located in the amygdala, hippocampus, and neocortex, these spherical foci consist of enlarged axons, dendrites, and synaptic terminals (containing straight filaments and paired helical filaments) associated with extracellular deposits of amyloid. Plaques represent sites of abnormal synaptic interactions. In aged non-human primates and individuals with AD, neurites in plaques are derived from a variety of transmitter systems, including cholinergic, monoaminergic, and peptidergic neurons (Kitt *et al.* 1984, 1985). Within individual plaques, neurites may arise from more than one transmitter system.

Amyloid is located in plaque cores (in proximity to degenerating neurites) and in the walls of cerebral blood vessels. Amyloid fibrils are composed, in substantial part, of a β-pleated sheet protein with a unique sequence (Price 1986; Wong *et al.* 1985). Recently, oligonucleotides corresponding to β-protein sequences have been used to isolate clones encoding the β-protein precursor from human brain expression libraries; the gene encoding the β-protein is highly conserved and is localized to human chromosome 21 (Goldgaber *et al.* 1987; Kang *et al.* 1987). In four pedigrees of familial AD, a link has been demonstrated between two anonymous DNA markers on chromosome 21 and the presence of familial AD. In Down's syndrome and in certain putative non-familial cases of AD, there may be a microduplication of a subsection of the long arm of chromosome 21 that contains the gene encoding the amyloid protein. A 3.5-kb mRNA for the β-protein is present in mammalian brain (as well as non-neural tissues), and this transcript encodes a protein consisting of 695 residues (Kang *et al.* 1987). This protein, which may be a glycosylated cell-surface receptor, is apparently cleaved to form the much smaller amyloid peptide (44 amino acids) that is deposited in brain (Kang *et al.* 1987).

ANIMAL MODELS

Studies of animal models provide an opportunity to examine certain degenerative disorders in ways not possible in humans. In certain animal diseases, specific populations of neurons are selectively destroyed. We briefly consider three examples: the parkinsonian syndrome produced by intoxication with 1-methyl-4-phenyl-1,2,3,6,tetrahydropyridine (MPTP) (Burns *et al.* 1983; Langston *et al.* 1984; Kitt *et al.* 1986); the motor neuron disease, Hereditary Canine Spinal Muscular Atrophy (HCSMA), occurring in Brittany spaniels (Sack *et al.* 1984); and aged non-human primates who show behavioural and pathological features similar to those occurring in aged humans and individuals with AD (Kitt *et al.* 1984, 1985).

Experimental parkinsonian syndrome

When systemically administered to humans and monkeys, MPTP produces an akinesia, rigidity, postural tremor, and flexed posture (Burns *et al.* 1983; Langston *et al.* 1984). After passing through the blood–brain barrier, MPTP binds to monoamine oxidase B, an enzyme enriched in certain regions, including the striatum. MPTP is then converted to 1-methyl-4-phenylpyridinium, which is taken up by a high-affinity dopamine uptake system in nerve terminals within the striatum. This toxin selectively damages the nigrostriatal dopaminergic system: at low levels, the toxin produces a chemical axotomy of dopaminergic neurons; at high levels, SNpc neurons are destroyed (Kitt *et al.* 1986). Surviving nigral neurons show reduced tyrosine hydroxylase-like immunoreactivity (Kitt *et al.* 1986), and dopaminergic markers are reduced in the striatum (Burns *et al.* 1983).

Hereditary canine spinal muscular atrophy (HCSMA)

HCSMA, occurring in Brittany spaniels, is an autosomal dominant motor neuron disease exhibiting three phenotypes—chronic, intermediate, and accelerated disease (Sack *et al.* 1984). All affected dogs develop weakness, fasciculations, and neurogenic atrophy. At autopsy, some motor neurons show chromatolysis, and, in some of these cells, CAT immunoreactivity appears to be reduced. Proximal motor axons contain neurofilament-filled axonal swellings (Cork *et al.* 1982), and fibre calibres are reduced in ventral roots. Axonal transport is impaired, i.e. reductions occur in the rate of slowly transported proteins, particularly neurofilament proteins. Eventually, neurons degenerate, and ventral roots and peripheral nerves show evidence of Wallerian degeneration. These pathological changes are similar to those occurring in lower motor neurons in ALS (Cork *et al.* 1982).

Aged monkeys

Aged monkeys exhibit a variety of cognitive/memory deficits, including reductions in short-term memory, difficulties with problem-solving, etc.

Moreover, aged non-human primates develop senile plaques resembling the plaques occurring in aged humans and in patients with AD (Selkoe *et al.* 1987). Late in the second decade of life, macaques develop axonal pathology manifested, in part, as neurite-rich cortical plaques; older animals have more plaques, and these plaques contain greater amounts of amyloid (Struble *et al.* 1985). Deposits show immunological cross-reactivity with amyloid from AD brain (Selkoe *et al.* 1987). Neurites in plaques are derived from axons and terminals of cholinergic, peptidergic, catecholaminergic, and gamma aminobutyric acid (GABA)ergic systems (Kitt *et al.* 1984, 1985), and axons/terminals in an individual plaque may be derived from more than one source. In aged macaques, trends exist for plaque densities to be a better predictor of impaired cognitive functions than chronological age (Struble *et al.* 1985).

CONCLUSION

Neurobiological approaches have enhanced our understanding of important features of a variety of degenerative disorders of the central nervous system. It is likely that some of these strategies can be used to clarify some of the processes occurring in AF-associated syndromes. For example, *in situ* hybridization and immunocytochemical studies suggest that neurons of the inferior olive use CRF as a transmitter (Young *et al.* 1986). Perhaps levels of CRF in cerebrospinal fluid are decreased in AF–MSA; if so, a radioimmunoassay may be of diagnostic value. Moreover, it has been shown that the pedunculopontine nucleus is a major non-motor cholinergic nucleus of the brainstem and that this nucleus is affected in several neurological diseases (Whitehouse *et al.* 1987); the cholinergic deficits in the brainstem in AF–MSA may result from lesions of this nucleus. Finally, recent molecular biological approaches have begun to demonstrate the responses of neurons in ganglia to axotomy (Hoffman *et al.* 1987); similar approaches can be used to examine ganglia in AF-associated syndromes. The above-described examples and the above-cited studies of AD, ALS, and PD illustrate new approaches that may be used in future investigations of AF syndromes.

Acknowledgements

The author thanks Drs Linda C. Cork, Cheryl A. Kitt, Lary C. Walker, John W. Griffin, Paul N. Hoffman, George H. Sack, Robert G. Struble, and Peter J. Whitehouse for helpful discussions.

This work was supported by grants from the US Public Health Service (NIH NS 10580, NS 15721, AG 03359, AG 05146) and funds from the Robert L. and Clara G. Patterson Trust and the Claster family.

REFERENCES

Adams, R. D., van Bogaert, L., and Van der Eecken, H. (1961). Dégénérescences nigro-striées et cérébello-nigro-striées. *Psychiat. Neurol.* **142**, 219.

Adams, R. D., van Bogaert, L., and van der Eecken, H. (1964). Striato-nigral degeneration. *J. Neuropathol. exp. Neurol.* **23**, 584–608.

Bannister, R., Gibson, M., Michaels, L., and Oppenheimer, D. (1981). Laryngeal abductor paralysis in multiple system atrophy. *Brain* **104**, 351–86.

Bannister, R. and Oppenheimer, D. R. (1972). Degenerative diseases of the nervous system associated with autonomic failure. *Brain* **95**, 457–74.

Bernheimer, H., Birkmayer, W., and Hornykiewicz, O. (1961). Verteilung des 5-Hydroxytryptamins (Serotonin) im Gehirn des Menschen und sein Verhalten bei Patienten mit Parkinson-Syndrom. *Klin. Wochenschr.* **39**, 1056–9.

Black, I. and Petito, C. (1976). Catecholamine enzymes in the degenerative neurological disease idiopathic orthostatic hypotension. *Science, NY* **192**, 910–12.

Burns, R. S., Chiueh, C. C., Markey, S. P., Ebert, M. H., Jacobowitz, D. M., and Kopin, I. J. (1983). A primate model of parkinsonism: selective destruction of dopaminergic neurons in the pars compacta of the substantia nigra by N-methyl-4-phenyl-1,2,3,6-tetrahydropyridine. *Proc. Nat. Acad. Sci., USA* **80**, 4546–50.

Castaigne, P., Laplane, D., Autret, A., Bousser, M. G., Gray, F., and Baron, J. C. (1977). Syndrome de Shy et Drager avec troubles du rhythme respiratoire et de la vigilance. *Revue neurol.* **133**, 455–6.

Commissiong, J. (1981). Evidence that the noradrenergic coerulospinal projection decussates at the spinal level. *Brain Res.* **212**, 145–51.

Cork, L. C., Griffin, J. W., Choy, C., Padula, C. A., and Price, D. L. (1982). Pathology of motor neurons in accelerated Hereditary Canine Spinal Muscular Atrophy. *Lab. Invest.* **46**, 89–99.

Corsellis, J. A. N. (1976). Pick's disease. In *Greenfield's neuropathology*, 3rd edn, pp. 817–21. Arnold, London.

de Lean, J. and Deck, J. H. (1976). Shy–Drager syndrome. Neuropathological correlation and response to levodopa therapy. *Can. J. neurol. Sci.* **3**, 161–73.

DeSouza, E. B., Whitehouse, P. J., Kuhar, M. J., Price, D. L., and Vale, W. W. (1986). Reciprocal changes in corticotrophin-releasing factor (CRF)-like immunoreactivity and CRF receptors in cerebral cortex of Alzheimer's disease. *Nature* **319**, 593–5.

Doba, N. and Reis, D. (1974). Role of the cerebellum and vestibular apparatus in regulation of orthostatic reflexes in the cat. *Circulation Res.* **34**, 9–18.

Evans, D., Lewis, P., Malhotra, O., and Pallis, C. (1972). Idiopathic orthostatic hypotension. Report of an autopsied case with histochemical and ultrastructural studies of the neuronal inclusions. *J. neurol. Sci.* **17**, 209–18.

Fichefet, J. P., Sternon, J. E., Franken, L., Demanet, J. C., and Vanderhaeghen, J. J. (1965). Etude anatomo-clinique d'un cas d'hypotension orthostatique idiopathique. *Acta cardiol.* **20**, 332–48.

Fischer, E. and Petri, C. (1969). The orthostatic hypotensioin syndrome of Shy–Drager: a clinical-pathological report. *Dan. med. Bull.* **16**, 189–92.

Forno, L. S. (1966). Pathology of parkinsonism: a preliminary report of 24 cases. *J. Neurosurg.* **24**, 266–71.

Forno, L. S. (1986). The Lewy body in Parkinson's disease. In *Parkinson's disease.*

Advances in neurology (ed. M. D. Yahr and K. J. Berrgmann), Vol. 45, pp. 35–43. Raven Press, New York.

Glazer, E. and Ross, L. (1980). Localisation of noradrenergic terminals in sympathetic preganglionic nuclei of the rat; demonstration by immunocytochemical localisation of dopamine-β-hydroxylase. *Brain Res.* **185**, 39–49.

Goldgaber, D., Lerman, M. I., McBride, O. W., Saffiotti, U., and Gajdusek, D. C. (1987). Characterization and chromosomal localization of a cDNA encoding brain amyloid of Alzheimer's disease. *Science* **235**, 877–80.

Graham, J. G. and Oppenheimer, D. R. (1969). Orthostatic hypotension and nicotine sensitivity in a case of multiple system atrophy. *J. Neurol. Neurosurg. Psychiat.* **32**, 28–34.

Griffin, J. W., Hoffman, P. N., Clark, A. W., Carroll, P. T., and Price, D. L. (1978). Slow axonal transport of neurofilament proteins: impairment by β,β'-iminodipropionitrile administration. *Science* **202**, 633–5.

Guard, O., Sindou, M., and Carrier, H. (1974). Syndrome de Shy–Drager; une nouvelle observation anatomo-clinique. *Lyon méd.* **231**, 1075–84.

Hassler, R. (1938). Zur Pathologie der Paralysis agitans und des postenzephalitischen Parkinsonismus. *J. Psychol. Neurol., Leipzig* **48**, 387.

Hoehn, M. M. and Yahr, M. D. (1967). Parkinsonism: onset, progression and mortality. *Neurology, Minneapolis.* **17**, 427–42.

Hoffman, P. N., Cleveland, D. W., Griffin, J. W., Landes, P. W., Cowan, N. J., and Price, D. L. (1987). Neurofilament gene expression: a major determinant of axonal caliber. *Proc. Nat. Acad. Sci., USA* **84**, 3472–6.

Hopkins, D. and Holstege, G. (1978). Amygdaloid projections to the mesencephalon, pons and medulla oblongata in the cat. *Exp. Brain Res.* **32**, 529–47.

Hornykiewicz, O. (1982). Brain neurotransmitter changes in Parkinson's disease. In *Movement disorders, neurology* (ed. C. D. Marsden and S. Fahn), Vol. 2, pp. 41–58. Butterworth Scientific, London.

Hughes, J. T. (1982). Pathology of amyotrophic lateral sclerosis. In *Human motor neuron diseases. Advances in neurology* (ed. L. P. Rowland), Vol. 36, pp. 61–74. Raven Press, New York.

Hughes, R. C., Cartlidge, N. E. F., and Millac, P. (1970). Primary neurogenic orthostatic hypotension. *J. Neurol. Neurosurg. Psychiat.* **33**, 363–71.

Iwata, M. and Hirano, A. (1978). Sparing of the Onufrowicz nucleus in sacral anterior horns. *Ann. Neurol.* **4**, 245–9.

Jager, W. A. den H. and Bethlem, J. (1960). The distribution of Lewy bodies in the central and autonomic nervous systems in idiopathic paralysis agitans. *J. Neurol. Neurosurg. Psychiat.* **23**, 283–90.

Jellinger, K. and Danielczyk, W. (1968). Striato-nigrale degneration. *Acta neuropathol.* **10**, 242–57.

Jellinger, K. and Tarnowska-Dziduszko, E. (1971). Die ZNS-Veränderungen bei den olivo-ponto-cerebellaren Atrophien. *Z. Neurol.* **199**, 192–214.

Johnson, R. H., Lee, G. de J., Oppenheimer, D. R., and Spalding, J. M. K. (1966). Autonomic failure with orthostatic hypotension due to intermediolateral column degeneration. *Quart. J. Med.* **35**, 276–92.

Kaiya, H. (1974). Spino-olivo-ponto-cerebello-nigral atrophy with Lewy bodies and binucleated nerve cells. *Acta neuropathol.* **30**, 263–9.

Kang, J., Lemairee, H-. G., Unterbeck, A., Salbaum, J. M., Masters, C. L.,

Grzeschik, K-. H., Multhaup, G., Beyreuther, K., and Müller-Hill, B. (1987). The precursor of Alzheimer's disease amyloid A4 protein resembles a cell-surface receptor. *Nature* **325**, 733–6.

Kemper, T. (1984). Neuroanatomical and neuropathological changes in normal aging and in dementia. In *Clinical neurology of aging* (ed. M. L. Albert), pp. 9–52. Oxford University Press, New York.

Kennedy, P. G. E. and Duchen, L. W. (1985). A quantitative study of intermediolateral column cells in motor neuron disease and the Shy–Drager syndrome. *J. Neurol. Neurosurg. Psychiat.* **48**, 1103–6.

Kidd (1963). Paired helical filaments in electron microscopy of Alzheimer's disease. *Nature* **197**, 192–3.

Kitt, C. A., Cork, L. C., Eidelberg, E., Joh, T. H., and Price, D. L. (1986). Injury of nigral neurons exposed to 1-methyl-4-phenyl-1,2,3,6,tetrahydropyridine: a tyrosine hydroxylase immunocytochemical study in monkey. *Neuroscience* **17**, 1089–103.

Kitt, C. A., Price, D. L., Struble, R. G., Cork, L. C., Wainer, B. H., Becher, M. W., and Mobley, W. C. (1984). Evidence for cholinergic neurites in senile plaques. *Science* **226**, 1443–5.

Kitt, C. A., Struble, R. G., Cork, L. C., Mobley, W. C., Walker, L. C., Joh, T. H., and Price, D. L. (1985). Catecholaminergic neurites in senile plaques in prefrontal cortex of aged nonhuman primates. *Neuroscience* **16**, 691–9.

Kluyskens, Y., Bossaert, L., Snoeck, J., and Martin, J. J. (1977). Idiopathic orthostatic hypotension and the Shy and Drager syndrome: physiological studies in four cases; pathological report of one case. *Acta cardiol.* **32**, 317–35.

Konigsmark, B. W. and Weiner, L. P. (1970). The olivopontocerebellar atrophies: a review. *Medicine, Baltimore* **49**, 227–41.

Konno, H., Yananotot, T., Iwasaki, Y., and Iizuka, H. (1986). Shy–Drager syndrome and amyotrophic lateral sclerosis: cytoarchitectonic and morphometric studies of sacral autonomic neurons. *J. neurol. Sci.* **73**, 193–204.

Kwak, S. (1985). Biochemical analysis of transmitters in the brains of multiple system atrophy. *No Shinkei* **37**, 691–4.

Langston, J. W., Forno, L. S., Rebert, C. S., and Irwin, I. (1984). Selective nigral toxicity after systemic administration of 1-methyl-4-phenyl-1,2,5,6-tetrahydropyrine (MPTP) in the squirrel monkey. *Brain Res.* **292**, 390–4.

Lewis, P. (1964). Familial orthostatic hypotension. *Brain* **87**, 719–28.

Lipkin, L. E. (1959). Cytoplasmic inclusions in ganglion cells associated with Parkinsonian states. *Am. J. Path.* **35**, 1117–33.

Lloyd, K., Davidson, L., and Hornykiewicz, O. (1975). The neurochemistry of Parkinson's disease—effect of L-dopa therapy. *J. Pharmacol. exp. Ther.* **195**, 453–64.

Lockwood, A. H. (1976). Shy–Drager syndrome with abnormal respirations and antidiuretic hormone release. *Arch. Neurol., Chicago* **33**, 292–5.

Loewy, A. (1981). Descending pathways to sympathetic and parasympathetic preganglionic neurones. *J. auton. nerv. Syst.* **3**, 265–75.

Loewy, A. and McKellar, S. (1981). Serotonergic projections from the ventral medulla to the intermediolateral cell column in the rat. *Brain Res.* **211**, 146–52.

Mannen, T., Iwata, M., Toyakura, Y., and Nagashima, K. (1977). Preservation of a certain motor neurone group of the sacral cord in amyotrophic lateral sclerosis: its clinical significance. *J. Neurol. Neurosurg. Psychiat.* **40**, 464–9.

Mark, G. (1969). Die idiopathische orthostatische Hypotonie. *Schweitz. med. Wochenschr.* **99**, 1877–86.

Moore, R. and Bloom, F. (1979). Central catecholamine neuron systems: anatomy and physiology of the norepinephrine and epinephrine systems. *Ann. Rev. Neurosci.* **2**, 113–68.

Mountjoy, C. Q., Roth, M., Evans, N. J. R., and Evans, H. M. (1983). Cortical neuronal counts in normal elderly controls and demented patients. *Neurobiol. Aging* **4**, 1–11.

Nick, J., Contamin, F., Escourolle, R., Guillard, A., and Marcantoni, J.-P. (1967). Hypotension orthostatique idiopathique avec syndrome neurologique complexe à prédominance extra-pyramidale. *Revue neurol.* **116**, 213–27.

Onufrowicz, B. (1900). On the arrangement and function of the cell groups of the sacral region of the spinal cord in man. *Arch. Neurol. Psychopathol.* **3**, 387–412.

Oppenheimer, D. R. (1980). Lateral horn cells in progressive autonomic failure. *J. neurol. Sci.* **46**, 393–404.

Price, D. L. (1986). New perspectives on Alzheimer's disease. *Ann. Rev. Neurosci.* **9**, 489–512.

Price, D. L., Whitehouse, P. J., and Struble, R. G. (1986). Cellular pathology in Alzheimer's and Parkinson's diseases. *Trends Neurosci.* **9**, 29–33.

Rajput, A. H. and Rozdilsky, B. (1976). Dysautonomia in parkinsonism: a clinico-pathological study. *J. Neurol. Neurosurg. Psychiat.* **39**, 1092–100.

Reznik, M. (1980). Le syndrome de Shy–Drager: confrontation anatomo-clinique. *Acta neurol. belg.* **80**, 271–86.

Ricardo, J. and Koh, E. (1978). Anatomical evidence for direct projections from the nucleus of the solitary tract to the hypothalamus, amygdala and other forebrain structures in the rat. *Brain Res.* **153**, 1–26.

Roessmann, U., van den Noort, S., and McFarland, D. E. (1971). Idiopathic orthostatic hypotension. *Arch. Neurol., Chicago* **24**, 503–10.

Rohmer, F., Warter, J. M., Coquillat, G., Schupp, C., and Maitrot, D. (1973). 'Maladie' de Shy et Drager; a propos d'une observation anatomoclinique. Revue de la littérature. *Ann. Med. intern.* **124**, 665–73.

Sack, G. H. Jr., Cork, L. C., Morris, J. M., Griffin, J. W., and Price, D. L. (1984). Autosomal dominant inheritance of Hereditary Canine Spinal Muscular Atrophy. *Ann. Neurol.* **15**, 369–73.

Saper, C., Loewy, A., Swanson, L., and Cowan, W. (1976). Direct hypothalamo-autonomic connections. *Brain Res.* **117**, 305–12.

Schober, R., Langston, J. W., and Forno, L. S. (1975). Idiopathic orthostatic hypotension: biochemical and pathologic observations in 2 cases. *Eur. Neurol.* **13**, 177–88.

Schwarz, G. A. (1967). The orthostatic hypotension syndrome of Shy-Drager. *Arch. Neurol. Chicago* **16**, 123–39.

Selkoe, D. J., Bell, D. S., Podlisny, M. B., Price, D. L., and Cork, L. C. (1987). Conservation of brain amyloid proteins in aged mammals and humans with Alzheimer's disease. *Science* **235**, 873–7.

Sharpe, J., Rewcastle, N., Lloyd, K., Hornykiewicz, O., Hill, M., and Tasker, R. (1973). Striatonigral degeneration. Response to levodopa therapy with pathological and neurochemical correlation. *J. neurol. Sci.* **19**, 275–86.

Shy, G. and Drager, G. (1960). A neurological syndrome associated with orthostatic hypotension. *Arch. Neurol., Chicago* **2**, 511–27.

Sigwald, J., Lapresle, J., Raverdy, P., and Recondo, J. (1964). Atrophie cérébelleuse familiale avec association de lésions nigériennes et spinales. *Presse méd.* **72**, 557–62.

Smith, O. A. and DeVito, J. L. (1984). Central neural integration for the control of autonomic responses associated with emotion. *Ann. Rev. Neurosci.* **7**, 43–65.

Spokes, E. and Bannister, R. (1981). Catecholamines and dopamine receptor binding in parkinsonism. In *Research progress in Parkinson's disease* (ed. F. C. Rose and R. Capildeo), pp. 195–204. Pitman, London.

Spokes, E., Bannister, R., and Oppenheimer, D. R. (1979). Multiple system atrophy with autonomic failure. Clinical, histological and neurochemical observations on four cases. *J. neurol. Sci.* **43**, 59–82.

Struble, R. G., Price, D. L. Jr., Cork, L. C., and Price, D. L. (1985). Senile plaques in cortex of aged normal monkeys. *Brain Res.* **361**, 267–75.

Sung, J. H. (1979). Autonomic neurons affected by lipid storage in the spinal cord in Fabry's disease: distribution of autonomic neurons in the sacral cord. *J. Neuropath. exp. Neurol.* **38**, 87–98.

Sung, J. H., Mastri, A. R., and Segal, E. (1979). Pathology of Shy–Drager syndrome. *J. Neuropath. exp. Neurol.* **38**, 353–68.

Szabo, J. (1962). Topical distribution of the striatal efferents in the monkey. *Exp. Neurol.* **5**, 21–36.

Szabo, J. (1967). The efferent projections of the putamen in the monkey. *Exp. Neurol.* **19**, 463–76.

Takei, Y. and Mirra, S. S. (1973). Striato-nigral degeneration: a form of multiple system atrophy with clincal parkinsonism. In *Progress in neuropathology*, Vol. 2. (ed. H. M. Zimmerman), pp. 217–51. Grune and Stratton, New York.

Tandan, R. and Bradley, W. G. (1985). Amytrophic lateral sclerosis: Part 1. Clinical features, pathology, and ethical issues in management. *Ann. Neurol.* **18**, 271–80.

Thapedi, I. M., Ashenhurst, E. M., and Rozdilsky, B. (1971). Shy–Drager syndrome: report of an autopsied case. *Neurology, Minneapolis* **21**, 26–32.

Troncoso, J. C., Hoffman, P. N., Griffin, J. W., Hess-Kozlow, K. M., and Price, D. L. (1985). Aluminium intoxication: a disorder of neurofilament transport in motor neurons. *Brain Res.* **342**, 172–5.

Vanderhaeghen, J. J., Périer, O., and Sternon, J. E. (1970). Pathological findings in idiopathic orthostatic hypotension: its relationship with Parkinson's disease. *Arch. Neurol., Chicago* **22**, 207–14.

Veening, J. G., Swanson, L. W., and Sawchenko, P. E. (1984). The organization of projections from the central nucleus of the amygdala to brainstem sites involved in central autonomic regulation: a combined retrograde transport–immunohistochemical study. *Brain Res.* **303**, 337–57.

Vuia, O. (1975). Striato-nigral degeneration and Shy–Drager syndrome (idiopathic orthostatic hypotension). *Clin. Neurol. Neurosurg.* **78**, 196–203.

Whitehouse, P. J., Vale, W. W., Zweig, R. M., Singer, H. S., Mayeux, R., Kuhar, M. J., Price, D. L., and DeSouza, E. B. (1987). Reductions in corticotrophin releasing factor-like immunoreactivity in cerebral cortex in Alzheimer's disease, Parkinson's disease, and progressive supranuclear palsy. *Neurology* **37**, 905–9.

Wolozin, B. L., Pruchnicki, A., Dickson, D. W., and Davies, P. (1986). A neuronal antigen in the brains of Alzheimer patients. *Science* **232**, 648–50.

Wilcox, C. S. and Aminoff, M. J. (1976). Blood pressure responses to noradrenaline and dopamine infusions in Parkinson's disease and the Shy–Drager syndrome. *Br. J. clin. Pharmacol.* **3**, 207–14.

Williams, A. (1981). CSF biochemical studies on some extrapyramidal diseases. In *Research progress in Parkinson's disease* (ed. F. C. Rose and R. Capildeo), pp. 170–80. Pitman, London.

Wong, C. W., Quaranta, V. and Glenner, G. G. (1985). Neuritic plaques and cerebrovascular amyloid in Alzheimer disease are antigenically related. *Proc. nat. Acad. Sci. USA* **82**, 8729–32.

Yamamura, Y., Ikuta, F., Oyanagi, S., Atsumi, T., and Tsukada, Y. (1973). Striatonigral degeneration with autonomic failure, with especial reference to its correlation with olivo-ponto-cerebellar atrophy. [In Japanese with English summary.] *J. Niigata. med. Ass.* **87**, 508–16.

Young, W. S. III, Walker, L. C., Powers, R. E., DeSouza, E. B., and Price, D. L. (1986). Corticotrophin-releasing factor mRNA is expressed in the inferior olives of rodents and primates. *Mol. Brain Res.* **1**, 189–92.

26. The Lewy body and autonomic failure

W. R. G. Gibb

INTRODUCTION

In 1817 James Parkinson speculated that the site of pathology in paralysis agitans was the upper cervical spinal cord and medulla oblongata. Nearly a century later Friederich Lewy described cellular degeneration with inclusion bodies in the dorsal motor nucleus of the vagus (Fig. 26.1), as well as in the nucleus basalis of Meynert, thalamus, and hypothalamus. Lewy believed that the pathology in the medulla was the most important finding for it seemed to correlate with disorders of 'vegetative function' such as sweating, excessive tears, and blue swollen limbs. The autonomic nervous system was also implicated by Lafora in 1913 who identified similar inclusions in cells of the oculomotor nucleus. It was Tretiakoff in 1919 who implied that 'corps de Lewy' and cell loss in the substantia nigra were responsible for symptoms of Parkinson's disease, although it was not until the work of Hassler in 1938 that the substantia nigra was established as the main site of cell loss. In time Lewy bodies were also found in sympathetic ganglia and other specific locations such as the cerebral cortex. The term Lewy body–Parkinson's disease denotes Lewy bodies and cell degeneration in a specific distribution, principally involving the substantia nigra, locus ceruleus, dorsal motor nucleus of the vagus, nucleus basalis of Meynert, raphe nuclei, and autonomic nervous system (Bethlem and Den Hartog Jager 1960).

It was a popular nineteenth-century concept that sufferers from paralysis agitans showed features indicative of 'autonomic disturbance', such as seborrhoea, siallorhoea, poor skin colour, and constipation. Persons with postencephalitic parkinsonian syndrome, surviving the 1917–25 pandemic of encephalitis lethargica, were said to exhibit 'vagotonia', possibly a result of hypothalamic inflammation, thus further encouraging the belief that a number of commonly occurring signs in Parkinson's disease might reflect some ill-defined autonomic abnormality. However, many of these signs can be attributed more appropriately to the consequences of akinesia, for example. In contrast,

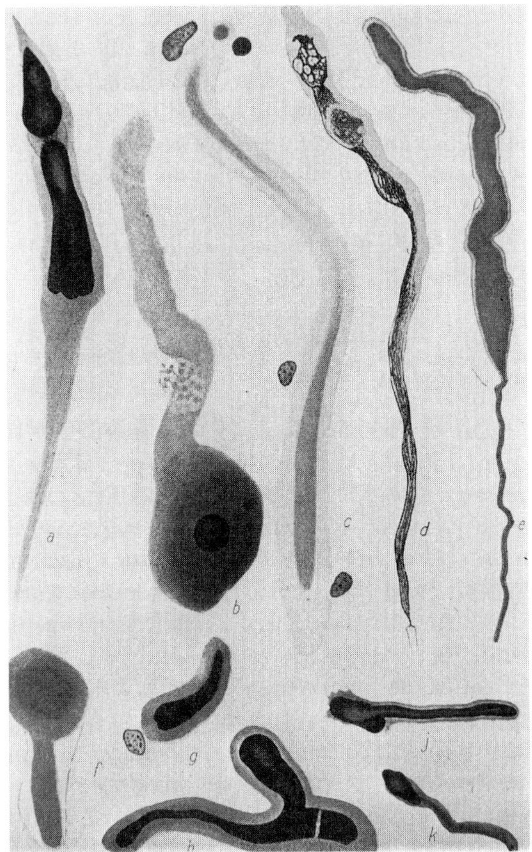

Fig. 26.1. Elongated bodies in the dorsal motor nucleus of the vagus in Parkinson's disease. (Taken from Lewy (1923).)

autonomic failure with symptoms of postural hypotension, sphincter disturbance, and sweating abnormalities, associated with pathological changes in the autonomic nervous system, is a relatively recent finding. Developments here began with the first pathological description by Shy and Drager of a parkinsonian syndrome complicated by autonomic failure. The lesions of striatal atrophy and loss of nigral cells, Purkinje cells, and intermediolateral column cells were consistent with the disorder now called multiple system atrophy (MSA) and not with Lewy body–Parkinson's disease. However, in 1965 severe postural hypotension was described in a woman, aged 71 years, who died 1 year later, after developing rest tremor, bradykinesia, and muscular rigidity (Fichefet *et al.* 1965; Vanderhaeghen *et al.* 1970). Lewy bodies were found in the substantia nigra as well as in cervical, thoracic, and lumbar sympathetic ganglia. Cells of anterior and lateral horns of the spinal cord were thought to be depleted, but Lewy bodies were not seen. In contrast to MSA the striatum and cerebellum were normal. With the publication of additional cases in the next few years it became clear (Graham and Oppenheimer 1969; Vanderhaeghen *et al.* 1970) that one pathological lesion in primary autonomic failure consisted of Lewy bodies and cell loss occurring in a similar distribution to that in Parkinson's disease. An alternative pathology, without Lewy bodies, was striatonigral degeneration, olivopontocerebellar atrophy (OPCA), and loss of preganglionic autonomic neurons in the spinal cord, which form the MSA spectrum.

AUTONOMIC FAILURE IN LEWY BODY–PARKINSON'S DISEASE

Following the report of Fichefet *et al.* (1965) a number of clinical studies endeavoured to quantitate the severity and prevalence of autonomic failure in Parkinson's disease. One consistent finding was that relatively minor degrees of postural hypotension were common, but were not associated with other features of autonomic failure. Recently, significant differences in supine pulse rate, postural hypotension, Valsalva response, and cold pressor diastolic rise were detected between 32 clinically diagnosed patients with Parkinson's disease and 10 controls (Goetz *et al.* 1986). However, the values represented relatively slight changes and fell within the normal range.

A few patients with Parkinson's disease develop dizziness related to postural hypotension and show a blood pressure fall of more than 20 mm Hg on standing (Kono *et al.* 1976; Rajput and Rozdilsky 1976, Cases 2 and 4; Oppenheimer 1980, Case 5). Reported pathological findings include Lewy bodies within sympathetic ganglia, possibly with cell loss, and cell loss in the lateral horns of the spinal cord. Cases similar to that of Fichefet *et al.* (1965), in which autonomic failure antedates Parkinson's disease, are uncommon. Three additional cases are reported in which parkinsonian features developed within 4 years of autonomic failure (Bannister and Oppenheimer 1972, Case 3; Schober *et al.* 1975, Case 2; Rajput and Rozdilsky 1976, Case 6). This contrasts with the relative frequency of autonomic failure as a presenting feature of MSA, not uncommonly antedating parkinsonian or cerebellar features by several months. In addition, in the context of Parkinson's disease, patients with autonomic failure, but no evidence of Parkinson's disease during life, are rare. Johnson *et al.* (1966), Case 1, described a 62-year-old man, who developed autonomic failure and died without evidence of Parkinson's disease 4 years later. Lewy bodies were present in the substantia nigra without detectable cell loss. They were also present in the intermediolateral columns and the cervical and thoracic sympathetic ganglia. The important difference between the degenerative changes in the substantia nigra of this case and that of Fichefet *et al.* was that the severity of nigral cell loss in this case was insufficient to produce parkinsonian features.

Vanderhaeghen *et al.* (1970, Case 2) and Roessman *et al.* (1971, Case 1) described similar patients that died 2 and 13 years, respectively, after first developing symptoms of autonomic failure. In the first case the substantia nigra did not show obvious cell loss, but in some areas microglia were increased and there was phagocytosis of melanin (Vanderhaeghen *et al.* 1970). In the second case cells were depleted in the substantia nigra, locus ceruleus, and dorsal vagal nucleus, where Lewy bodies were also present (Roessman *et al.* 1971). In neither case were the putamina and pontine nuclei confirmed to be normal, and one showed astrocytic reaction and neuronal loss in the inferior olives (Roessman *et al.* 1971). In view of the relatively infrequent finding of autonomic failure in Lewy body–Parkinson's disease, the possibility of dual pathology (see below) with MSA and Lewy bodies should be carefully considered in cases with short clinical histories. Two other cases, men aged 83 years and 70 years with 0.5 and 5-year histories, respectively, had autonomic failure without Parkinson's disease or obvious nigral cell loss, but Case 7 showed definite cell loss in the locus ceruleus (Oppenheimer 1980, Cases 7 and 8). The striatum, pontine nuclei, and Purkinje cells were confirmed to be normal.

LEWY BODY–PARKINSON'S DISEASE

Morphology of Lewy bodies

The Lewy body is seen in neuronal cytoplasm (Fig. 26.2(a)), but may be found in nerve cell processes (Fig. 26.2(b)) and a few lie free in the neuropil, after their release from degenerating cells. The classical Lewy body in the substantia nigra and locus ceruleus is a spherical intracytoplasmic inclusion, 5–25 μm in diameter, with a dense eosinophilic core, a body with or without concentric laminations, and a surrounding halo. More commonly, Lewy bodies in the substantia nigra and locus ceruleus have a simple structure consisting of a body and halo alone (Fig. 26.2(b)). Other neuronal changes in Lewy body–Parkinson's disease, including pale staining inclusions without haloes, are not as specific for the disease. The morphology of the Lewy body varies according to its location. Those in the autonomic nervous system, including the hypothalamus, dorsal vagal nucleus, and sympathetic ganglia, are more often in nerve cell processes and their appearances are almost unique to these locations. Some are elongated and serpiginous (Vanderhaeghen *et al.* 1970); others are large, irregularly rounded, pale bodies with or without central condensations, resembling Lewy bodies (Fig. 26.2(c)). In the

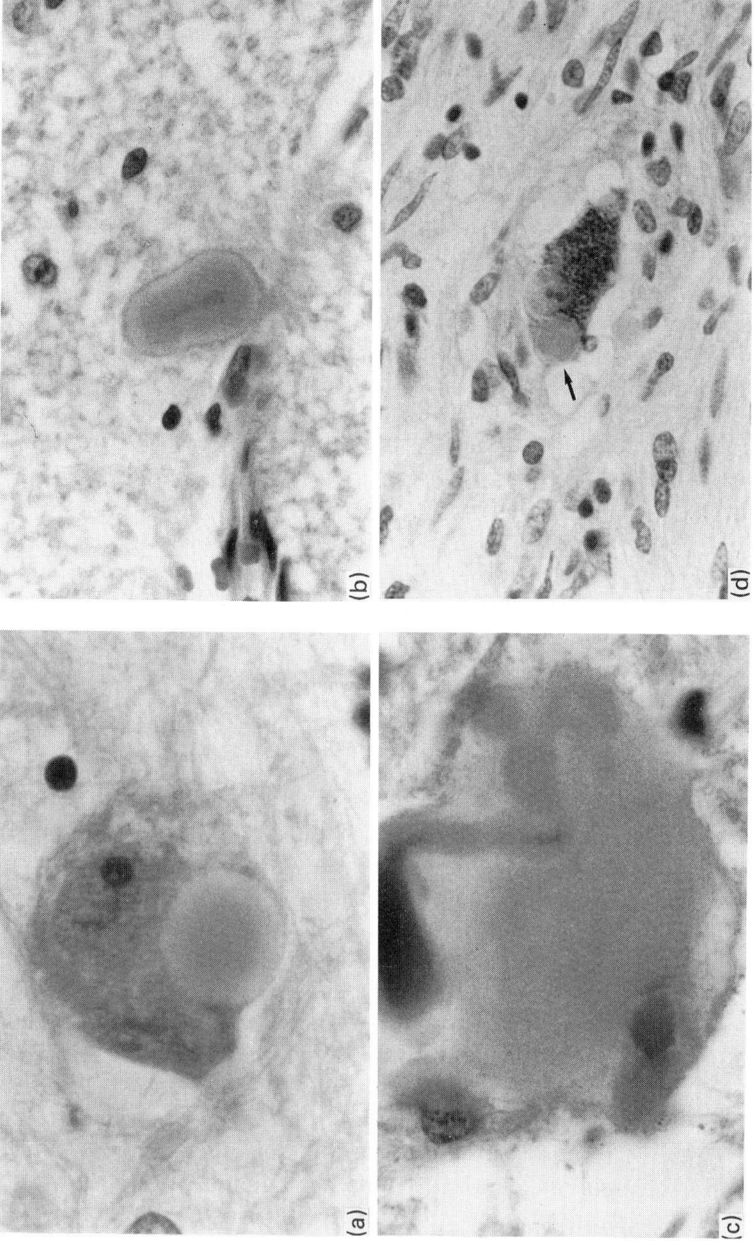

Fig. 26.2. (a) Lewy body with halo in non-pigmented neuron of the substantia nigra. H & E, ×800. (b) Lewy body with darker core, body, and halo in the locus ceruleus, probably in a nerve-cell process. H & E, ×400. (c) Complex Lewy body in the dorsal motor nucleus of the vagus. H & E, ×625. (d) Round Lewy body (arrow) in melanized neuron of the superior cervical ganglion. H & E, ×400.

dorsal vagal nucleus and sympathetic ganglia simple rounded intraneuronal Lewy bodies similar to those in the midbrain are least common (Fig. 26.2(d)), but in the myenteric plexus of the oesophagus they are more common than other forms (Qualman *et al.* 1984).

Ultrastructurally, the Lewy body consists of filamentous material, the classical brainstem form having a dense core of granular material, surrounded by an outer zone of radially orientated filaments 7–20 nm in diameter, which extend peripherally to melanin granules or dense core vesicles (Duffy and Tennyson 1965). Considerable variation in filament profiles and packing density explain the laminations seen by light microscopy. In sympathetic ganglia a few Lewy bodies are ultrastructurally similar to those in the brainstem, but granular forms, which are found in nerve cell processes, are more common. These have a dense core with a peripheral zone of coarse ill-defined granules mixed with vesicles and filaments (Forno and Norville 1976).

Antibodies raised against neurofilament polypeptides were first used to investigate the Lewy body by Goldman *et al.* (1983). Four polyclonal antisera reacted with many nigral Lewy bodies, some of which stained homogeneously, while others showed peripheral staining only. Monoclonal antibodies recognizing neurofilament protein have also produced identical reactions towards the periphery of Lewy bodies in both the substantia nigra and stellate ganglia (Forno *et al.* 1983). Lewy bodies therefore contain components of neurofilament protein, but it is not clear whether they contain constituents of other cytoskeletal proteins.

Distribution of Lewy bodies

The distribution of Lewy bodies and cell loss in Lewy body–Parkinson's disease is specific to certain cell populations (Bethlem and Den Hartog Jager 1960) (Table 26.1). These include nuclei in the diencephalon and brainstem, some of which are pigmented, non-pigmented, cholinergic, or monoaminergic. Lewy bodies and cell loss are never restricted to one or two locations, but many sites are involved in any one case. The distribution of greatest cell loss changes little, thus in part explaining why Parkinson's disease is the most common manifestation of the pathology, the diagnosis of which depends on finding moderate-to-severe cell loss with Lewy bodies in the substantia nigra. The infrequency of autonomic failure in Lewy body disease is a reflection of the often mild or insignificant degeneration and cell loss in intermediolateral columns of the spinal cord (Oppenheimer 1980). In contrast, cases associated with autonomic failure show substantial cell loss at this site. Many consider that Lewy bodies and nerve cell degeneration in the nucleus basalis of Meynert are responsible for some cases of dementia in Parkinson's disease (Perry *et al.* 1985), while Lewy bodies in the cerebral cortex are

Table 26.1. Main distribution of Lewy bodies in idiopathic Lewy body–Parkinson's disease

Brainstem	
	Substantia nigra
	Locus ceruleus
	Raphe nuclei
Diencephalon	
	Nucleus basalis of Meynert
	Thalamus
Limbic lobe and cerebral cortex	
	Parahippocampal and cingulate gyri
	Temporal and frontal lobes
Autonomic nervous system	
	Hypothalamus
	Edinger–Westphal nucleus
	Dorsal motor nucleus of the vagus
	Intermediolateral nucleus
	Sympathetic and parasympathetic ganglia

also associated with dementia (Kosaka *et al.* 1984). The consequences of Lewy bodies and cell loss at other locations are not known.

The cell groups affected in Parkinson's disease are not known to share any peculiar, inherent characteristic, although the Lewy body is always found when cell loss is present at these sites. In fact cell loss has been documented for most locations in which the Lewy body is found so that it has often been considered a marker of cell degeneration. One peculiarity of Parkinson's disease is the selective involvement of the autonomic nervous system, in addition to other pigmented and cholinergic neurons. For example, in a regional study of the medulla in Parkinson's disease, Eadie (1963) found Lewy bodies in the cholinergic dorsal vagal nucleus; in contrast the adjacent hypoglossal nucleus was spared. A number of authors have described degeneration of neurons of the oculomotor nucleus, but it is the cholinergic visceral motor neurons of the Edinger–Westphal nucleus that are lost, which are structurally similar to those of the dorsal vagal nucleus, not the juxtaposed somatic motor neurons of the principal oculomotor nucleus. Neurons of the salivatory nuclei supplying parasympathetic fibres accompanying the seventh and ninth cranial nerves may also be affected.

In a study of the hypothalamus Langston and Forno (1978) found Lewy bodies in 13 hypothalamic nuclei of 30 patients with Lewy bodies in the substantia nigra. The tuberomamillary, lateral, and posterior nuclei were most severely and frequently affected in 79, 86, and 83 per cent, respectively. The arcuate, supraoptic, anterior, and medial preoptic nuclei were less affected, and the tuberoinfundibular region which contains most dopamine was relatively spared. Matzuk and Saper (1985) examined seven brains containing Lewy bodies in the substantia nigra and found that the number of melanin-pigmented cells in the periventricular and arcuate nucleus was no fewer than in five controls, thus supporting the view that in Parkinson's disease important hypothalamic neuroendocrine defects are absent and that basal levels of prolactin are normal.

Lewy bodies occur in sympathetic ganglia at the cervical, thoracic, lumbar, or sacral levels in patients with Parkinson's disease with or without autonomic failure. Bethlem and Den Hartog Jager (1960) found them in five of six patients and Forno and Norville (1976) identified them in the stellate ganglion in eight of 10 cases. Lewy bodies can also be found in the parasympathetic myenteric plexus of the oesophagus (Qualman *et al.* 1984), but as yet there is no evidence that at this site, or in other parasympathetic ganglia, that Lewy bodies and nerve-cell degeneration have important physiological consequences. The occurrence of Lewy bodies in peripheral autonomic ganglia means that occasionally they may be identified in surgical specimens taken during life. One example was their finding in the oesophagus of patients treated surgically for achalasia (Qualman *et al.* 1984). Another example was the finding of Lewy bodies in sympathetic ganglia removed at lumbar sympathectomy from a patient with leg cramps, who developed classical parkinsonian features 3 years later (Stadlan *et al.* 1965).

Spherical eosinophilic cytoplasmic inclusions can be found in the adrenal medulla (Den Hartog Jager 1970) situated in a zone adjacent to the adrenal cortex. These adrenal bodies bear no structural resemblance to Lewy bodies for they are dense, rounded, 0.5–15 μm in diameter, and homogeneous without a filamentous component. Furthermore, they lack specificity for Lewy body–Parkinson's disease, for they cannot always be found and they often occur in Alzheimer's disease and various controls. They are reported in one case of MSA without Lewy bodies, but they are not thought to be relevant to autonomic failure.

Cell loss in the autonomic nervous system

The location of cell depletion responsible for symptoms of autonomic failure is believed to be the intermediolateral columns. Oppenheimer (1980) found that intermediolateral cells are reduced in cases of Lewy body–Parkinson's disease complicated by autonomic failure, compared to uncomplicated cases, but not to the extent seen in MSA with autonomic failure. Quantitative analysis of cells in sympathetic ganglia has not been done, but it is also plausible that substantial cell loss may occur in some cases (Rajput and Rozdilsky 1976, Case 6). The consequence of autonomic-tract lesions at other sites is uncertain. Degeneration of the Edinger–Westphal nucleus might cause detectable alterations of the pupil responses to light or convergence and hypothalamic pathology might relate to common 'autonomic disturbances', such as seborrhoea.

THE PREVALENCE OF LEWY BODIES IN MULTIPLE SYSTEM ATROPHY

Striatonigral degeneration (SND) which is one of the principal findings in MSA was first described in detail by Adams *et al.* (1964). In Case 3 mild gliosis was reported in the putamen and caudate nucleus, but Lewy bodies were also present in the substantia nigra (Adams *et al.* 1964). In retrospect these striatal changes were probably not as unequivocal as the obvious macroscopic shrinkage and destruction of the putamen observed in three other patients. While the classification of this case is in doubt, the question of the frequency of Lewy bodies in MSA was raised—an important point if the Lewy body is to be considered useful in the diagnosis and separation of these disorders. Indeed, Lewy bodies were reported in elderly persons over 60 years (Woodard 1962) and might therefore represent a degenerative change of little importance.

A personal survey of the literature reveals 80 pathologically reported cases in which SND, with or without cell loss in intermediolateral columns of the spinal cord, was the predominant finding. Multiple brainstem Lewy bodies were reported in patients with autonomic failure, aged 58 and 51 years (Thapedi *et al.* 1971). In a third patient with autonomic failure, aged 61 years, a single nigral Lewy body was combined with severe cell loss (Yamamura *et al.* 1974). Lewy bodies were also found in the substantia nigra of three patients with an apparent pure parkinsonian syndrome. A total of six cases compares well with the prevalence of Lewy bodies in normal individuals over the age of 50 years (see below), but the age-specific prevalence of Lewy bodies may be increased in the sixth decade (Table 26.2). Some 23 cases reporting OPCA as the main finding were also surveyed. One case, aged 59 years, with Lewy bodies was found in a group of OPCA cases, from which familial cases were excluded. Kaiya (1974) reported a 58-year-old man with cerebellar signs, a parkinsonian syndrome, and autonomic failure in whom Lewy bodies were present in the substantia nigra and intermediolateral columns. Another case was that of a man aged 61 years in whom Lewy bodies were found in the substantia nigra and elsewhere (Kobayashi *et al.* 1979). In a fourth case, of unstated age, degenerative changes and Lewy bodies were found in the intermediolateral columns and sympathetic ganglia (Yoshimura *et al.* 1980). These four cases

Table 26.2. Age-specific prevalence of pathologically reported cases of striatonigral degeneration and olivopontocerebellar atrophy with Lewy bodies

Age group (years)	*Lewy body cases/total cases examined*		
	*SND**	*OPCA*	*Total†*
40–9	0/5	0/1	0/6
50–9	5/40 (12.5%)	3/13	8/53 (15.1%)
60–9	1/28 (3.6%)	1/8	2/36 (5.6%)
70–9	0/7	0/1	0/8

* Mean age, 58.9 years.
† Mean age, 57.9 years.

combine with the cases of SND to give a prevalence of 15.1 per cent in the sixth decade and 5.6 per cent in the seventh decade (Table 26.2).

For many years it has been recognized that cerebral Lewy bodies may be found in persons dying without Parkinson's disease. The first large post-mortem study to report the number of Lewy body-positive cases in each decade was from three California State Mental Hospitals, where 400 consecutive unselected cases were investigated (Woodard 1962). Lewy bodies were present in either the substantia nigra, oculomotor nucleus, locus ceruleus, or dorsal vagal nucleus of 27 cases aged 60–89 years, equivalent to a prevalence of 11.8 per cent of those aged over 60 years. However, seven (26 per cent) of the 27 cases with Lewy bodies had parkinsonian manifestations. The exclusion of parkinsonian cases was not always guaranteed in other similar studies (Table 26.3). Combining data from five studies gives a prevalence of 1.8 per cent in the fifties, rising thereafter to 10.7 per cent in the sixties, figures that may overestimate the prevalence of non-parkinsonian individuals by as much

Table 26.3. Age-specific prevalence of incidental Lewy-body disease. Lewy bodies generally located in the substantia nigra or locus ceruleus

Age group (years)	*Lewy-body cases/ total cases examined*	*Prevalence (per cent)*
50–9	3/167	1.8
60–9	29/270	10.7
70–9	38/304	12.5
80–9	18/99	18.2
90–9	2/12	16.7

Data taken from Woodard (1962), Hamada and Ishii (1963), Hirai (1968), Forno and Alvord (1971), and Tomonaga (1983).

as one-quarter, because of the inclusion of early parkinsonian cases as in Woodard's (1962) study. Forno (1969) commented that cell depletion was usually intermediate between that of controls and Parkinson's disease, making it a reasonable assumption that cases of 'incidental Lewy body disease' are in a preclinical phase, corresponding to a period of falling striatal dopamine (Bernheimer *et al.* 1973).

There are a number of obvious drawbacks to comparing reported estimations of incidental Lewy-body disease and the prevalence of case reports of Lewy bodies occurring in MSA. In addition, the prevalence of Lewy bodies in parkinsonian MSA patients should, in theory, be compared with the combined prevalence of incidental Lewy body disease and Lewy body–Parkinson's disease. The results show (Tables 26.2 and 26.3) that the frequency of Lewy bodies in MSA is similar to that in controls, as would be expected on the basis of an incidental association between Lewy bodies and MSA. However, in the sixth decade the prevalence of Lewy bodies in MSA may be slightly high.

We have recently compared the age-specific prevalence of Lewy bodies in 43 cases of MSA with the prevalence rates obtained in 273 controls without Parkinson's disease (Gibb and Lees 1987). One to four unilateral sections, of 7 μm thickness, of substantia nigra were examined. The number of cases in the MSA group was relatively small, but the frequency of Lewy bodies was slightly greater (not statistically significant) than in the controls (Table 26.4). One small factor helping to account for this discrepancy could be the selection and premature death of patients with MSA and Lewy bodies, and therefore a twofold cause for nigral cell loss. Consequently, this slight difference is still compatible with a chance association of Lewy bodies with MSA.

Table 26.4. Age-specific prevalence of Lewy bodies in cases of multiple system atrophy (43), arbitrarily divided into those with mainly SND and those with OPCA, and in 'control' cases

Age group (years)	*Lewy-body cases/total cases examined*			
	SND	*OPCA**	*Total with MSA*	*Controls*
30–9	0	0/1	0/1	0/17
40–9	0/3	0/1	0/4	0/27
50–9	1/8	1/7	2/15 (13.3%)	2/53 (3.8%)
60–9	2/12	0/3	2/15 (13.3%)	3/64 (4.7%)
70–9	0/6	0/1	0/7	4/43 (9.3%)
80–9	0/1	0	0/1	5/39 (12.8%)

* Two cases of OPCA of unknown age have been included in the fifties (the mean age for the OPCA group).

Acknowledgement

This work was supported by a grant from the Medical Research Council.

REFERENCES

Adams, R. D., Bogaert, van L., and Eecken, H. V. (1964). Striato-nigral degeneration. *J. Neuropathol. exp. Neurol.* **24**, 584–608.

Bannister, R. and Oppenheimer, D. R. (1972). Degenerative diseases of the nervous system associated with autonomic failure. *Brain* **95**, 457–74.

Bernheimer, H., Birkmayer, W., Hornykiewicz, O., Jellinger, K., and Seitelberger, F. (1973). Brain dopamine and the syndromes of Parkinson and Huntington. *J. neurol. Sci.* **20**, 415–55.

Bethlem, J. and Den Hartog Jager, W. A. (1960). The incidence and characteristics of Lewy bodies in idiopathic paralysis agitans (Parkinson's disease). *J. Neurol. Neurosurg. Psychiat.* **23**, 74–80.

Den Hartog Jager, W. A. (1970). Histochemistry of adrenal bodies in Parkinson's disease. *Arch. Neurol.* **23**, 528–33.

Duffy, P. E. and Tennyson, V. M. (1965). Phase and electron microscopic observations of Lewy bodies and melanin granules in the substantia nigra and locus coeruleus in Parkinson's disease. *J. Neuropathol. exp. Neurol.* **24**, 398–414.

Eadie, M. J. (1963). The pathology of certain medullary nuclei in parkinsonism. *Brain* **86**, 781–92.

Fichefet, J. P., Sternon, J. E., Franken, L., Dermanet, J. C., and Vanderhaeghen, J. J. (1965). Étude anatomo-clinique d'un cas d'hypotension orthostatique 'idiopathique'. *Acta cardiol.* **20**, 332–48.

Forno, L. S. (1969). Concentric hyalin intraneuronal inclusions of Lewy type in the brains of elderly persons (50 incidental cases). Relationship to Parkinsonism. *J. Am. geriat. Soc.* **17**, 557–75.

Forno, L. S. and Alvord, E. C. (1971). The pathology of parkinsonism. In *Recent advances in Parkinson's disease* (ed. F. H. McDowell and C. H. Markham), pp. 120–61. Blackwell, Oxford.

Forno, L. S. and Norville, R. L. (1976). Ultrastructure of Lewy bodies in the stellate ganglion. *Acta neuropathol.* **34**, 183–97.

Forno, L. S., Strefling, A. M., Sternberger, L. A., Sternberger, N. H., and Eng, L. F. (1983). Immunocytochemical staining of neurofibrillary tangles and the periphery of Lewy bodies with a monoclonal antibody to neurofilaments. *J. Neuropathol. exp. Neurol.* **42**, 342.

Gibb, W. R. G. and Lees, A. J. (1987). The significance of the Lewy body in the diagnosis of idiopathic Parkinson's disease. (In press).

Goetz, C. G., Lutge, W., and Tanner, C. M. (1986). Autonomic dysfunction in Parkinson's disease. *Neurology* **36**, 73–5.

Goldman, J. E., Yen, S-H., Chiu, F-C., and Peress, N. S. (1983). Lewy bodies of Parkinson's disease contain neurofilament antigens. *Science* **221**, 1082–4.

Graham, J. G. and Oppenheimer, D. R. (1969). Orthostatic hypotension and nicotine sensitivity in a case of multiple system atrophy. *J. Neurol. Neurosurg. Psychiat.* **32**, 28–34.

Hamada, S. and Ishii, T. (1963). The Lewy body in the brain of the aged. *Adv. neurol. Sci.* **7**, 184–6.

Hirai, S. (1968). Ageing of the substantia nigra. *Adv. neurol. Sci.* **12**, 845–9.

Johnson, R. H., Lee, de J., Oppenheimer, D. R., and Spalding, J. M. K. (1966). Autonomic failure with orthostatic hypotension due to intermediolateral column degeneration. *Quart. J. Med.* **35**, 276–92.

Kaiya, H. (1974). Spino-olivo-ponto-cerebello-nigral atrophy with Lewy bodies and binucleated nerve cells: a case report. *Acta neuropathol.* **30**, 263–9.

Kobayashi, H., Mukouyama, M., Muroga, T., Mano, U., Takayanagi, T., Sofue, I., and Matsuyama, H. (1979). A case of olivopontocerebellar atrophy, Parkinson syndrome and Lewy bodies in the substantia nigra and locus coeruleus. *Adv. neurol. Sci.* **23**, 599.

Kono, C., Matsubara, M., and Inagaki, T. (1976). Idiopathic orthostatic hypotension with numerous Lewy bodies in the sympathetic ganglia. Report of a case. *Neurol. Med.* **4**, 568–70.

Kosaka, K., Yoshimura, M., Ikeda, K., and Budka, H. (1984). Diffuse type of Lewy body disease: progressive dementia with abundant cortical Lewy bodies and senile changes of varying degree—a new disease! *Clin. Neuropathol.* **3**, 185–92.

Langston, J. W. and Forno, L. S. (1978). The hypothalamus in Parkinson's disease. *Ann. Neurol.* **3**, 129–33.

Lewy, F. H. (1923). *Die Lehre von Tonus und der Bewegung.* Springer, Berlin.

Matzuk, M. M. and Saper, C. B. (1985). Preservation of hypothalamic dopaminergic neurons in Parkinson's disease. *Ann. Neurol.* **18**, 552–5.

Oppenheimer, D. R. (1980). Lateral horn cells in progressive autonomic failure. *J. neurol. Sci.* **46**, 393–404.

Perry, E. K., Curtis, M., Dick, D. J., Candy, J. M., Atack, J. R., Bloxham, C. A., Blessed, G., Fairbairn, A., Tomlinson, B. E., and Perry, R. H. (1985). Cholinergic correlates of cognitive impairment in Parkinson's disease: comparisons with Alzheimer's disease. *J. Neurol. Neurosurg. Psychiat.* **48**, 413–21.

Qualman, S. J., Haupt, H. M., Young, P., and Hamilton, S. R. (1984). Esophageal Lewy bodies associated with ganglion cell loss in achalasia. Similarity to Parkinson's disease. *Gastroenterology* **87**, 848–56.

Rajput, A. H. and Rozdilsky, B. (1976). Dysautonomia in parkinsonism: a clinicopathological study. *J. Neurol. Neurosurg. Psychiat.* **39**, 1092–100.

Roessman, U., Noort, van den S., and McFarland, D. E. (1971). Idiopathic orthostatic hypotension. *Arch. Neurol.* **24**, 503–10.

Schober, R., Langston, J. W., and Forno, L. S. (1975). Idiopathic orthostatic hypotension. Biochemical and pathological observation in two cases. *Eur. Neurol.* **13**, 177–88.

Stadlan, E. M., Duvoisin, R., and Yahr, M. (1965). The pathology of parkinsonism. In *Proceedings of the Fifth International Congress of Neuropathologists*, Zurich. Excerpta Medica International Congress Series, no. 100, pp. 569–71. Excerpta Medica, Amsterdam.

Thapedi, I. M., Ashenhurst, E. M., and Rozdilsky, B. (1971). Shy–Drager syndrome. Report of an autopsied case. *Neurology* **21**, 26–32.

Tomonaga, M. (1983). Neuropathology of the locus coeruleus: a semiquantitative study. *J. Neurol.* **230**, 231–40.

Vanderhaeghen, J-J., Perier, O., and Sternon, J. E. (1970). Pathological findings in idiopathic orthostatic hypotension. *Arch. Neurol.* **22**, 207–14.

Woodard, J. S. (1962). Concentric hyaline inclusion body formation in mental disease. Analysis of twenty-seven cases. *J. Neuropathol. exp. Neurol.* **21**, 442–9.

Yamamura, Y., Ohama, E., Yoshimura, N., Atsumi, T., Oyanagi, S., and Ikuta, F. (1974). Striato-nigral degeneration, a form of multiple system atrophy allied to olivopontocerebellar atrophy. *Adv. neurol. Sci.* **18**, 89–105.

Yoshimura, M., Shimada, H., Nakura, H., and Tomonaga, M. (1980). Two autopsy cases of Lewy type–Parkinson's disease with Shy–Drager syndrome. *Trans. Soc. Pathol. Jap.* **69**, 432.

27. The quantitation of intermediolateral column neurons in autonomic failure, diabetic autonomic neuropathy, and motor neuron disease

Peter G. E. Kennedy

INTRODUCTION

The intermediolateral column (ILC) neurons in the lateral horns of the grey matter of the thoracic spinal cord are the preganglionic neurons of the sympathetic nervous system. In searching for a neuroanatomical basis for the severe autonomic failure which occurs in conditions such as autonomic failure (AF) and diabetic autonomic neuropathy, it occurred to several workers that ILC cells might be abnormal and/or depleted, although a cause-and-effect relationship between the clinical and pathological observations could not be assumed. The author subscribes to the view (Graham and Oppenheimer 1969; Bannister and Oppenheimer 1972; Oppenheimer 1980) that AF can be divided into two groups. In the first group, AF occurs by itself or in association with clinical parkinsonism. In these cases Lewy inclusion bodies are demonstrable histologically—hence the term 'Lewy-body disease'. In the second group AF occurs in association with multiple system atrophy (MSA), a term which embraces a spectrum of degenerative diseases of the CNS which includes olivopontocerebellar atrophy and striatonigral degeneration.

There is now considerable neuropathological evidence that the number of ILC cells is markedly diminished both in AF and MSA and in AF with Lewy-body disease and, in a number of studies, the degree of ILC cell loss has been quantitated (Johnson *et al.* 1966; Graham and Oppenheimer 1969; Bannister and Oppenheimer 1972; Oppenheimer 1980). More recently, ILC cells have been examined quantitatively in other conditions in which neuronal degeneration occurs elsewhere in the nervous system such as diabetic autonomic neuropathy (Duchen *et al.*

1980) and motor neuron disease (MND) (Kennedy and Duchen 1985). The purpose of this chapter is to provide an overview of these various studies, and in particular to discuss critically the methodology of ILC counting and the significance of the ILC-cell loss in relation to the clinical dysautonomic features. A detailed account of the general neuropathology of AF is given in Chapter 25A.

CRITICAL ASSESSMENT OF ILC CELL-COUNTING TECHNIQUES

Although ILC-cell loss has been clearly documented in cases of AF, the number of published quantitative studies in relatively small and, even in these, precise details of the cell-counting techniques and criteria have not always been provided. The most extensive and important study to date is that of Oppenheimer (1980) in which he clearly and critically defined both the rationale and problems involved in ILC cell counting. The following considerations are a reiteration of those of Oppenheimer and are presented in the light of our own observations (Kennedy and Duchen 1985).

Anatomical definition of a lateral horn

The lateral horn is recognized anatomically as a triangular region of the grey matter of the thoracic spinal cord which points laterally into the white columns. When counting cells within this area, the boundaries of the triangle have to be visualized subjectively, and this may be particulary difficult when the shape of this 'imaginary' triangle shows variations from section to section. In our own studies this has on occasion proved very problematical, but the difficulty has been surmounted to some extent by the use of a straight eye-piece graticule which helps to define the borders. The neurons of the ILC give rise to the fibres of the preganglionic sympathetic outflow. Most of the ILC cells are located within the lateral horns, but some cells with the appearance of ILC neurons may lie outside the defined area; thus the terms 'lateral horn' and 'ILC' are not strictly synonymous (Oppenheimer 1980). It seems reasonable to count only cells within the lateral horns and exclude those which lie outside it. Cells which are on the borders of the triangle can be included, but the criteria for inclusion should be consistent.

Difficulties may also arise as a result of anatomical variations of the first thoracic segment (T1), which may have the appearance of either the thoracic or cervical cord; in the latter case ILC cells may be evident in the absence of a lateral horn. For this reason Oppenheimer (1980) suggested that counts should be performed on the T1 to T12 segments inclusive when the T1 appearance is 'thoracic' and on T2 to L1 segments inclusive in the event of a 'cervical' T1 segment. Most previous studies have counted ILC cells in all of the paraffin-embedded thoracic cord segments, and most have grouped together counts in the upper (T1–T4), middle (T5–T9), and lower (T9–T12 or L1) thirds, cell counts being higher in the upper thoracic segments.

Assessment of cell numbers

Only cells which are definitely identifiable as neuronal in type and which are contained within the lateral horns should be counted. Only cells which contain a clearly visible prominent nucleolus should be classified as neurons, and for this reason the sections have to be routinely stained for visualization of neuronal RNA, e.g. with cresyl fast violet. Each section contains two lateral horns and, therefore, allows two separate cell counts. There is a remarkable variability in cell numbers in the lateral horns such that ILC cell numbers in serial or even the same section may differ by as much as fivefold (Oppenheimer 1980; Kennedy and Duchen 1985). This is one of the major reasons why quantitative studies of ILC cells are so important, as a non-quantitative random assessment of a cell column which is so liable to irregular clustering can be easily misleading. This difficulty is exacerbated by the very small numbers of cells in each lateral horn. The question arises as to whether it is preferable to count large numbers of cells in a small number of cases or count smaller numbers of cells in more cases. An accurate assessment is more likely with increasing numbers of cell counts, and for this reason the former strategy was adopted (Kennedy and Duchen 1985). The numbers of serial sections and spinal cord blocks which have been used also vary considerably in different studies, and this should also be taken into account.

In comparing the results of different studies, it is important to take into account not only the cell-counting technique but also the thickness of the cord sections examined since cell numbers will obviously be greater in thicker sections. While most studies have used 20 μm thick sections, others have used 8–10 μm sections. The method of fixation should also be considered. In our own experience, 20 μm thick sections from celloidin-fixed material are difficult to study since cell morphology may not be accurately visualized.

Blinding of studies

When looking for differences in cell counts in pathological cases compared with controls it is obviously preferable to carry out the studies blind. This point has been addressed before (Oppenheimer 1980; Kennedy and Duchen 1985) and has been considered by some authors to be somewhat impractical. The greatest problem in our own experience is that the distinctive pathological features of the various cases are immediately apparent as soon as the sections are examined. For example, sections of the cord showing the striking loss of anterior horn cells in MND may sometimes be easily distinguished from those showing loss of ILC cells in AF.

Statistical analysis

The pathological cases under examination should obviously be compared with control tissues obtained from age- and sex-matched cases in whom the spinal cords are normal. In his study of cases of AF Oppenheimer (1980) considered that the loss of ILC cells in these cases compared with controls was so striking that statistical analysis of the results was not necessary. In view of the marked reductions observed in this and many other studies (see below), this view seems quite reasonable. However, when attempting to define less obvious losses of ILC cells the case for formal statistical analysis is far stronger and, in the author's opinion, becomes mandatory.

Conclusions

Counting ILC cells in large numbers of serial sections and obtaining a mean cell number per section does seem to be a valid method of assessing ILC cell numbers, but it is essential to be aware of the numerous technical factors which may lead to differences between the results of various studies on the same condition. It is important to obtain as many individual cell counts as possible to obtain meaningful data which may be subjected to statistical analysis. A consistent well-defined method should be used in any individual study. However, even when the cell-counting methods are standardized, the techniques serve only to compare one spinal cord with another and do not represent absolute cell counts.

STUDIES OF ILC CELLS IN AUTONOMIC FAILURE

There have now been a number of studies which have documented ILC cell loss in cases of AF. Indeed, the first neuropathological description of this condition by Shy and Drager (1960) mentioned loss of ILC cells in the spinal cord. While most of these studies have based their conclusions on morphological criteria without quantitation, a small number of studies have applied quantitative methods, although technical details have seldom been given. The advantages of cell counting have been discussed above, and the following comments will be limited to published work in which cell-counting procedures have been employed.

The first quantitative study of ILC cells in AF was that of Johnson *et al.* (1966) in which multiple cell counts were performed on the spinal lateral horns of two individuals who had died with this condition. ILC cell numbers were reduced by about 90 per cent compared with controls in one case, and by about 70 per cent of controls in the other. It was considered likely that the autonomic failure was a consequence of ILC-cell loss. Similar quantitative observations have been repeatedly confirmed by several further studies, including those of Graham and Oppenheimer (1969, one case), Roessmann *et al.* (1971, one case), Bannister and Oppenheimer (1972, four cases), Evans *et al.* (1972, one case), Guard *et al.* (1974, one case), de Lean and Deck (1976, one case), Spokes *et al.* (1979, three of four cases), Sung *et al.* (1979, two of four cases), Oppenheimer (1980, 21 cases including 11 cases which had been previously reported), and Kennedy and Duchen (1985, two cases). Taking all of these studies into consideration, the overall reduction of ILC cells is in the region of 75 per cent, i.e. only about 25 per cent of cells remain. Typical cell counts for 20 μm thick sections are shown in Table 27.1 in which the result of three separate studies (seven cases) are shown. It can be seen that the cell numbers, not surprisingly, are greater than those obtained from 8–10 μm thick sections of this condition (Tables 27.2 and 27.3). Cell numbers in the upper third of the spinal cords are always greater than those in the middle and lower thirds both in controls and cases of AF. Numbers are also reduced in all three spinal cord levels in AF cases compared with controls.

Particular mention should be made of the study by Oppenheimer (1980), which is the largest and most definitive report so far published. The cases examined included 16 cases of MSA with autonomic failure, three cases of MSA without autonomic failure, five cases of autonomic failure showing Lewy bodies in the brainstem, three cases of Parkinson's disease without autonomic failure, and normal controls. The results are shown in Fig. 25.2 (p. 458). As can be seen, there was a very strong positive correlation between loss of lateral horn cells and autonomic failure with a very marked loss of ILC cells in case of AF with MSA, and cases of AF with Lewy bodies. The cell counts in uncomplicated Parkinson's disease were no different from control cases and, interestingly, the cases of MSA without autonomic failure showed a reduction of ILC cells of only about half that of controls. A recent report also documented significant loss of ILC neurons in the lateral horns of three patients dying with AF and idiopathic Parkinson's disease with Lewy bodies (Mizutani, T., personal communication).

Although the primary purpose is to consider preganglionic sympathetic neurons, it is of interest that the number of sacral

Table 27.1. Cell counts, with standard errors, showing mean numbers of lateral horn cells in 20 μm sections in patients with autonomic failure

Level	*Controls*	*Bannister and Oppenheimer (1972)*				*Johnson* et al. *(1966)*		*Graham and Oppenheimer (1969)*
		Case 1	*Case 2*	*Case 3*	*Case 4*	*Case 1*	*Case 2*	
T1–4	15.8 ± 1.0 (48)	4.9 ± 0.3 (40)	4.3 ± 0.4 (40)	6.5 ± 0.5 (40)	4.6 ± 0.7 (36)	1.3 ± 0.3 (36)	4.3 ± 0.5 (36)	4.2 ± 0.6 (48)
T5–8	9.2 ± 0.7 (48)	1.9 ± 0.2 (40)	1.2 ± 0.2 (40)	2.5 ± 0.2 (40)	0.8 ± 0.2 (36)	1.0 ± 0.2 (36)	1.9 ± 0.2 (48)	1.3 ± 0.2 (48)
T9–L1	9.5 ± 0.7 (48)	2.7 ± 0.4 (40)	2.0 ± 0.3 (40)	3.4 ± 0.4 (40)	2.3 ± 0.4 (36)	2.0 ± 0.3 (36)	2.7 ± 0.3 (48)	1.3 ± 0.2 (48)

Figures in brackets show the number of counts made at each level.
Reprinted, with slight modification, with permission from Bannister and Oppenheimer (1972).

Table 27.2. Mean cell counts, with standard errors (SE) of lateral horns per 8 μm section of each thoracic segment of spinal cord. Seven controls and two patients with Shy–Drager syndrome (S–D) are pooled respectively

Thoracic segments	*I*	*II*	*III*	*IV*	*V*	*VI*	*VII*	*VIII*	*IX*	*X*	*XI*	*XII*
Controls (*N*=7)												
Mean	6.1	7.7	6.3	4.7	4.3	3.2	3.5	3.2	3.5	4.4	4.9	5.5
SE	(1.2)	(0.8)	(1.0)	(1.4)	(0.4)	(0.7)	(0.6)	(0.5)	(0.6)	(1.1)	(0.7)	(0.8)
S–D (*N*=2)												
Mean	3.9	2.8	2.4	1.6	1.4	1.3	1.1	1.4	1.3	1.7	1.5	1.4
SE	(0.4)	(0.9)	(0.1)	(0.1)	(0.1)	(0.1)	(0.1)	(0.1)	(0.4)	(0.5)	(0.4)	(0.6)

Reprinted, with permission from Sung *et al.* (1979).

Table 27.3. Number of cells in the intermediolateral columns of thoracic spinal cord

Case	*Age (years)*	*Sex*	*Diagnosis*	*Mean cell counts in*		
				Upper third (T2–4)	*Middle third (T6–8)*	*Lower third (T10–12)*
1	58	Male	Cerebral haemorrhage	5.8 ± 0.8 (95)*	3.5 ± 0.8 (94)	3.1 ± 1.0 (97)
2	49	Male	Cerebral glioma	5.6 ± 1.5 (79)	3.8 ± 1.6 (80)	2.9 ± 1.0 (100)
3	61	Female	Cerebral glioma	5.3 ± 1.0 (82)	3.7 ± 1.0 (81)	3.1 ± 0.7 (98)
4	68	Male	Motor neuron disease	4.2 ± 1.0 (148)	3.4 ± 1.1 (99)	2.8 ± 1.3 (95)
5	38	Female	Familial motor neuron disease	4.2 ± 1.1 (98)	3.3 ± 1.0 (96)	2.6 ± 1.1 (95)
6	50	Male	Motor neuron disease	5.6 ± 1.7 (164)	4.2 ± 1.1 (150)	3.3 ± 1.1 (162)
7	62	Male	Motor neuron disease	3.9 ± 1.2 (96)	2.7 ± 0.9 (94)	1.8 ± 0.9 (94)
8	58	Male	Motor neuron disease	5.2 ± 1.7 (191)	3.4 ± 1.2 (141)	2.7 ± 0.9 (150)
9	43	Female	Multiple system atrophy	1.6 ± 0.7 (90)	1.3 ± 0.9 (81)	1.1 ± 0.6 (95)
10	58	Male	Multiple system atrophy	1.4 ± 0.8 (101)	1.2 ± 0.6 (98)	1.0 ± 0.7 (93)

* Mean number of neurons ± standard deviation in one lateral horn in a 10 μm section. The figure in brackets shows the number of cell counts performed, each section providing two cell counts. Reprinted with permission from Kennedy and Duchen (1985).

parasympathetic preganglionic neurons has also been shown to be significantly reduced in cases of MSA (Sung *et al.* 1979; Konno *et al.* 1986). The study by Konno *et al.* (1986) is the only one to date which has quantitated the loss of cells in the inferior intermediolateral nucleus (IML) which are the parasympathetic preganglionic neurons supplying the bladder and rectum. Using techniques similar to those described above, a marked depletion of these neurons was demonstrated in five cases of MSA with AF compared with controls (Fig. 27.1) (see also later). A significant reduction of neurons in the nucleus of Onuf and sacral somatic neurons was also detected in the MSA cases.

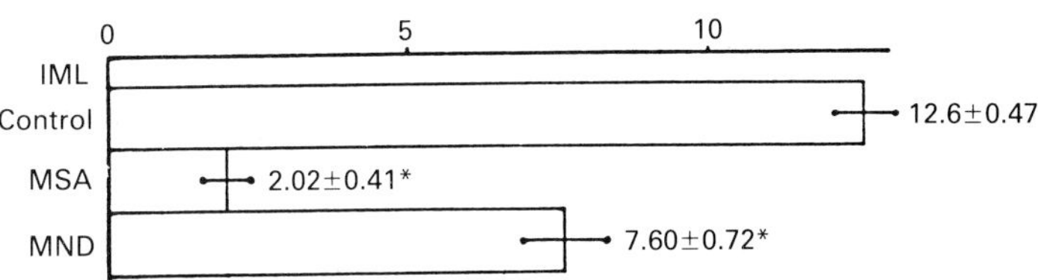

Fig. 27.1. The mean numbers of neurons per section in each sacral intermediolateral nucleus (IML) of the control, multiple system atrophy (MSA), and motor neuron disease (MND) spinal cords. The horizontal scale indicates the mean number of neurons per section. Values are the mean ±standard error. The differences between the control and disease groups were analysed. *, $p < 0.001$ (Student's t-test). (Reprinted with permission from Konno *et al.* (1986).)

It is abundantly clear from the quantitative data, as well as data derived from numerous non-quantitative studies, that there is a significant positive correlation between loss of ILC cells and the progressive autonomic failure associated with MSA or Lewy-body disease. The question obviously arises, however, whether this loss is the primary cause of the autonomic failure. Several lines of evidence suggest that it is unlikely to be the only cause. Although loss of ILC cells may well be implicated in, for example, postural hypotension and anhidrosis, it could not account for some of the other features of autonomic failure such as sphincter disturbances. The loss of neurons in the nucleus of Onuf and the IML in the sacral cord is far more likely to account for these features. Moreover, it has been noted above that a 50 per cent reduction of ILC cells occurred in three individuals with MSA who did not have autonomic failure. Conversely, two cases of MSA with autonomic failure have been reported in whom ILC-cell loss did not occur (Hughes *et al.* 1970; Evans *et al.* 1972), and in the case of Evans *et al.* formal cell counting was performed. The observations cast doubt on the essential role of ILC-cell loss in producing dysautonomic features and, in these two patients, the autonomic failure must have been caused by a lesion or lesions elsewhere in the sympathetic nervous system. In this context it is possible that the autonomic failure is not secondary to the ILC-cell loss *per se*. In the more usual cases, i.e. those with ILC-cell loss, the loss of cells may be due to a 'chain' degeneration occurring in some other region of the autonomic system. A further possibility is that there may be hitherto undetected biochemical or pharmacological defects in groups of sympathetic neurons which have not been observed to be morphologically abnormal (see Chapter 25A). Clearly, such information would be difficult to obtain with current technology. It is possible that future advances in our ability to investigate the biochemical, physiological, and pharmacological functions of autonomic neurons in patients and post-mortem material will shed light on this question.

STUDIES OF ILC-CELL LOSS IN DIABETIC AUTONOMIC NEUROPATHY

A quantitative assessment of ILC cells in the spinal cords of individuals dying with diabetic autonomic neuropathy was carried out by Duchen *et al.* 1980). The techniques employed were similar to those of Oppenheimer (1980) described above, but 10 μm thick sections rather than 20 μm thick sections were used. The results of this study are shown in Table 27.4. It can be seen that there was a considerable reduction in the numbers of ILC cells in four of the five cases of diabetes with severe autonomic failure. The loss in these cases was evident mainly in the upper and middle regions of the thoracic cords. Although both control and diabetic cords showed a lower number of ILC cells in the lower segments, the degree of cell loss in these regions of the pathological cords was less marked, possibly related to the greater difficulty in assessing cell numbers in this region. A feature of particular interest is that the patient

Table 27.4. Number of nerve cells in intermediolateral columns of spinal cord in cases of diabetic autonomic failure

	Normal controls		*Patients with diabetic autonomic failure aged*				
	Case 1	*Case 2*	♂44 *years*	♂45 *years*	♀47† *years*	♂52 *years*	♂30 *years*
T2–3	7.0*	Damaged	4.0	3.8	4.7	4.4	8.5
	9.9	—	3.4	3.7	4.4	5.4	7.8
T5–6	9.5	6.8	3.5	3.7	3.8	3.8	5.5
	6.7	8.0			3.8	3.2	6.0
T10–11	5.2	6.7	4.8	4.9	4.5	3.8	4.9
	4.3	7.0	5.8	4.8	4.1	3.6	5.2

* Mean number of cells in 10 μm paraffin section. Cells counted in 20 serial sections from two blocks at each level in most cases.

† This patient was female; all other diabetic patients in the table were male.

Reprinted with permission from Professor L. W. Duchen, Department of Neuropathology, Institute of Neurology, National Hospital, London, WC1.

who had normal ILC cell counts had clinical evidence of severe autonomic failure. This anomaly may relate in part to the relatively young age (30 years) of this patient, making a comparison with the other older cases somewhat difficult. However, this finding suggests that the spinal ILC-cell loss may have been secondary to the peripheral autonomic pathology. The latter includes structural abnormalities of sympathetic neurons and ganglia, inflammatory changes in autonomic ganglia and nerve fibres, and demeyelination in autonomic nerves (Duchen *et al.* 1980). Such a mechanism of 'retrograde loss' of ILC cells is certainly consistent with the reported pathology of diabetic autonomic neuropathy, but it is not know whether the degeneration in diabetic autonomic failure crosses the synapse between the preganglionic fibre and the sympathetic ganglion cell.

STUDIES OF ILC CELLS IN MOTOR NEURON DISEASE

A number of post-mortem studies have considered that spinal ILC cells are not depleted in individuals dying with MND (Bertrand and Van Bogaert 1925; Brownell *et al.* 1970; Hughes 1982). However, cell-counting techniques have not been employed in any of these reports. It is of interest that a recent report has documented mild but significant abnormalities of autonomic function in patients with MND when compared with controls (Steiner *et al.* 1984). A 'decentralization' type of end-organ supersensitivity in MND patients was considered likely although evidence of widespread autonomic failure was not detected. Further, neuronal degeneration in MND affects not only the anterior horns and pyramidal tracts but also in some cases the anterolateral and posterior columns (Brownell *et al.* 1970) and Clarke's column (Averback and Croker 1982). In view of this widespread involvement of the spinal cord in MND, and the fact that neurons of the anterior horns and ILC are both cholinergic, we considered it possible that the neuronal degeneration in MND might also affect cells of the ILC.

The techniques used in this study (Kennedy and Duchen 1985) were the same as those of Oppenheimer (1980). The cases examined were five cases of MND, three control cases consisting of individuals in whom the spinal cords and roots were normal, and two cases of AF. The results are shown in Table 27.3 (see also Fig. 27.2). It can be seen that the number of ILC cells in the MND cases was slightly but consistently reduced in all three regions of the thoracic sympathetic outflow. This reduction, however, failed to reach statistical significance, $p > 0.1$ (Student's *t*-test) for pooled counts of the whole cord, $p > 0.05$ for pooled counts in upper third of cord, and $p > 0.1$ for pooled counts in middle and lower thirds. As has already been indicated, the ILC counts in the AF cases were

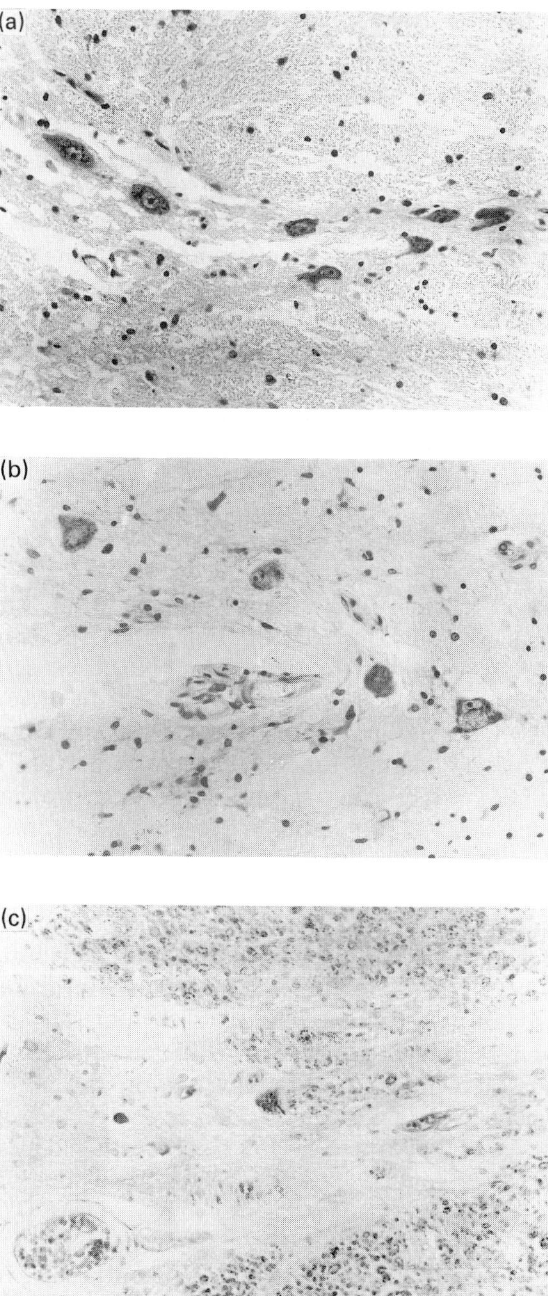

Fig. 27.2. Lateral grey horns in 10-μm paraffin sections of thoracic cords of (a) normal case (T6 level stained with cresyl fast violet), (b) a case of motor neuron disease (T4 level stained with cresyl fast violet), and (c) a case of MSA with autonomic failure (T4 level stained with luxol fast blue–cresyl violet). Note the moderate depletion of ILC neurons in (b) and marked depletion of these cells in (c) compared with the normal case. The normal cord section contains the greatest number of neurons even though it is obtained from a slightly lower thoracic segment. All magnifications are ×165.

significantly reduced ($p < 0.001$ for all regions of the cord). Nevertheless, there was a clear trend towards reduction of ILC cells in the MND cases. Interestingly, the patient with the shortest duration of disease (7 months) showed the highest cell counts, whereas the patient with the longest disease duration (7 years) had the lowest counts, but the significance of this observation is not clear. It should also be mentioned that obvious morphological abnormalities of the ILC cells were not seen in any of the cases studied. Furthermore, none of the MND cases had clinical evidence of autonomic failure, although formal testing of autonomic function had not been performed. It is possible that, had these been carried out, abnormalities similar to those reported by Steiner *et al.* (1984) may have been detected.

It is relevant to point out that Konno *et al.* (1986) detected a significant reduction in the numbers of sacral preganglionic parasympathetic neurons in the IML in patients with MND compared with controls (Fig. 27.1). Not surprisingly, this reduction was not as marked as that found in cases of AF with MSA. The absence of sphincter involvement in MND is consistent with the normal cell counts which were observed in the nucleus of Onuf and only a modest loss of IML neurons. These important findings provide yet further evidence that the neuronal degeneration in MND is more widespread than may have been thought in the past, and the data shown in Fig. 27.1 show remarkable similarities to our own in the lateral horns (Table 27.3).

Overall, our findings in MND cases, as well as those of Konno *et al.* (1986), are consistent with the mild clinical autonomic abnormalities documented by Steiner *et al.* (1984). However, the latter were thought to be a reflection of defects at several anatomical levels; this makes it highly unlikely that the slight loss of ILC cells could be entirely responsible for the abnormalities. Moreover, the extent to which the autonomic abnormalities in MND cases are primary defects or mainly secondary to chronic neurological disease is not known. These questions should be addressed in future studies in this group of patients.

Acknowledgements

I thank Professors L. W. Duchen and D. I. Graham for helpful discussions, and Dr D. R. Oppenheimer for critical reading of the manuscript.

REFERENCES

Averback, P. and Croker, P. (1982). Regular involvement of Clarke's nucleus in sporadic amyotrophic lateral sclerosis. *Arch. Neurol.* **39**, 155–6.

Bannister, R. and Oppenheimer, D. R. (1972). Degenerative diseases of the nervous system associated with autonomic failure. *Brain* **95**, 457–74

Bertrand, I. and Van Bogaert, L. (1925). Rapport sur la sclérose latérale amyotrophique (anatomie pathologique). *Rev. Neurol., Paris* **1**, 779–806.

Brownell, B., Oppenheimer, D. R., and Hughes, J. T. (1970). The central nervous system in motor neurone disease. *J. Neurol. Neurosurg. Psychiat.* **33**, 338–57.

de Lean, J. and Deck, J. H. (1976). Shy–Drager syndrome. Neuropathological correlation and response to levodopa therapy. *Can. J. neurol. Sci.* **3**, 161–73.

Duchen, L. W., Anjorin, A., Watkins, P. J., and MacKay, J. D. (1980). Pathology of autonomic neuropathy in diabetes mellitus. *Ann. intern. Med.* **92**, 301–3.

Evans, D. J., Lewis, P. D., Malhotra, O., and Pallis, C. (1972). Idiopathic orthostatic hypotension. Report of an autopsied case with histochemical and ultrastructural studies of the neuronal inclusions. *J. neurol. Sci.* **17**, 209–18.

Graham, J. G. and Oppenheimer, D. R. (1969). Orthostatic hypotension and nicotine sensitivity in a case of multiple system atrophy. *J. Neurol. Neurosurg. Psychiat.* **32**, 28–34.

Guard, O., Sindon, M., and Carrier, H. (1974). Syndrome de Shy–Drager; une nouvelle observation anatomo-clinique. *Lyon Méd.* **231**, 1075–84.

Hughes, J. T. (1982). Pathology of amyotrophic lateral sclerosis. In *Human motor neurone diseases* (ed. L. P. Rowland), pp. 61–74. Raven Press, New York.

Hughes, R. C., Cartlidge, N. E. F., and Millac, P. (1970). Primary neurogenic orthostatic hypotension. *J. Neurol. Neurosurg. Psychiat.* **33**, 363–71.

Johnson, R. H., Lee, G. de J., Oppenheimer, D. R., and Spalding, J. M. K. (1966). Autonomic failure with orthostatic hypotension due to intermediolateral column degeneration. *Q. J. Med.* **35**, 276–92.

Kennedy, P. G. E. and Duchen, L. W. (1985). A quantitative study of intermediolateral column cells in motor neuron disease and Shy–Drager syndrome. *J. Neurol. Neurosurg. Psychiat.* **48**, 1103–6.

Konno, H., Yamamoto, T., Iwasaki, Y., and Iizuka, H. (1986). Shy–Drager syndrome and amyotrophic lateral sclerosis. Cytoarchitectonic and morphometric studies of sacral autonomic neurons. *J. neurol. Sci.* **73**, 193–204.

Oppenheimer, D. R. (1980). Lateral horn cells in progressive autonomic failure. *J. neurol. Sci.* **46**, 393–404.

Roessmann, U., van den Noort, S., and McFarland, D. E. (1971). Idiopathic orthostatic hypotension. *Arch. Neurol., Chicago* **24**, 503–10.

Shy, G. M. and Drager, G. A. (1960). A neurological syndrome associated with orthostatic hypotension—a clinico-pathologic study. *Arch. Neurol., Chicago* **2**, 511–27.

Spokes, E. G. S., Bannister, R., and Oppenheimer, D. R. (1979). Multiple system atrophy with autonomic failure—clinical, histological and neurochemical observations on four cases. *J. neurol. Sci.* **43**, 59–82.

Steiner, T. J., Sethi, K. D., and Rose, F. C. (1984). Autonomic function in motor neurone disease (MND). In *Research progress in motor neurone disease* (ed. F. C. Rose), pp. 180–8. Pitman, London.

Sung, J. H., Mastri, A. R., and Segal, E. (1979). Pathology of Shy–Drager syndrome. *J. Neuropathol. exp. Neurol.* **38**, 359–68.

28. Neuropeptides in the spinal cord in multiple system atrophy

P. Anand

INTRODUCTION

Although a number of diseases may cause secondary damage to autonomic fibres (see Chapter 1), primary autonomic failure (AF) results from an unexplained selective neuronal degeneration. It may occur either alone or with two different degenerations of the nervous system—Parkinson's disease and multiple system atrophy (MSA). The best classification of AF syndromes is pathological, but is still controversial on crucial points, e.g. whether loss of spinal cord intermediolateral column cells, which form the final common pathway of thoracic autonomic outflow, occurs in all cases of AF (see Chapter 25A). A major difficulty has been the quantitative assessment of autonomic neurons, even in normal subjects.

The discovery that neuropeptides are present in autonomic pathways in the spinal cord thus provided a new approach to pathological studies of AF syndromes. Various peptides are selectively present in human spinal cord autonomic pathways (Anand 1984; Anand and Bloom 1984). In addition, peptides may act not only as neurotransmitters or modulators, but also as neurotrophic agents (Anand *et al.* 1985; Burnstock 1982).

This chapter demonstrates that neuropeptides are preferentially present in central autonomic pathways in mammalian spinal cord, and that they may provide a new key to the classification and aetiology of multiple system degenerations.

SELECTIVE MARKERS OF SPINAL-CORD AUTONOMIC PATHWAYS

Classical neuroanatomical tracing techniques have failed to identify clearly the autonomic pathways in thoracic and sacral spinal cord. Autonomic neurons are not easily distinguished in conventional histological materials and silver impregnation methods lack sensitivity in demonstrating fine fibres in degeneration studies (Morgan *et al.* 1981). Nevertheless, Pick (1970) reviewed the classical studies and constructed a scheme of autonomic connections—a modified diagram is shown in Fig. 28.1.

There is an impressive number of different peptide-containing fibres and terminals around autonomic efferents in a number of species, including man. These include oxytocin in the rat and monkey (Swanson and McKellar 1979), vasopressin and oxytocin in man (Jenkins *et al.* 1984), CCK in the rat (Schroder 1983), a-PP (NPY) in the rat (Hunt *et al.* 1981), VIP in man (Anand *et al.* 1983) and cat (Kawatani *et al.* 1983; Honda *et al.* 1983; Gibson *et al.* 1984*a*), substance P and met-encephalin in man (LaMotte and de Lanerolle 1981), somatostatin in the rat (Senba

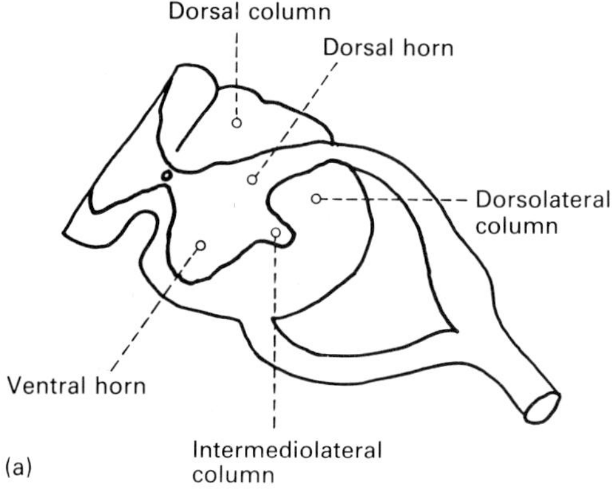

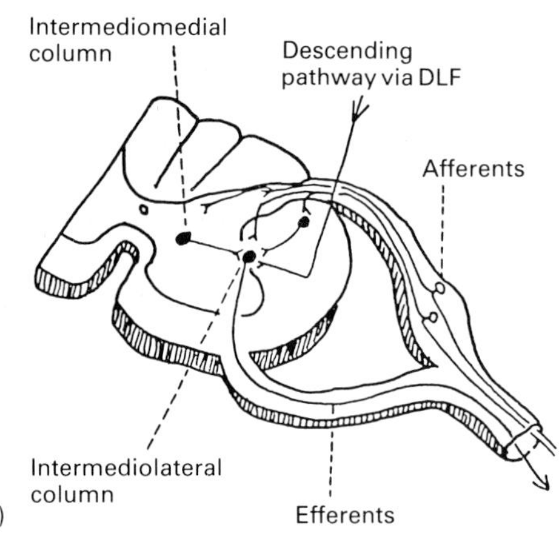

Fig. 28.1. (a) Transverse section of human thoracic spinal cord showing the regions microdissected for peptide analysis. (b) A diagrammatic representation of some autonomic pathways in human spinal cord. DLF, dorsolateral funiculus.

et al. 1982), leu-encephalin in rat (Senba *et al.* 1982), and calcitonin gene-related peptide (CGRP) in a number of species (Gibson *et al.* 1984*b*).

The fibres and terminals to the autonomic efferents may come from a number of sources, including the pelvic primary afferents (Mawe *et al.* 1984), local interneurons, cell bodies in the dorsolateral funiculus, intermediomedial nucleus (see Pick 1970), and supraspinal descending pathways (see Nathan and Smith 1958). A number of studies have demonstrated peptides marking all these sources, which will be reviewed in turn.

The pelvic primary afferents selectively contain vasoactive intestinal peptide (VIP) (Anand *et al.* 1983; Kawatani *et al.* 1983; Honda *et al.* 1983), PHI/PHM (Anand *et al.* 1984), as well as a number of peptides in common with somatic afferents such as substance P (de Groat *et al.* 1983).

In the rat, cell bodies in the dorsolateral funiculus contain substance P (Barber *et al.* 1979; Senba *et al.* 1982) and VIP (Fuji *et al.* 1983), which themselves receive afferents containing substance P (Barber *et al.* 1979) and fibres staining for encephalin, neurotensin, CCK (Gibson *et al.* 1981; Senba *et al.* 1982). Fibres containing substance P (S. J. Gibson, personal communication) and CCK (Schroder 1983) connect the dorsolateral funiculus to the intermediolateral column.

Connecting the intermediomedial region with the intermediolateral region in the thoracic cord, but significantly not in cervical cord, are fibres containing substance P, somatostatin, and neurotensin (Senba *et al.* 1982): this is also observed in the sacral region of rat (S. J. Gibson, personal communication).

Descending pathways to the intermediolateral columns in thoracic and sacral regions have been shown to contain oxytocin in rat and monkey (Swanson and McKellar 1979) and vasopressin and oxytocin in man (Jenkins *et al.* 1984).

Finally, the sacral preganglionic neurons have themselves been shown to contain leu-encephalin in the cat (de Groat *et al.* 1983), and a-PP (NPY) and met-encephalin in the rat (Hunt *et al.* 1981).

VIP MARKS PELVIC AFFERENTS IN SACRAL CORD

The studies of neuropeptides in pelvic-nerve afferent fibres illustrate how they may selectively mark autonomic pathways. A VIP-containing system has been discovered in the post-mortem human sacral spinal cord (Figs. 28.2 and 28.3) (Anand *et al.* 1983) and an investigation of VIP distribution in six mammalian species showed that the monkey and cat sacral cord appeared to be excellent models for that of the human

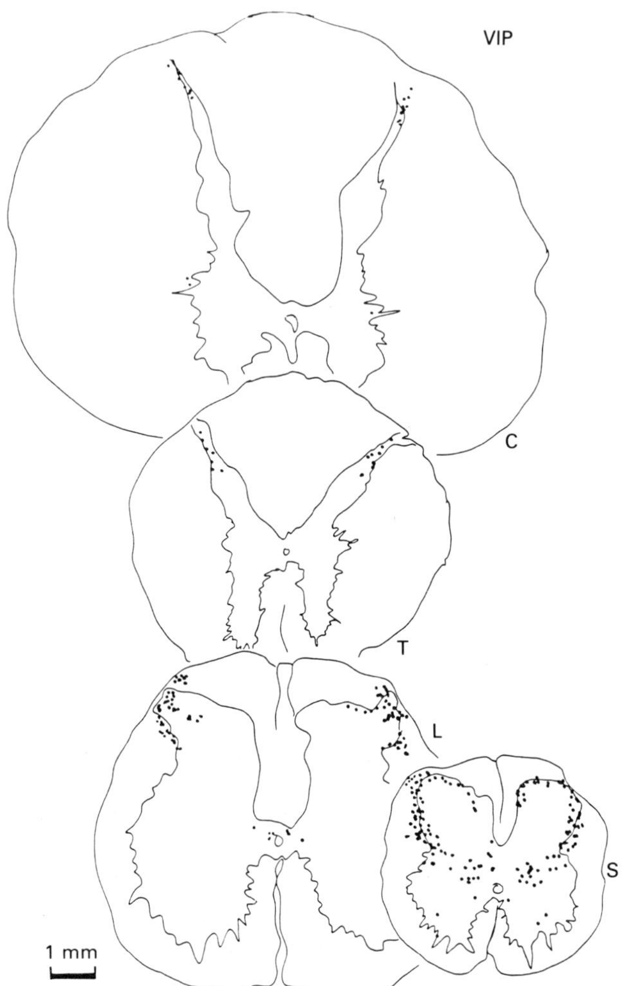

Fig. 28.2. Distribution of VIP fibres and terminals in the cervical (C), thoracic (T), lumbar (L), and sacral (S) human spinal cord. The map was constructed using camera lucida.

(Gibson *et al.* 1984*a*). In man and the other species, PHI-like immunoreactivity co-located with VIP in the sacral cord. It was considered likely, given that VIP and PHI/PHM are derived from a common precursor molecule, that they marked the same population of neurons (Anand *et al.* 1984).

A striking similarity was observed between the immunocytochemical localization of VIP in human and cat sacral cord and the central termination of fibres from the pelvic nerve of the cat, as labelled by retrograde horseradish peroxidase tracing. Dorsal rhizotomy in the cat

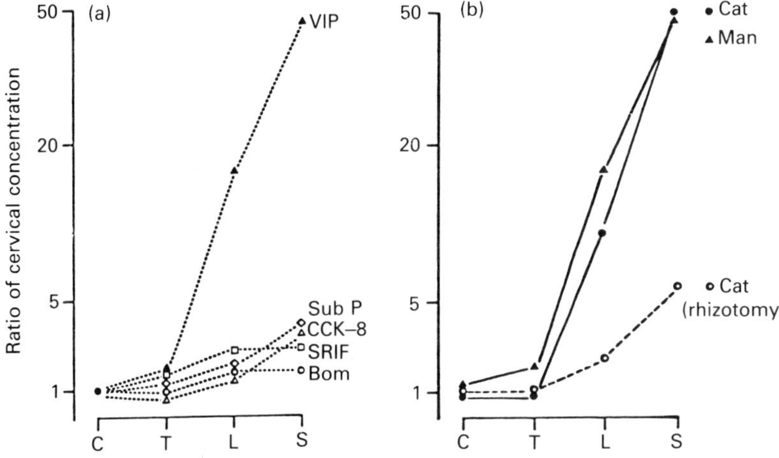

Fig. 28.3. (a) Dorsal regional concentration of substance P (Sub P), VIP, somatostatin (SRIF), bombesin (Bom), and CCK-8 as ratios of their dorsal cervical concentrations. (b) VIP in the dorsal cord regions of normal man (solid triangles) and cat (solid circles) as a ratio of the dorsal cervical concentrations. After unilateral lumbosacral rhizotomies in the cat, there is a marked decrease in lumbar and sacral concentrations of VIP (open circles). C, cervical; T, thoracic; L, lumbar; S, sacral.

established that the source of the distinctive VIP-containing system in the sacral cord was the sacral dorsal roots (Gibson *et al.* 1984*a*) (Fig. 28.3). de Groat's group combined dye-tracing experiments with histochemistry to demonstrate that VIP and substance P were located in visceral afferent perikarya in the sacral dorsal root ganglia and their terminals in the sacral autonomic nucleus (Kawatani *et al.* 1983). At the ultrastructural level, Honda *et al.* (1983) found the VIP-like immunoreactivity in cat sacral cord in dense-core vesicles within axonal enlargements containing both dense-core and small clear round vesicles. They too concluded that, although substance P, somatostatin, and CCK-like immunoreactivity may be located in some visceral as well as other afferent fibres, VIP appeared to be preferentially contained in pelvic visceral afferent fibres. In support, 4 weeks after pelvic-nerve transection in the cat there was a marked depletion of VIP from the ipsilateral sacral dorsal horn (Gibson *et al.* 1986).

A study of stimulation-provoked release of VIP from cat sacral cord is in accord with the anatomical findings. Pelvic nerve stimulation induced a 495 per cent (approx 45 pmol/l/10 min) increase of VIP-like immunoreactivity into spinal-cord superperfusate (Fig. 28.4) (Blank *et al.* 1984). In contrast sciatic nerve stimulation in the same model produced only a 135 per cent increase of VIP in the superperfusate (approx 1.5 to 2.8 pmol/l/10 min), suggesting that pelvic-nerve stimulation is the more adequate stimulus for VIP release.

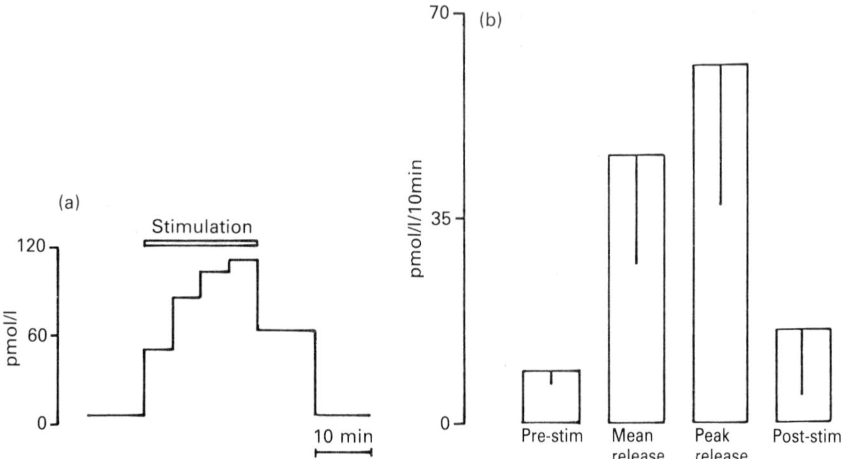

Fig. 28.4. (a) Release of VIP-like immunoreactivity into spinal cord superperfusate during a 20-min period of pelvic-nerve stimulation in one cat. (b) Results of the VIP-like immunoreactivity in cat spinal cord superperfusate following stimulation of the pelvic nerve (pmol/1/10 min, $n=4$). Columns show mean $\pm$SEM. On account of the wide variation in release, the data was log-transformed before applying Student's paired t-test, which showed the release to be significant ($p < 0.01$).

SPINAL-CORD NEUROPEPTIDES IN AF WITH MSA

A study has been undertaken of post-mortem spinal-cord peptide concentrations in four clinically and neuropathologically established cases of AF with MSA (Anand *et al.* 1987). The peptides studied were substance P, somatostatin, VIP, calcitonin gene-related peptide (CGRP), as well as newly discovered peptides not previously examined regionally in human spinal cord—galanin, and substance K, which belongs to the tachykinin family as does substance P. The regions dissected, shown in Fig. 28.1, were the dorsal, ventral, and lateral horns, the dorsal columns, and the dorsolateral white matter: only thoracic spinal cord was available for examination. The results are shown in Fig. 28.5, with the exception of VIP whose levels were below the detection limit (less than 0.8 pmol/g), in accord with a previous study (Anand *et al.* 1983). The neuropeptide depletion appears most marked in MSA dorsal cord regions, particularly for substance P and substance K. There appears to be almost complete loss of substance P and substance K immunoreactivity in the dorsal and dorsolateral columns. All neuropeptides measured are depleted in the dorsal horn, and substance P significantly reduced in ventral horn as well.

Although substance P-containing fibres are present in several known projections to preganglionic cell bodies, substance P immunostaining is

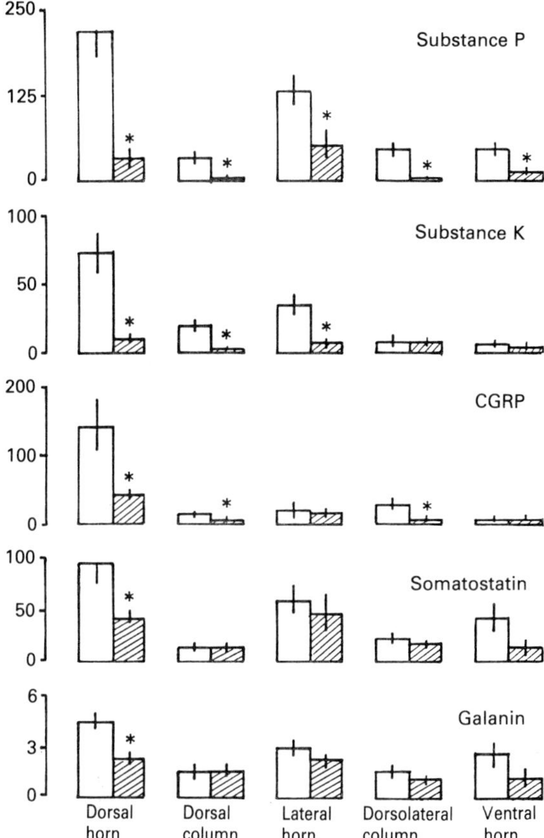

Fig. 28.5. Regional concentrations of neuropeptides (pmol/g) in control and MSA (hatched columns) spinal cord. Asterisk (*) denotes a statistically significant difference in concentration between control and MSA specimens of a particular region ($p < 0.05$, Student's unpaired *t*-test).

not apparent within cell bodies of thoracic autonomic efferents. The depletion of substance P thus provides a new marker to study neuronal fibre loss or dysfunction in the dorsal and lateral horns in syndromes of AF. In agreement with the general depletion of substance P, a 50 per cent reduction of substance P has been found in the cerebrospinal fluid of MSA patients, with normal levels in parkinsonian subjects (Williams 1981).

The depletion of substance P, substance K, and CGRP in dorsal regions in MSA spinal cord was both unexpected and intriguing, and further studies are necessary to establish its significance. None of the cases had any sensory symptoms or clinical evidence of somatic sensory neuropathy. Could it be that the peptide depletion occurred exclusively in visceral afferents? Or even in non-sensory pathways in dorsal cord? The findings in the dorsal column made it unlikely that the peptide depletion was restricted to non-sensory pathways. Otsuka *et al.* (1978) found decreased concentrations of substance P in the dorsal horn in motoneuron disease (which spares sensory and autonomic pathways), but they reported normal levels in the dorsal columns. Whereas substance K and CGRP may coexist with substance P in some primary sensory neurons, somatostatin and galanin are confined to different primary afferents; this may be relevant to their preservation in the dorsal column of MSA spinal cord.

There is evidence that skin flares are produced by release of substance P or CGRP (or indeed both) from sensory unmyelinated fibre terminals in skin. Histamine-induced skin flares were therefore studied in patients with AF and MSA (Anand *et al.* 1987). Skin flares were found to be intact in these patients, in support of the view that the substance P and CGRP depletion may occur mainly or exclusively in visceral afferents. On the other hand, it is possible that substance P and CGRP are sufficient but not essential to the production of flares in human skin, or that there is much redundancy in the system.

It is now feasible and necessary to examine other cord regions, and measure neuropeptides (e.g. vasopressin) selectively present in central autonomic pathways or in preganglionic sympathetic and parasympathetic neurons: combined with peptide immunocytochemistry, this would help clarify the syndromes associated with autonomic failure. A comparison with changes in classical transmitters would also be of interest. Although no studies appear to have reported levels of classical neurotransmitters in MSA spinal cord, widespread depletion of dopamine, noradrenalin, and choline acetyltransferase activity have been found in the brain regions of cell loss and fibre termination in MSA cases (see Chapter 25B).

It has been postulated that defects of neurotrophic agent synthesis, transport, or release (thereby of postsynaptic effects) may be responsible for the 'chain' pattern of cell loss in AF and MSA. Kwak (1985) reported markedly reduced concentrations of substance P in the basal ganglia, particularly the substantia nigra, in AF with MSA, and found that this reduction is relatively selective. With new techniques, including mRNA *in situ* hybridization, it is possible to examine the hypothesis that reduced substance P or other neurotrophic peptide synthesis in specific neurons may be a causative or permissive factor in AF with MSA and other progressive 'chain' degenerations. It is of interest that a decrease of substance P-immunoreactive terminals around motoneurons has been reported in the ventral horn of the spinal cord in motoneuron disease (Patten and Croft 1984).

To conclude, we have in neuropeptides new tools to investigate AF syndromes, and they promise new therapeutic approaches to progressive degenerative disorders.

REFERENCES

Anand, P. (1984). The role of neuropeptides in the pathophysiology of the peripheral nervous system. MD thesis, Cambridge University.

Anand, P., Bannister, R., McGregor, G. P., Ghatei, M. A., Mulderry, P. K., and Bloom, S. R. (1987). Marked depletion of dorsal spinal cord substance P and CGRP with intact skin flare responses in multiple system atrophy. *J. Neurol. Neurosurg. Psychiat.* (In press).

Anand, P. and Bloom, S. R. (1984). Neuropeptides are selective markers of spinal cord autonomic pathways. *Trends Neurosci.* **7**, 267–8.

Anand, P., Gibson, S. J., McGregor, G. P., Blank, M. A., Ghatei, M. A., Bacarese-Hamilton, A. J., Polak, J. M., and Bloom, S. R. (1983). A VIP-containing system concentrated in the lumbosacral region of human spinal cord. *Nature* **305**, 143–5.

Anand, P., Gibson, S. J., Yiangou, Y., Christofides, N. D., Polak, J. M., and Bloom, S. R. (1984). PHI-like immunoreactivity co-locates with the VIP-containing system in human lumbosacral spinal cord. *Neurosci. Lett.* **46**, 191–6.

Anand, P., Polak, J. M., and Bloom, S. R. (1985). Review article: Aspects of neuronal and hormonal peptides. *Clin. Physiol.* **5**, 110–20.

Barber, R. P., Vaughn, J. E., Slemmon, J. R., Salvaterra, P. M., Robert, E., and Leeman, S. E. (1979). The origin, distribution and synaptic relationship of substance P axons in rat spinal cord. *J. comp. Neurol.* **184**, 331–52.

Blank, M. A., Anand, P., Lumb, B. M., Morrison, J. F. B., and Bloom, S. R. (1984). Release of VIP-like immunoreactivity from cat urinary bladder and sacral spinal cord during pelvic nerve stimulation. *Dig. Dis. Sci.* **29**, 115.

Burnstock, G. (1982). Neuropeptides as trophic factors. In *Systemic role of regulatory peptides* (ed. S. R. Bloom, J. M. Polak, E. Lindenlaub), pp. 422–43. Schattauer, Stuttgart.

de Groat, W. C., Kawatani, M., Hisamitsu, T., Lowe, I., Morgan, C., Roppolo, J., Booth, A. M., Nadelhaft, I., Kuo, D., and Thor, K. (1983). The role of neuropeptides in the sacral autonomic reflex pathways of the cat. *J. auton. nerv. Syst.* **7**, 339–50.

Fuji, K., Senba, E., Heda, Y., and Tohyama, M. (1983). VIP containing neurons in the spinal cord of the rat and their projections. *Neurosci. Lett.* **37**, 51–5.

Gibson, S. J., Polak, J. M., Anand, P., Blank, M. A., Morrison, J. F. B., Kelly, J. S., and Bloom, S. R. (1984*a*). The distribution and origin of VIP in the spinal cord of six mammalian species. *Peptides* **5**, 201–7.

Gibson, S. J., Polak, J. M., Anand, P., Blank, M. A., Yiangou, Y., Su, H. C., Terenghi, G., Katagiri T., and Bloom, S. R. (1986). A VIP/PHI containing pathway links urinary bladder and sacral cord. *Peptides* **7**, 205–19.

Gibson, S. J., Polak, J. M., Bloom, S. R., Sabate, I. M., Mulderry, P., Ghatei, M. A., McGregor, G. P., Morrison, J., Kelly, J. S., Evans, R. M., and Rosenfeld, M. G. (1984*b*). Calcitonin gene-related peptide immunoreactivity in the spinal cord of man and eight other species. *J. Neurosci* **4**, 3101–11.

Honda, C. N., Rethelyi, M., and Petrusz, P. (1983). Preferential immunohistochemical localization of VIP in the sacral spinal cord of the cat: light and electron microscopic observations, *J. Neurosci.* **3**, 2183–96.

Hunt, S. P., Emson, P. C., Gilbert, M., Goldstein, M., and Kimmel, J. R. (1981). Presence of avian pancreatic polypeptide-like immunoreactivity in catecholamine and met-enkephalin containing neurons within the central nervous system. *Neurosci. Lett.* **21**, 125–30.

Jenkins, J. S., Ang, V. T. Y., Hawthorn, J., Rossor, M. N., and Iversen, L. L. (1984). Vasopressin, oxytocin and neurophysins in the human brain and spinal cord. *Br. Res.* **291**, 111–17.

Kawatani, M., Lowe, I. P., Nadelhaft, I., Morgan, C., and de Groat, W. C. (1983). VIP in visceral afferent pathways to the sacral spinal cord of the cat. *Neurosci. Lett.* **42**, 311–16.

Kwak, S. (1985). Biochemical analysis of transmitters in the brains of multiple system atrophy. *N. Shinkei* **37**, 691–4.

LaMotte, C. C. and de Lanerolle, N. C. (1981). Human spinal neurons: innervation by both substance P and enkephalin. *Neuroscience* **6**, 713–23.

Mawe, G. M., Bresnahan, J. C., and Beattie, M. S. (1984). Primary afferent projections from dorsal and ventral roots to autonomic preganglionic neurons in the cat spinal cord: light and electron microscopic observations. *Br. Res.* **290**, 152–7.

Morgan, C., Nadelhaft, I., and de Groat, W. C. (1981). The distribution of visceral primary afferents from the pelvic nerve to Lissauer's tract and the spinal grey matter and its relationship to the sacral parasympathetic nucleus. *J. comp. Neurol.* **201**, 415–40.

Nathan, P. W., and Smith, M. C. (1958). The centrifugal pathway for micturition within the spinal cord. *J. Neurol. Neurosurg. Psychiat.* **21**, 177–89.

Otsuka, M., Kanazawa, I., Sugita, H., and Toyokura, Y. (1978). Substance P in the spinal cord and serum of amyotrophic lateral sclerosis. In *Amyotrophic lateral sclerosis* (ed. T. Tsubaki and Y. Toyokura), pp. 405–11. University Park Press, Baltimore.

Patten, B. M. and Croft, S. (1984). Spinal cord substance P in amyotrophic lateral sclerosis. In *Research progress in motor neurone disease* (ed. F. C. Rose), pp. 283–9. Pitman, London.

Pick, J. (1970). *The autonomic nervous system*, pp. 61–72. Lippencott, Philadelphia.

Schroder, H. D. (1983). Localization of CCK-like immunoreactivity in the rat spinal cord, with particular reference to the autonomic innervation of the pelvic organs. *J. comp. Neurol.* **217**, 176–86.

Senba, E., Shiosaka, S., Hara, Y., Inagaki, S., Sakanaka, M., Takatsuki, K., Kawai, Y., and Tohyama, M. (1982). Ontogeny of the peptidergic system in the rat spinal cord: immunohistochemical analysis. *J. comp. Neurol.* **208**, 54–66.

Swanson, L. W. and McKellar, S. (1979). The distribution of oxytocin- and neurophysin-stained fibres in the spinal cord of the rat and monkey. *J. comp. Neurol.* **188**, 87–106.

Williams, A. (1981). CSF biochemical studies on some extrapyramidal diseases. In *Research progress in Parkinson's disease* (ed. F. C. Rose and R. Capildeo), pp. 170–80. Pitman, London.

29. Assessing the peripheral ganglia in autonomic failure

Margaret R. Matthews

INTRODUCTION

Elucidating the cause or causes of the autonomic failure which occurs in multiple system atrophy (MSA), in some cases of Parkinson's disease, or rarely as an isolated phenomenon (pure autonomic failure (PAF)) is proving remarkably difficult. The craniosacral, parasympathetic autonomic functions may be involved as well as the sympathetic. Clinical testing suggests that the cause is more efferent or central than afferent; and the effects are fairly symmetrical and slowly progressive, without apparent involvement of the higher centres of autonomic integration. Peripheral adrenoceptors are present and responsive; indeed in some patients there is evidence of hypersensitivity, both of the decentralization and the denervation type, suggesting a partial postganglionic lesion. Some peripheral sympathetic nerve endings are still present, however, and are charged with noradrenalin, though it may be subnormal in amount, and this can be released by appropriate drug treatment (see Chapter 31). The indications are that surviving ganglionic neurons are not being recruited reflexly—hence the profound fall of blood pressure which occurs on passive tilting or on the assumption of the erect posture. These and other observations suggested that the primary defect was in the preganglionic, intermediolateral neurons, or in the preganglionic–postganglionic interaction, if not located more centrally.

Neuropathological studies of over 50 cases, many of them reviewed and reported by Oppenheimer (see Chapter 25A), have lent extensive support to the first of these possibilities, by showing that there is in almost all cases examined considerable loss of neurons from the intermediolateral nucleus (IML) of the spinal cord, amounting at thoracic levels to 75 per cent or more of control numbers. The situation is not entirely straightforward, however. At least one case, substantiated by cell counts, showed no significant loss of neurons from the intermediolateral columns. Not all the preganglionic sympathetic neurons are necessarily in the IML, however; in experimental animals neurons in the intercalated (IC) and intermediomedial (IMM) groups also become retrogradely labelled by tracers injected into the adrenal glands or into prevertebral sympathetic ganglia. Loss of neurons from the intermediomedial nucleus could contribute to the extent of preganglionic denervation which may occur in human autonomic failure, and this possibility adds point to studies such as that of Low *et al.* (1978) in which differential size counts were made of axons in ventral roots in addition to neuron counts in the IML.

There are also some reports of changes in sympathetic ganglia. Here it is important to note the distinction between two types of autonomic failure, one occurring in cases of multiple system atrophy, and the other as a clinically pure autonomic failure, sometimes associated with Parkinson's disease. In the second, but not the first, type it is characteristic to find Lewy bodies or hyaline, fibrillar inclusions in the pigmented neurons of the brainstem (substantia nigra and locus ceruleus), with or without neuronal loss, and also in sympathetic ganglia, suggesting the possibility of a somewhat different aetiology. In one case of autonomic failure with Parkinson's disease, Rajput and Rozdilsky (1976) reported marked neuronal loss and degeneration in sympathetic ganglia, together with Lewy bodies, with only minimal loss of neurons in the IML.

In a study of four cases of autonomic failure Petito and Black (1978) found in the superior cervical ganglion that levels of choline acetyltransferase (CAT), the transmitter-synthesizing enzyme of the preganglionic nerve endings, lay within the normal range in all three cases in which it was measured, and they observed moderate neuron loss in the IML in only two cases, but they made no formal counts, and there must be reservations about the precise diagnostic group of their cases. Tyrosine hydroxylase (TOH) activity in the superior cervical ganglia was reported to be within normal limits but dopamine β-hydroxylase activity was low or undetectable; both these enzymes are involved in the biosynthesis of noradrenalin by the adrenergic neurons. Control studies indicated that post-mortem changes in enzyme activity should have been negligible. Petito and Black interpreted these findings as showing that, if there were cell loss in the IML, it had been compensated by intraganglionic sprouting from terminals of surviving IML neurons. In sympathetic ganglia Petito and Black found evidence of focal phagocytosis of ganglion cells in three cases (subjects 2–4), some increase of satellite cells in all, and perivascular mononuclear infiltration in three cases (1, 2, and 4), with Lewy-like hyaline interstitial bodies in case 3, which at electron microscopy were seen to be 'enlarged, swollen axons filled with proliferated filaments' with focal accumulations of mitochondria, typical of dystrophic axons. There was also some evidence suggesting loss of unmyelinated postganglionic axons. Petito and Black concluded that in a subpopulation of cases the primary failure may be in the ganglionic neurons, and that '*some* of the histological changes in the spinal cord intermediolateral columns . . . result from faulty retrograde regulation by diseased adrenergic neurones'. This might indeed be possible, especially in the group which involves 'Lewy-body disease' of pigmented and autonomic neurons. The peculiarity of the normal level of ganglionic TOH, coupled with low or absent dopamine β-hydroxylase (DBH), both of which enzymes are regulated transsynaptically, suggests to this author that surviving ganglionic neurons may be compensating for any neuronal loss in terms of TOH activity, which is a cytoplasmic enzyme, but that DBH, which is enclosed in the noradrenalin-forming nerve secretory granules, and is subject to a more rapid turnover, may also be leaving the ganglion along the postganglionic axons as soon as it is formed, to service the transmitter functions of hard-driven axon terminals, thus remaining at paradoxically low levels within the ganglion. Another possibility is that the normal reserve of inactive TOH is all in the active state (TOH activity can increase without synthesis of new protein), whereas the same two alternative states may not exist in the case of DBH. In the face of such ambiguities it is clearly important to look carefully at the sympathetic ganglia for any further evidence which may throw light on the pathological processes involved.

Why is it so difficult to be sure about the underlying changes? There are various reasons, some of which are common to all neuropathological studies while others are peculiar to the autonomic nervous system. First, the basic defect may be biochemical, metabolic, or regulatory, and may not express itself in gross structural terms. Second, the condition may be well advanced before it presents clinically. This is perhaps particularly true of the autonomic system. At the somatic neuromuscular junction a single nerve terminal innervates a muscle fibre, giving rise to suprathreshold activation; denervation, or silencing of motoneurons, is likely to be seen early as disturbance of power or tone, even if it is later compensated by collateral sprouting. Here also, an upper motor neuron lesion is clearly distinguishable from a lower motor neuron lesion by alterations of tone and of reflex excitability, etc. In the autonomic nervous system there is no clear functional demarcation between an upper (higher centres) and a lower motor neuron (IML) lesion. There are both divergence and convergence of preganglionic neurons on to ganglionic neurons; the latter receive multiple inputs which have the characteristic that they are subthreshold, requiring coincidence of several inputs to bring the neuron to the threshold for firing. The peripheral effectors are smooth or cardiac muscle and gland cells, neuroeffector contacts are typically not close, and electrotonic coupling in the effector organ is frequent or typical. The interstitial dropping-out of peripheral nerve endings may be initially compensated by diffusion of transmitter, since fewer nerve endings mean less high-affinity re-uptake, by increased receptor density, and by electronic coupling, until the changes have become extreme. Moreover, collateral sprouting of preganglionic nerves in the ganglia (cf. Liestøl *et al.* 1986) and also of postganglionic nerves in the periphery are further able to compensate to a remarkable extent. A slowly progressive change may thus not become clinically evident until the underlying pathological changes are severe, as in the case of IML neuron loss in postural hypotension (Oppenheimer 1980).

By this time, secondary trophic and degenerative changes may well have occurred, involving not only neurons but also satellite or Schwann cells, supporting tissues, and vasculature. As far as the neurons are concerned, these secondary changes are likely to be transneuronal in character, but could be either anterograde or retrograde. (See Cowan (1970) for a wide-ranging review and discussion.) Since that review was written, much more has become known about retrograde trophic influences on neurons, and this knowledge has derived largely from studies in the autonomic nervous system, relating to nerve growth factor and, more recently, to ciliary neurotrophic factors, which govern the development and maintenance of peripheral ganglion cells (for example, see Elliott and Lawrenson 1981); but other such factors are currently being isolated from sources which include central nervous tissues, and a similar control may be expected to apply in the case of the preganglionic neurons. Briefly, a neuron receives from its target a factor or factors necessary for its continued survival and maintenance; this is released from the target upon activation, is taken up by the nerve endings, and retrogradely transported to the cell body, where it takes effect. Anterograde influences are also important, as is well exemplified by the striated muscle fibre: trophic maintenance is influenced by activation and, in its absence, cell shrinkage and a varying degree of dedifferentiation may occur. Whether in the long term this may lead to neuronal death is uncertain: it depends strongly on age, on the type of neuron, and the presence or absence of other inputs.

From the time of onset of autonomic failure a patient may survive for many years. The availability of biopsy is strictly limited, for example, to the peripheral autonomic terminals as seen in muscle or skin biopsies, since the removal of ganglia would be too destructive; the possibility of early biopsy is virtually ruled out by the lateness of presentation. Post-mortem changes may preclude the finer aspects of the eventual analysis, and agonal changes, involving intense nervous discharges, may also have supervened, as the terminal event is often apparently asphyxial.

DESIDERATA FOR STUDYING THE GANGLIA POST-MORTEM

Early chilling of the body and early post-mortem

The advantages of early chilling and early post-mortem are obvious, but they are not always easy to attain. It may be noted encouragingly, however, that small peptide molecules are not rapidly autolysed post-mortem: Pioro *et al.* (1984) found that post-infarction differences in levels of substance P and encephalin in the nigrostriatal system could still be demonstrated immunohistochemically even when post-mortem had been delayed for up to 67 hours. In a situation at or close to the ideal, Allen *et al.* (1984) were able to chart the comparative distribution of neuropeptide Y (NPY) in human spinal cords removed within 24 h post-mortem, where chilling had been begun within 2 hours after death.

Extensive sampling within the autonomic system

Sampling should be bilaterally symmetrical, so that equivalent specimens may be appropriately fixed for different histological investigations, and should ideally include paravertebral sympathetic ganglia from all levels and the coeliac–superior mesenteric ganglion complex. If the sympathetic chains can be removed entire, for storage and future reference, so much the better. Desirably, cranial parasympathetic ganglia should also be obtained, if possible, e.g. ciliary and pterygopalatine, and at an early post-mortem pieces of gut wall for enteric ganglia. Peripheral tissues normally rich in autonomic endings should also be sampled, including an iris, if eye removal is permitted, and cardiac muscle, skeletal muscle (for sampling of arterioles), and (in the male) vas deferens.

Appropriate fixation

Probably the most generally useful fixation schedules are, for tissues from one side, 4 per cent formaldehyde, freshly prepared from paraformaldehyde powder, in 0.1 M sodium phosphate buffer at pH 7.4, and for the other side, 3 per cent glutaraldehyde, freshly diluted from 25 per cent stock solution stored at 4°C, in the same 0.1 M phosphate buffer, pH 7.4. The formaldehyde-fixed specimens can be used for paraffin-embedding and conventional histology (recommended for the superior cervical ganglion (SCG) for neuron counts) and for cryostat or frozen sections, for immunohistochemistry. The glutaraldehyde fixation prepares tissues for electron microscopy. Large or densely-encapsulated specimens should be halved lengthwise with a sharp razor blade to facilitate penetration. Tissues should be fixed for a minimum of 4 hours.

Appropriate range of investigations on paraformaldehyde-fixed tissues

1. Conventional light microscopy of 10–15 μm paraffin sections stained with haematoxylin and eosin for general cytology, thionin or cresyl violet for assessment of Nissl material, a silver stain such as the Glees and Marsland technique for morphology of neurons and nerve fibres, and such other specific techniques as may be suggested by the findings.

It must be stressed that serial sectioning (evenly spaced sections of constant thickness) throughout the entire specimen is essential for neuron counts (Konigsmark 1970), which are of considerable relevance and importance in this condition. Of the sympathetic ganglia, the superior cervical ganglion (SCG) is the best-defined, with a neuron population which is relatively constant within a species (Ebbesson 1963; Gabella 1976). In the author's experience, haematoxylin and eosin provides the most useful stain for such counts, which must be based upon the nucleus, not the nucleolus, since sympathetic neurons may have more than one nucleolus. (Sometimes, though less often, they are binucleate also.)

2. Enzyme histochemistry, e.g. acetylcholinesterase histochemistry on frozen or cryostat sections. This enzyme is present both at the preganglionic nerve terminal and in the ganglionic neurons.

3. Immunohistochemistry, on frozen or cryostat sections, for some or all of the following, according to availability of antibodies: tyrosine hydroxylase (TOH), dopamine β-hydroxylase (DBH), various neuropeptides (e.g. encephalin, substance P (SP), calcitonin gene-related peptide (CGRP), neuropeptide Y (NPY), vasoactive intestinal peptide (VIP), somatostatin, etc.).

Appropriate range of investigations on glutaraldehyde-fixed tissues

Here one may employ not only electron microscopy of selected areas, but also the examination in their own right of 1-μm sections from the resin-embedded blocks, stained with toluidine blue or with a mixture of methylene blue and Azur II, which give remarkable clarity of information about the state of neurons and of associated nerve fibres, blood vessels, connective tissue, nature and location of cellular infiltrates, and so on.

In practice, for various reasons, not all of these investigations may be possible or practicable, preservation may be poor, and very little material may be available in any one case.

EXPERIMENTAL RESULTS

The following account is based upon the examination of control material obtained through the courtesy of Dr David Oppenheimer, and material from subjects dying with autonomic failure who had been in the care of Sir Roger Bannister. The material falls into three categories:

1. Various sympathetic ganglia from six subjects with multiple system atrophy, confirmed by autopsy findings in the brainstem, of whom two are represented only by paraffin-embedded specimens. No Lewy bodies were found in any of these ganglia.
2. SCGs, and in one case other ganglia, from two subjects with clinically pure autonomic failure, showing Lewy bodies. One of the SCGs was formaldehyde-fixed and cut serially for cell counting; the other was fixed for electron microscopy.
3. SCGs from three subjects dying of other causes, all female, aged 16, 64, and 98 years; causes of death were, respectively, road accident, cerebral vascular accident, and empyema. These were osmium- or glutaraldehyde-fixed and resin-embedded for electron microscopy. None of these ganglia showed Lewy bodies.

Light microscopy

The ganglia of subjects with MSA were well populated with neurons which, in sections stained with haematoxylin and eosin, appeared within the range seen in the control ganglia in respect of size, general cytological appearance, and packing density in the neuropil. Almost all neurons had conspicuous aggregates of lipofuscin granules. Nissl material was however relatively scanty. In silver-stained preparations many neurons were seen to have well preserved dendritic arborizations (Fig. 29.1). Some of these dendritic patterns were perhaps unusually complex and profuse, and some processes unusually stout, but no gross distortions were observed. Some of the smaller neurons showed no stainable arborizations; but failure to stain processes in this material cannot necessarily be taken to imply their absence.

The use of 1-μm resin-embedded sections from comparable mid-ganglion levels (Fig. 29.2) permitted semiquantitative cytological comparisons. In SCGs of three control subjects, the mean packing density of neurons in areas of neuropil averaged 7.1 nucleated neuronal profiles in the area of a standard photoframe graticule at ×325 magnification (range of means 5.6–8.3). In SCGs of three subjects with MSA the corresponding average was 8.9 nucleated neuronal profiles (range of means 6.8–10.4). This is not suggestive of severe neuronal loss, but might indicate compaction consequent on reduction of other elements in

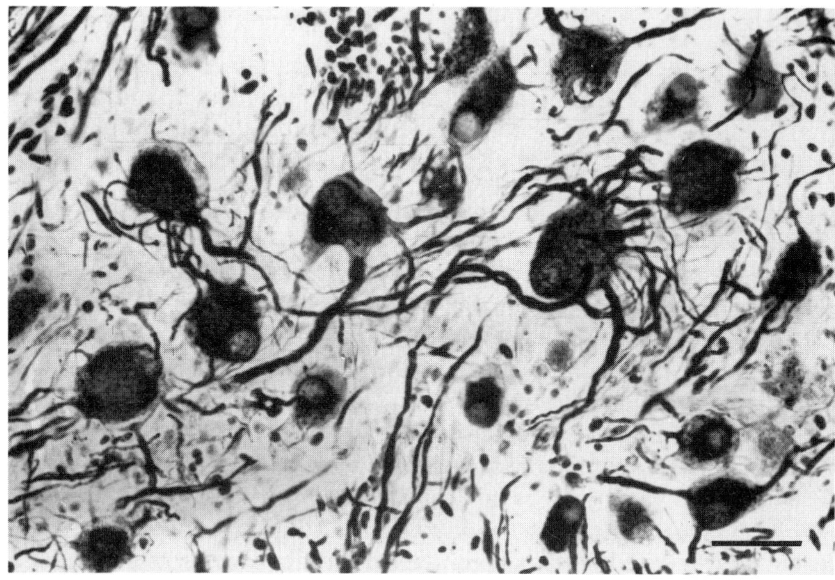

Fig. 29.1. Neurons of a thoracic sympathetic ganglion from a subject with MSA. Silver preparation (Glees and Marsland). Scale bar, 50 μm.

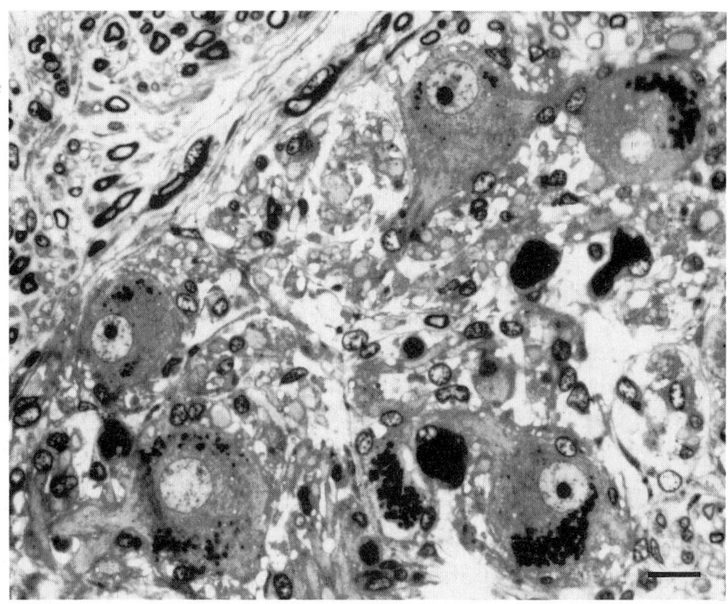

Fig. 29.2. 1-μm section of an Araldite-embedded thoracic ganglion of a subject with MSA, stained with methylene blue and Azur II. Most of the neurons have eccentric nuclei and contain arcs or masses of darkly-stained lipofuscin bodies, but also contain some distinct Nissl material (intermediate grey clumps). Scale bar, 20 μm.

the neuropil, such as preganglionic nerve fibres and extent of dendritic trees.

Nucleated neuronal profiles (NNP) in these 1-μm sections were assessed for various features (sample size 45–320, median 137). These included the presence of distinct Nissl granules, the incidence of lipofuscin bodies, the degree of nuclear eccentricity, and the size range of the neuron population. In the three control subjects, a mean of 91 per cent (range 84–95 per cent) showed distinct Nissl granules. In all three subjects with MSA, fewer neurons (37, 46, and 72 per cent of NNP) showed distinct Nissl granules. In the youngest control subject only 35 per cent of NNP showed heavy clumps or masses of lipofuscin bodies, but the incidences in the other two were 87 and 84 per cent. In the subjects with MSA, the mean incidence per NNP of massed lipofuscin bodies was 84 per cent (range 78–93 per cent). The proportion of NNP showing centrally situated, rather than eccentric, nuclei was likewise similar in the two groups (control mean 15 per cent, range 11–24 per cent; MSA mean 13 per cent, range 8–18 per cent). The mean diameters of the five to eight largest and smallest neurons were compared, for two subjects from each group, and were not found to differ markedly (*smallest NNP*: control youngest 15.6 μm, oldest 22.3 μm; MSA 21.1 and 21.1 μm; *largest NNP*: control youngest 41.3, oldest 44.3 μm; MSA 45.3, 51.4 μm).

Thus, in the MSA group of subjects with autonomic failure, the principal observed difference from the controls lay in the reduced incidence of distinct Nissl granules in the neuronal cell bodies. No consistent abnormalities were noted in the vasculature or in adventitial cells in the ganglia, but in one of the MSA subjects there was some perivenular lymphocytic infiltration, part of a generalized distribution associated with a longstanding leukaemic condition (Waldeström macroglobulinaemia).

In sympathetic ganglia from the two subjects with pure autonomic failure the packing densities of nucleated neuronal profiles in the neuropil were strikingly reduced, to means of 3.4 and 2.2 per standard graticule area, and the overall impression was of heavy depopulation of neurons, with scattered evidence of neuronophagia, in all ganglia studied. Lewy bodies were seen in both subjects, with mean incidences of 1.1 and 1.25 per NNP; these were sometimes in neuronal somata and sometimes in enlarged neuronal processes. In the surviving neurons, however, the mean incidence of visible Nissl granules was high (92 and 93 per cent of NNP) and the proportions of NNP which showed massed lipofuscin bodies (82 per cent in each case) were similar to those reported above for the MSA and control subjects. In these ganglia, therefore, the salient and distinctive features were the evidence of loss of neurons and the presence of Lewy bodies. In one of these subjects an entire SCG was available for neuron-counting in serial paraffin sections. Counts of all neuronal nuclei in every fiftieth section, of 10-μm thickness (cf. Ebbesson 1963), with application of correction factors according to the formula of Konigsmark (1970), yielded an estimate of 214 002 neurons in the entire ganglion. This is to be compared with the mean figure of approximately 937 000 (range 760 370–1 041 652) obtained from four ganglia by Ebbesson (1963), and suggests a loss of over 75 per cent of neurons, which is much greater than might be expected to occur even with age in normal subjects.

Histochemistry and immunohistochemistry

In frozen sections of a thoracic ganglion from one of the subjects with pure autonomic failure specific acetyl cholinesterase activity was demonstrable, after prolonged incubation, with a normal distribution in surviving neuronal cell bodies and in the neuropil but not in nerve bundles (Fig. 29.3). Immunofluorescence microscopy by standard procedures in ganglia of one subject with MSA and one with pure autonomic failure showed that traces of persistent varicose nerve trails immunoreactive for substance P or CGRP and for encephalin could be demonstrated in the coeliac ganglion, and less abundantly in thoracic and lumbar paravertebral ganglia (Fig. 29.4) (cf. del Fiacco *et al.* 1984). The substance P, and also CGRP, are attributable to sensory collateral branches (cf. Matthews and Cuello 1984) and the encephalin probably to preganglionic nerve fibres (Schultzberg *et al.* 1983). The cell bodies of

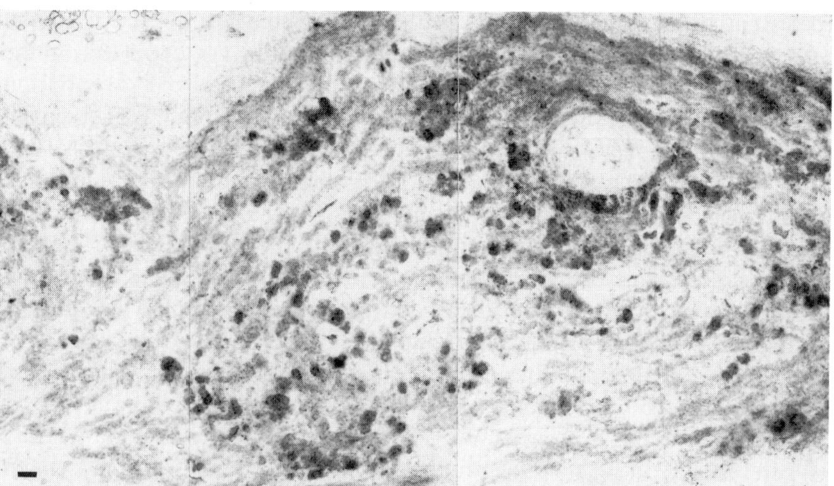

Fig. 29.3. Acetylcholinesterase staining of a number of scantily-distributed surviving neurons and of neuropil, but not of nerve bundles, in a thoracic ganglion from a subject with pure autonomic failure. (Fine dark granules are artefacts of prolonged reaction time.) Scale bar, 100 μm.

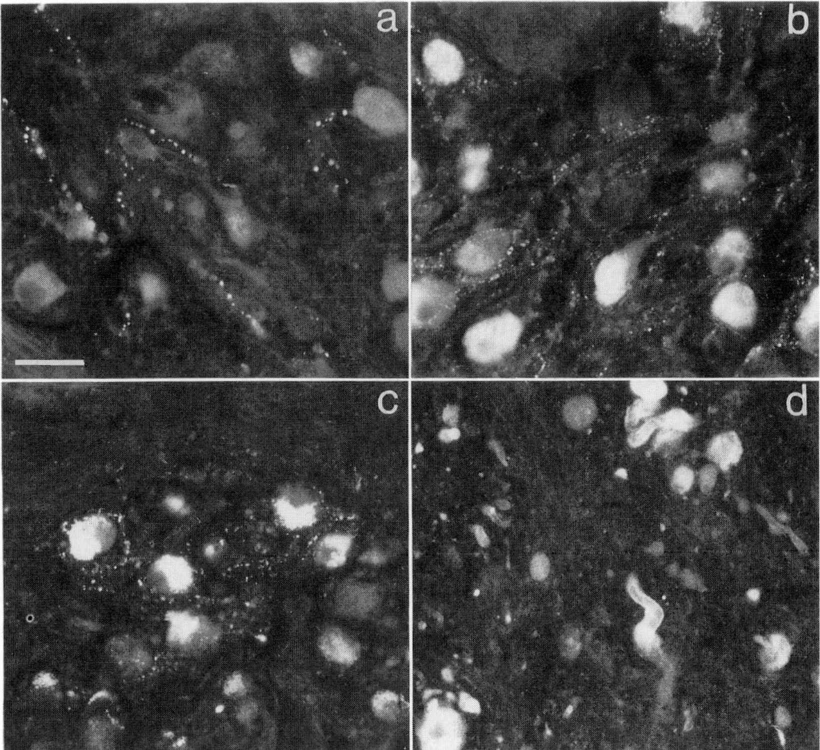

Fig. 29.4. Immunofluorescent staining for neuropeptides in the coeliac ganglion: (a) encephalin, (b) substance P, (c) CGRP, all from a case of MSA; (d) neuropeptide Y in dystrophic neurites, from a case of pure autonomic failure. Scale bars, 50 μm. Some neurons in (b) and (c) show intensely autofluorescent lipofuscin masses.

some neurons were seen to be encephalin-immunoreactive, and most neurons showed weak immunoreactivity for TOH. In the coeliac ganglion of the subject with pure autonomic failure NPY was also demonstrable in some neurons, including dystrophic neurites, in some small cells, possibly SIF cells (the catecholamine-rich 'small intensely fluorescent' cells) and in occasional varicose sprays or trails. Catecholamine fluorescence was barely detected after the aqueous formaldehyde fixation which had been used; low initial levels and post-mortem diffusion may both have influenced this finding.

Electron microscopy

Not all the material was sufficiently well preserved to be informative. Questions which were addressed included general neuronal cytology (Fig. 29.5), the presence and type of synapses, the completeness of satellite cell cover of the neurons (a question raised earlier by Petito and Black 1978), and the state of the pre- and postganglionic nerve fibres.

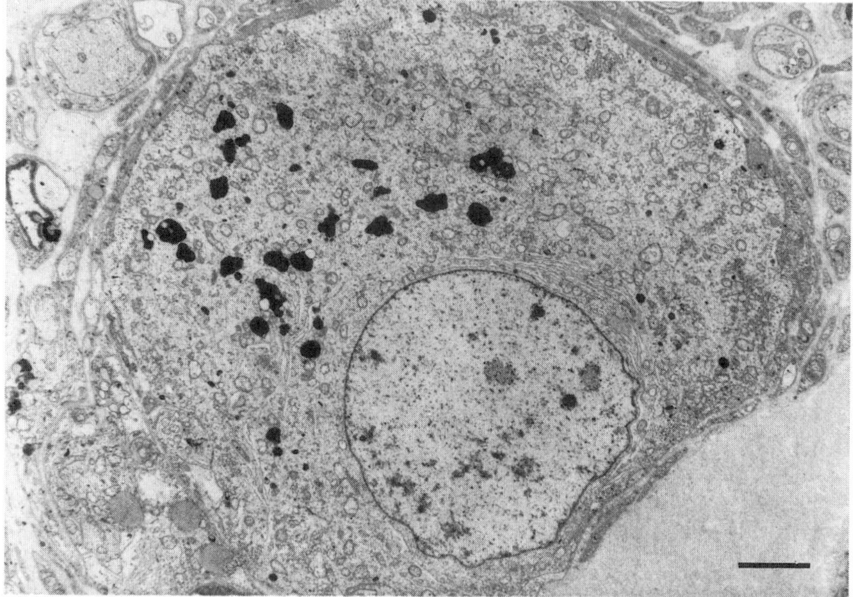

Fig. 29.5. Electron micrograph of a typical neuron from the SCG of a subject with MSA. At the lower right the satellite sheath of the neuron is very thin and in places deficient (cf. Fig. 29.11). Scale bar, 5 μm.

In the youngest control subject, synapses were readily localizable with an incidence of approximately 6 to 10 per grid square of side 100 μm; they were of cholinergic preganglionic type (Fig. 29.6; Matthews 1983) and were mostly axo-dendritic. In the subjects with MSA similar synapses were present (Fig. 29.7), occurring in clusters in areas of dendritic neuropil, but were much less frequent and were difficult to find, with a tendency to be greatly expanded and depleted of vesicles (Fig. 29.8). This appearance was not necessarily just a post-mortem artefact, since it appeared equally in ganglia fixed within 8 h and over 36 h post-mortem: it recalled the appearance of nerve endings heavily overstimulated by black widow spider venom (Clark *et al.* 1972; Duchen *et al.* 1981), and could possibly have reflected intense sympathetic discharges in surviving preganglionic endings in the ante-mortem period. In addition, occasional synapses were seen containing tubular vesicles with a relatively electron-dense content (Fig. 29.9): these resemble a type of adrenergic nerve ending and could be intrinsic synapses, which can increase markedly in incidence in denervated (and presumably in partly denervated) ganglia (Ramsay and Matthews 1985).

Neuro–neuronal attachment plaques were seen both in control and in MSA ganglia (Figs. 29.9 and 29.10).

Neuron–satellite relations did not seem to differ markedly between

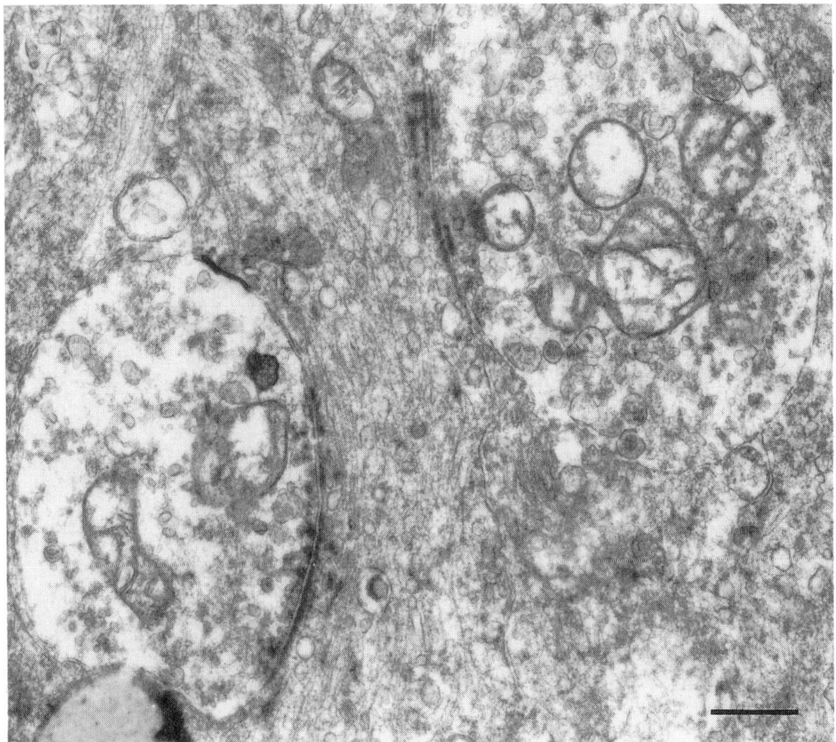

Fig. 29.6. Two synapses on opposite faces of the same dendrite, from the SCG of a control subject aged 16. Scale bar, 0.5 μm.

control and MSA ganglia. In both, neurons or their dendrites could show short, sometimes multiple, regions of their surfaces devoid of satellite cell cover (Figs. 29.10 and 29.11); these appeared at least as frequent in the MSA ganglia. If there was any difference, it may have resided in a tendency for the enveloping satellite cell processes to be thinner in the MSA ganglia. Further study, of material better matched as to age and preservation, would be required to clarify this question.

In one MSA subject, the pre- and postganglionic nerve fibres were sufficiently well preserved for ultrastructural study. Among the preganglionic nerve fibres there was evidence of loss of axons, in the form of collagen-filled Schwann cell channels; myelinated fibres were few and heavily myelinated, and other Schwann-axon units contained each only one or two unmyelinated axons (Fig. 29.12). The indications of fibre loss are consistent with the findings of Oppenheimer (see Chapter 25A) in the intermediolateral nucleus and of Low *et al.* (1978) (see Chapter 30) in the ventral roots. Some of the unmyelinated axons were singly ensheathed and of relatively large diameter, up to 4 μm, which suggests

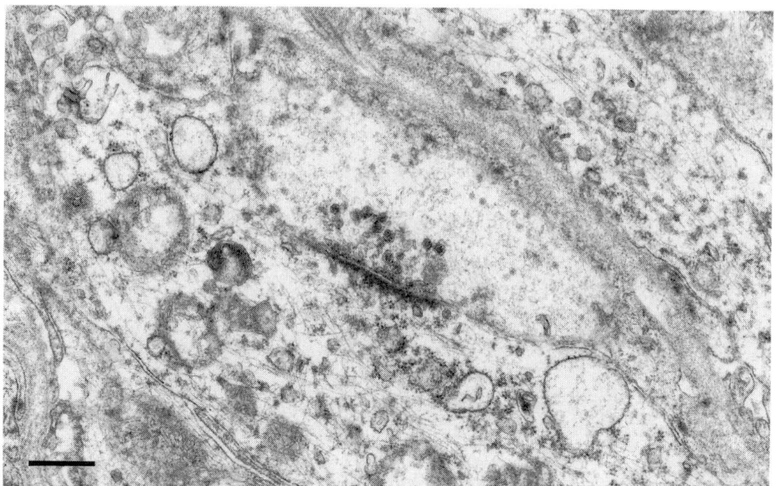

Fig. 29.7. Axodendritic synapse from the SCG of a subject with MSA. The presynaptic profile is heavily depleted of synaptic vesicles and shows evidence of numerous coated vesicles, suggesting recent extensive liberation of transmitter. Scale bar, 0.5 μm.

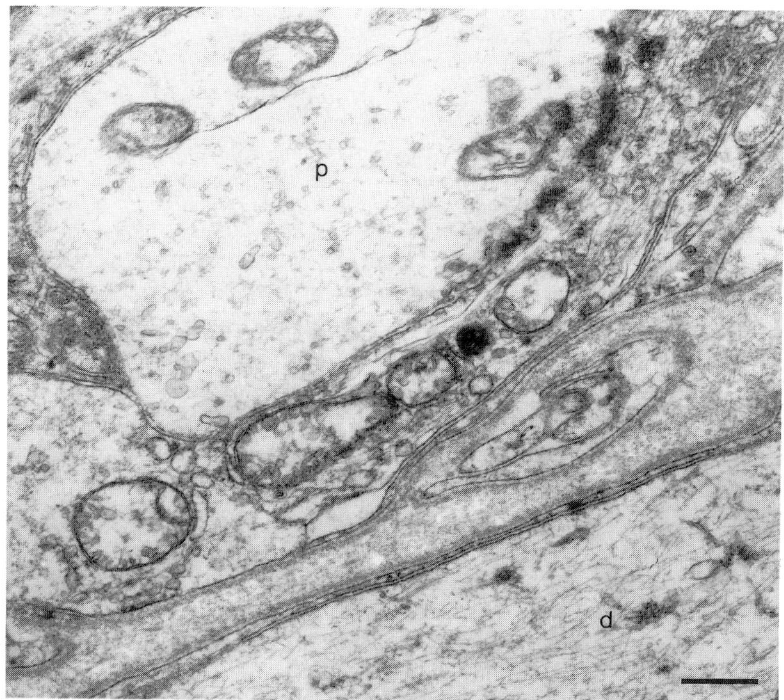

Fig. 29.8. Axodendritic synapse from the SCG of another subject with MSA. The presynaptic profile (p) appears swollen and is heavily depleted of synaptic vesicles. The dendritic shaft (d) in the lower part of the figure has a very thin but continuous satellite ensheathment. Scale bar, 0.5 μm.

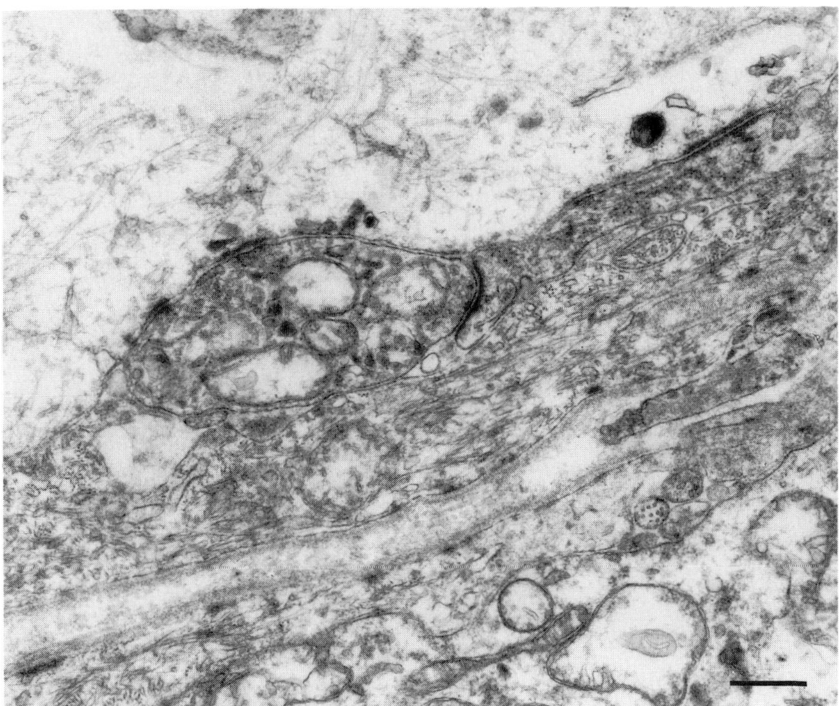

Fig. 29.9. Two synapses of possible adrenergic type from the same presynaptic profile, one axodendritic and the other probably axosomatic, from the SCG of a subject with MSA (same ganglion as Fig. 29.7). On the right the dendrite is linked with the presumptive soma by an attachment plaque. Scale bar, 0.5 μm.

possible demyelination, or hypertrophy without accompanying myelination. Among the postganglionic fibres in the internal carotid trunk there was also some suggestion of fibre loss, in the form of collagen-filled channels in Schwann cells, and here also there was a wide range of diameters of unmyelinated axons, suggesting possible denervation atrophy of some neurons and hypertrophy of others (Fig. 29.13). The number of fibres per Schwann unit was not unduly high, ranging mostly from 2 to 6; thus, there was little evidence of axon-sprouting at this level.

In one of the subjects with pure autonomic failure, although preservation of the interneuronal neuropil was poor, information was obtained on the nature of the Lewy bodies in these sympathetic neurons (Fig. 29.14): a mass of densely fibrillar material with an amorphous denser core was surrounded by a rim of dense-cored vesicles, which were associated with the marginal filaments of the mass (cf. Forno and Nerville 1976). Figure 29.15 shows an example of densely packed lysosomal bodies seen in one of the neurons: as was noted earlier, the surviving neurons, apart from those containing Lewy bodies, did not look grossly abnormal.

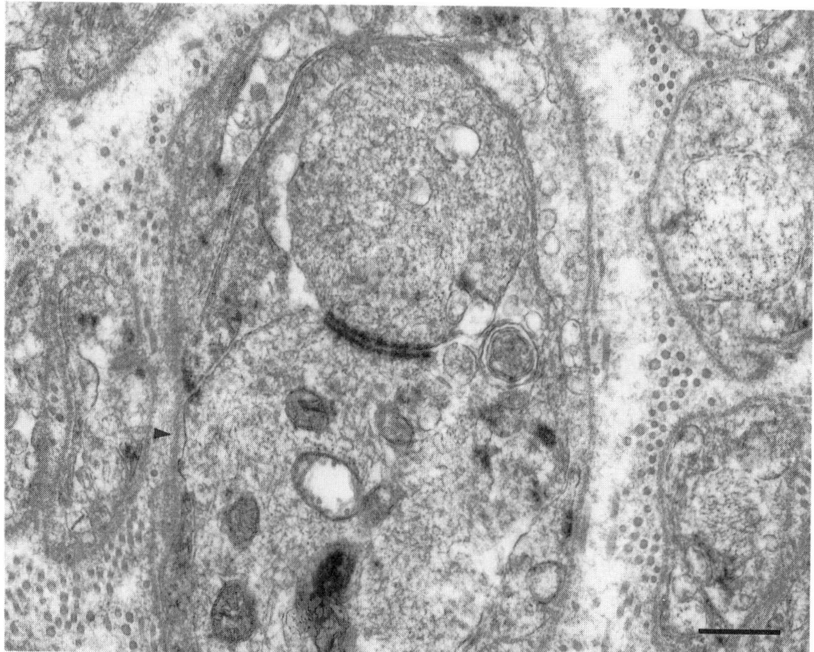

Fig. 29.10. Attachment plaque between two dendritic profiles, from the SCG of a control subject aged 16. At arrowhead, the satellite sheath of one of the profiles is deficient over a short distance. Scale bar, 0.5 μm.

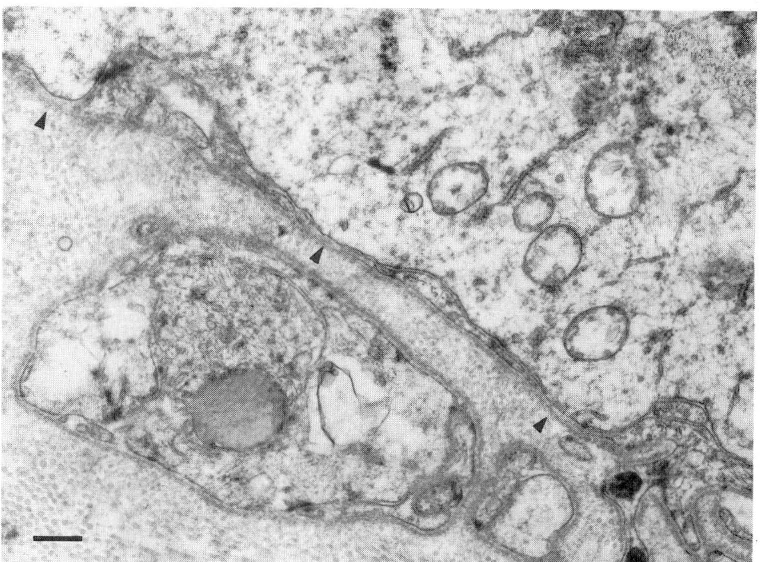

Fig. 29.11. Arrowheads indicate short deficiencies in the satellite sheath of a neuron, from the SCG of a subject with MSA. Scale bar, 0.5 μm.

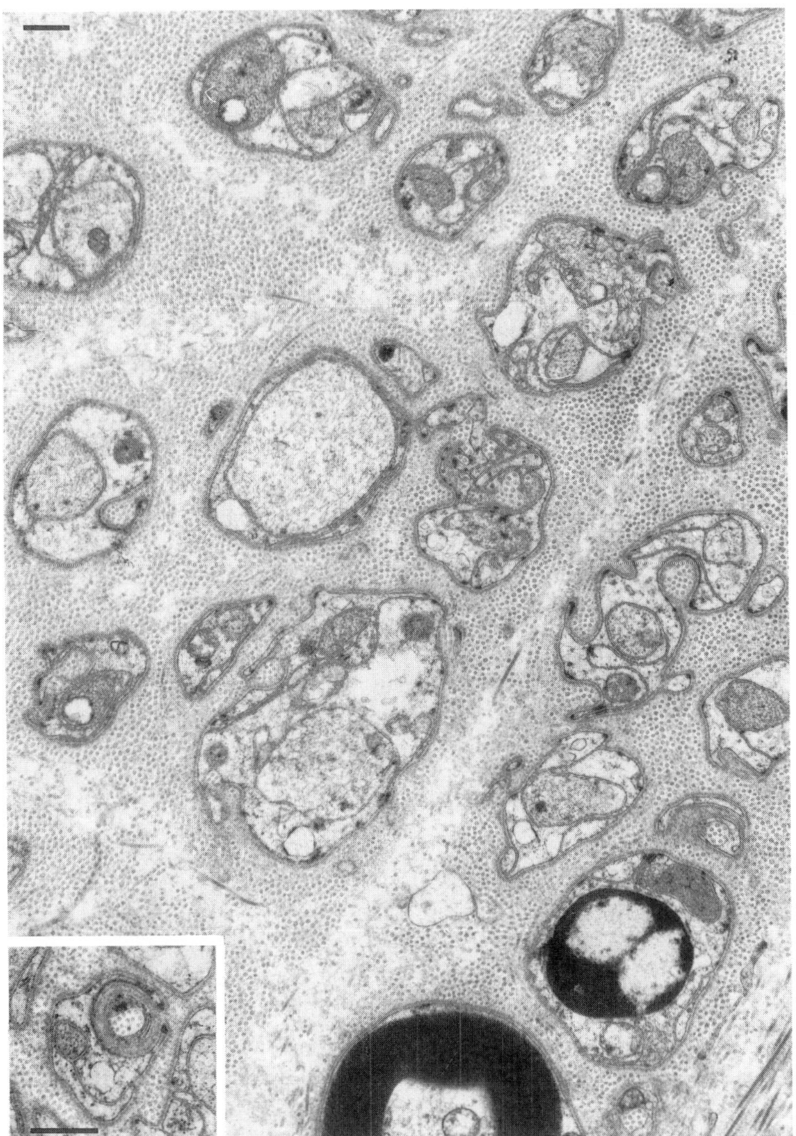

Fig. 29.12. Unmyelinated axons, and part of a myelinated axon, from the cervical sympathetic trunk of a subject with MSA, taken close to the SCG. Schwann-axon profiles are widely separated by dense endoneurial collagen. Most of the Schwann profiles contain only one or two axons, which are of 0.6 to 4 μm diameter; even large axons are unmyelinated in this field. The small numbers of axons per Schwann unit, and the occurrence of collagen-filled channels in the Schwann cells, sometimes lined by basal lamina, suggest appreciable loss of axons. Inset: Schwann unit containing one small axon and a collagen-filled channel, lined by reduplicated basal lamina. Scale bars, 1 μm.

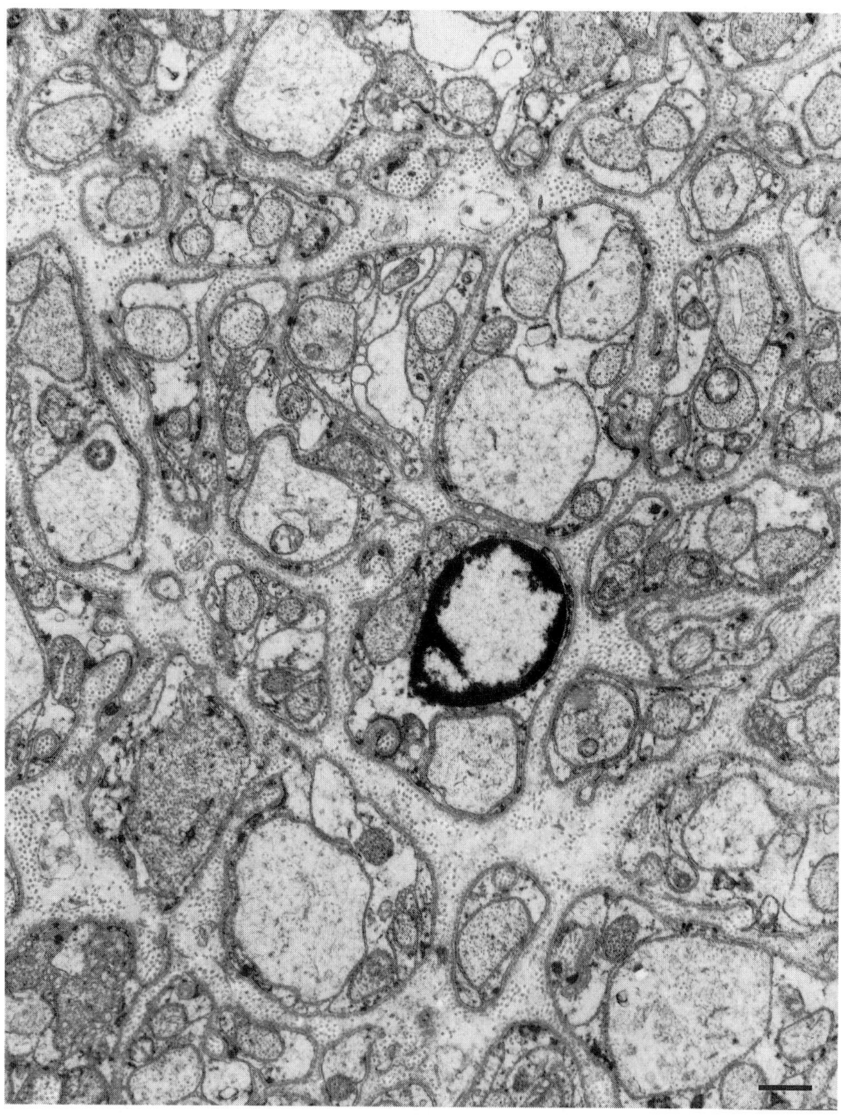

Fig. 29.13. Postganglionic axons from the internal carotid nerve of the same subject as in Fig. 29.12. Schwann-axon profiles are closely packed with little intervening collagen. The axons are unmyelinated, but are of very non-uniform size ranging in diameter from about 0.5 to over 3 μm; this might represent hypertrophy in some axons and atrophy in others. There are also some collagen-filled channels in Schwann cells, suggesting fibre loss. Scale bar, 1 μm.

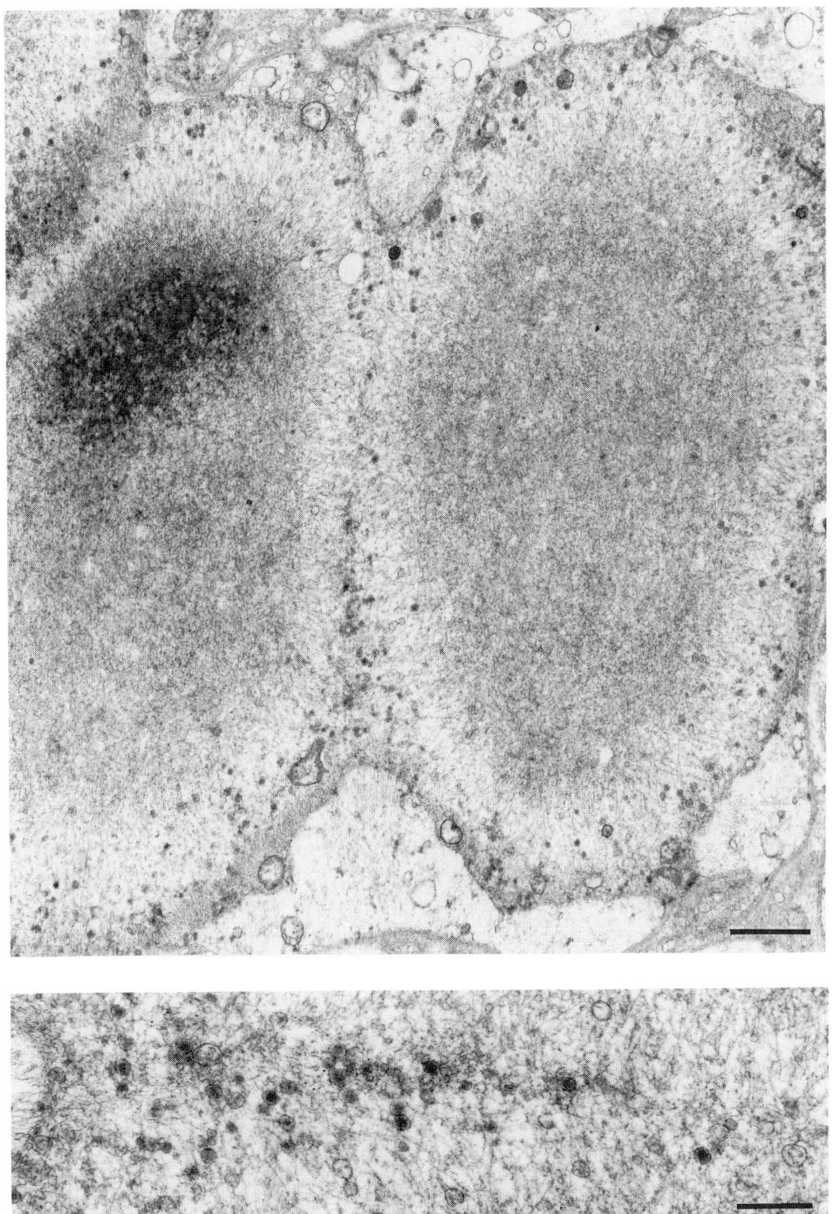

Fig. 29.14. Electron micrograph of two Lewy bodies filling adjacent neuronal profiles, possibly axons, from the SCG of a subject with pure autonomic failure. Scale bar, 2 μm. Below is shown at higher magnification part of the periphery of the Lewy bodies, where dense-cored vesicles are associated with the margins of the fibrillary mass. Scale bar, 0.5 μm.

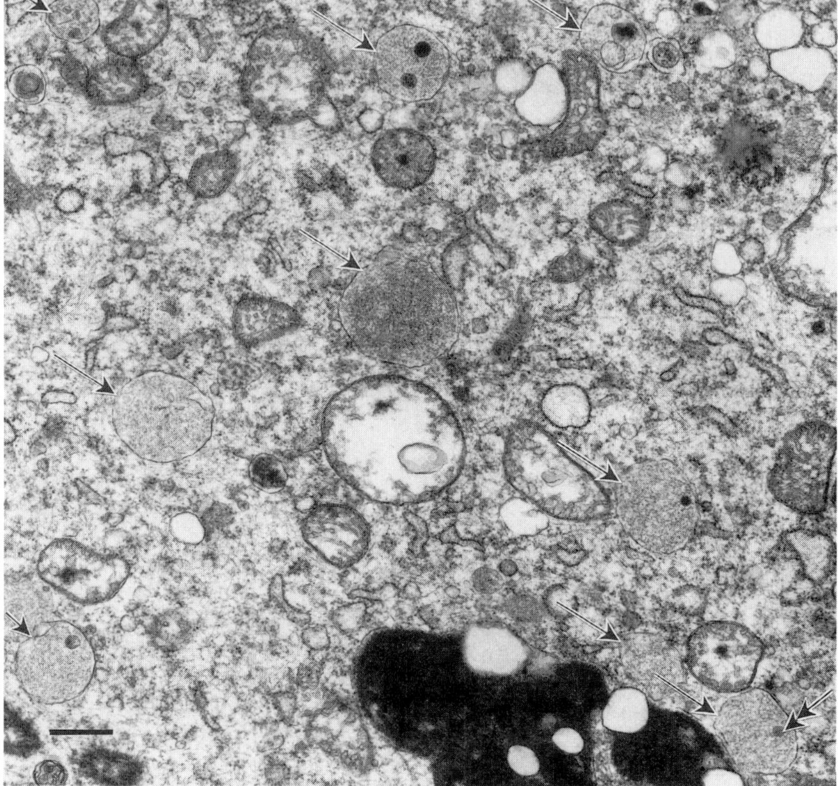

Fig. 29.15. A mass of lysosomal elements (arrows), some primary, some enclosing cytoplasmic constituents, including apparent dense-cored vesicles (double arrow), from a neuron in the same ganglion as Fig. 29.14. This suggests active resorption of vesicles. Many residual lipofuscin bodies were present in the same neuron, one of which is shown at the lower edge of the figure. Scale bar, 0.5 μm.

SUMMARY AND CONCLUSIONS

This preliminary study has indicated a clear difference in ganglionic pathology and, hence, presumably in underlying mechanisms of causation of the autonomic failure, between multiple system atrophy and pure autonomic failure. In MSA the neurons of sympathetic ganglia are not severely reduced in number and do not appear grossly abnormal, except that considerably fewer of them may show distinguishable Nissl granules than in control subjects. This relative lack of Nissl material might indicate a denervation atrophy of long standing. There is confirmatory evidence of the loss of preganglionic nerve fibres, which has already been extensively documented, and there is evidence which suggests a severe deficiency of preganglionic nerve endings in the ganglia and possible overdriving of surviving endings.

In pure autonomic failure, on the other hand, the packing density of ganglionic neurons is severely reduced; and counts in one complete superior cervical sympathetic ganglion have indicated a surviving neuron population of about 214 000, which is less than 25 per cent of the figures reported for normal ganglia and corresponds with the proportional loss of IML neurons at which autonomic failure occurs (Chapter 25A). Some of the surviving ganglionic neurons show Lewy bodies, and some show evidence of intense lysosomal activity, but almost all of the remainder show well-defined Nissl granules and do not appear grossly abnormal for the age of the subject.

It therefore seems reasonable to assume, as a working hypothesis, that these two forms of autonomic failure result, respectively, from the loss of preganglionic and of ganglionic neurons. This might in due course prove too simple a view. The initial causes of the loss of neurons are still obscure, though in the case of 'Lewy body disease' it may be surmised that it is the same metabolic dysfunction which causes the fibrillar accumulations that leads to neuronal death. It remains to be confirmed whether there is comparable loss of ganglionic neurons in the autonomic failure which may occur in Parkinson's disease (cf. Rajput and Rozdilsky 1976). The ramifications of the secondary consequences remain likewise to be unravelled. As Oppenheimer (1980) has shown, subjects with pure autonomic failure may also exhibit some loss of IML neurons, which can be quite as severe as that found in subjects with multiple system atrophy. This could be a retrograde neuronal death, consequent upon target deprivation and related to the profundity and duration of the latter. Indeed, the loss of IML neurons in multiple system atrophy might itself be due to disruption of the retrograde trophic influence exerted upon them by the ganglionic neurons, which might in its turn arise, for example, from dysfunction of the ganglionic excitatory synapse without overtly evident changes in the ganglionic neurons. Experiments are in progress to test some of these possibilities.

Acknowledgements

This work is supported by a grant from the Medical Research Council. Thanks are due to Mr P. Belk for technical assistance, Mr B. Archer, Mr T. Barclay, and Mr C. Beesley for photographic work, and Miss J. Ballinger for secretarial assistance. Generous gifts of primary antibodies from A. C. Cuello (SP, Enk, TOH) and J. M. Polak (CGRP, NPY) are gratefully acknowledged. The author thanks Drs D. R. Oppenheimer, J. R. Ponsford, M. Rossi, N. D. Francis, and F. Scaravilli for obtaining ganglia, and Professor L. W. Duchen for access to paraffin-embedded material.

REFERENCES

Allen, J. M., Gibson, S. J., Adrian, T. E., Polak, J. M., and Bloom, S. R. (1984). Neuropeptide Y in human spinal cord. *Brain Res.* **308**, 145–8.

Clark, A. W., Hurlbut, W. R., and Mauro, A. (1972). Changes in the fine structure of the neuromuscular junction of the frog caused by black widow spider venom. *J. Cell Biol.* **52**, 1–14.

Cowan, W. M. (1970). Anterograde and retrograde transneuronal degeneration in the central and peripheral nervous system. In *Contemporary research methods in neuroanatomy* (ed. W. J. H. Nauta and S. O. E. Ebbesson), pp. 217–49. Springer, Berlin.

Del Fiacco, M., Levanti, M. C., Brotzu, G., and Montisci, R. (1984). Substance P-like immunoreactivity in human sympathetic ganglia. *Brain Res.* **321**, 143–6.

Duchen, L. W., Gomez, F., and Queiroz, L. S. (1981). The neuromuscular junction of the mouse after black widow spider venom. *J. Physiol., London* **316**, 279–91.

Ebbesson, S. O. E. (1963). A quantitative study of human superior cervical sympathetic ganglia. *Anat. Rec.* **146**, 353–6.

Elliott, K. and Lawrenson, G. (Eds.) (1981). *Development of the autonomic nervous system.* Ciba Foundation Symposium, Vol. 83. Pitman Medical, London.

Forno, L. S. and Nerville, R. L. (1976). Ultrastructure of Lewy bodies in the stellate ganglion. *Acta neuropathol., Berlin* **34**, 183–97.

Gabella, G. (1976). *Structure of the autonomic nervous system.* Chapman and Hall, London.

Konigsmark, B. W. (1970). Methods for the counting of neurons. In *Contemporary research methods in neuroanatomy* (ed. W. J. H. Nauta and S. O. E. Ebbesson), pp. 315–40. Springer, Berlin.

Liestøl, K., Maehlen, J., and Njå, A. (1986). Selective synaptic connections: significance of recognition and competition in mature sympathetic ganglia. *Trends Neurosci.* **9**, 21–4.

Low, P. A., Thomas, J. E., and Dyck, P. J. (1978). The splanchnic autonomic outflow in Shy-Drager syndrome and idiopathic orthostatic hypotension. *Ann. Neurol.* **4**, 511–14.

Matthews, M. R. (1983). The ultrastructure of junctions in sympathetic ganglia of mammals. In *Autonomic ganglia* (ed. L.-G. Elfvin), pp. 27–66. John Wiley, Chichester.

Matthews, M. R. and Cuello, A. C. (1984). The origin and possible significance of substance P immunoreactive networks in the prevertebral ganglia and related structures in the guinea-pig. *Phil. Trans. R. Soc. Lond.* **B306**, 247–76.

Oppenheimer, D. R. (1980). Lateral horn cells in progressive autonomic failure. *J. neurol. Sci.* **46**, 393–404.

Petito, C. K. and Black, I. B. (1978). Ultrastructure and biochemistry of sympathetic ganglia in idiopathic orthostatic hypotension. *Ann. Neurol.* **4**, 6–17.

Pioro, E. P. J., Hughes, J. T., and Cuello, A. C. (1984). Loss of substance P and enkephalin immunoreactivity in the human substantia nigra after striato-pallidal infarction. *Brain Res.* **292**, 339–47.

Rajput, A. H. and Rozdilsky, B. (1976). Dysautonomia in Parkinsonism: a clinicopathological study. *J. Neurol. Neurosurg. Psychiat.* **39**, 1092–100.

Ramsay, D. A. and Matthews, M. R. (1985). Denervation-induced formation of adrenergic synapses in the superior cervical sympathetic ganglion of the rat and the enhancement of this effect by postganglionic axotomy. *Neuroscience* **16**, 997–1026.

Schultzberg, M., Hökfelt, T., Lundberg, J. M., Dalsgaard, C.-J., and Elfvin, L.-G. (1983). Transmitter histochemistry of autonomic ganglia. In *Autonomic ganglia* (ed. L.-G. Elfvin), pp. 205–33. John Wiley, Chichester.

30. Structure and function of pre- and postganglionic neurons in pure autonomic failure and multisystem atrophy with autonomic failure

Phillip A. Low and Robert D. Fealey

IMPORTANCE OF SPLANCHNIC SYMPATHETIC OUTFLOW IN THE MAINTENANCE OF POSTURAL NORMOTENSION

The splanchnic mesenteric capacitance bed is a large-volume, low-resistance system of great importance in the maintenance of postural normotension (Rowell *et al.* 1972) comprising approximately 25–30 per cent of total blood volume. The splanchnic veins are densely innervated and are markedly baroreflex-responsive, responding to a reduction in pulse pressure by α-mediated venoconstriction (Thirlwell and Zsoter 1972).

The sympathetic nerve supply to the mesenteric bed is mainly by the greater splanchnic nerve. This is a predominantly cholinergic preganglionic nerve with its cell body in the intermediolateral column (mainly T4 to T9) and synapses at the coeliac ganglion from whence postganglionic fibres go on to supply effector cells. There is much research and clinical evidence to support the importance of the sympathetic outflow in the maintenance of postural normotension (Low *et al.* 1975; Low 1984). Bilateral splanchnicectomy regularly results in orthostatic hypotension while neither bilateral lumbar sympathectomy (denervating the legs) nor cardiac denervation cause orthostatic hypotension (White and Smithwick 1944; Wilkins *et al.* 1951). Orthostatic hypotension regularly occurs in spinal-cord lesions above T4 (decentralizing the splanchnic outflow) but is absent in lesions below T9 (Guttmann and Whitteridge 1947; Pollock *et al.* 1951; Fealey *et al.* 1984).

MORPHOMETRY OF THE NORMAL SPLANCHNIC SYMPATHETIC OUTFLOW

Because of the above considerations we studied the splanchnic outflow in fresh autopsy material of 12 persons aged 4.5 to 79 years who had died of disorders not affecting the splanchnic outflow (cardiac arrest, automobile accident, suicide, pulmonary embolus). Tissue was harvested within 4–6 hours of death. The spinal cord was celloidin-embedded to avoid cellular shrinkage (as in paraffin-embedded tissues). The predominant cell type within the intermediolateral column had the staining characteristics of motor neurons with coarse and irregular Nissl substance. The nucleus was large and often eccentric and neurons were oval, polygonal, spindle, or club-shaped (Fig. 30.1). The mean preganglionic cell counts in the intermediolateral column at the T6, T7, and T8 spinal-cord segments were 5002, 5004, and 4654, respectively (Low *et al.* 1977). There was no significant sex difference. Most cells ranged in diameter from 6 to 23 μm (Fig. 30.2) with the major peak at 12–13 μm. There was a progressive reduction of preganglionic neuron numbers with age. In adults 370 preganglionic neurons (8 per cent) were lost per

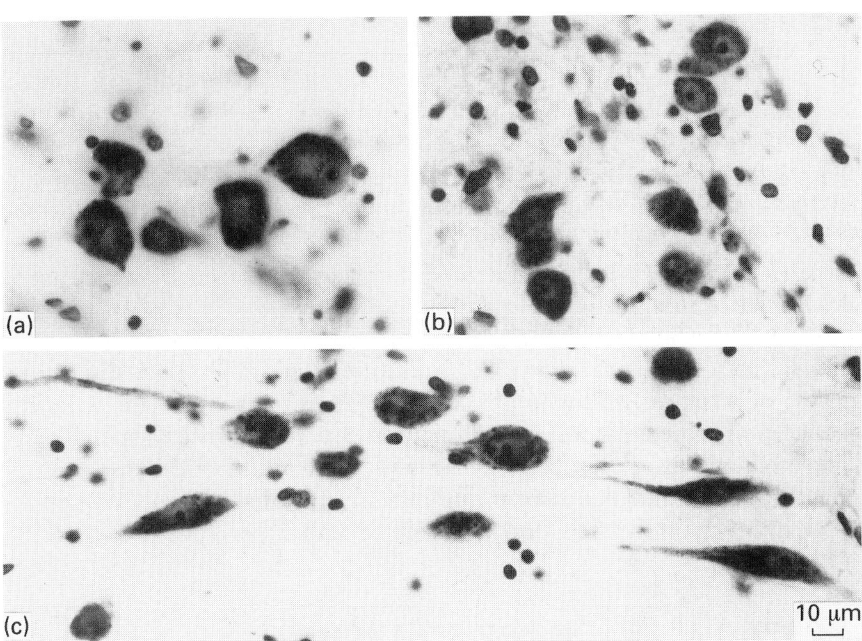

Fig. 30.1. Representative preganglionic sympathetic neurons in the intermediolateral column of normal man. (a) Nuclei are eccentrically placed; (b) neurons are mainly small and polygonal; (c) neurons are more spindle-shaped. Celloidin-embedded, cresyl violet stained, 20-μm sections. (Taken with permission from Low *et al.* (1977).)

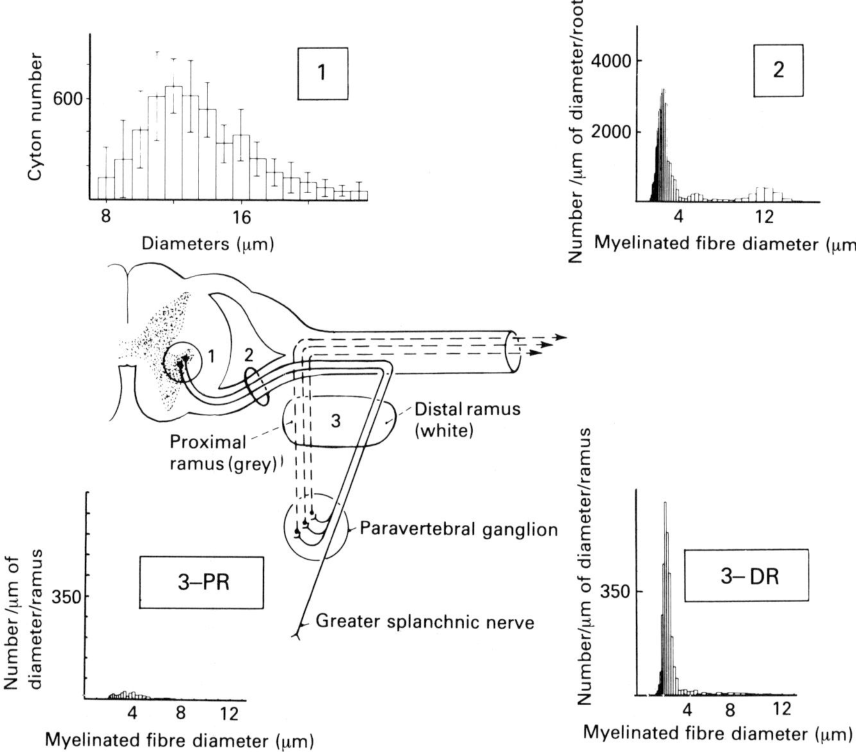

Fig. 30.2. Diameter histograms for T7 intermediolateral column neurons (1), ventral spinal root (2), grey ramus (3-PR), and white ramus (3-DR) of normal man. (Taken with permission from Low (1984).)

decade (Fig. 30.3). No significant differences in neuron numbers were found between segments.

Morphometric studies were also done on the corresponding ventral spinal root (Low and Dyck 1977) and autonomic rami (Low and Dyck 1978) of a representative segment (T7). There was good concordance between intermediolateral-column neuron counts and ventral spinal-root preganglionic-axon numbers (0.81) and with autonomic rami counts (0.95). The preganglionic axon numbers in ventral spinal root and rami underwent a similar attrition with age (8 and 5 per cent, per decade, respectively).

MORPHOMETRY OF THE SPLANCHNIC SYMPATHETIC OUTFLOW IN MULTIPLE SYSTEM ATROPHY (MSA) AND PURE AUTONOMIC FAILURE (PAF)

All published reports on MSA with a single exception agree that there is a marked reduction in preganglionic sympathetic neurons qualitatively

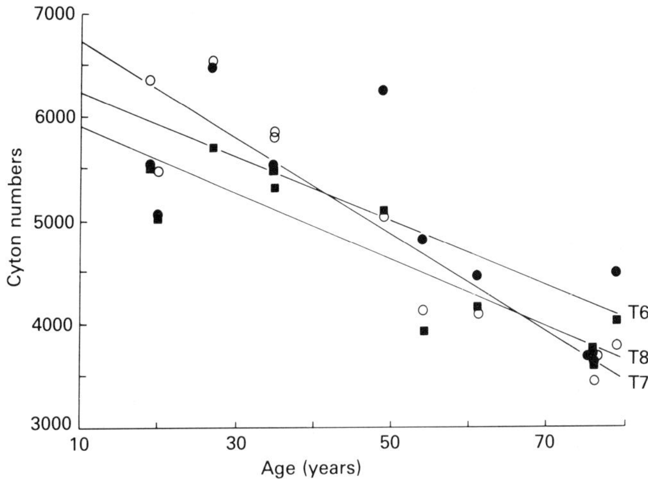

Fig. 30.3. Alteration in numbers of neurons with age for T6 (open circles), T7 (closed circles), and T8 (closed squares). (Taken with permission from Low *et al.* (1977).)

and quantitatively; this subject is reviewed in Chapter 25A. In our study on two patients with MSA and one with PAF (Low *et al.* 1978), we measured preganglionic neuron sizes as well and related our neuron counts to axonal counts (Fig. 30.4). In the patients with MSA the T7 preganglionic neuron numbers were 10 and 24 per cent of age-matched controls. Their corresponding preganglionic axon numbers were 10 and 33 per cent of controls. Abnormalities in the preganglionic axons were milder in the patient with PAF. The preganglionic neurons and axons were 52 and 41 per cent of normal, respectively. The diameter distribution of neurons and axons were not different to controls.

Of interest was an associated reduction in larger myelinated axons (alpha and gamma motoneuron axons) in patients with MSA. Reductions of alpha motoneurons have been reported (Thapedi *et al.* 1971; Sung *et al.* 1979) and sacral motoneurons are particularly severely affected (Sung *et al.* 1979; Konno *et al.* 1986), findings that are particularly relevant to the clinical findings of weak external anal sphincters in patients with MSA (Sakuta *et al.* 1978).

Pathological changes in the postganglionic neuron in autonomic ganglia have been described in MSA (Thapedi *et al.* 1971) but are usually absent (Johnson *et al.* 1966; Schwartz 1967). We have reported morphometric studies on the splanchnic sympathetic outflow in MSA, PAF (Low *et al.* 1978), in amyloid neuropathy and Tangier disease (Low *et al.* 1978), in familial dysautonomia (Dyck *et al.* 1978), and in diabetic autonomic neuropathy (Low *et al.* 1975; Low 1984). Based on the correlation between orthostatic hypotension and preganglionic neuron numbers with age and in disorders where the brunt of the pathology

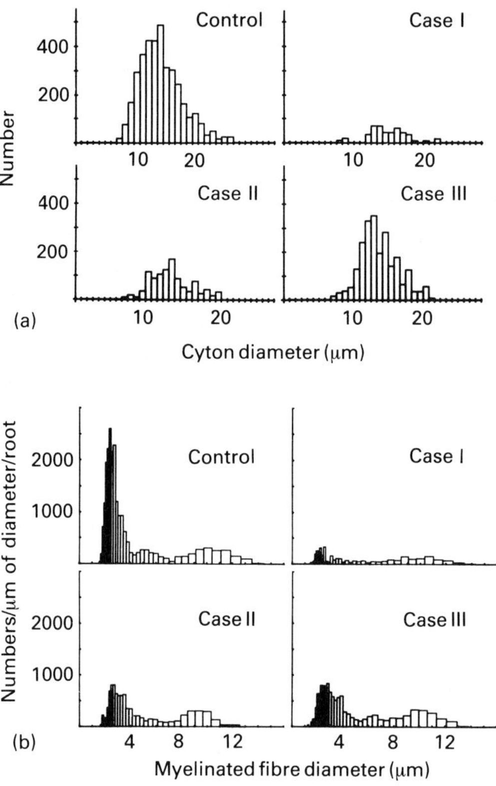

Fig. 30.4. Diameter histograms of (a) intermediolateral column neurons and (b) ventral spinal root myelinated fibres in a control, two patients with MSA (Cases I and II), and a patient with PAF (case III). (Modified with permission from Low *et al.* (1978).)

falls on the preganglionic system we suggested that orthostatic hypotension does not occur until an attrition of at least 50 per cent of preganglionic neurons have occurred. This observation does not apply to disorders such as PAF and the peripheral autonomic neuropathies where there is an additional postganglionic lesion.

IS PAF A POSTGANGLIONIC DISORDER?

There is recent pharmacological evidence of postganglionic adrenergic failure in PAF leading to the suggestion that PAF is a postganglionic disorder and MSA a preganglionic disorder (Ziegler *et al.* 1977; Polinsky *et al.* 1981). Our morphometric study also suggested that the preganglionic neuron was more severely affected in MSA. To pursue this question we studied 97 consecutive patients with PAF or MSA (38 PAF; 59 MSA) seen at the Mayo Autonomic Reflex and Thermoregulatory

Sweat Laboratories over a 3.5-year period. These patients had severe generalized autonomic failure as indicated by the finding of orthostatic hypotension, widespread anhidrosis on the thermoregulatory sweat test (TST; Fig. 30.5) (Fealey *et al.* 1985), and impairment of heart period responses to deep breathing and the Valsalva manoeuvre. Postganglionic sudomotor and vasomotor functions were studied using the Quantitative Sudomotor Axon Reflex Test (Q-SART) and supine plasma noradrenalin, respectively. The methodology for Q-SART has been previously described (Low *et al.* 1983, 1986). One population of eccrine sweat glands are stimulated by the iontophoresis of 10 per cent acetylcholine and the evoked sweat response dynamically recorded from a second population of sweat glands (Fig. 30.6) by a sudorometer. In early experiments intradermal acetylcholine was also injected to check if the reduced response was due to reduced access to sweat glands in chronically anhidrotic patients. We found excellent concordance between intradermal and iontophoresed responses so that later experiments were done with iontophoresis alone. Since axon reflex sudomotor function varies

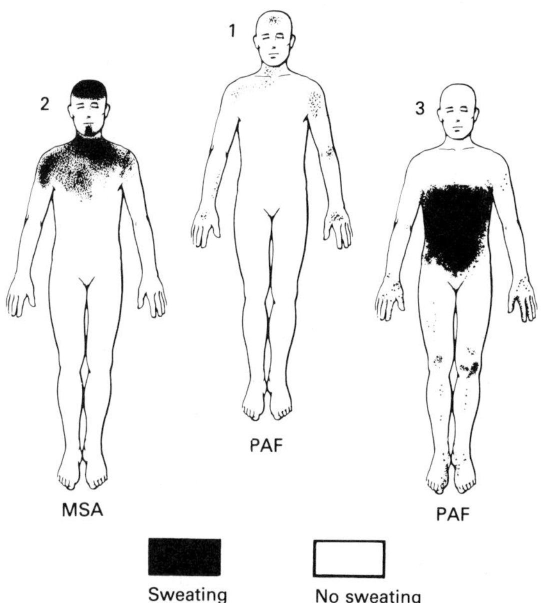

Fig. 30.5. Thermoregulatory sweat test results showing characteristic anhidrosis in MSA and PAF. Exemplified is the widespread anhidrosis seen in most patients with PAF (case 1) and MSA (case 2) as well as the occasional case of PAF with strikingly preserved segments of sweating (case 3).

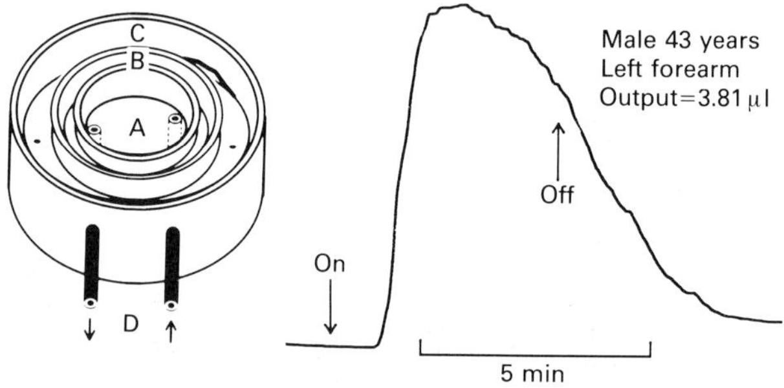

Fig. 30.6. Multicompartmental sweat cell (left) and evoked sweat response (right). The capsule is strapped on to skin and acetylcholine (compartment C), is iontophoresed using a constant current generator with the anode connected to compartment C. Axon reflex evoked sweat response in compartment A is evaporated off by a stream of nitrogen at a controlled flow rate and quantitated dynamically by a sudorometer. Compartment B and associated ridges prevent diffusion and leakage of acetylcholine.

with sex (Low *et al.* 1983; Ahmed and Le Quesne 1986), the results were expressed as a sex-matched percentile of control values ($n=100$). Postganglionic failure occurred at the forearm in 45 per cent (Fig. 30.7) and at the foot in 61 per cent of PAF patients (Fig. 30.8) providing clear evidence that sympathetic sudomotor fibres are also involved.

However, abnormalities were not confined to the postganglionic axon. The TST and Q-SART have similar sensitivity so that it is possible to define the site of the sudomotor lesion (pre- or postganglionic) from the combined use of the two tests on the same patient. Postganglionic function was completely normal in some patients with anhidrosis on TST indicating a preganglionic lesion in these patients. More commonly, there was combined pre- and postganglionic involvement in PAF (Cohen *et al.* 1987).

Plasma noradrenalin (NA) results from a spillover of noradrenalin from sympathetic postganglionic nerve terminals and the supine value is an index of net sympathetic activity (Ziegler *et al.* 1977; Polinsky *et al.* 1981), being affected by the rate of noradrenalin secretion and clearance (Esler *et al.* 1980). Supine plasma free noradrenalin values were significantly reduced in PAF ($p<0.001$) but not in MSA (Fig. 30.9). Plasma noradrenalin increment on standing were reduced in both PAF and MSA (Fig. 30.10) ($p<0.001$) and the difference was not significant.

Although there is clear evidence for postganglionic sympathetic failure in PAF, we think the disorder should be considered a combined pre- and postganglionic autonomic failure rather than a pure postganglionic disorder for the following reasons:

1. There is preganglionic failure morphologically (Johnson *et al.* 1966; Low *et al.* 1978).

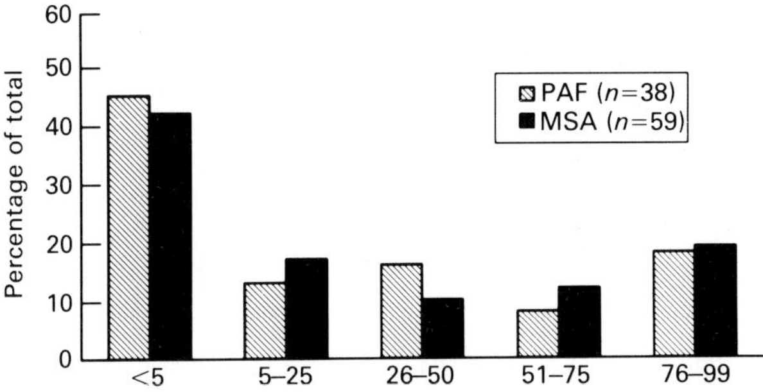

Fig. 30.7. Quantitative sudomotor axon reflex sweat test (Q-SART) results expressed as a percentile of control data for the forearm in patients with pure autonomic failure (PAF) and multiple system atrophy (MSA).

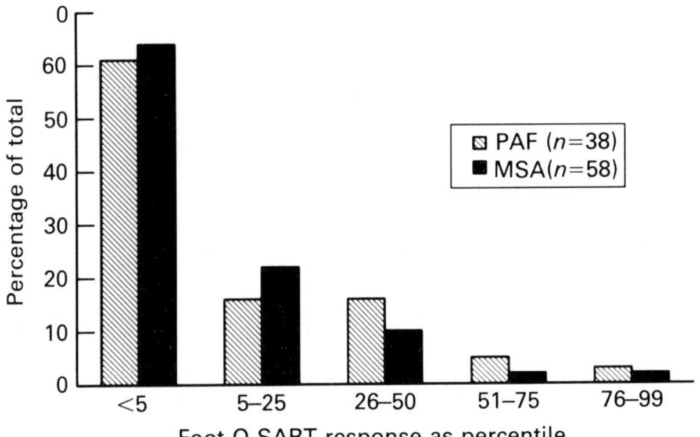

Fig. 30.8. Quantitative sudomotor axon reflex sweat test (Q-SART) results expressed as a percentile of control data for the foot in patients with pure autonomic failure (PAF) and multiple system atrophy (MSA).

2. There is evidence of preganglionic sudomotor failure using the criterion of a normal Q-SART responses over anhidrotic skin on TST.
3. There is a significant subset of PAF patients with normal supine noradrenalin which fails to rise on standing, a pattern suggestive of failure of preganglionic sympathetic activation (Ziegler *et al.* 1977).
4. Considering the degree of orthostatism and anhidrosis, these patients have less postganglionic sympathetic failure than the postganglionic autonomic neuropathies, e.g. acute panautonomic neuropathy where the Q-SART and supine noradrenalin values are uniformly reduced (Low *et al.* 1983).
5. Some cases of PAF have generalized anhidrosis and entirely normal postganglionic sympathetic function.

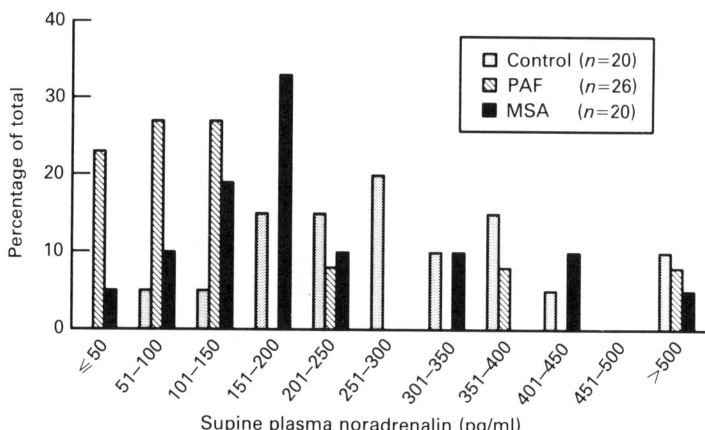

Fig. 30.9. Supine plasma noradrenalin in control subjects and patients with pure autonomic failure (PAF) and multiple system atrophy (MSA).

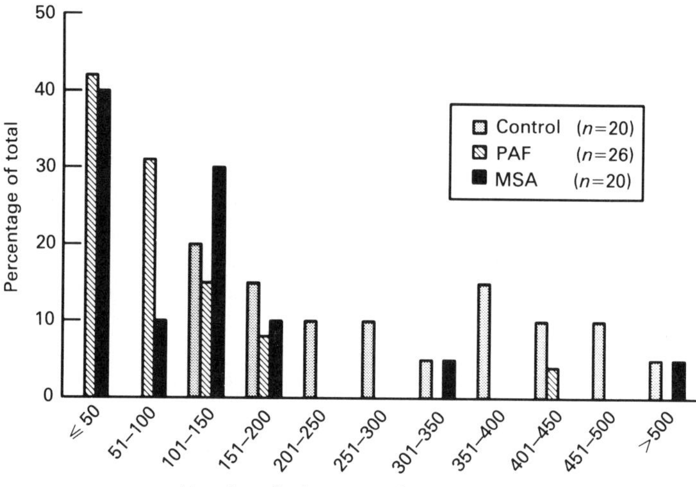

Fig. 30.10. Plasma noradrenalin increment in control subjects and patients with pure autonomic failure (PAF) and multiple system atrophy (MSA).

IS MSA A PREGANGLIONIC DISORDER?

Apart from its association with involvement of other central nervous structures, especially striatonigral and olivopontocerebellar, MSA is usually but not invariably associated with a normal resting supine noradrenalin. Compared to disorders with a similar degree of autonomic failure such as acute panautonomic neuropathy (Low *et al.* 1984) or diabetic autonomic neuropathy (Christensen 1972), the reduction in supine noradrenalin is much less, suggesting a preganglionic site. The significantly reduced noradrenalin response to standing in MSA is thought to indicate a failure to activate central sympathetic pathways (Ziegler *et al.* 1977). These findings are consonant with published reports of a marked reduction in preganglionic sympathetic neurons (Low *et al.* 1978; Oppenheimer, see Chapter 25A), including morphometric studies (Low *et al.* 1978; Oppenheimer, see Chapter 25A).

Although MSA patients appear to be a relatively homogeneous group with only a minor subset with postganglionic adrenergic failure, the latter has been well demonstrated pharmacologically (Steiner *et al.* 1974) and by using catecholamine fluorescence and electron microscopy of muscle blood vessels (Bannister *et al.* 1981).

In contrast to adrenergic failure, where there is separation between PAF and MSA, postganglionic sudomotor failure occurred as frequently in MSA as it did in PAF occurring at the forearm in 42 per cent (Fig. 30.7) and at the foot in 64 per cent of MSA patients (Fig. 30.8). Our data lends some support to the hypothesis that the postganglionic sympathetic sudomotor failure in MSA is due to a transsynaptic effect. If the mechanism is transsynaptic, the degree of postganglionic sudomotor failure should vary with the severity of autonomic failure. (Grading of autonomic failure followed the following critieria: (1) mild—orthostatic symptoms and blood-pressure drop but patient is able to maintain activities of daily living without medication or a body support stocking; (2) moderate—the patient requires medications and/or body support stocking but is able to maintain activities of daily living; (3) severe—severely limited in spite of medications; cannot remain on his/her feet for 1 hour at a time.) In fact, there was a significant regression with severity, percentage of anterior body surface anhidrosis on TST, and with supine plasma noradrenalin in MSA supporting the hypothesis. The greater percentage of postganglionic failure in the foot than in the forearm suggests a length-dependent transsynaptic mechanism. The insignificant regression with duration of disease is not surprising since all cases were chronic.

Although there is good statistical separation between groups of patients with PAF and MSA using supine plasma noradrenalin, there is also considerable overlap, so that supine plasma noradrenalin cannot be relied on to always separate the individual patient with PAF from MSA (Fealey *et al.* 1985). Patients with PAF often have normal supine plasma noradrenalin (Fig. 30.9). Moreover, some patients with MSA have reduced noradrenalin (Fig. 30.9; Bannister *et al.* 1977). The most reliable way to diagnose MSA is still the demonstration of central nervous system involvement on examination (Thomas and Schirger 1970). Finally, the occasional patient will progress from apparent PAF to MSA.

PERIPHERAL NEUROPATHY IN MSA AND PAF

Somatic peripheral-nerve involvement in MSA has also been reported (Low *et al.* 1978; Galassi *et al.* 1982; Toghi *et al.* 1982). We analysed the clinical neuropathic profile in the first 62 patients in our series (Table 30.1). Clinical neuropathy occurred in two of 26 patients with PAF and seven of 36 patients with MSA. In addition to the neuropathy, patient 1 had bilateral Adie's pupils. The neuropathy was a mild or asymptomatic distal sensorimotor polyneuropathy. Sensory symptoms were absent except in a single patient who complained of distal numbness and tingling. Electrophysiologic studies were undertaken when distal weakness, hypo- or areflexia, or hypaesthesiae were present, and the abnormalities were uniformly relatively mild consisting of distal motor-unit changes of chronic partial denervation, reduction of motor and sensory action potentials with relatively preserved conduction velocities without excessive dispersion. A sural-nerve biopsy was done in one patient and showed a mild reduction in myelinated-fibre density. Nine per cent of teased single-nerve fibres showed segmental remyelination and 2 per cent showed axonal degeneration.

Table 30.1. Peripheral neuropathy in pure autonomic failure and multiple system atrophy with autonomic failure

Patient	*Diagnosis*	*Symptoms*	*Signs*	*EMG*
1	MSA	−	+	+
2	MSA	−	+	+
3	MSA	−	+	+
4	MSA	+	−	+
5	MSA	−	−	+
6	MSA	+	+	+
7	MSA	−	+	nd
8	PAF	−	+	nd
9	PAF	−	+	+

+, Present; −, absent; nd, not done.

CONCLUSION

Generalized autonomic failure occurs in both MSA and PAF. However, while PAF is characterized by combined postganglionic sudomotor and adrenergic failure, postganglionic adrenergic denervation is less common in MSA while the preganglionic neuron is more severely affected. We speculate that the postganglionic sympathetic sudomotor failure in MSA may be due to a transsynaptic effect since the degree of postganglionic sudomotor failure increases with the severity of autonomic failure, the percentage of anhidrosis of anterior body surface on TST, and the degree of reduction in supine plasma noradrenalin.

Somatic neuropathy is more common in MSA and is usually mild or asymptomatic. The more frequent occurrence of somatic neuropathy seems to be in keeping with the more widespread involvement of neurologic and autonomic systems in MSA than in PAF clinically and neuropathologically (Oppenheimer, see Chapter 25A). These studies suggest that multiple system atrophy extends to involve the peripheral nervous system as well. Indeed, the number of systems involved in MSA continues to grow as investigators evaluate more systems. From the clinical standpoint, the neurologic examination seeking multisystem involvement continues to be a more reliable discriminator of MSA from PAF than nuances of the degree or site of autonomic failure.

Acknowledgements

This work was supported in part by grants from NINCDS (NS14304, R01 NS22302), MDA, Mayo, and Mogg funds.

REFERENCES

Ahmed, M. E. and Le Quesne, P. M. (1986). Quantitative sweat test in diabetics with neuropathic foot lesions. *J. Neurol. Neurosurg. Psychiat.* **49**, 1059–62.

Bannister, R., Crowe, R., Eames, R., and Burnstock, G. (1981). Adrenergic innervation in autonomic failure. *Neurology* **31**, 150–6.

Bannister, R., Sever, P. S., and Gross, M. (1977). Cardiovascular reflexes and biochemical responses in progressive autonomic failure. *Brain* **100**, 327–44.

Christensen, N. J. (1972). Plasma catecholamines in long-term diabetics with and without neuropathy and in hypothysectomized subjects. *J. clin. Invest.* **51**, 779–87.

Cohen, J., Low, P. A., Fealey, R. D., Sheps, S., and Jiang, N-S. (1987). Peripheral somatic, adrenergic and sudomotor function in idiopathic orthostatic hypotension and multiple system atrophy with autonomic failure. *Ann. Neurol.* (In press.)

Dyck, P. J., Kawamura, Y., Low, P. A., Shimono, M., and Solovy, J. S. (1978). The number and sizes of reconstructed peripheral autonomic sensory and motor neurones in a case of dysautonomia. *J. Neuropathol. exp. Neurol.* **37**, 741–55.

Esler, M., Jackman, G., Kelleher, D., Skews, H., Jennings, G., Bobik, A., and Korner, P. (1980). Norepinephrine kinetics in patients with idiopathic autonomic insufficiency. *Circulation Res.* **46** (Suppl. 1), 147–8.

Fealey, R. D., Schirger, A., and Thomas, J. E. (1985). Orthostatic hypotension. In *Clinical medicine* (ed. J. A. Spittell, Jr), Vol. 7, pp. 1–12. Harper and Row, Philadelphia.

Fealey, R. D., Szurszewski, J. H., Merritt, J. L., and DiMagno, E. P. (1984). Effect of traumatic spinal cord transection on human upper gastrointestinal motility and gastric emptying. *Gastroenterology* **87**, 69–75.

Galassi, G., Nemni, R., Baraldi, A., Gibertoni, M., and Colombo, A. (1982). Peripheral neuropathy in multiple system atrophy with autonomic failure.

Neurology **32**, 1116–21.

Guttman, L. and Whitteridge, D. (1947). Effects of bladder distension on autonomic mechanisms after spinal cord injuries. *Brain* **70**, 361–404.

Johnson, R. H., Lee, G. de J., Oppenheimer, D. R., and Spalding, J. M. K. (1966). Autonomic failure with orthostatic hypotension due to intermediolateral column degeneration. A report of two cases with autopsies. *Quart. J. Med.* **35**, 276–92.

Konno, H., Yamamoto, T., Iwasaki, Y., and Iizuka, H. (1986). Shy–Drager syndrome and amyolateral sclerosis. *J. neurol. Sci.* **73**, 193–204.

Low, P. A. (1984). Quantitation of autonomic function. In *Peripheral neuropathy*, 2nd edn. (ed. P. J. Dyck, P. K. Thomas, E. H. Lambert, and R. Bunge), pp. 1139–66. Saunders, Philadelphia.

Low, P. A., Caskey, P. E., Tuck, R. R., Fealey, R. D., and Dyck, P. J. (1983). Quantitative sudomotor axon reflex in normal and neuropathic subjects. *Ann. Neurol.* **14**, 573–80.

Low, P. A. and Dyck, P. J. (1977). Splanchnic preganglionic neurons in man: II. Preganglionic ventral root fibers. *Acta neuropathol.* **40**, 219–26.

Low, P. A. and Dyck, P. J. (1978). Splanchnic preganglionic neurons in man: III. Morphometry of myelinated fibers of rami communicantes. *J. Neurolpathol. exp. Neurol.* **37**, 734–40.

Low, P. A., Okazaki, H., and Dyck, P. J. (1977). Splanchnic preganglionic neurons in man: I. Morphometry of preganglionic cytons. *Acta neuropathol.* **40**, 55–61.

Low, P. A., Thomas, J. E., and Dyck, P. J. (1978). The splanchnic autonomic outflow in Shy–Drager syndrome and idiopathic orthostatic hypotension. *Ann. Neurol.* **4**, 511–14.

Low, P. A., Walsh, J. C., Huang, C. Y., and McLeod, J. G. (1975). The sympathetic nervous system in diabetic neuropathy. A clinical and pathological study. *Brain* **98**, 341–56.

Low, P. A., Zimmerman, B. R., and Dyck, P. J. (1986). Comparison of distal sympathetic with vagal function in diabetic neuropathy. *Muscle Nerve* **9**, 592–6.

Polinsky, R. J., Kopin, I. J., Ebert, M. H., and Weise, V. (1981). Pharmacologic distinction of different orthostatic hypotension syndromes. *Neurology* **31**, 1–7.

Pollock, L., Boshes, B., Chor, H., Finkelman, I., Arieff, A., and Brown, M. (1951). Defects in regulatory mechanisms of autonomic function in injuries to the spinal cord. *J. Neurophysiol.* **14**, 85–93.

Rowell, L. B., Detry, J. M., Blackman, J. R., and Wyass, C. (1972). Importance of the splanchnic bed in human blood pressure regulation. *J. appl. Physiol.* **32**, 213.

Sakuta, M. T., Nakanishi, T., and Toyokura, Y. (1978). Anal muscle electromyograms differ in amyotrophic lateral sclerosis and Shy–Drager syndrome. *Neurology* **28**, 1289–93.

Schwartz, G. A. (1967). The orthostatic hypotension syndrome of Shy–Drager. A clinicopathologic report. *Arch. Neurol.* **16**, 123.

Steiner, J. A., Low, P. A., Huang, C. Y., West, M., Uther, J. B., Allsop, J. L., and Chalmers, J. P. (1974). L-dopa and the Shy–Drager syndrome. *Med. J. Aust.* **2**, 133–6.

Sung, J. H., Mastri, A. R., and Segal, E. (1979). Pathology of Shy–Drager syndrome. *J. Neuropathol. exp. Neurol.* **38**, 353–68.

Thapedi, I. M., Ashenhurst, E. M., and Rozdilsky, B. (1971). Shy–Drager syndrome. *Neurology* **21**, 26–32.

Thirlwell, M. P. and Zsoter, T. T. (1972). The effect of propranolol and atropine on venomotor reflexes in man. *J. Med.* **3**, 65.

Thomas, J. E. and Schirger, A. (1970). Idiopathic orthostatic hypotension. A study of its natural history in 57 neurologically affected persons. *Arch. Neurol.* **22**, 289–93.

Toghi, H., Tabuchi, M., Tomonaga, M., and Izumiyama, N. (1982). Selective loss of small myelinated and unmyelinated fibers in Shy–Drager syndrome. *Acta neuropathol.* **57**, 282–6.

White, J. C. and Smithwick, R. H. (1944). *The autonomic nervous system, anatomy, physiology and surgical application*, 2nd ed. Macmillan, London.

Wilkins, R. W., Culbertson, J. W., and Inglefinger, F. J. (1951). The effect of splanchnic sympathectomy in hypertensive patients upon estimated hepatic blood flow in the upright as contrasted with the horizontal position. *J. clin. Invest.* **30**, 312.

Ziegler, M., Lake, C., and Kopin, I. (1977). The sympathetic nervous system defect in primary orthostatic hypotension. *New Engl. J. Med.* **296**, 293–7.

31. Histochemical studies in autonomic failure

A. Sympathetic terminals in autonomic failure

Roger Bannister

Defective sympathetic reflexes underly the postural hypotension of autonomic failure (AF) but there remains uncertainty about the precise site of the lesion in the sympathetic pathways. The problem of the site of the lesion is also of clinical importance because the extent of peripheral denervation determines the supersensitivity to pressor drugs which are often used in treatment (Davies *et al.* 1978). The plasma noradrenalin is low in many cases of autonomic failure and fails to rise on tilting, suggesting a defect of release of noradrenalin from sympathetic vascular endings (Ziegler *et al.* 1977; Bannister *et al.* 1977).

In deltoid muscle from five patients with pure autonomic failure (PAF), Kontos *et al.* (1975) found no catecholamine fluorescence in perivascular nerves. These patients also failed to show any constrictor response to forearm arterioles to intra-arterial infusion of tyramine, but were supersensitive to noradrenalin. Rubenstein *et al.* (1978) reported preliminary findings of a similar lack of fluorescence in one case of PAF but found fluorescence in two cases of AF with multiple system atrophy (MSA). Nanda *et al.* (1976) found that in three cases of AF with MSA, perivascular catecholamine fluorescence was absent from the palmaris longus and quadriceps biopsies. However, it was present in three other patients, one with AF and MSA and two with apparent PAF. One of the patients with PAF appeared to have a unique defect of noradrenalin release, identified by the lack of response to tyramine but normal catecholamine staining (Nanda *et al.* 1977). The findings suggested failure of noradrenalin release, though noradrenalin synthesis and storage were normal.

We analysed the results of muscle biopsies studied by catecholamine fluorescence and electron microscopy in 10 patients with autonomic failure, in whom the defects of cardiovascular reflexes were known (Bannister *et al.* 1981). Six had AF with MSA and four had PAF. The specimens were studied by electron microscopy by Dr R. Eames and special histochemical techniques by Dr R. Crowe (Falk *et al.* 1962; Axelsson *et al.* 1973).

In the control human biopsies and in animal tissues, green varicose fluorescent adrenergic nerve fibres were observed on the adventitial side of the media of arteries (Fig. 31.1(a), (b)) and veins (diam. 20–200 μm). The larger vessels in the human tissues (diam. 250–300 μm) appeared to be either sparsely innervated or not innervated at all. In most of the arteries autofluorescence was observed in the intima, elastic and collagen fibres. In sections of control tissue examined, more than 85 per cent of the vessels showed some positive fluorescence for catecholamine-containing nerves whereas in the cases of AF only 2–7 per cent of the arteries and veins (Diam. 40–150 μm) were innervated by adrenergic nerves (Fig. 31.1(c), (f)). In these vessels, the number of fluorescent nerve bundles observed was approximately 35 per cent of those observed in vessels in the control biopsies. There was no obvious difference in the intensity of fluorescence in the nerves that were observed.

The electron microscopic studies were technically more difficult and insufficient numbers of nerve profiles were available for quantitative analysis. Prolonged searching was necessary to find vessels of a size (100 μm) in which catecholamine fluorescence is normally present and a region where a varicosity was seen in cross-section. In two control biopsies, large granular, small clear, and small granular (adrenergic) vesicles were seen in proportions comparable to those described in other sympathetic nerves (Furness 1973; Burnstock 1975*a,b*) and no preparations showed a scanty population of vesicles such as occurred in the cases of autonomic failure. In one patient with PAF, the sympathetic nerve terminals showed normal general morphology but contained only scanty vesicles, both of the small dense and small clear types (Fig. 31.2). This was the most severe abnormality found. In the cases of AF with MSA there were less severe changes although the small dense vesicles were also much reduced in number (Fig. 31.3). In different patients the changes ranged between severe (Fig. 31.2) and moderate (Fig. 31.3). The specimens in the two cases of PAF in which satisfactory electron microscopic material was available were pre-treated with 5-hydroxydopamine but the controls and the three cases of AF with MSA were not so treated. The low number of small dense vesicles in PAF is therefore likely to be significant but the problem of sampling errors makes the study of more patients necessary. Lack of fluorescence cannot of course be taken to indicate absence of adrenergic nerves; it may simply mean that noradrenalin levels in intact nerves are below the levels detectable with the formaldehyde method. Despite these problems, our results suggest that marked reduction of catecholamine fluorescence is a feature of all moderate or severe cases of AF irrespective of the coexistence of

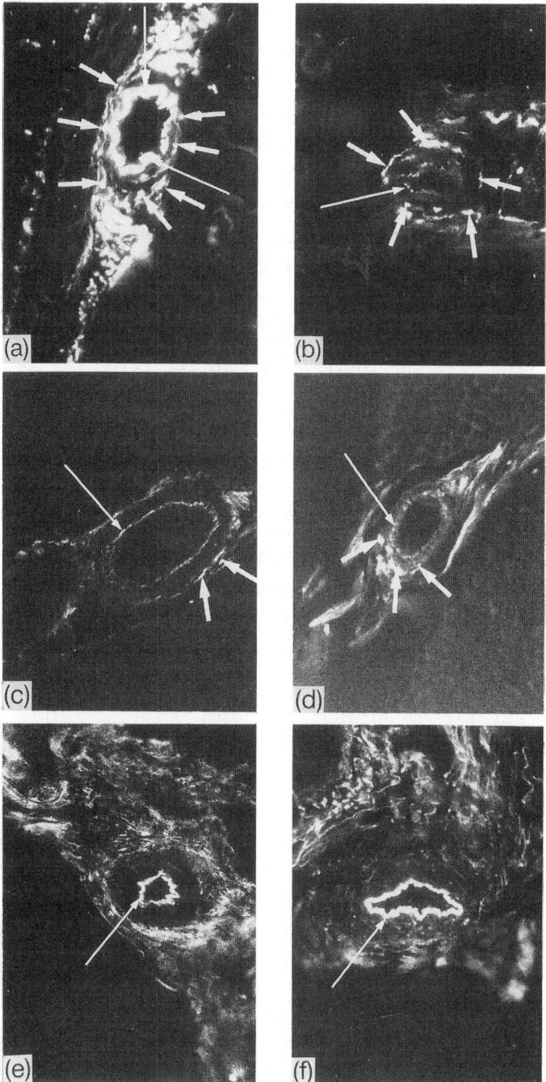

Fig. 31.1. Catecholamine fluorescent nerves associated with blood vessels of human quadriceps muscle. (a) and (b) Control tissue. Note adrenergic nerves on the adventitial side of the media (thick white) of the arteries. Autofluorescence (thin white) can be seen in the intima. Fluorescent micrograph (a) ×180; (b) ×174. (c)–(f) Tissue from patients with autonomic failure. (c) and (d) Note few adrenergic nerves are present on the adventitial-medial border (thick white) of the arteries. Autofluorescence can be seen in the intima (thin white). Fluorescent micrograph. (c) ×134; (d) ×188. (e) and (f) Note lack of adrenergic nerves in the arteries although autofluorescence can be seen, especially in the intima. Fluorescent micrograph. (e) and (f) ×134. (Taken with permission from Bannister *et al.* (1981).)

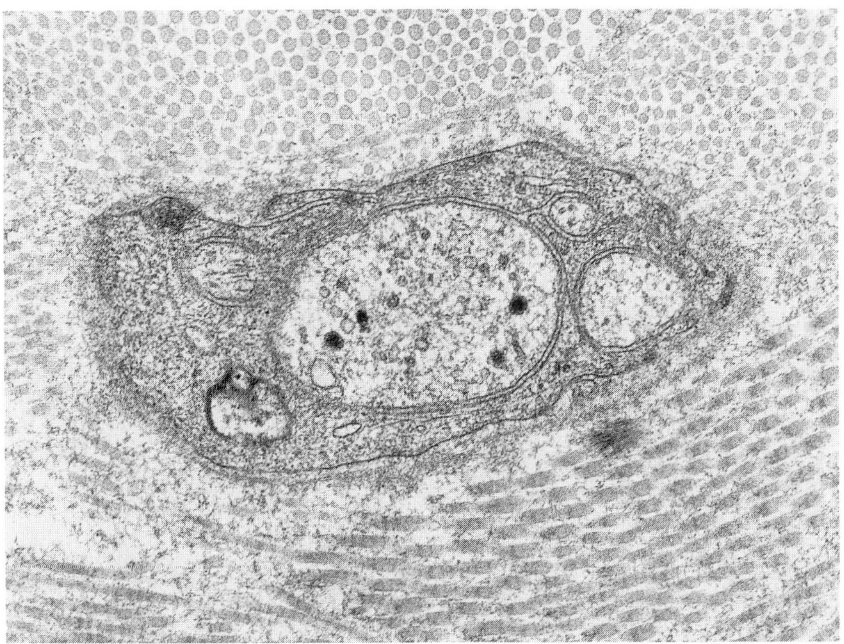

Fig. 31.2. From patient with pure autonomic failure. Electron micrograph showing high-powered views of nerve ending close to blood vessel. The ending shows a marked reduction in the number of vesicles of all three types. ×28 500; 5-OHD incubated. (Taken with permission from Bannister *et al.* (1981).)

central lesions in multiple system atrophy which reduce central sympathetic impulse traffic. These results are consistent with the failure of tyramine to release detectable amounts of noradrenalin after an infusion rate which causes a pressor response, in contrast with a 50 per cent rise in plasma noradrenalin in normal subjects (Bannister *et al.* 1979). These observations are also consistent with the fact that small doses of fludrocortisone, insufficient to increase body weight or plasma volume, increase the sensitivity of vascular receptors to exogenous (intravenous) noradrenalin infusion (Davies *et al.* 1978, 1979). Our results suggest that patients with PAF had more extreme degeneration of adrenergic nerves than patients with AF and MSA but it would be necessary to study a larger number of biopsies to establish this quantitatively, with allowance made for the progression of the disease. Since the catecholamine fluorescence was much reduced, even in the most mildly affected patients, it seems probable that the pathological changes start as soon as or even before symptoms are clinically apparent.

Since these studies, further types of autonomic failure with specific defects located to the sympathetic terminals have been described. Klein *et al.* (1980), while confirming the lack of perivascular noradrenergic

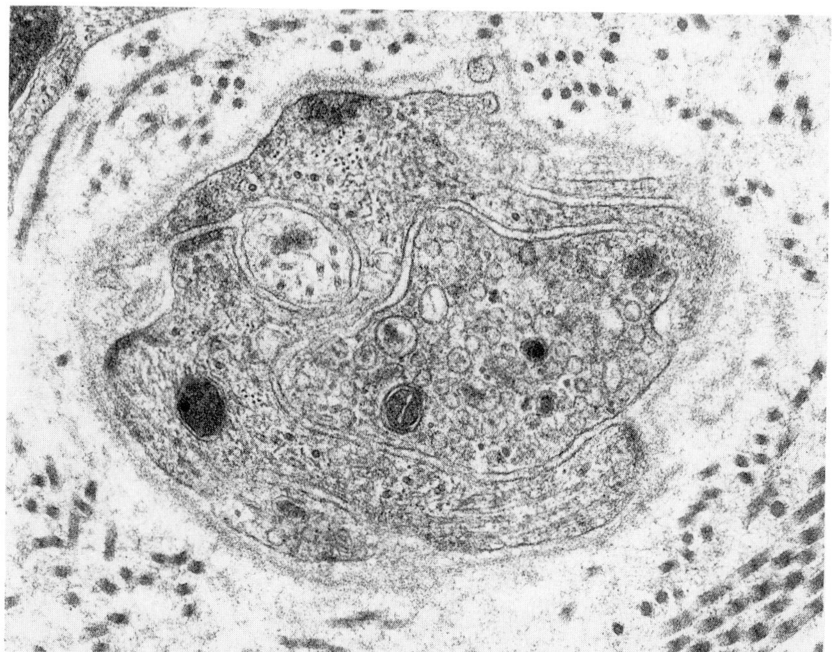

Fig. 31.3. From a patient with autonomic failure and multiple system atrophy. Electron micrograph showing high-powered view of nerve endings close to small blood vessels. Schwann cell partly enclosing adrenergic axon which contains reduced numbers of vesicles of all three types and a single mitochondrion. ×37 500. (Taken with permission from Bannister *et al.* (1981).)

vesicles in three cases of pure autonomic failure, described two patients with low levels of circulating noradrenalin but with a hyperadrenergic response to standing, with normal noradrenalin perivascular stores on catecholamine histochemistry and electron microscopy. They proposed a possible blunting of the response of the α-receptor of smooth muscle. Robertson *et al.* (1986) and, more recently, Man in't Veld *et al.* (1987) described a genetically determined deficiency of dopamine β hydroxylase, the enyzme converting dopamine to noradrenalin. Man in't Veld *et al.*'s patient had ptosis and skeletal muscle hypotonia from childhood but eventually developed obvious orthostatic hypotension. Physiological and pharmacological stimuli of sympathetic neurotransmitter release caused an increase of plasma dopamine rather than plasma noradrenalin (Fig. 31.4). No biopsy was taken of perivascular nerve endings. We have studied a pair of siblings who were unrelated but both have the HLA A32 antigen. Now in their thirties they have, since they were teenagers, shown features of autonomic failure without other neurological symptoms. Their plasma noradrenalin and adrenalin levels were undetectable but their dopamine levels were very much elevated. This

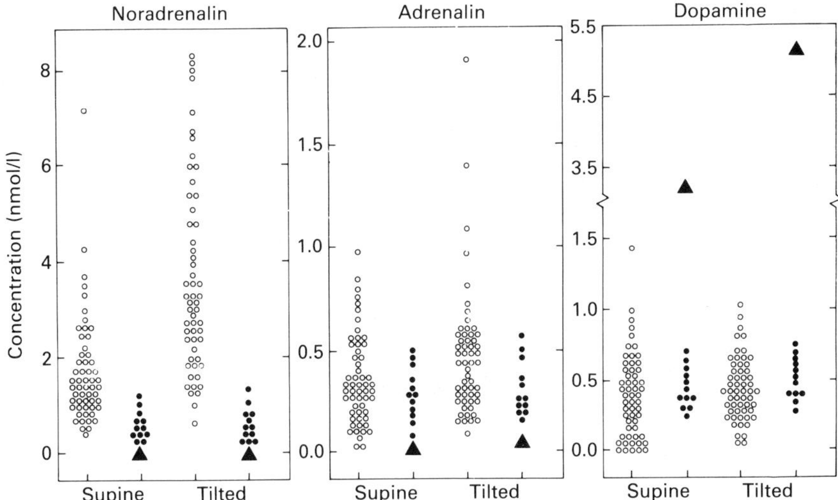

Fig. 31.4. Basal and stimulated (5 min 60° head-up tilt) concentrations of plasma catecholamines. (●) Patients with chronic autonomic failure; (○) age- and sex-matched controls; (▲) patient with dopamine β hydroxylase deficiency. (Taken with permission from Man in't Veld *et al.* (1987).)

sharply distinguishes them from patients with pure autonomic failure (PAF) in whom dopamine can hardly be detected in the plasma even when noradrenalin and adrenalin levels are extremely low. These two patients have congenital DβH deficiency but, like other patients, have responded to L-dihydroxyphenylserine (L-DOPS) which by-passes the defect. Clearly autonomic failure patients exist in whom selective enzymatic lesions either of noradrenalin synthesis, release, re-uptake, or receptor blockade cause a sympathetic efferent lesion, with clinical features of autonomic failure. They are difficult to distinguish clinically from the main group in which the lesion is thought to be preganglionic and ganglionic. Clearly homogeneity of sympathetic efferent lesions cannot be assumed and now that the techniques for precise study are available we must await with interest the recognition of further subtypes of autonomic failure whose existence we at present can only predict on theoretical grounds.

B. Amyotrophy in multiple system atrophy

Roger Bannister, Marjorie Ellison, and John Morgan-Hughes

INTRODUCTION

Muscle wasting was reported in the original description by Shy and Drager of two cases of the syndrome which now bears their name, autonomic failure with multiple system atrophy (MSA). Since then there have been no systematic studies of muscle biopsy changes but a few isolated reports of electromyographic studies and nerve and muscle biopsies (Galassi *et al.* 1982; Toghi *et al.* 1982; Montagna *et al.* 1983). However, loss of anterior horn cells has been reported in half the neuropathological reports of multiple system atrophy (see Chapter 25A). In the hope of throwing some light on this aspect of the curiously selective degeneration of neurons in MSA, the opportunity was taken of a previous investigation into the catecholamine fluorescence and electron microscopy of muscle blood vessels (Bannister *et al.* 1981) to study striated muscle, taking advantage of modern histochemical techniques.

MUSCLE BIOPSY FINDINGS

The biopsies of the quadriceps femoris muscle were examined in 10 patients with MSA, using a battery of histochemical reactions. Fibre diameters were measured with a digitized pit pad on an image analyser. Three patients showed atrophy of Type 2a and Type 2b fibres, one patient showed selective Type 2b atrophy, and in a fifth case the Type 1 and Type 2b fibres were atrophic (Figs. 31.5 and 31.6). The variations in selective fibre-type atrophy could not be correlated with the clinical features of the patients nor with their age. The muscle biopsy appearances and fibre-diameter histograms were entirely normal in the remaining five cases, except that one case showed early grouping of the Type 1 muscle fibres. Again this patient was not in any other way atypical of the entire group. The morphometric changes were not related to age, as the patients with the selective fibre-type atrophy were generally younger than those with normal fibre diameters.

A biopsy was taken from only one patient with pure autonomic failure (PAF). The patient was a man of 68 who had had postural hypotension for 20 years, without other significant neurological symptoms or signs apart from impotence. His muscle biopsy was studied by the same histochemical techniques as used for the patients with MSA and there were no abnormalities.

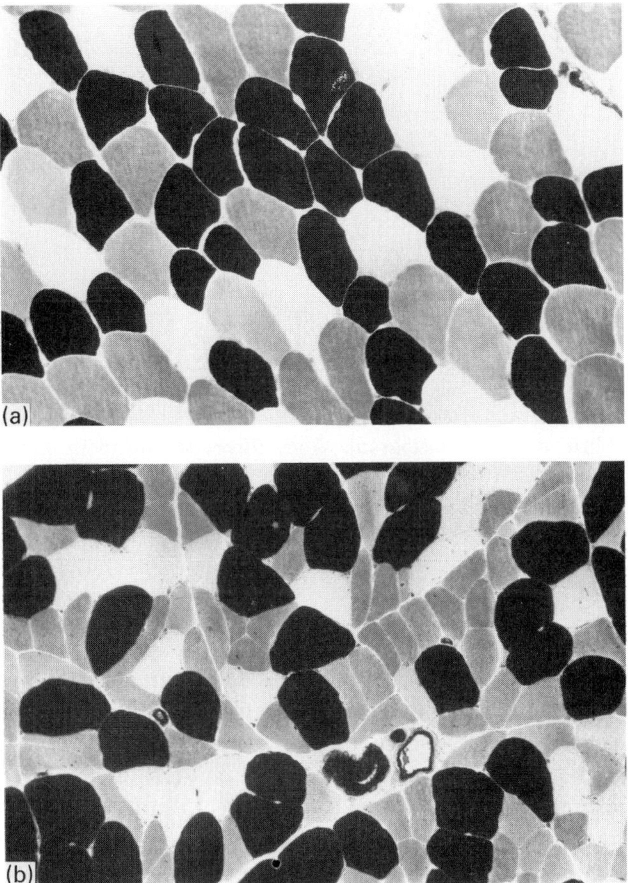

Fig. 31.5. (a) Transverse sections of the vastus lateralis muscle from (a) a normal human control and (b) a patient with multiple system atrophy stained with the ATPase reaction at pH 4.35. The Type 1 fibres are dark, the Type 2a fibres are light, and the Type 2b fibres are intermediate. Note the presence of Type 2a and Type 2b muscle-fibre atrophy in the patient.

DISCUSSION

The pattern of histochemical muscle fibre responses in human quadriceps is well established (Mahon *et al.* 1984; Dorriguzzi *et al.* 1986). The type of selective fibre atrophy seen in half the patients with MSA is quite abnormal. It is unlike the large-group atrophy or small-group atrophy seen in motoneuron disease, a disease with which, in some clinical respects, it might be thought to have some similarities (Dubowitz 1981: Jennekens 1982). Nor is there a suggestion of type grouping with large clusters of different fibre types, adjacent to each other, as occurs in regeneration as a result of sprouting. Perhaps a closer parallel is the

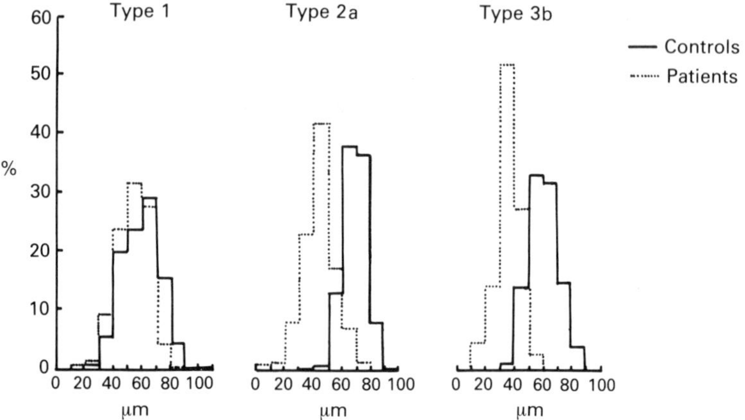

Fig. 31.6. Fibre diameter histograms from three patients with multiple system atrophy to show selective atrophy of the Type 2a and Type 2b fibres (interrupted line). Three age-matched controls are shown for comparison (continuous lines). Between 400 and 450 muscle fibres were measured in each case.

selective fibre-type atrophy which sometimes occurs in myasthenia gravis (Aström and Adams 1981). Selective fibre atrophy itself is a rather non-specific type of change, seen in a range of diverse disease pathologies from steroid or alcoholic myopathy to collagen vascular disease.

It could be argued that in multiple system atrophy there is a preferential selective involvement of Type 2a and 2b neurons by a process that in general seems to spare Type 1 neurons and is not associated with sprouting and reinnervation. The morphological appearances of the anterior horn cells giving rise to each type of motor unit is not known. The number of neurons which need to be affected to produce changes of this type may be small, in that up to 1000 muscle fibres in the human quadriceps may be innervated from a single neuron. In multiple system atrophy the anterior horn cells have not been systematically counted in the same way as intermediolateral column cells and so mild reductions in the number of these cells may have been missed.

These histochemical findings are consistent with several reports of electromyographic signs of degeneration in MSA (see Chapter 30 and Montagna *et al.* 1983). Reports of nerve biopsies in MSA are rare but Toghi *et al.* (1982) found selective loss of small myelinated and unmyelinated fibres in three cases of MSA by comparison with control patients with olivopontocerebellar degeneration without autonomic dysfunction. Galassi *et al.* (1982) described loss of both large and small fibres in a sural-nerve biopsy in a single case of MSA. An anterior tibial-muscle biopsy showed chronic neurogenic changes with large fields of atrophic fibres of the same histological type.

Clearly, further studies will be needed before it is possible to comment firmly on the type of process responsible for the selective fibre-type involvement in multiple system atrophy and, in particular, whether in pure autonomic failure there may be changes of a similar type though less marked than those in multiple system atrophy.

REFERENCES

Aström, K. E. and Adams, R. D. (1981). Pathology of human skeletal muscle. In *Disorders of voluntary muscle* (ed. J. N. Walton), pp. 151–208. Churchill Livingstone, Edinburgh.

Axelsson, S., Bjorklund, A., and Falck, B. (1973). Glyoxylic acid; a new fluorescence method for the histochemical demonstration of biogenic monoamines. *Acta physiol. scand.* **87**, 57–62.

Bannister, R., Crowe, R., Eames, R., and Burnstock, G. (1981). Adrenergic innervation in autonomic failure. *Neurology, Minneapolis* **31**, 1501–6.

Bannister, R., Davies, B., Holly, E., Rosenthal, T., and Sever, P. (1979). Defective cardiovascular reflexes and supersensitivity to sympathomimetic drugs in autonomic failure. *Brain* **102**, 163–76.

Bannister, R., Sever, P., and Gross, M. (1977). Cardiovascular reflexes and biochemical responses in progressive autonomic failure. *Brain* **100**, 327–44.

Burnstock, G. (1975*a*). Innervation of vascular smooth muscle: histochemistry and electronmicroscopy. In *Physiological and pharmacological control of blood pressure.* IUPS Symposium, October 1974. *Clin. exp. Pharmacol. Physiol.* Suppl. 2, 7–20.

Burnstock, G. (1975*b*). Control of smooth muscle activity in vessels by adrenergic nerves and circulating catecholamines. In *Smooth muscle pharmacology and physiology*, Vol. 50, pp. 251–64. INSERM, Paris.

Davies, B., Bannister, R. and Sever, P. (1978). Pressor amines and monoamine oxidase inhibitors for treatment of postural hypotension in autonomic failure. *Lancet* **i**, 172–5.

Davies, B., Bannister, R., and Sever, P. (1979). The pressor actions of noradrenaline angiotensin II and saralasin in chronic autonomic failure treated with fludrocortisone. *Br. J. clin. Pharamacol.* **8**, 253–60.

Dorriguzzi, C. P., Palmucci, L., Mongini, T., Leone, M., Gagnor, E., Gagliano, A., and Schiffer, D. (1986). Quantitative analysis of quadriceps muscle biopsy. *J. neurol. Sci.* **72**, 201–9.

Dubowitz, V. (1981). Histochemistry of muscle disease. In *Disorders of voluntary muscle* (ed. J. N. Walton), pp. 261–95. Churchill Livingstone, Edinburgh.

Falk, B., Hillarp, N. A., and Thiem, G. (1962). Fluorescence of catecholamines and related compounds condensed with formaldehyde. *J. Histochem. Cytochem.* **10**, 348–54.

Furness, J. B. (1973). Arrangement of blood vessels and their relation with adrenergic nerves in the rat mesentery. *J. Anat.* **115**, 437–64.

Galassi, G., Nemni, R., Baraldi, A., Gibertoni, M., and Columbo, A. (1982).

Periperhal neuropathy in multiple system atrophy with autonomic failure. *Neurology, NY* **32**, 1116–20.

Jennekens, F. G. I. (1982). Muscle histochemistry. In *Skeletal muscle pathology* (ed. F. L. Mastaglia and J. N. Walton), pp. 204–34. Churchill Livingstone, London.

Klein, R. L., Baggett, J. McM., Thureson, K. Å., and Langford, H. G. (1980). Idiopathic orthostatic hypotension: circulating noradrenaline and ultrastructure of saphenous vein. *J. auton. nerv. Syst.* **2**, 205–22.

Kontos, H. A., Richardson, D. W., and Narvell, J. E. (1975). Norepinephrine depletion in idiopathic orthostatic hypotension. *Ann. intern. Med.* **82**, 336–41.

Mahon, M., Toman, A., Willan, P. L. T., and Bagnall, K. M. (1984). Variability of the histochemical and morphometric data from needle biopsy specimens of human quadriceps. *J. neurol. Sci.* **63**, 85–100.

Man in't Veld, A. J., Boomsma,, H., Moleman, P., and Schalekamp, M. A. D. H. (1987). Congenital dopamine-beta-hydroxylase deficiency. *Lancet* **i**, 183–8.

Montagna, P., Martinelli, P., Rizzuto, N., Salviati, A., Rasi, F., and Lugaresi, E. (1983). Amyotrophy in Shy–Drager syndrome. *Acta neurol. belg.* **83**, 142–57.

Nanda, R. N., Boyle, R. C., Gillespie, J. S., Johnson, R. M., and Keogh, H. J. (1976). Adrenergic innervation of peripheral blood vessels in patients with neurogenic orthostatic hypotension. *J. Neuropathol. appl. Neurobiol.* **2**, 49.

Nanda, R. N., Boyle, R. C., Gillespie, J. S., Johnson, R. M., and Keogh, H. J. (1977). Idiopathic orthostatic hypotension from failure of noradrenaline release in a patient with vasomotor innervation. *J. Neurol. Neurosurg. Psychiat.* **40**, 11–19.

Rubenstein, A. E., Yahr, M. D., and Mytilineou, C. (1978). Peripheral adrenergic hypersensitivity in orthostatic hypotension; the effects of denervation versus decentralization. *Neurology, Minneapolis* **28**, 376.

Robertson, D., Goldberg, M. R., Onrot, J., Hollister, A. S., Wiley, R., Thompson, J. G., and Robertson, R. M. (1986). Isolated failure of autonomic noradrenergic neurotransmission: evidence for impaired β-hydroxylation of dopamine. *New Engl. J. Med.* **214**, 1494–7.

Toghi, H., Tabuchi, M., Tomonaga, M., and Izumiyana, N. (1982). Selective loss of small myelinated and unmyelinated fibres in Shy–Drager syndrome. *Acta neuropathol., Berlin* **57**, 282–6.

Ziegler, M. C., Lake, C. R., and Kopin, I. J. (1977). The sympathetic nervous system defect in primary orthostatic hypotension. *New Engl. J. Med.* **296**, 293–7.

32. Management of postural hypotension

Roger Bannister and Christopher Mathias

GENERAL PRINCIPLES

Treatment of postural hypotension due to autonomic failure is fraught with difficulties, many caused by inaccurate localization of the sites of the lesions. Treatment requires targeting; as Ehrlich commented on chemotherapy 'we must learn to aim and aim in a chemical sense'. In autonomic failure, treatment has to be directed to overcoming precisely identified defects. Some principles of management are, however, common to all patients.

Cerebral blood flow

First, it is important not to be overconcerned about a low standing blood pressure if the patient is without symptoms. Patients can sometimes tolerate a standing systolic blood pressure as low as 70 mm Hg without dizziness or syncope, probably because their cerebral blood flow is maintained at an adequate level because of the capacity of their cerebral circulation for autoregulation. There have been several studies attempting to clarify whether in autonomic failure there is a reduced fall of cerebral blood flow for a standard fall of mean arterial pressure. It is not to be expected that such a heterogeneous group of patients would respond identically and autoregulation was thought to persist in autonomic failure by Skinhoj *et al.* (1971), Caronna and Plum (1973), and Nanda *et al.* (1976). However, Meyer *et al.* (1973) and Shinohara and Gotoh (1973) reported that autoregulation was lost. Thomas and Bannister (1980) studied five patients with autonomic failure (AF) and multiple system atrophy (MSA) and found that autoregulation was preserved down to a systolic blood pressure close to 60 mm Hg which is well below the 80 mm Hg at which autoregulation fails in normal subjects. The results in a further three patients with pure autonomic failure (PAF) showed a similar trend. A shift of autoregulation to the left in AF almost certainly occurs and the reason some have failed to record it is probably that when cerebral blood flow was measured during tilt the arterial pressure may have been transiently much lower than the recorded pressure. We found evidence of this in one patient with AF who developed syptoms of cerebral ischaemia when his systolic pressure fell transiently to 40 mm Hg and the clearance curve changed, implying a transient fall in flow (Fig. 32.1). The change in autoregulation may be the result of prolonged exposure to lower than normal arterial pressure, causing some changes in the response of normally innervated vessels, or because the cerebral vessels, like muscle vessels, are partially or completely sympathectomized in autonomic failure. It has been suggested that the major sympathetic innervation is to the extra-parenchymal vessels, the intraparenchymal vessels being under myogenic and metabolic control. If this is so, the sympathetic innervation at the lower level of autoregulation may normally reduce cerebral blood flow by constricting extraparenchymal vessels. Whatever the explanation, it is certain that patients with autonomic failure have a remarkable tolerance to low blood pressure without developing postural hypotensive symptoms.

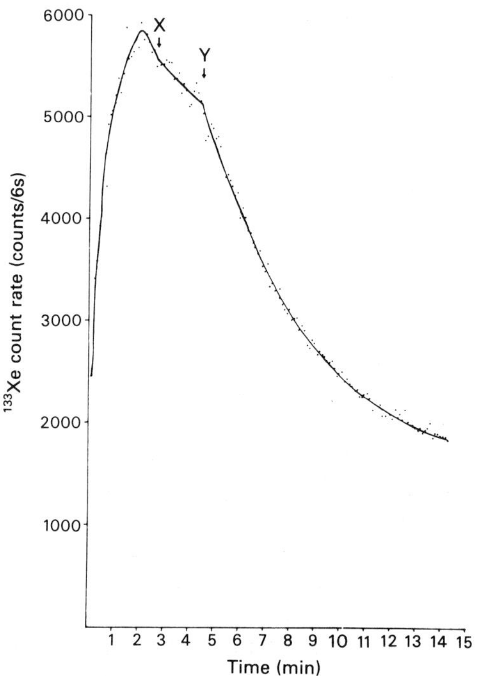

Fig. 32.1. Cerebral ^{133}Xe count rates/6 s in patient G.K. with pure autonomic failure tilted to 45°. At point X, the blood pressure fell suddenly to a systolic pressure of 40 mm Hg. The rate of ^{133}Xe clearance decreased and the patient developed symptoms of cerebral ischaemia. At point Y, the tilt table was lowered, blood pressure rose, and the rate of clearance increased. (Taken with permission from Thomas and Bannister (1980).)

Recumbent hypertension

A second principle which has to be considered in treatment is the tendency of patients to develop recumbent hypertension owing principally to defective baroreceptor reflexes, supersensitivity, and treatment with drugs such as fludrocortisone. Clearly, this may result in a reactive increase of cerebrovascular resistance leading to the likelihood of cerebral ischaemic symptoms when such patients stand suddenly. Some patients, if nursed recumbent for long periods develop persistent and severe hypertension and run the risk of developing complications such as papilloedema and cerebral haemorrhage.

Control of blood volume

A third principle is that, although loss of baroreflexes determines the immediate response of blood pressure to standing, control of blood volume, determined by low-pressure receptors and the kidney, through antidiuretic hormone and the renin–angiotensin–aldesterone mechanism, is the long-term and more important adjustment to postural hypotension in autonomic failure.

Limitations of treatment

All methods of treatment, directly or indirectly, aim either at reducing the vascular volume into which pooling occurs on standing or increasing the volume of blood available for pooling. A reduction of the volume into which the blood may pool by pressor drugs has its limitations. Unless the drugs increase the responsiveness of vessels to small amounts of noradrenalin which can still be liberated, they will aggravate the tendency to recumbent hypertension. An increase in blood volume runs the risks of overloading the circulation and leading to cardiac failure and peripheral oedema. Many patients with autonomic failure have defects of renal preservation of sodium when recumbent and are sensitive to sodium depletion which leads to a reduction of extracellular fluid volume. Though we are aware that many patients continue to receive a variety of treatments in different medical centres, it is probable that any treatment with pressor drugs which temporarily enables a patient to become more mobile will improve the patient's other homeostatic responses to standing. These include an increase in extracellular fluid volume and improved myogenic tone. Hence, a sustained improvement may be erroneously attributed to a particular form of treatment when it might, under controlled conditions, be possible to withdraw or replace it with a safer method.

Testing of drugs

There have been a series of reports of treatment with many different drugs, usually given empirically for a short uncontrolled trial, often in patients with an inadequately precise diagnosis of autonomic failure. It may reasonably be asked whether any pressor drug is effective when so many different treatments have been proposed. It is also reasonable to question whether the effects of drugs can be monitored when the lack of baroreceptor reflexes in autonomic failure leads to such marked fluctuations with changes of posture over the course of 24 hours so that adequate maintenance of blood pressure is as difficult as targeting in a video space game. In any attempt to measure the benefit of a drug in autonomic failure, the standing and recumbent blood pressure must be taken under standard conditions, preferably four times a day by trained staff. As the blood pressure of these patients usually continues to fall when they stand, the duration of standing has to be recorded. We aim to record the blood pressure 2 minutes after the onset of standing because arterial recording has shown that any fall in blood pressure will then be clearly apparent. Prior to drug treatment it is advisable to have an equilibrium period of a week on a standard daily sodium diet of 150 mmol, with monitoring of position and physical activity during the day and measurement of head-up tilt at night. It is also advisable to measure the haematocrit, plasma proteins, urea, creatinine, and electrolytes every 3 days, weigh the patient on accurate scales twice daily, measure day and night fluid balance and urinary sodium and potassium excretion, and measure blood pressure four times a day before meals.

Drug combinations

Since patients with autonomic failure have lesions at more than one site, it should always be considered whether a combination of drugs may be more effective than a single drug. For example, drugs with central, ganglionic, and postganglionic effects may have synergistic actions. At the sympathetic terminals drugs which increase noradrenalin release may be combined with drugs which reduce re-uptake of the transmitter or increase the sensitivity of receptors.

APPROACHES TO TREATMENT (Table 32.1)

Advice on factors which influence blood pressure

A number of factors have been now defined, which can considerably lower blood pressure and thus enhance the postural fall and therefore the symptoms accompanying postural hypotension. The pathophysiological mechanisms accounting for a number of these have been worked

Table 32.1. Approaches to treatment

I	Advice on factors which influence blood pressure
	1. Straining during micturition and defaecation
	2. Diurnal changes in blood pressure
	3. Exposure to a warm environment
	4. The effects of food
	5. Effects of drugs with vasoactive properties
II	Head-up tilt at night
III	External support
IV	Cardiac pacing
V	Drugs (see Table 32.2)

out and in a number of situations avoidance measures can be instituted. Patients should therefore be advised on these factors.

Straining during micturition and defaecation

A number of patients suffer from either urinary bladder problems or from constipation. Straining might result in a Valsalva manoeuvre being performed. This can result in a substantial reduction in blood pressure without the recovery mechanisms which normally come into play. Episodes of hypotension in some situations may be particularly dangerous, as patients may lose consciousness while propped against a lavatory wall and may not fall to the ground and thus correct their blood pressure.

Diurnal changes in blood pressure

The supine blood pressure in patients with autonomic failure is lowest in the morning and rises gradually during the day. This has been confirmed by non-invasive measurements and also by using continuous ambulatory intra-arterial blood pressure recording (see Fig. 32.2). The circadian changes in blood pressure are the reverse of those in normal subjects, in whom the blood pressure falls during sleep and rises prior to awakening. The low level of blood pressure in the morning appears to be the result of nocturnal polyuria and natriuresis, which can result in a substantial overnight weight loss, at times over 1 kilogram. The reduction in extracellular fluid volume is likely to contribute to the low blood pressure as it is improved by administration of desmopressin (see below). The low blood pressure aggravates the symptoms of postural hypotension in the morning, and some patients find it extremely difficult to conduct their normal activities for a few hours after waking. Methods of preventing morning postural hypotension are described below.

Exposure to a warm environment

Patients exposed to tropical or subtropical temperatures tend to have greater symptoms for a variety of reasons. They often lack the ability to

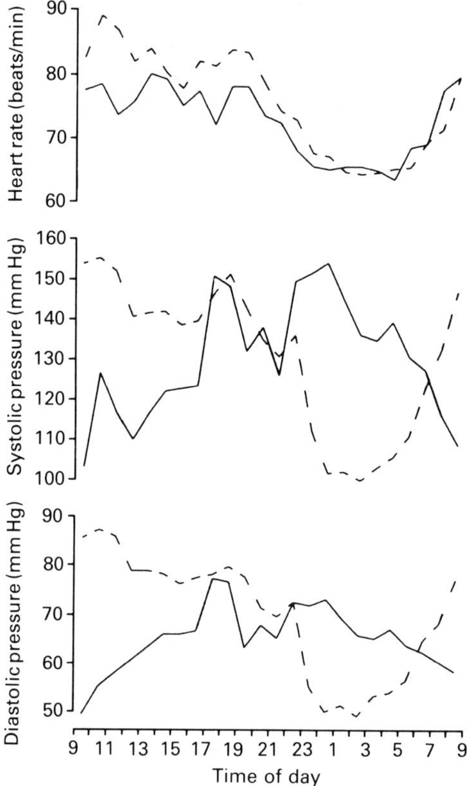

Fig. 32.2. Overall trend in heart rate, systolic and diastolic pressures of six subjects with autonomic failure (———) compared with those derived from a matched group of six subjects with normal or elevated blood pressure (– – – –). Lines join pooled hourly means. (Taken with permission from Mann *et al.* (1983).)

sweat, and their core temperature can therefore rise. Uncompensated vasodilatation often ensues and the blood pressure can fall. Adequate precautions should therefore be taken by patients travelling to warm countries, with awareness of the possible worsening of postural hypotension.

The effects of food

The majority of patients with autonomic failure have substantial postprandial hypotension. This occurs soon after food ingestion and may last for up to three hours after a standard meal. The supine blood pressure can be lowered to levels of 80/50 mm Hg even in the supine position and therefore they often get increased symptoms of postural hypotension. Carbohydrate appears to be the major component causing the hypotension, and this may be linked to the release of insulin and other gastrointestinal hormones which have vasodilatory properties. Vasodilatation in the gut, not compensated for by defective sympathetic reflexes, is the probable cause of the reduction in pressure. The pathophysiology of this important condition is described in Chapter 20. It is likely, that alcoholic drinks with their potential to cause vasodilatation, will lower blood pressure in these patients.

Effect of drugs with vasoactive properties

Both the patient and the physician should be aware that drugs with vasoactive properties, even if only a minor action of the agent, may result in substantial vascular changes, because of supersensitivity. The responses to pressor agents, particularly sympathomimetic agents have already been described (see Chapter 16). Vasopressor responses may occur to a variety of agents acting on receptors other than adrenoceptors. Agents used via the intraocular or intranasal route, which include sypathomimetics, β-adrenoceptor blockers, and anticholinergic agents, may be sufficiently absorbed to exert systemic effects which include supine hypertension and bradycardia. The reverse, marked hypotension, may also occur with drugs which have vasodilatatory properties. An example is provided by the agent glyceryl trinitrate, which is routinely used sublingually in patients with angina pectoris. This drug, even when given with patients in the suprine position, can result in severe hypotension.

Head-up tilt at night

The first line of treatment in a patient with autonomic failure is to attempt to increase the patient's blood volume by the use of head-up tilt at night. This method of treatment was first proposed by Maclean and Allen (1940). Figure 32.3 (Bannister *et al.* 1969) shows the change in lying and standing blood pressure and body weight in a patient placed in the head-up position at night. The increase of 2.6 kg in body weight points to a progressive increase in extracellular fluid volume, which was reversed on the one night when the patient slept flat. The effect of this procedure was studied further in one patient in whom water and sodium balance were followed on a 90 mmol per day sodium diet. As shown in Fig. 32.4 (Sever and Bannister, unpublished) the patient was losing more sodium and water during the night than during the day for each of 5 days until head-up tilt at night was introduced, when the nocturnal loss of sodium and water was reversed over the subsequent 5 days. This postural salt and water retention is enhanced by fludrocortisone (Wilson *et al.* 1969). Head-up body tilt at night is likely to operate by reducing renal arterial pressure and promoting renin release with consequent angiotensin II formation, aldosterone stimulation, and thus increasing

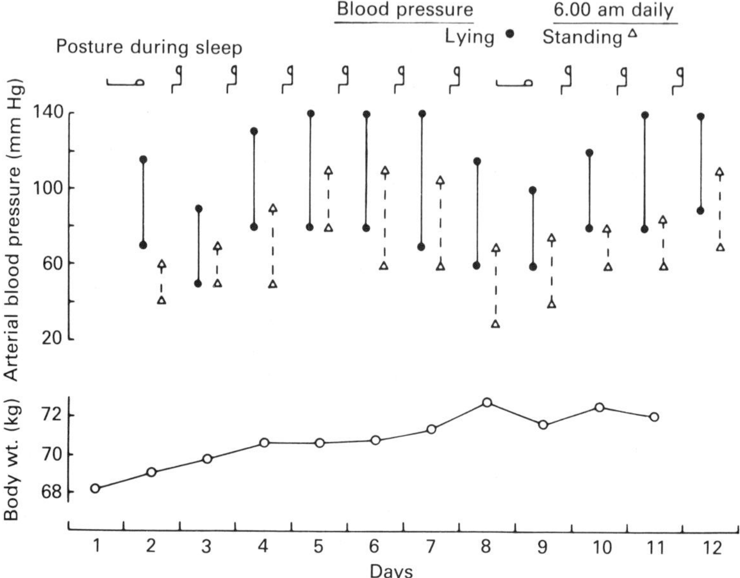

Fig. 32.3. The change in the early-morning blood pressure (lying and standing) in a patient (H) with autonomic failure and MSA studied when he slept in the sitting position for 10 days with one interruption. The changes in blood volume and body weight are also shown. (Taken with permission from Bannister *et al.* (1969).)

blood volume for patients with autonomic failure who can still release renin (Bannister *et al.* 1977). The excessive nocturnal polyuria was studied by Wilcox *et al.* (1977) and there are more complex defects of renal sodium conservation in autonomic failure. Many patients with pure autonomic failure, with incapacitating postural hypotension until the introduction of head-up tilt, have been maintained satisfactorily for years solely by this form of treatment.

External support

A simple method of treatment is to reduce the volume into which blood may pool on standing by external support for the trunk and legs by a custom-fitted elastic counter-pressure garment (Sheps 1976). This treatment, however, reduces the useful myogenic response to stretch which is present even in partially denervated vessels. It is therefore physiologically unsound and leaves the patient vulnerable to hypotension if he gets up without the garment. It is sometimes necessary as a temporary expedient, for example after a patient has been recumbent for a few days because of an intercurrent infection, and in some patients, when drugs prove ineffective, may be of value in long-term treatment. Figure 32.5 shows a tracing from such a patient with a brachial artery catheter. His blood pressure could be maintained when

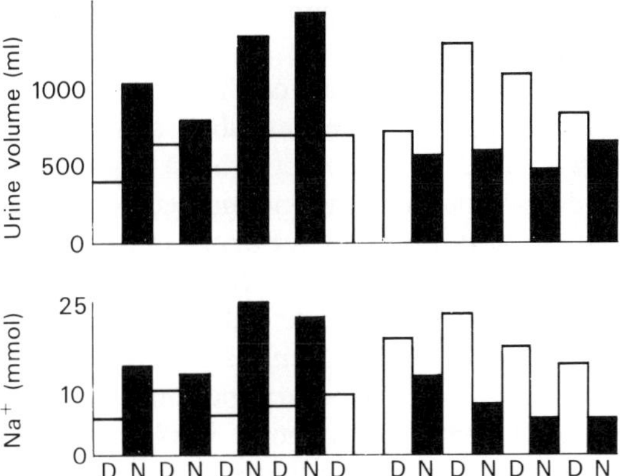

Fig. 32.4. Diurnal changes in water and sodium excretion in a patient with autonomic failure and multiple system atrophy during 5 days lying flat at night and 5 days of head-up tilt at night. D=day; N=night.

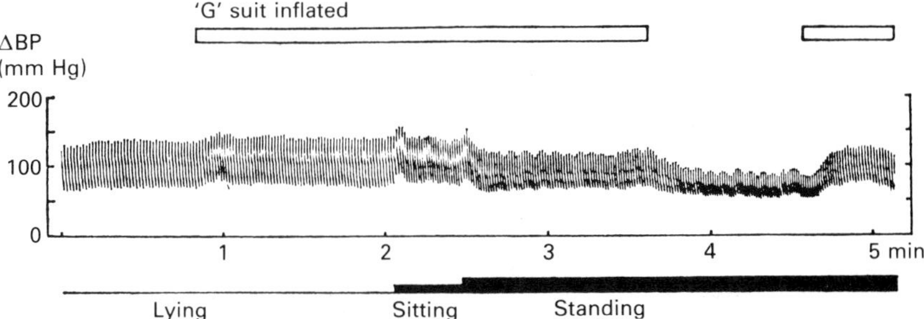

Fig. 32.5. The effect of an antigravity suit on the changes of brachial arterial blood pressure (ΔBP) which occur on sitting and standing on a patient with pure autonomic failure. (Taken with permission from Bannister *et al.* (1969).)

he was sitting or standing, provided an inflated antigravity suit was used to protect him against pooling of blood in the extremities. Without this support his blood pressure fell continuously and he would eventually lose consciousness.

Cardiac pacing

There have been reports of benefits obtained by implantation of a cardiac pacemaker, and elevation of heart rate during postural change. The benefit noted by Moss *et al.* (1980) occurred in a patient who apparently had an incomplete autonomic lesion, and therefore had the potential to vasoconstrict at times. In patients with more severe lesions, with very low plasma noradrenalin levels at rest and in response to tilt, there appeared to be no benefit. Beneficial effects of tachypacing are unlikely in patients who have maximal arteriolar and venodilatation, as cardiac output is dependent upon venous return which is often considerably reduced in such patients. Occasionally, cardiac pacing may be needed to prevent excessive bradycardia, in response to elevation of blood pressure by drugs. We have described a patient in whom atrial demand pacing was needed to protect against vagal overactivity in the presence of a severe sympathetic autonomic neuropathy (Bannister *et al.* 1986). In this patient administration of drugs to raise the blood pressure resulted in severe bradycardia and consequent dysrhythmias (see Fig. 32.6). Assessment was initially made with atropine, which raised the heart rate but resulted in unacceptable side-effects. Atrial pacing was performed, initially with a temporary pacemaker which was clearly beneficial, and later with permanent implantation. This enabled effective use of pressor agents without the fear of development of either cardiac arrest or a serious dysrhythmia (see Fig. 32.7).

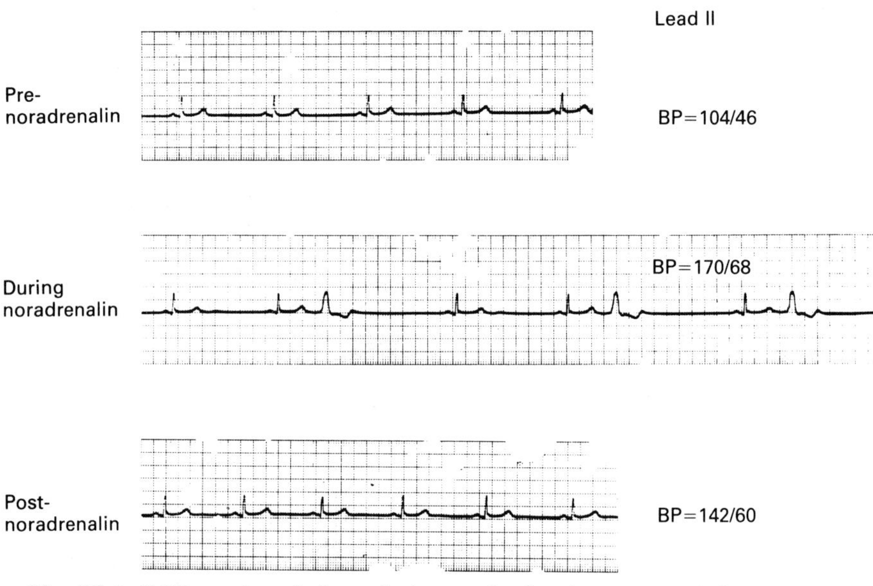

Fig. 32.6. ECG tracings before, during, and after intravenous infusion of noradrenalin. Sinus bradycardia and coupled beats occur when the blood pressure (BP) is elevated to 170/68 mm Hg. This is reversed when the BP returns to normal. (Taken with permission from Bannister *et al.* (1986).)

DRUGS IN POSTURAL HYPOTENSION

A variety of agents have been used to raise supine blood pressure and so reduce postural hypotension. In Table 32.2 an attempt has been made to classify these agents on the basis of their main actions in helping postural hypotension. They are described below.

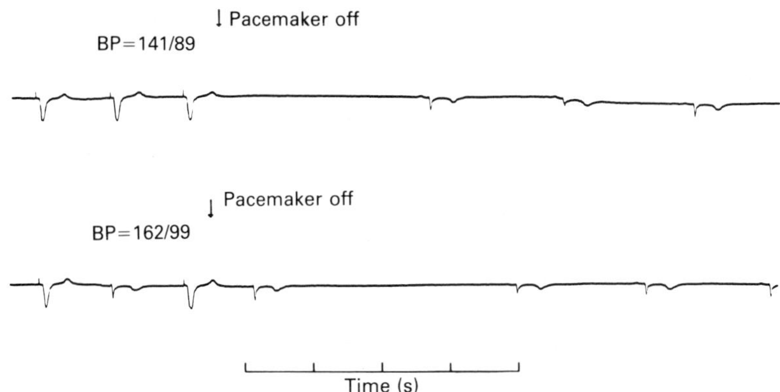

Fig. 32.7. ECG tracings, initially with the pacemaker on (upper trace). There are pacemaker triggered complexes followed by a pause and then sinus bradycardia. During noradrenalin infusion (lower trace) with the BP elevated, there are alternating pacemaker-induced and intrinsic complexes. Following exclusion of the pacemaker there is a longer pause before endogenous rhythm takes over. The elevation in BP appears to enhance sinus node suppression. (Taken with permission from Bannister *et al.* (1986).)

Vasoconstriction

A variety of drugs have been used which cause vasoconstriction by direct effects either upon adrenoceptors or other receptors responsible for constriction of vascular smooth muscle. These drugs may act either directly (phenylephrine, noradrenalin) or indirectly to cause release of noradrenalin and thus constriction (tyramine). The majority of these agents act upon resistance vessels, but there are semi-selective agents, such as dihydroergotamine, which act predominantly upon the venous capacitance vessels.

Historically, the first vasoconstrictor drugs to be reported to cause an improvement in standing blood pressure in autonomic failure were phenylephrine, with a direct sympathomimetic action and, to a lesser and variable extent, ephedrine, with a mainly indirect sympathomimetic action (Barnett and Wagner 1958; Parks *et al.* 1961). The reduced response to ephedrine and an increased pressor response to phenylephrine suggested that in their patients with autonomic failure there was a postganglionic sympathetic lesion. The response was correlated with changes of hand blood flow but hand blood flow does not necessarily reflect forearm flow and even flow in one forearm may not reflect muscle flow in the other forearm and still less in the critically involved circulations in the splanchnic area and legs (Bannister *et al.* 1967). These drugs were reinvestigated using lower-body negative pressure by Bannister *et al.* (1969) who showed that the beneficial effect of phenylephrine on postural hypotension in one out of three patients

Table 32.2. Drugs used in the treatment of postural hypotension

Site of action	*Drugs*	*Predominant action*
Vessels: vasoconstriction		
Adrenoceptor mediated:		
Resistance vessels	Ephedrine	Indirectly acting sympathomimetic
	Midodrine, phenylephrine, methylphenidate	Directly acting sympathomimetics
	Tyramine	Release of noradrenalin
	Clonidine	Postsynaptic α-adrenoceptor agonist
	Yohimbine	Presynaptic α_2-adrenoceptor antagonist
Capacitance vessels	Dihydroergotamine	Direct action on α-adrenoceptors
Vessels: prevention of vasodilatation		
	Propanolol	Blockade of β_2-receptors
	Indomethacin	Blockade of prostaglandins
	Metoclopramide	Blockade of dopamine
Vessels: prevention of postprandial hypotension		
	Caffeine	Blockade of adenosine receptors
	SMS 201–995	Blockade of vasodilator peptides
Heart: stimulation		
	Pindolol	Intrinsic sympathetic action (I.S.A.)
	Xamoterol	
Plasma volume expansion	Fludrocortisone	1. Mineralocorticoid effects 2. Increased plasma volume (large dose) 3. Sensitization of α-receptors to noradrenalin (small dose)
Kidney: reducing diuresis	Desmopressin	Action: V_2-receptors of renal tubules

with AF and MSA was marred by the accompanying recumbent hypertension, which raised serious doubts as to the usefulness of this drug. The problem was reinvestigated later, using single doses and repeated doses of ephedrine with similar conclusions (Davies *et al.* 1978).

Another pressor drug reported to be beneficial in patients with autonomic failure is midodrine (Schirger *et al.* 1981). This is an α-agonist with constrictor effects on both arterioles and venous capacity vessels, without apparent effect on the heart. Several of the patients studied were also taking fludrocortisone and, in one, metoprolol was used in addition to attempt to reduce the recumbent hypertension. Like other drugs, in which early encouraging results have been reported, midodrine requires a rigorously controlled trial.

One potential future advance may be the utilization of devices which are closely linked to blood pressure control and postural change and which administer short-acting drugs such as noradrenalin when needed. One such device is that of Polinsky *et al.* (1983). They used an electromechanical device, utilizing the arterial transducer, to record blood pressure from one arm while controlling the rate of an intravenous infusion of noradrenalin into the opposite arm (see Fig. 32.9). Advances in this approach using either implantable devices or mini-infusion pumps, linked to a non-invasive method of measuring blood pressure might be the way ahead in severely impaired patients in whom multiple drug therapy has failed.

Drugs acting as vasoconstrictors can be broadly divided as follows:

1. Directly acting agents. A variety of agents have been used which act directly on α-adrenoceptors. These include agents such as phenylephrine, methylphenidate, and midodrine. These drugs are α-agonists which in some trials have been reported to be of benefit. A factor to be kept in mind is the potential of these agents to cause severe constriction in peripheral vessels. This might be a disadvantage especially in the elderly who are more likely to have peripheral vascular abnormalities.
2. Indirectly acting agents. Ephedrine acts by both releasing noradrenalin and also by acting directly on adrenoceptors. This drug may have a role in patients with incomplete lesions, where a combination of its direct effects and the release of noradrenalin may be of benefit. As with this and with other agents the potential to cause supine hypertension is always present. The value of the drug in patients with severe sympathetic lesions is probably minimal.

Drugs releasing noradrenalin predominantly

Tyramine is an agent which raises blood pressure by the release of noradrenalin at the sympathetic nerve endings. In some patients with autonomic failure there may be sufficient intact nerve endings for this to

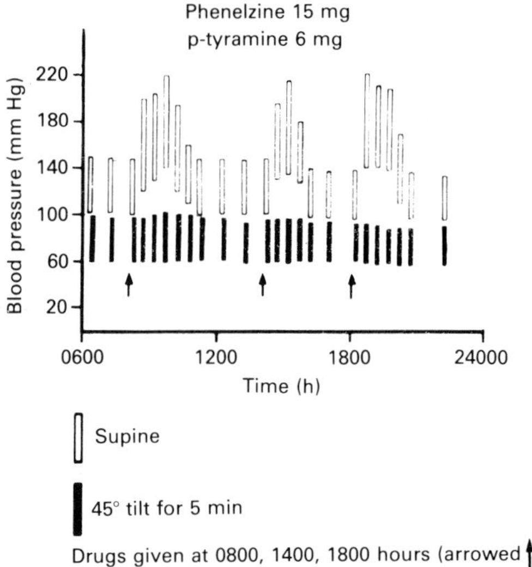

Fig. 32.8. Blood pressure and heart rate before and after treatment of a patient with pure autonomic failure with phenelzine and *p*-tyramine. (Taken with permission from Davies *et al.* (1978).)

be achieved, and the effects of tyramine can be potentiated by the concurrent administration of a monoamine-oxidase inhibitor as used by Diamond *et al.* (1970) and Nanda *et al.* (1970). A number of foods contain p-tyramine, such as cheese and this may have been partially responsible for the erratic responses, except that these were also obtained using chemically pure p-tyramine. Studies with the combination of p-tyramine and phenelzine in our unit resulted in marked fluctuation of blood pressure, with pronounced supine hypertension which was potentially hazardous (Fig. 32.8; Davies *et al.* 1978). It appeared that the improvement in postural hypotension caused by this combination was less effective than that caused by phenylephrine or ephedrine alone.

α_2-Adrenoceptor agonist: clonidine

Clonidine is an α_2-adrenoceptor agonist, which is highly lipophilic and has actions both centrally and peripherally. Its central actions, which result in withdrawal of sympathetic tone are responsible for the fall in supine blood pressure in both normal subjects and in hypertensive patients. In tetraplegics, therefore, with a decentralized sympathetic nervous system clonidine does not lower resting blood pressure; however, it is capable of attenuating the pressor response to bladder stimulation indicating that it may have effects either on spinal sympathetic neurons or on presynaptic α_2-receptors in the periphery (Mathias *et al.* 1979). When given intravenously to tetraplegics there is an initial pressor response (Mathias and Frankel, unpublished observations) which results

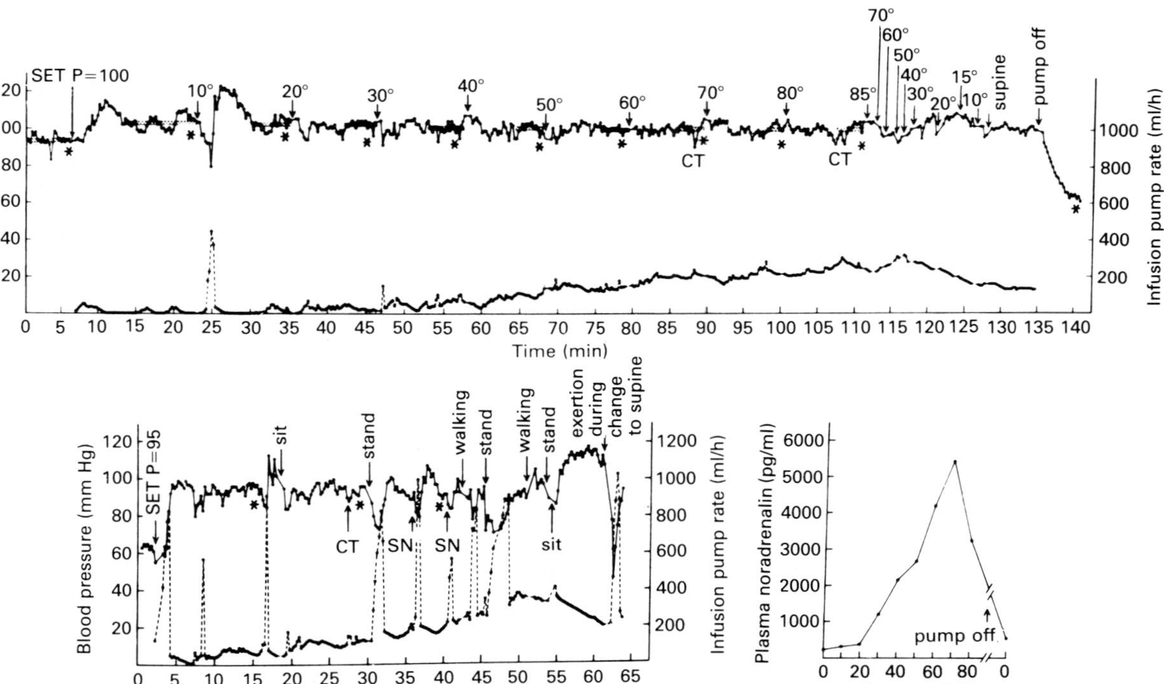

Fig. 32.9. Mean blood pressure (●——●), noradrenalin infusion rate (●– –●), and plasma noradrenalin levels during clinical trial of sympathetic neural prosthesis. The shaded area in the upper graph represents the average mean blood pressure (±SEM) during that interval. The * indicates points at which blood samples were obtained. CT, clear throat; SN, sneeze. (Taken with permission from Polinsky *et al.* (1983).)

from its normally transient peripheral postsynaptic effects causing vasoconstriction. These are probably a combination of both α_1- and α_2-receptor effects. These effects are probably the basis for the observations of the benefit of clonidine in some patients with autonomic failure (Robertson *et al.* 1981). In four of their patients with low supine plasma noradrenalin levels and supersensitivity to phenylephrine oral clonidine (0.4 mg b.i.d.) was beneficial and provided long-term improvement in postural hypotension in two patients. Our own experience with the use of clonidine in autonomic failure patients has not been as favourable as that of Robertson *et al.* and it may be that the drug is only of benefit in those with complete lesions involving postganglionic fibres where there is extreme pressor sensitivity to α-adrenoceptor agents.

Presynaptic α_2-adrenoceptor antagonist: yohimbine

Yohimbine is an α_2-adrenoceptor antagonist which can act both centrally and peripherally. The blockade of presynaptic α_2-adrenoceptors may facilitate the release of noradrenalin at nerve terminals. The drug has been used in single doses with benefit in six patients with autonomic failure where it was likely that they had partial lesions, thus resulting in accentuation of noradrenalin release. The drug may, therefore, have a role in certain patients with autonomic failure and incomplete lesions. It has not been evaluated in the long term and it may not have any advantages over ephedrine.

Predominantly venoconstrictor agents with direct action on α-receptors: dihydroergotamine

Dihydroergotamine has a long history in treatment of postural hypotension, since reports by Mellander and Nordenfelt (1970) and Nordenfelt and Mellander (1972). It acts as a direct α-agonist, stimulating venous capacity vessels, though resistance vessels may even show slight dilatation when normally innervated. It increases central blood volume by about 120 ml with only a slight rise in venous pressure. Nordenfelt and Mellander (1972) studied patients with intact sympathetic function but liable to syncope ('sympathotonic' orthostatic hypotension) and their results are not applicable to AF. When there is sympathetic denervation as in autonomic failure, dihydroergotamine almost certainly causes constriction of resistance vessels (Bevegard *et al.* 1974). It is highly effective after venous injection and abolishes postural hypotension almost completely for half an hour even in severe cases of progressive autonomic failure. It also prevents the fall in pressure during phase II of the Valsalva manoeuvre, but this benefit is obtained at the price of severe recumbent hypertension. The effectiveness of intravenous dihydroergotamine was confirmed by Jennings *et al.* (1979), in two patients with PAF and two with AF and MSA. They showed reduction of the excessive fall of central blood volume on standing. An oral dose of 30 mg daily was needed in three out of four patients to improve their postural hypotension and the addition of fludrocortisone resulted in further improvement.

The major disadvantage with dihydroergotamine is its poor bioavailability. One approach has been to combine it with oral glyceryl trinitrate, which was reported to increase its bioavailability (Bobik *et al.* 1981) and thus increase its efficacy. Repeat studies however using such a combination in our patients with autonomic failure did not provide any evidence of beneficial effect, when dihydroergotamine with placebo was compared against dihydroergotamine in combination with 0.5 mg of glyceryl trinitrate. In some patients there may have even been a fall in blood pressure, presumably because of the vasodilator effects of glyceryl trinitrate. Increasing the daily oral dose of dihydroergotamine may be of benefit in some patients, keeping in mind the potential complication of peripheral vasoconstriction. Dihydroergotamine can also be given parenterally, either subcutaneously or intramuscularly, as in the prevention of thromboembolic complications. It has been used intramuscularly in patients with autonomic failure resulting from alcoholism and diabetes with benefit (Hoeldtke *et al.* 1986). Other ergot derivatives have also been assessed in patients with autonomic failure. Ergotamine tartrate can be given orally, and has been used in doses of 2 to 5 mg daily with some benefit in patients with autonomic failure (Chobanian *et al.* 1983).

Prevention of vasodilatation

A variety of drugs have been used on the premise that blood-pressure control can be improved by preventing vasodilatatory mechanisms.

β-adrenoceptor blockade: propanolol

Propanolol was introduced in the treatment of autonomic failure on the grounds, despite the obvious α-adrenoceptor defect, that β-agonist induced vasodilatation might also contribute to the orthostatic hypotension (Abboud and Eckstein 1966) and should be reversed by the β-adrenoceptor blocking properties of propranolol. It may also act on presynaptic β-receptors and so reduce the release of noradrenalin. A third effect might result from the β-blocking effect by increasing adrenal release of noradrenalin and adrenalin which occurs on exercise in normal individuals treated with β-receptor blocking drugs (Irving *et al.* 1974). Chobanian *et al.* (1977) reported beneficial effects in four patients with a diagnosis of pure autonomic failure on oral propranolol in doses of 40 to 240 mg daily, but as they were already taking 0.3 to 0.5 mg fludrocortisone daily and had an excessive salt intake, no clear conclusion can be drawn. They later withdrew propranolol in one patient because it caused severe recumbent hypertension and they reported that in two patients episodes of syncope still occurred in the early morning when orthostatic intolerance was most severe. In practice, propranolol has not proved sufficiently encouraging for other trials to be reported, possibly because of its cardiac β-blocking effects. Propranolol, however, has been shown to be effective in the treatment of hyper-bradykinism, a rare cause of orthostatic hypotension (Streeten *et al.* 1972).

Other forms of orthostatic hypotension have been treated with propranolol. Some patients who have not been studied in detail physiologically or pharmacologically, appear to have no autonomic defect but have orthostatic tachycardia leading to postural hypotension due to a decreased output. The tachycardia is probably emotionally determined and is accompanied by a mounting sense of anxiety when standing, associated with overbreathing, increasing bouts of vagally induced bradycardia, and may eventually lead to syncope. Propranolol reduces the initial tachycardia and benefits such patients. Some patients with AF or diabetes and with sparing of cardiac sympathetic efferents but impaired sympathetic tone to the arterial bed have a compensatory tachycardia and deteriorate if this compensatory mechanism is blocked by propranolol.

Prostaglandin synthetase inhibitors: indomethacin and flurbiprofen

Indomethacin was first proposed on the theoretical basis that some prostaglandins are potent vasodilators and their effect may be inhibited by indomethacin, though indomethacin has several other effects on vascular responses. Kochar and Itskovitz (1978) reported improvement in four patients with postural hypotension due to AF and MSA. However, the diagnosis was uncertain in one of them in that the standing blood pressure was within the normal range for her age and, in all, the diagnosis of AF and MSA was based on clinical features without the benefit of physiological tests. Davies *et al.* (1980) showed that oral indomethacin (50 mg t.d.s.) increased sensitivity to infused noradrenalin and angiotensin II in four patients with AF and MSA but the pressor effect was only significant on recumbent blood pressure, probably because the hydrostatic stresses on standing require compensatory constriction of different blood vesels in different vascular beds. Inhibition of prostaglandin synthesis may be a factor because urinary prostaglandin excretion was greater than in normal subjects and was decreased by indomethacin. The lack of improvement in the standing blood pressure might also have been due to a decrease in plasma renin activity due to indomethacin. Abate *et al.* (1979) studied 12 patients with postural hypotension and Parkinson's disease both after intravenous infusion of indomethacin and after a dose of 50 mg daily for five days and reported improvement. Insufficient information was given about the clinical and physiological state of the patients but the postural fall suggests some may have had AF with Parksinson's disease or early MSA; details of frequency, time, and duration of standing before blood-pressure measurement were not stated. Watt *et al.* (1981) have shown benefit from the combined effect of fludrocortisone and flurbiprofen in PAF. Since both prostaglandin inhibitors and fludrocortisone have pressor effects, we have decided in some cases failing to respond to fludrocortisone alone to add indomethacin since both substances appear to increase smooth muscle sensitivity to noradrenalin and, in larger doses, may increase blood volume.

Dopamine antagonists: metoclopramide

Metoclopramide a dopamine antagonist has been used in the treatment of autonomic failure, on the basis that metoclopramide blocks the vasodilator effects of dopamine. In a single patient with postural hypotension after an extensive sympathectomy, Kuchel *et al.* (1980) reported an improvement in the postural hypotension. They postulated that this was the result of the drug inhibiting the vasodilator and natriuretic effects of the excess dopamine released. However, caution is necessary in patients with supersensitivity of central dopamine receptors who may be vulnerable to the extrapyramidal side-effects.

Drugs preventing postprandial hypotension (see Chapter 20)

Dilatation within the splanchnic circulation following a meal is probably the cause of the marked postprandial fall in blood pressure in autonomic failure patients. Splanchnic vasodilatation may result from the release of vasodilatatory neuropeptides. Drugs such as indomethacin and dihydroergotamine seem to have minimal effects in preventing post-prandial hypotension. Recently, two other agents have been used with benefit.

Caffeine

Caffeine is a methylxanthine which occurs naturally and raises blood pressure in normal subjects. This is thought to be by increasing sympathetic nervous activity or by activating the renin–angiotensin system. In 12 patients with autonomic failure caffeine prevented the fall in pressure induced by a standard meal (Onrot *et al.* 1985). This occurred both acutely and when it had been administered over a period of 7 days. The prevention of hypotension was not related to activation of the renin–angiotensin system nor to stimulation of sympathoadrenal activity. It may be therefore that blockade of vasodilatatory adenosine receptors was responsible although suppression of vasodilatatory gut peptides was not excluded. Two cups of coffee could be expected to contain between 200 and 250 mg of caffeine and the authors suggested that this would provide sufficient caffeine to help reduce postprandial hypotension.

Somatostatin analogues

These agents, especially the new one (SMS 201-995) have the potential to prevent the release of a variety of peptides, including those released following food ingestion. This was first used in patients with autonomic failure as a result of diabetes and alcoholism and prevented postprandial hypotension (Hoeldtke *et al.* 1986). This has now been confirmed by our group in seven patients with chronic autonomic failure who were challenged with a glucose meal (unpublished). SMS 201–995 is so far only available for subcutaneous use, which limits its use, but advances are being made in relation to its oral administration which could be of particular benefit in such patients.

Drugs acting on the heart

Pindolol

Pindolol has additional partial β-agonist adrenoceptor activity (so-called intrinsic sympathomimetic activity) which should cause less reduction in resting heart rate than a pure β-blocker might be expected to cause. The initial encouraging report was by Frewin *et al.* (1980) on two patients with diabetic autonomic neuropathy who probably had supersensitivity to noradrenalin. It was followed by Man in't Veld and Schalekamp (1981), who showed benefits in three patients with AF, two of whom had amyloidosis and one following acute autonomic neuropathy. They argued that when receptor occupancy is low, as is assumed in the post-ganglionic lesion of AF, there was a strong possibility that even a partial β-agonist would act as a full agonist and its agonist effect would be enhanced by denervation hypersensitivity and lack of baroreflexes. They also raised the possibility that pindolol might have an effect on β-receptors in veins and, like dihydroergotamine, might increase venous tone. They showed that the improvement in postural hypotension was due to an improvement in cardiac output but vascular resistance was unchanged. Their patients had an increase in cardiac rate. However, this enthusiasm was premature. Davidson and Smith (1981) reported no benefit from pindolol in three patients with autonomic neuropathy and two with amyloid. Davies *et al.* (1981) reported briefly on five patients studied under standard conditions after a control period. Pindolol was given in an adequate dose gauged by the heart-rate response to intravenous isoprenaline but did not increase blood pressure or cause symptomatic benefit at any dose level. The trend was towards decrease in lying and standing pressures. Pindolol did not have a chronotropic action and there was instead a tendency for the pulse rate to decrease with increasing doses of pindolol. Two patients had raised jugular venous pressure after 3 days on 15 mg daily and frank cardiac failure after 45 mg daily for 3 days. Pindolol causes a rightward shift of the isoprenaline dose-response curve so that, although in theory pindolol acts more as a sympathetic agonist than competitive antagonist, its β-blocking action was still pronounced. In our patients there was evidence of increased receptor numbers and denervation supersensitivity to noradrenalin. The view put forward by Man in't Veld and Schalekamp (1981) that their patients responded because of the partial agonist effect of pindolol may therefore not be the only explanation.

Prenalterol and xamoterol

Two other β-blockers with β_1-adrenoceptor partial agonist effects have been assessed in autonomic failure. Prenalterol was found to be effective (Goovaerts *et al.* 1984). More recently, xamoterol has also been shown in a larger number of patients to benefit postural hypotension (Mehlsen and Trap-Jensen 1985). These drugs, unlike pindolol which has the potential to cause cardiac failure should be less likely to induce this complication.

Plasma volume expansion and reducing natriuresis

Fludrocortisone

Fludrocortisone is the most commonly used drug treatment and has multiple pharmacological effects (Chobanian *et al.* 1979). In an initial dose of 0.1 mg daily, in some patients with autonomic failure, fludrocortisone approaches most closely to the ideal of a drug which increases effective vasoconstriction on standing, by augmenting the action of noradrenalin released by normal sympathetic efferent activity but without aggravating recumbent hypertension. In normal subjects fludrocortisone sensitizes vascular receptors to pressor amines (Raab *et al.* 1950; Schmidt *et al.* 1966). Studies by Tobian and Redleaf (1958) indicated that fludrocortisone may also increase the fluid content of vessel walls, so increasing their resistance to stretching.

In a study of four patients with AF and MSA, 0.1 mg of fludrocortisone daily did not increase body weight but caused a shift to the left of the noradrenalin infusion sensitivity curve and a significant rise in standing blood pressure (Davies *et al.* 1979). This effect may be less apparent in patients with pure autonomic failure (Chobanian *et al.* 1979). We speculated whether fludrocortisone might either increase the number of α-receptors or change their structure, or decrease the clearance rate by the uptake $_2$ mechanism by smooth muscle of blood vessels. Davies *et al.* (1982) and Bannister *et al.* (1981) have shown that there is an increase in the α-receptors of platelets and β-receptors of lymphocytes in autonomic failure and these changes are increased further after treatment with fludrocortisone (see Chapter 19). In autonomic failure there is also an increase in the pressor response to angiotensin II which is not affected by fludrocortisone, indicating a probable change in angiotensin vascular receptors as well as α-adrenoceptors (Davies *et al.* 1979).

In a higher dose fludrocortisone can, with careful supervision, expand the blood volume, improve cardiac output, and so reduce postural hypotension. Patients with AF have a normal or slightly low plasma volume when supine but this does not, as in normal subjects, fall on standing, probably because the lowered arterial pressure compensates for the raised hydrostatic pressure in the legs on standing. Patients with AF lose twice as much body weight as control subjects when on a low-sodium diet, with a corresponding increase in their postural hypotension. The resting plasma renin activity in AF is usually low, with a reduced rise on standing, though this is increased by sodium restriction or by dopamine infusion. This suggests that renin synthesis and storage are intact but release may be defective. Aldosterone secretion is usually reduced in autonomic failure but the defect is likely to be the result of a chronic reduction of angiotensin stimulation of aldosterone secretion, rather than an adrenal defect. The dose of fludrocortisone likely to increase the blood volume by replacing aldosterone levels without overloading the circulation requires delicate and continuous adjustment, in contrast to a patient with Addison's disease, probably because of the baroreflex defect. As with other forms of treatment, each patient shows variations in response which are the result of the different types of lesion present in each patient.

Desmopressin

Desmopressin (DDAVP) is a vasopressin-like agent which specifically acts upon the V_2-receptors on the renal tubules, which are responsible for the antidiuretic effects of vasopressin. It has virtually no activity on the V_1-receptor, which is responsible for the vasoconstriction induced by vasopressin. In patients with autonomic failure, nocturnal polyuria, overnight weight loss, and the subsequent reduction in extracellular fluid volume and probably intravascular volume accounts for the low morning blood pressures and for the increased severity of symptoms from postural hypotension. Intramuscular DDAVP prevents nocturnal polyuria, reduces overnight weight loss, and raises the supine blood pressure in the morning, thus improving symptoms resulting from postural change (Mathias *et al.* 1986) (Fig. 32.10). Because of the lack of direct vascular effects of DDAVP an increased tendency to supine hypertension is not present. Studies with intranasal DDAVP indicate that it is equally effective in the short term and also in the long term: doses between 5 and 40 μg given at bedtime as a single dose are of benefit both in relation to preventing nocturia (which can be a problem especially in those with bladder involvement) and also morning postural hypotension.

DDAVP, however, has the potential to cause side-effects. Some patients are exquisitely sensitive to its action and hyponatraemia can readily ensue. This is best evaluated by determining the patients responses to intramuscular DDAVP in a hospital environment and under close supervision. Small doses of intranasal DDAVP can then be administered in appropriate doses, again under careful supervision to ensure that hyponatraemia does not occur before stabilization on an out-patient basis. In some patients natriuresis continues as before and occasionally is in excess and DDAVP needs to be combined with

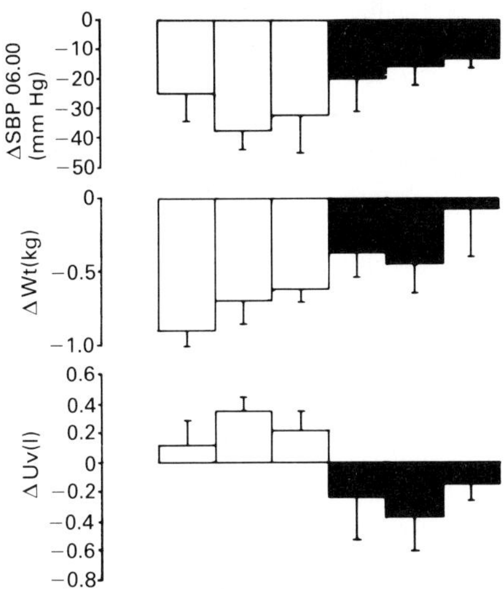

Fig. 32.10. Desmopressin (DDAVP) in the treatment of autonomic failure. From above, morning postural hypotension, difference between sitting and lying systolic pressure (ΔSBP), change in body weight overnight (ΔWt), and change in urine volume between night and day (ΔUv). The open rectangles show the changes during a 3-day control period and the closed rectangles the changes after 2 μg i.m. of DDAVP each evening for 3 days. The mean results in five patients with autonomic failure show after DDAVP a reduction in postural hypotension, and the gain in extracellular and intravascular fluid volume as measured by the reduction in nocturnal weight loss and nocturnal urinary volume.

fludrocortisone and sodium supplements to ensure that the patient remains in sodium balance. We have treated patients with intranasal DDAVP for over a year with no long-term side-effects and with monitoring of osmolality and plasma sodium levels on a 6-weekly or 2-monthly basis.

REFERENCES

Abate, G., Polimeni, R. M., Cuccurollo, F., Puddo, P., and Lenzi, S. (1979). Effects of indomethacin on postural hypotension in parkinsonism. *Br. med. J.* **ii**, 1466–8.

Abboud, F. W. and Eckstein, J. W. (1966). Active reflex vasodilatation in man. *Fed. Proc. Fed. Am. Soc. exp. Biol.* **25**, 1611–17.

Bannister, R., Ardill, L., and Fentem, P. (1967). Defective autonomic control of blood vessels in idiopathic orthostatic hypotension. *Brain* **90**, 725–46.

Bannister, R., Ardill, L., and Fentem, P. (1969). An assessment of various methods of treatment of idiopathic orthostatic hypotension. *Quart. J. Med.* **38**, 377–95.

Bannister, R., Boylston, A. W., Davies, I. B., Mathias, C. J., Sever, P. S., and Sudera, D. (1981). Beta-receptor numbers and thermodynamics in denervation supersensitivity. *J. Physiol., London* **319**, 369–77.

Bannister, R., da Costa, D. F., Hendry, C. H., Jacobs, J., and Mathias, C. J. (1986). Atrial demand pacing to protect against vagal overactivity in sympathetic autonomic neuropathy. *Brain* **109**, 345–56.

Bannister, R., Sever, P., and Gross, M. (1977). Cardiovascular reflexes and biochemical responses in progressive autonomic failure. *Brain* **100**, 327–44.

Barnett, A. J. and Wagner, G. R. (1958). Severe orthostatic hypotension: case report and description of response to sympatheticomimetic drugs. *Am. Heart. J.* **56**, 412–24.

Bevegard, S., Castenfors, J., and Lindblad, L.-E. (1974). Haemodynamic effects of dihydroergotamine in patients with postural hypotension. *Acta med. scand.* **196**, 473–7.

Bobik, A., Jennings, G., Skews, H., Esler, M., and McLean, A. (1981). Low oral bioavailability of dihydroergotamine and first-pass extraction in patients with orthostatic hypotension. *Clin. Pharmacol. Ther.* **30**, 673–9.

Caronna, J. J. and Plum, F. (1973). Cerebrovascular regulation in preganglionic and postganglionic autonomic insufficiency. *Stroke* **4**, 12–19.

Chobanian, A. V., Tifft, C., Faxon, D. P., Creager, M. A., and Sackel. H. (1983). Treatment of orthostatic hypotension with ergotamine. *Circulation* **67**, 602–9.

Chobanian, A. V., Volicer, L., Liang, C. S., Kershaw, G., and Tifft, C. (1977). Use of propranolol in the treatment of idiopathic orthostatic hypotension. *Trans. Ass. Am. Physns.* **90**, 324–34.

Chobanian, A. V., Volicer, L., Tifft, C., Gavras, H., Liang, C., and Faxon, D. (1979). Mineralocorticoid-induced hypertension in patients with orthostatic hypotension. *New Engl. J. Med.* **301**, 68–73.

Davidson, A. C. and Smith, S. E. (1981). Pindolol in orthostatic hypertension. *Br. med. J.* **282**, 1704(c).

Davies, B., Bannister, R., Hensby, C., and Sever, P. (1980). The pressor actions of noradrenaline, angiotensin II in chronic autonomic failure treated with indomethacin. *Br. J. clin. Pharmacol.* **10**, 223–9.

Davies, B., Bannister, R., Mathias, C., and Sever, P. (1981). Pindolol in postural hypotension; the case for caution. *Lancet* **i**, 982–3(c).

Davies, B., Bannister, R., and Sever, P. (1978). Pressor amines and monoamine-oxidase inhibitors for treatment of postural hypotension in progressive autonomic failure. Limitations and hazards. *Lancet* **i**, 172–5.

Davies, B., Bannister, R., Sever, P., and Wilcox, C. S. (1979). The pressor actions of noradrenaline, angiotensin II and saralasin in chronic autonomic failure treated with fludrocortisone. *Br. J. clin. Pharmacol.* **8**, 253–60.

Davies, B., Sudera, D., Sagnella, E., Marchese-Saviotti, E., Mathias, C., Bannister, R., and Sever, P. (1982). Increased numbers of alpha-receptors in sympathetic denervation supersensitivity in man. *J. clin. Invest.* **69**, 779–84.

Diamond, M. A., Murray, R. H., and Schmid, P. G. (1970). Idiopathic postural hypotension; physiologic observations and report of a new mode of therapy. *J. clin. Invest.* **49**, 1341–8.

Frewin, D. B., Leonello, P. P., Pentall, R. K., Hughes, L., and Harding, P. E. (1980). Pindolol in orthostatic hypotension; possible therapy? *Med. J. Aust.* **1**, 128.

Goovaerts, J., Ver faillie, C., Fagard, R., and Knochaert, D. (1984). Effect of prenalterolol on orthostatic hypotension in the Shy–Drager syndrome. *Br. med. J.* **288**, 817–18.

Hoeldtke, R. D., O'Dorisio, T. M., and Boden, G. (1986). Treatment of autonomic neuropathy with a somatostatin analogue. S.M.S.-201.995. *Lancet* **ii**, 602–5.

Irving, M. H., Britton, B. J., Wood, W. G., Padgham, C., and Carruthers, M. (1974). Effects of beta adrenergic blockade on plasma catecholamines in exercise. *Nature, London* **248**, 531–3.

Jennings, G., Esler, M., and Holmes, R. (1979). Treatment of orthostatic hypotension with dihydroergotamine. *Br. med. J.* **ii**, 307–8.

Kochar, M. S. and Itskovitz, H. D. (1978). Treatment of idiopathic orthostatic hypotension (Shy–Drager syndrome) with indomethacin. *Lancet* **i**, 1011–14.

Kuchel, O., Buu, N. T., Gutkowska, J., and Genest, J. (1980). Treatment of severe orthostatic hypotension by metoclopramide. *Ann. intern. Med.* **93**, 841–3.

Maclean, A. R. and Allen, E. V. (1940). Orthostatic hypotension and orthostatic tachycardia. Treatment with the 'head-up' bed. *J. Am. med. Ass.* **115**, 2162–7.

Man in't Veld, A. J. and Schalekamp, M. A. D. H. (1981). Pindolol acts as beta-adrenoceptor agonist in orthostatic hypotension: therapeutic implications. *Br. med. J.* **282**, 929–31.

Mann, S., Altman, D. G., Raftery, E. B., and Bannister, R. (1983). *Circulation* **68**, 477–83.

Mathias, C. J., Fosbraey, P., da Costa, D. F., Thorley, A., and Bannister, R. (1986). Desmopressin reduces nocturnal polyuria, reverses overnight weight loss and improves morning postural hypotension in autonomic failure. *Br. med. J.* **293**, 353–4.

Mathias, C. J., Reid, J. L., Wing, L. M. H., Frankel, H. L., and Christensen, N. J. (1979). Antihypertensive effects of clonidine in tetraplegic subjects devoid of central sympathetic control. *Clin. Sci.* **57**, 425–6.

Mehlsen, J. and Trap-Jensen, J. (1985). Use of xamoterol, a new selective beta-adrenoceptor partial agonist, in the treatment of postural hypotension. *Proc.*

Cardiovasc. Pharmacotherapy Int. Symp. Geneva. Abs 73. ICI.

Mellander, S. and Nordenfelt, I. (1970). Comparative effects of dihydroergotamine and noradrenaline on resistance, exchange and capacity functions in the peripheral circulation. *Clin. Sci.* **31**, 183–201.

Meyer, J. S., Shirmazu, K., Fukuuchi, Y., Ohuchi, T., Okamolo, S., Koto, A., and Friesson, A. D. (1973). Cerebral dysautoregulation in central neurogenic orthostatic hypotension (Shy–Drager syndrome). *Neurology, Minneapolis* **23**, 262–73.

Moss, A. J., Glaser, W., and Topol, E. (1980). Atrial tachypacing in the treatment of a patient with primary orthostatic hypotension. *New Engl. J. Med.* **302**, 1456–7.

Nanda, R. N., Johnson, R. H., and Keogh, H. J. (1976). Treatment of neurogenic orthostatic hypotension with a monoamine oxidase inhibitor and tyramine. *Lancet* **ii**, 1164–7.

Nordenfelt, I. and Mellander, S. (1792). Central haemodynamic effects of dihydroergotamine in patients with orthostatic hypotension. *Acta. med. scand.* **191**, 115–20.

Onrot, J., Goldberg, M. R., Biaggioni, I., Hollister, A. S., Kincaid, D., and Robertson, D. (1985). Haemodynamic and humoral effects of caffeine in autonomic failure. Therapeutic implications for post-prandial hypotension. *New Engl. J. Med.* **313**, 549–54.

Onrot, J., Goldberg, M. R., Biaggioni, I., Wiley, R. G., Hollister, A. S., and Robertson, D. (1987). Oral yohimbine in human autonomic failure. *Neurology* **37**, 215–20.

Parks, V. J., Sandison, A. G., Skinner, S. L., and Whelan, R. F. (1961). Sympathomimetic drugs in orthostatic hypotension. *Lancet* **i**, 1133–6.

Polinsky, R. J., Samaras, G. M., and Kopin, I. J. (1983). Sympathetic neural prosthesis for managing orthostatic hypotension. *Lancet* **i**, 901–4.

Raab, W., Humphreys, R. J., and Lepeschkin, F. (1950). Potentiation of pressor effects of norepinephrine and ephinephrine in man by desoxycorticosterone acetate. *J. clin. Invest.* **29**, 1397.

Reid, J. L. (1981). The clinical pharmacology of clonidine and related central hypotensive drugs. *Br. J. clin. Pharmacol.* **12**, 295–302.

Robertson, D., Goldberg, M. R., Hollister, A. S., Wode, D., and Robertson, R. M. (1981). Clonidine raises blood pressure in idiopathic orthostatic hypotension. *Circulation* **64**, Abstr. 7.

Schirger. P. G., Sheps, S. G., Thomas, J. E., and Fealey, R. D. (1981). Midodrine—a new agent in the management of idiopathic orthostatic hypotension and Shy–Drager syndrome. *Proc. Staff Meet. Mayo Clin.* **56**, 429–33.

Schmidt, P. G., Eckstein, J. W., and Abboud, F. M. (1966). Effect of 9-alpha-fluorohydrocortisone on forearm vascular responses to norepinephrine. *Circulation* **34**, 620–6.

Sheps, S. G. (1976). The use of an elastic garment in the treatment of idiopathic orthostatic hypotension. *Cardiology* **61**, Suppl. 1, 271–9.

Shinohara, Y. and Gotoh, F. (1973). Autoregulation of cerebral circulation in orthostatic hypotension. (Abstr.) *Stroke* **4**, 372–3.

Skinhoj, E., Oleson, J., and Strandgaard, S. (1971). In *Brain and blood flow* (ed. R. W. Ross Russell), pp. 351–3. Pitman, London.

Streeten, D. H. P., Kerr, L. P., Kerr, C. C., Prior, J. C., and Dalakos, T. G. (1972).

Hyperbradykinism: a new orthostatic syndrome. *Lancet* **ii**, 1048–53.

Thomas, D. J. and Bannister, R. (1980). Preservation of autoregulation of cerebral blood flow in autonomic failure. *J. neurol. Sci.* **44**, 205–12.

Tobian, L. and Redleaf, P. D. (1958). Ionic composition of the aorta in renal and adrenal hypertension. *Am. J. Physiol.* **192**, 325–30.

Watt, S. J., Tooke, J. E., Perkins, C. M., and Lee, M. (1981). The treatment of idiopathic orthostatic hypotension: a combined fludrocortisone–flurbiprofen regime. *Q. Jl Med.* **50**, 205–12.

Wilcox, C. S., Aminoff, M. J., and Slater, J. D. H. (1977). Sodium homeostasis in patients with autonomic failure. *Clin. Sci. mol. Med.* **53**, 321–8.

Wilson, R. J., Mills, I. H., and De Bono, E. (1969). Cardiovascular reflexes and the control of aldosterone production and sodium excretion. *Proc. R. Soc. Med.* **62**, 1257–9.

33. The treatment of multiple system atrophy: striatonigral degeneration and olivopontocerebellar degeneration

A. J. Lees

INTRODUCTION

Problems of classification continue to bedevil the multiple system degenerations and, in common with many other regions of neurological taxonomy, the literature broadly falls into those who prefer to 'lump' and those who prefer to 'split'. Other schisms, however, can be discerned with separate disease entities being claimed on the basis of somewhat speculative genetic, pathological, or biochemical distinctions. Time may prove that multiple system atrophy is indeed a heterogeneous disorder caused by several different biochemical abnormalities. At the present time three separate clinical presentations of multiple system atrophy with autonomic failure are generally accepted as discussed elswhere in this book (see Chapters 1 and 25):

1. Cerebellar presentation with or without ophthalmoplegia. These patients may also have corticospinal tract signs, peripheral neuropathy, retinal abnormalities, and mild extrapyramidal features (the olivopontocerebellar form of multiple system atrophy).
2. A parkinsonian presentation usually with rigidity and bradykinesia with the later development of mild corticospinal signs and evidence of cerebellar degeneration on neuroimaging (the striatonigral form of multiple system atrophy).
3. Autonomic failure presentation with impotence, incontinence of urine, and postural hypotension with the later appearance of cerebellar, extrapyramidal, and corticospinal tract signs.

TREATMENT OF CEREBELLAR SYMPTOMS

Attempts to treat the cerebellar ataxia of multiple system degeneration have so far proved fruitless. Occasional successes have been reported with cholinergic drugs, 5-hydroxytryptophan, isoniazid, baclofen, and propanolol. For the large majority of patients these drugs prove to be ineffective. One intriguing observation is the apparent temporary exacerbation of ataxia by cigarette smoking (Spillane 1955; Graham and Oppenheimer 1969; Johnsen and Miller 1986). The tobacco sensitivity takes the form of an acute increase in unsteadiness of gait and less commonly slurring of speech; extrapyramidal symptoms are not made worse and only one patient had increased orthostatic hypotension. Spillane injected nicotine tartrate intravenously in two of his patients documenting changes identical to those occurring with smoking. The exact mechanism for this effect is unclear but a direct effect on the central nervous system is more probable than a secondary effect due to autonomic changes. Nicotine is known to increase the release of acetylcholine in many areas of the brain and probably also releases noradrenalin, dopamine, 5-hydroxytryptamine, and other neurotransmitters. Nicotinic systems may therefore play a role in cerebellar function. Johnsen and Miller (1986) suggested that trials with the nicotinic antagonist dihydro-β-erythroidine might be worthwhile in the cerebellar degenerations.

TREATMENT OF THE PARKINSONIAN SYMPTOMS

Striatonigral degeneration is frequently clinically indistinguishable from idiopathic Parkinson's disease and may be considerably underdiagnosed. Of the first 50 parkinsonian brains collected by The Parkinson's Disease Society Brain Bank approximately 15 per cent had multiple system degeneration at post-mortem. Helpful distinguishing clues, however, include the relative infrequency of a rest tremor, a greater tendency to symmetry of physical signs, the rather more malignant course, and the less reliable response to L-dopa therapy. Some of these cases will develop corticospinal tract signs and less commonly mild cerebellar signs. Computerized axial tomography frequently reveals striking cerebellar atrophy and brainstem atrophy which is not usually found in Parkinson's disease. Pastakia and colleagues (1986) demonstrated associated striking putaminal atrophy on the T1 magnetic resonance imaging (MRI) scans and abnormally decreased signal density in various brainstem structures on the T2 weighted sequences and it seems probable that advanced in MRI technology will improve the accuracy of clinical diagnosis of parkinsonian plus syndromes in the future. In striatonigral degeneration there is a severe depletion of nigral cells with a concomitant reduction in striatal dopamine. In contrast to Parkinson's disease, however, there is believed to be a severe supranigral lesion with involvement of central cholinergic systems (Spokes *et al.* 1979). If one reviews the therapeutic effects of levodopa on histologically proven cases of the striatonigral form of degeneration (see Table 33.1), the results are disappointing. Of the 21 patients in the literature only one patient derived sustained improvement with dyskinesias whereas another six derived initial benefit lasting for up to six months. Eight of these patients also had clinical autonomic failure and in only two of these did transient benefit in extrapyramidal clinical features occur. If one reviews therapeutic results in presumed cases of multiple system atrophy, however, the picture is a little brighter. Aminoff and colleagues (1973) treated five cases of multiple system atrophy with autonomic failure with L-dopa (1.25–3.50 g) and four of the five got worse with respect to their parkinsonian disabilities although two had some modest increase in the level of their standing blood pressure and three in their lying blood pressure. Sharpe and colleagues (1973) treated a 58-year-old man with small doses of L-dopa and a monoamine oxidase inhibitor in an attempt to produce anti-parkinsonian benefit and a controlled rise in his postural hypotension. Worthwhile benefit occurred with respect to tremor and rigidity but only minimal improvement in bradykinesia. Goetz *et al.* (1984) reported that 16 of 19 patients treated with L-dopa obtained definite improvement in rigidity and bradykinesia and postural tremor was helped in two. Ten of the patients experienced drug-induced chorea and five had hallucinations. Lang and colleagues (1986) reported three patients with parkinsonian syndrome and cerebellar atrophy on CT scan which they thought was multiple system atrophy who have derived sustained benefit from L-dopa preparations with the emergence of on–off oscillations. Modest rises in standing blood pressure have occasionally been reported with L-dopa though severe increase in orthostatic hypotension may also occur.

Results with the newer synthetic ergolenes bromocriptine, lisuride, and pergolide have been even more disappointing. Goetz and colleagues (1984) using doses of 10–80 mg daily of bromocriptine reported benefit in five patients who had responded to L-dopa and one patient who had failed to respond to L-dopa. Williams *et al.* (1979) also reported temporary benefit in an occasional patient; others have had more disappointing results (Gautier and Durand 1977). In a controlled trial with lisuride (mean dose 2.4 mg daily) only one of seven patients with MSA with autonomic failure derived modest improvement in parkinsonian features and another who had been deriving considerable benefit from levodopa treatment before the study began failed to respond at all to large doses of lisuride. Severe psychiatric side-effects occurred in six patients with nightmares, isolated visual hallucinations, and toxic confusional states of the sort which have more recently been encountered when using lisuride in ambulatory pump systems in Parkinson's disease (Lees and Bannister 1981). A trial of pergolide by the

Table 33.1. The therapeutic effects of levodopa on histologically proven cases of striatonigral degeneration (± autonomic failure) (all patients had severe rigidity and bradykinesia

				Clinical features						*Levodopa treatment*			
Reference	*Sex*	*Age at onset (y)*	*Duration of disease (y)*	*Tremor*	*Dysarthria*	*Pyramidal signs*	*Cerebellar signs*	*Postural hypotension*	*Sphincter dysfunction*	*Duration at onset (y)*	*Max. dosage (mg/day)*	*Results*	*Adverse effects*
Izumi *et al.* 1971	M	51	2			+				1	6400	No effect	None
	F	53	3							2	2600	No effect	None
Greet *et al.* 1971	F	73	4	+						3	1200	Marked benefit for 6 months	None
Bannister and Oppenheimer 1972	F	48	6		+	+		+		3	3000	No effect	Severe postural hypotension
Rajput *et al.* 1972	F	56	7		+				+	7	5000	No effect	None
		63	7		+	+	+			7	5000	No effect	Severe postural hypotension
Trotter 1973	F	66	8	+		+				4	8000	Modest benefit for 3 months	Orofacial dyskinesia
Sharpe *et al.* 1973	F	41	6	+	+	+				5	6000	Modest benefit for 2 months	Nausea
Takei and Mirra 1973	F	66	2		+					1	3000	No effect	None
Schober *et al.* 1975	F	53	3	+	+	+		+	+	1	2000* 3000	Modest benefit for 6 months	Rise in erect **pressure**
Michel *et al.* 1976	M	61	3		+	+			+	2	3000	No effect	none
	F	61	2		+	+			+	1	600* 3000	No effect	None
Boudin *et al.* 1976	F	59	7		+	+			+	3	600* 5000	No effect	None
	F	56	4		+	+			+	2	800* 4000	Modest benefit for 6 months	Orofacial dyskenesia

Table 33.1. (*cont.*)

Reference	*Sex*	*Age at onset (y)*	*Duration of disease (y)*	*Clinical features*						*Levodopa treatment*			
				Tremor	*Dysarthria*	*Pyramidal signs*	*Cerebellar signs*	*Postural hypotension*	*Sphincter dysfunction*	*Duration at onset (y)*	*Max. dosage (mg/day)*	*Results*	*Adverse effects*
DeLean and Deck 1976	M	54	6	+		+		+	+	4	1000	Modest benefit for 3 months	Rise in erect blood pressure
Rajput and Rozdilsky 1976	M	46	5	+	+	+		+	+	4	750*	No effect	Severe postural hypotension
Fève *et al.* 1977	F	61	4	+						1	3000	Marked benefit for 3 years	Dyskinesias
Spokes *et al.* 1979	M	70	9		+	+	+	+	+			No effect	None
	M	49	9		+	+		+	+			No effect	None
	M	51	4	+	+	+		+	+			No effect	None
	F	53	5	+	+	+		+	+			No effect	None

* In combination with a peripheral dopa decarboxylase inhibitor.

author in four patients with MSA with autonomic failure also failed to produce worthwhile responses.

A severe reduction in the levels of noradrenalin in the central nervous system also occurs in both Parkinson's disease and multiple system degeneration but so far trials with drugs known to enhance or antagonize noradrenalin seem to be without substantial effect in either disorder. Administration of threo-3,4-dihydroxyphenylserine(L-threo-DOPS), a non-physiological amino acid which can be converted by dopa decarboxylase to noradrenalin was shown by Birkmayer more than 20 years ago to increase standing blood pressure. In the belief that some of the refractory symptoms of Parkinson's disease such as freezing, poor balance, and dysarthria might be due to noradrenalin deficiency caused by severely lowered dopamine-β-hydroxylase activity, Narabayashi and colleagues (1986) have administered first DL-threo-DOPS and then more recently L-threo-DOPS to a large number of patients with parkinsonian syndrome. These authors have shown clear penetration of L-threo-DOPS into the central nervous system but it is not yet known whether the agent is able to increase the level of noradrenalin. Among the patients treated were six patients with multiple system atrophy and autonomic failure and 20 with a condition labelled as pure akinesia by Narabayashi. This latter syndrome consists of severe akinesia with hypotonia and freezing without tremor or rigidity but with the late emergence of supranuclear ophthalmoplegia in some patients. No post-mortem data is as yet available but it is possible that some of these cases may turn out to have multiple system atrophy. Of the six patients with multiple system atrophy and autonomic failure, three showed a slight improvement, one was unchanged, one was worse, and one was impossible to rate. In contrast, in the pure akinesia group two showed marked improvement, three moderate improvement, eight slight improvement, four no change, one worsened, and two were impossible to rate. The authors concluded that two-thirds of the cases with pure akinesia were benefited with dramatic improvement in freezing in two individuals, moderate in one, and relatively slight in six. Modest pressor effects were also reported in those patients with low blood pressure before medication and in one patient with syncope considerable functional improvement occurred. Striking antidepressant effects were also noted in a proportion of patients. A number of physicians in Western Europe and the United States of America have also urged this drug on small numbers of parkinsonian patients but with generally rather disappointing results but it seems clear from Narabayashi's study (Narabayashi *et al.* 1986) that patient selection is of the utmost importance and that the drug probably only substantially benefits hypotonic freezing. The author (Lees and Bannister, unpublished observations) has given DL-threo-DOPS in doses 1–1.5 g per day to four patients with multiple system atrophy, two of whom had marked gait problems with freezing. No clear benefit occurred in any of the four after treatment periods lasting up to 6 weeks. One patient went into acute retention of urine during drug therapy; another temporarily improved but this was not maintained. No significant elevations in blood pressure were recorded.

No systematic trials with anticholinergic drugs have been carried out in multiple system atrophy but general clinical experience would point to little or marginal benefit.

MULTIPLE SYSTEM ATROPHY WITH GLUTAMATE DEHYDROGENASE DEFICIENCY

A deficiency of the enzyme glutamate dehydrogenase (GDH) in white cells, fibroblasts, and platelets has been reported in certain patients presenting with multiple system atrophy (Plaitakis *et al.* 1980). The classical clinical picture of these patients is with mixed cerebellar and parkinsonian features together with a mild supranuclear gaze disturbance, mild peripheral sensory neuropathy, and sometimes widespread motor neuron involvement. Some patients have severe dysarthria and in others the predominant clinical feature may change, for example, from a presentation with a cerebellar syndrome, through a bradykinetic–rigid parkinsonian syndrome, to a picture which terminates with severe widespread amyotrophy and fasciculations. The one patient with low GDH levels who had come to post-mortem was found to have lipofuscinosis. It has also been suggested by Plaitakis that dysfunction of the enzyme is not merely a marker but underlies the pathogenesis of the disorder, deficiency of GDH allowing toxic amounts of glutamate, an excitotoxic transmitter to accumulate in the nervous system and produce gradual death of neurons containing glutamate receptors. Plaitakis's observation of impaired glutamate tolerance in GDH-deficient patients awaits independent confirmation. Leucine activates GDH and treatment with a leucine-rich diet or dietary supplementation with a mixture of the branch chain amino acids, leucine, valine, and isoleucine, which delivers 10 g of L-leucine daily has been attempted in the treatment of GDH-deficient cases. An apparent arrest of progression was observed in four patients by Plaitakis *et al.* (1983) using this treatment and Duvoisin also noted sustained partial improvement in a further patient for three years. These encouraging observations suggest that this treatment is worthy of further assessment.

REFERENCES

Aminoff, M. J., Wilcox, C. S., Woakes, M. M. and Kremer, M. (1973). Levodopa therapy for parkinsonism in the Shy–Drager syndrome. *J. Neurol. Neurosurg. Psychiat.* **36**, 350–3.

Bannister, R. and Oppenheimer, D. R. (1972). Degenerative diseases of the nervous system associated with autonomic failure. *Brain* **95**, 457–74.

Boudin, G., Guillard, A., Mikol, J. and Galle, P. (1976). Dégénerescence striato-nigrique—à propos de l'étude clinique, thérapeutique et anatomique de 2 cas. *Rev. Neurol., Paris* **132**, 137–56.

DeLean, J. and Deck, J. H. (1976). Shy–Drager syndrome—neuropathological correlation and response to levodopa therapy. *Can. J. neurol. Sci.* **3**, 167–77.

Fève, J. R., Mussini, J. M., Mathé, J. F., Cler, J.-L. and Nombalais, M.-F. (1977). Dégénerescence striato-nigrique—étude clinique et anatomique d'un cas ayant réagi tres favorablement à la L-dopa. *Rev. Neurol., Paris* **133**, 271–8.

Gautier, J.-C. and Durand, J.P. (1977). Traitement des syndromes parkinsoniens par la bromocriptine. *Nouv. Presse Méd.* **6**(3), 171–4.

Goetz, C. G., Tanner, C. M., and Klawans, H. L. (1984). The pharmacology of olivopontocerebellar atrophy. *Adv. Neurol.* **41**, 143–8.

Graham, J. G. and Oppenheimer, D. R. (1969). Orthostatic hypotension and nicotine sensitivity in a case of multiple system atrophy. *J. Neurol. Neurosurg. Psychiat.* **32**, 28–34.

Greer, M., Collins, G. H., and Anton, A. H. (1971). Cerebral catecholamines after levodopa therapy. *Arch. Neurol.* **25**, 461–7.

Izumi, K., Inoue, N., Shirabe, T., Miyazaki, T., and Kuroiwa, Y. (1971). Failed levodopa therapy in striato-nigral degeneration. *Lancet* **i**, 1355.

Johnsen, J. A. and Miller, V. T. (1986). Tobacco intolerance in multiple system atrophy. *Neurology* **36**, 986–8.

Lang, A. E., Birnbaum, A., Blair, R. D. G., and Kierans, C. (1986). Levodopa dose-related fluctuations in presumed olivopontocerebellar atrophy. *Movement Disorders* **1**, 93–102.

Lees, A. J. and Bannister, R. (1981). The use of lisuride in the treatment of multiple system atrophy with autonomic failure (Shy–Drager syndrome). *J. Neurol. Neurosurg. Psychiat.* **44**, 347–51.

Michel, D., Tommasi, M., Laurent, B., Trillet, M. and Schott, B. (1976). Dégénerescence striato-nigrique—á propos de 2 observations anatomocliniques. *Rev. Neurol., Paris* **132**, 3–22.

Narabayashi, H., Kondo, T., Yokochi, F., and Nagatsu, T. (1986). Clinical effects of L-threo-3,4-dihydroxyphenylserine in parkinsonism and pure akinesia. *Adv. Neurol.* **45**, 593–602.

Pastakia, B., Polinsky, R., Dichiro, G., Simmons, J. T., Brown, R., and Wener, L. (1986). Multiple system atrophy (Shy–Drager syndrome): MR imaging. *Radiology* **159**, 499–502.

Plaitakis, A., Berl, S., and Yahr, M. D. (1983). The treatment of GDH-deficient olivopontocerebellar atrophy with branched chain aminoacids. *Neurology* **33** (Suppl. 2), 78.

Plaitakis, A., Nicklas, W., and Desnick, R. J. (1980). Glutamate dehydrogenase deficiency in three patients with spinocerebellar syndrome. *Ann. Neurol.* **7**, 297–303.

Rajput, A., Kazi, K. A., and Rozdilsky, B. (1972). Striatonigral degeneration—response to levodopa therapy. *J. neurol. Sci.* **16**, 331–41.

Rajput, A. H. and Rozdilsky, B. (1976). Dysautonomia in Parkinsonism—a clinico-pathological study. *J. Neurol. Neurosurg. Psychiat.* **39**, 1092–100.

Schober, R., Langston, J. W., and Forno, L. S. (1975). Idiopathic orthostatic hypotension. Biochemical and pathologic observations in 2 cases. *Eur. Neurol.* **13**, 177–88.

Sharpe, J. A., Rewcastle, N. B., Lloyd, K. G., Hornykiewicz, O., Hill, M. and Tasker, R. (1973). Striato-nigral degeneration response to levodopa therapy with pathological and neurochemical correlation. *J. neurol. Sci.* **19**, 275–86.

Spillane, J. D. (1955). The effect of nicotine on spinocerebellar ataxia. *Br. med. J.* **2**, 1345–51.

Spokes, E. G. S., Bannister, R., and Oppenheimer, D. R. (1979). Multiple system atrophy with autonomic failure. Clinical histological and neurochemical observations in 4 cases. *J. neurol. Sci.* **43**, 59–82.

Takei, Y. and Mirra, S. A. (1973). A form of multiple system atrophy with clinical Parkinsonism. In *Progress in neuropathology* (ed. H. M. Zimmerman), Vol. 2, pp. 217–51. Grune and Stratton, New York.

Trotter, J. (1973). Striato-nigral degeneration. Alzheimer's disease and inflammatory changes. *Neurology* **23**, 1211–16.

Williams, A. C., Nutt, J., Lake, C. R., Pfeiffer, R., Teychenne, P. E., Ebert, M. and Calne, D. B. (1979). Actions of bromocriptine in the Shy–Drager and Steel–Richardson–Olszewski syndromes. In *Dopaminergic ergots and motor control* (ed. K. Fuxe and D. B. Calne), pp. 271–83. Pergamon Press, Oxford.

Part III

Other autonomic dysfunction syndromes

34. Autonomic dysfunction in peripheral nerve disease

J. G. McLeod

INTRODUCTION

The autonomic nervous system is affected to some extent in many peripheral neuropathies, although the clinical manifestations may be mild. When small-diameter myelinated and unmyelinated fibres in afferent and efferent nerves are pathologically involved by the disease process (e.g. diabetes, amyloid) or when segmental demyelination affects myelinated autonomic fibres in the vagus or sympathetic pathways (e.g. Guillain–Barré syndrome, diabetes), autonomic disturbances will be present. The clinical features of this autonomic dysfunction may range from the frequent mild impairment of sweating on the extremities to the more serious postural hypotension.

The mechanisms and manifestations of autonomic dysfunction in peripheral nerve diseases are summarized in this chapter. A more complete list of references is available in a recent review (McLeod and Tuck 1987).

HISTOLOGY OF THE AUTONOMIC NERVOUS SYSTEM

Sympathetic nervous system

The sympathetic chain, white rami, and splanchnic nerve in man consist of myelinated and unmyelinated fibres. The fibre diameter distribution of myelinated fibres is similar in all three nerves (McLeod 1980) (Fig. 34.1). Most of the fibres are in the range 2–6 μm but there is another distinct group of larger fibres with a peak at about 12 μm; the large myelinated fibres and some of the smaller myelinated fibres are afferent. Internodal lengths in the sympathetic chain and in the white rami are shorter in relation to fibre diameter than those in the peripheral nervous system (Fig. 34.1). Morphometric analysis of the preganglionic neurons in the spinal cord of man and of the sympathetic preganglionic fibres in

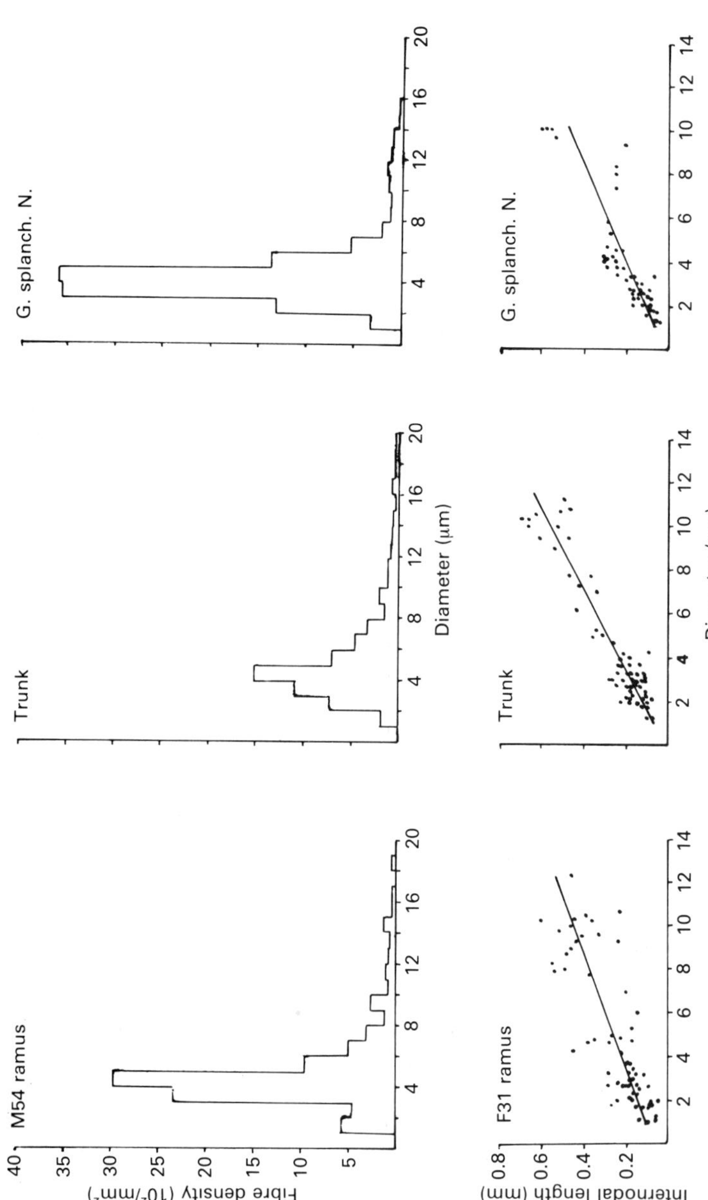

Fig. 34.1. Control subjects. Above: diameter distribution of myelinated fibres in white ramus, sympathetic trunk, and greater splanchnic nerve. Below: relationship between internodal length and diameter of myelinated fibres in white ramus, trunk, and greater splanchnic nerve. (From McLeod (1980).)

the ventral roots has shown that the preganglionic fibres range in diameter from 1.5 to 4.7 μm with a peak at 2.5 μm. There is progressive reduction of numbers of both cells and fibres with age.

Parasympathetic nervous system

The histological structure of the vagus nerve has been studied in man. Only a small proportion (about 20 per cent) of the afferent and efferent fibres in the cervical vagus are myelinated and most of these are 3 μm or less in diameter.

The carotid sinus nerve has been studied in different animal species including man and contains myelinated fibres which range in diameter from 2 to 12 μm, most of these being in the 2–5 μm diameter range; it also contains many unmyelinated fibres. Afferent fibres from the aortic-arch receptors are both myelinated and unmyelinated; the myelinated fibres in the cat range from 2 to 10 μm, although most are in the 2–6 μm range.

MANIFESTATIONS OF AUTONOMIC DYSFUNCTION IN PERIPHERAL NERVE DISEASES

Impaired sweating of the extremities is common and probably results from degeneration of cholinergic postganglionic sympathetic unmyelinated fibres that travel with the peripheral nerves to innervate sweat glands, or to degeneration or demyelination of preganglionic sympathetic efferent fibres. Hyperhidrosis may be seen in partial nerve injuries that cause causalgia or when there is pressure on the nerve roots such as occurs in malignancy and in some toxic neuropathies. When sweating is impaired in the extremities, excessive compensatory sweating may occur on trunk and face.

Orthostatic postural hypotension results from damage to the small-diameter myelinated and unmyelinated fibres in afferent and efferent nerves in the baroreflex pathways. Postural hypotension, therefore, most commonly occurs in diseases such as diabetes and amyloidosis in which the small fibres degenerate and in the Guillain–Barré syndrome in which segmental demyelination affects the myelinated autonomic fibres in the vagus and sympathetic pathways. Orthostatic hypotension is most likely to occur when fibres in the splanchnic vascular bed are pathologically involved since the latter plays an important part in human blood-pressure regulation (Low *et al.* 1975*a*; McLeod 1980). Orthostatic hypotension is uncommon in dying-back neuropathies which initially affect predominantly the large diameter fibres of the longest nerves. Impaired heart-rate control results from vagal impairment in patients with autonomic neuropathy, particularly diabetes. Bladder dysfunction, impotence, and pupillary abnormalities are other clinical manifestations of autonomic dysfunction in peripheral nerve disease.

AUTONOMIC DISORDERS WITH NO ASSOCIATED PERIPHERAL NEUROPATHY (Table 34.1)

Acute and subacute autonomic neuropathy

Young and his colleagues (1969) were the first to describe a pure pandysautonomia with subacute onset over a period of weeks followed by complete recovery. The condition differed from other neurological causes of autonomic dysfunction because somatic motor and sensory function were normal. Since their description, other cases of acute or subacute pandysautonomia and cases of pure cholinergic dysautonomia have been described (Chapter 35). The aetiology of the condition

Table 34.1. Causes of peripheral autonomic dysfunction

Disorders with no associated peripheral neuropathy

1. Acute and subacute autonomic neuropathy
   a. Pandysautonomia
   b. Cholinergic dysautonomia
2. Botulism

Disorders associated with peripheral neuropathy

1. Autonomic dysfunction clinically important
   a. Diabetes
   b. Amyloidosis
   c. Acute inflammatory neuropathy
   d. Acute intermittent porphyria
   e. Familial dysautonomia (Riley–Day syndrome; HMSN III)
   f. Chronic sensory and autonomic neuropathy
2. Autonomic dysfunction usually clinically unimportant
   a. Alcohol-induced neuropathy
   b. Toxic neuropathies (vincristine sulphate, acrylamide, heavy metals, perhexiline maleate, organic solvents)
   c. HMSN I, II, and V
   d. Malignancy
   e. Vitamin B_{12} deficiency
   f. Rheumatoid arthritis
   g. Chronic renal failure
   h. Systemic lupus erythematosus
   i. Mixed connective tissue disease
   j. Fabry's disease
   k. Chronic inflammatory neuropathy

remains uncertain but it is possible that it is a selective form of the Guillain–Barré syndrome; a number of reported cases have followed acute infective illnesses.

Botulism

Botulism is characterized by muscle paralysis, acute autonomic dysfunction, and gastrointestinal symptoms caused by absorption from the alimentary tract of toxins produced by strains of *Clostridium botulinum.* The toxin impairs the release of acetylcholine from nerve terminals; electrophysiological features are similar to those seen in the Eaton–Lambert syndrome (Oh 1977). Acute autonomic dysfunction may be present without associated muscular weakness; in this circumstance the condition may be difficult to distinguish clinically from acute autonomic neuropathy.

AUTONOMIC NEUROPATHY ASSOCIATED WITH PERIPHERAL SENSORIMOTOR NEUROPATHY (Table 34.1)

The autonomic nervous system is affected in many peripheral neuropathies, although the clinical manifestations may be mild (McLeod 1980; Krone *et al.* 1983). Autonomic dysfunction is clinically important in the neuropathies associated with diabetes, amyloid disease, porphyria, Riley–Day syndrome, and in the Guillain–Barré syndrome and some cases of chronic sensory and autonomic neuropathy. In most of the other conditions described below it is usually of little clinical importance.

Hereditary neuropathies

Charcot–Marie–Tooth disease (hereditary motor and sensory neuropathies (HMSN) Types I and II)

Jammes (1972) tested autonomic function in four patients with probable dominantly inherited hypertrophic Charcot–Marie–Tooth disease (HMSN Type I). Sweating over the extremities was reduced and reflex and local vasomotor responses to heating and cooling were impaired. There was evidence of denervation supersensitivity to adrenalin. There were also abnormalities of the blood-pressure and heart-rate response to change in posture and there were abnormalities of pupillary reactions and tear production consistent with sympathetic and parasympathetic lesions. It was concluded that there was impairment of the autonomic nervous system in Charcot–Marie–Tooth disease and that the postganglionic sympathetic fibres were predominantly involved.

Minor abnormalities have been noted by other workers in patients with autosomal dominant hypertrophic Charcot–Marie–Tooth disease (HMSN Type I). In one patient with hypertrophic Charcot–Marie–Tooth disease giant nerve fibres were seen in the myenteric plexus of a specimen of bowel taken at laparotomy. Bird *et al.* (1984) found abnormalitites of the pupillary light reflex and some impairment of heart-rate control, both findings suggesting parasympathetic nerve fibre damage. In our own studies of 11 patients with HMSN Type I and four with HMSN Type II, no significant abnormalities were found on autonomic testing except for abnormal sweat tests.

The impairment of sweating is consistent with the abnormalities of unmyelinated fibres seen in the sural nerve. Descriptions of the pathology of autonomic nerves in autopsy material are difficult to find. In the earlier literature changes have been described in progressive hypertrophic neuropathy but it is not clear whether these were cases of Charcot–Marie–Tooth disease, Déjérine–Sottas disease, or in some cases possibly chronic inflammatory neuropathy. Degenerating axons in onion bulb formations have also been noted in the sympathetic trunk in Refsum's disease.

Friedreich's ataxia

Autonomic function studies have been carried out in our laboratory on 16 patients with Friedreich's ataxia. The sweat test was normal and there was no evidence of postural hypotension or impairment of baroreflex function. In this condition there is a reduction in the number of large-diameter myelinated fibres in the peripheral nerve but small myelinated and unmyelinated fibres remain relatively intact (Dyck and Lambert 1968). Assuming that the pathological findings are similar in the autonomic nervous system, it is not surprising that autonomic function is normal. Abnormalities of sympathetic function have been described in other forms of spinocerebellar degeneration (Tamura *et al.* 1986).

Familial dysautonomia (Riley–Day syndrome)

See Chapter 2.

Amyloid disease

Autonomic dysfunction is common in primary amyloid disease. The autonomic disturbances may become disabling, frequently accompanying and often preceding the motor and sensory manifestations of peripheral neuropathy. Impotence, postural hypotension, abnormalities of sweating, impaired response to Valsalva manoeuvre, and impaired vasomotor responses to cold and inspiratory gasp are prominent features (Low *et al.* 1983). Autonomic dysfunction is attributable to the predominant loss of unmyelinated and small myelinated fibres in the peripheral nerves and to the reduction in the number of cells in the intermediolateral columns (Low *et al.* 1981). Widespread deposition of amyloid in the autonomic nerves and ganglia has been frequently noted.

Fabry's disease

Impaired autonomic function has been described in Fabry's disease (Cable *et al.* 1982).

Inflammatory neuropathies

Acute inflammatory neuropathy (Guillain–Barré syndrome)

Disturbances of autonomic function are well recognized in the Guillain–Barré syndrome. Tachycardia, which may remain fixed and unresponsive to postural change, has been reported by a number of workers (Tuck and McLeod 1982). Elevated or fluctuating arterial blood pressure has been documented as well as postural hypotension (Tuck and McLeod 1982; Fagius and Wallin 1983).

Abnormalities of the heart rate and of the blood pressure response to Valsalva manoeuvre have been described. The heart-rate response to elevated arterial blood pressure induced by intravenous injection of phenylephrine may be impaired (Fig. 34.2) and the sweat test is commonly abnormal (Fig. 34.3). The nature of the abnormalities of autonomic function is variable and depends upon the site of the

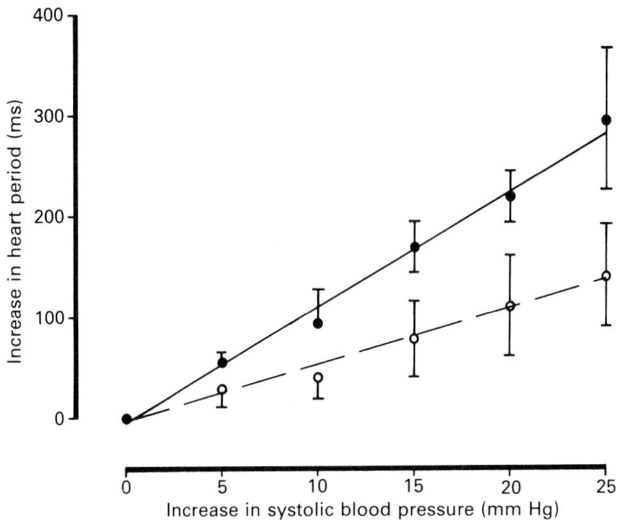

Fig. 34.2. Relationship of increase in heart period to increase in systolic blood pressure in control subjects (closed circles) and in patients with Guillain–Barré syndrome (open circles) following intravenous phenylephrine. Vertical bars represent ±1 SE. (From Tuck and McLeod (1982).)

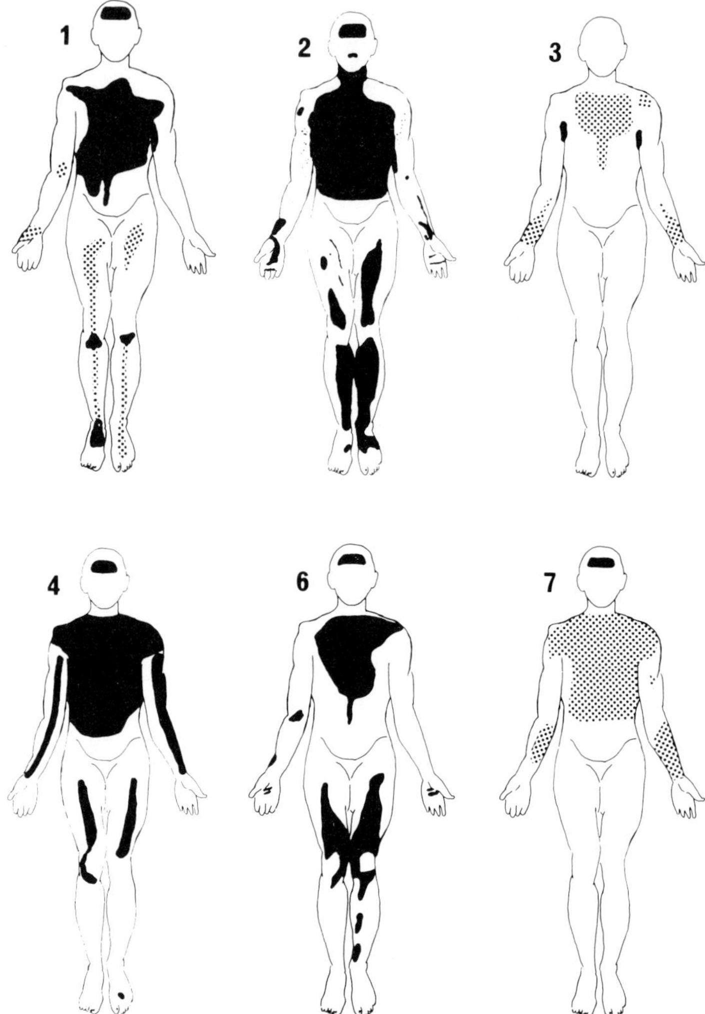

Fig. 34.3. Patterns of sweating in the Guillain–Barré syndrome. Black areas indicate regions of normal sweat production; spotted areas are those in which sweating was patchy. (From Tuck and McLeod (1982).)

demyelinating lesions which may occur in the afferent fibres in the vagus and glossopharyngeal nerves, in the arterial baroreceptors, in the efferent parasympathetic fibres in the vagus nerves, and in the sympathetic nerves that innervate the heart and control sweating and vasomotor tone. Pathological studies have demonstrated demyelinating lesions in the glossopharyngeal and vagus nerves and in the sympathetic chains and white rami. The severity of the involvement of the autonomic nervous system does not appear to be related to the degree of motor or sensory disturbance (Tuck and McLeod 1982). In most patients the consequences of involvement of the autonomic nervous system are not serious but on some occasions they can be life-threatening. Postural hypotension may lead to syncope and irreversible brain damage in a paralysed patient who is inadvertently left in a sitting position or who requires an anaesthetic; sudden death due to cardiac arrhythmias or to asystole may also occur.

Chronic inflammatory neuropathy

In chronic inflammatory demyelinating polyradiculoneuropathy, postural hypotension and other symptoms of autonomic nervous system dysfunction are very uncommon. These findings are in contrast to those in acute inflammatory neuropathy in which the more severe disturbance of autonomic function are presumed to be related to acute conduction block and possibly more extensive involvement of unmyelinated fibres in the acute stages.

Metabolic disorders

Diabetes

Autonomic neuropathy is commonly associated with diabetic peripheral neuropathy. It is considered in detail in Chapters 36–39.

Porphyria

Postural hypotension may occur in acute intermittent and variegate porphyria, although hypertension is more common and may precede the manifestation of peripheral neuropathy (Stewart and Hensley 1981; Yeung Laiwah *et al.* 1985). Persistent tachycardia may be an early feature of an attack and may also precede the onset of neuropathy. Autonomic function studies have demonstrated abnormalities of sympathetic and parasympathetic function (Stewart and Hensley 1981; Yeung Laiwah *et al.* 1985).

Chronic renal failure

Autonomic dysfunction, manifested by postural hypotension, impaired response to the Valsalva manoeuvre and to induced hypotension, and abnormal heart-rate and blood-pressure responses to standing up from the supine position have been demonstrated in patients on chronic haemodialysis and there is also an impaired baroreceptor response to rise in blood pressure (Ewing and Winney 1975; Nies *et al.* 1979). However, autonomic neuropathy does not appear to be the only explanation for the sustained hypotension that occurs in some haemodialysis patients (Nies *et al.* 1979). The precise mechanism of the autonomic dysfunction remains unclear but, since efferent sympathetic function appears to be normal (Nies *et al.* 1979), the most likely sites of primary damage are the baroreceptors or their afferent fibres or central nervous system connections.

Vitamin B_{12} deficiency

Orthostatic hypotension may be the initial manifestation of pernicious anaemia. It usually responds well to replacement therapy. The pathological findings in the peripheral neuropathy of vitamin B_{12} deficiency are those of axonal degeneration but this alone is unlikely to cause postural hypotension which may possibly be due to some central mechanism (McCombe and McLeod 1984).

Alcohol and nutritional disorders

Postural hypotension is common in patients with Wernicke's encephalopathy and is probably the result of impaired sympathetic outflow at central or peripheral levels. Clinical manifestations of autonomic dysfunction are unusual in uncomplicated alcoholic peripheral neuropathy (Low *et al.* 1975*b*), although postural hypotension may occur in patients who are severely affected (Novak and Victor 1974).

Low *et al.* (1975*b*) found no evidence of postural hypotension in 12 patients with clinical and electrophysiological evidence of peripheral neuropathy. Duncan *et al.* (1980) examined 20 chronic alcoholic men with varying degrees of peripheral and central nervous system damage, none of whom were found to have postural hypotension. These findings indicate that peripheral sympathetic vasomotor control is relatively well preserved in alcoholics until the peripheral neuropathy reaches an advanced stage, even though abnormal sweat tests indicate that there is early involvement of postganglionic sympathetic efferent fibres (Low *et al.* 1975*b*).

The Valsalva ratio was abnormal in two of nine patients studied by Low *et al.* (1975*b*). In contrast to patients with diabetic neuropathy, the relationship between blood pressure and heart period was similar to that of controls, although there was some distortion of the sigmoid curves and reduction of mean gain and heart period range that was not statistically significant (Fig. 34.4). These findings were consistent with some degree of sympathetic and vagal damage but could also have been attributed to hypertension and the age of the patients. Duncan *et al.* (1980) have since provided definite evidence of vagal damage in chronic alcoholics by demonstrating impaired heart rate responses to Valsalva manoeuvre, deep breathing, change in posture, neck suction, and atropine. Novak and Victor (1974) reported hoarseness and weakness of the voice and dysphagia as clinical manifestations of vagal neuropathy in four patients with severe alcoholic neuropathy.

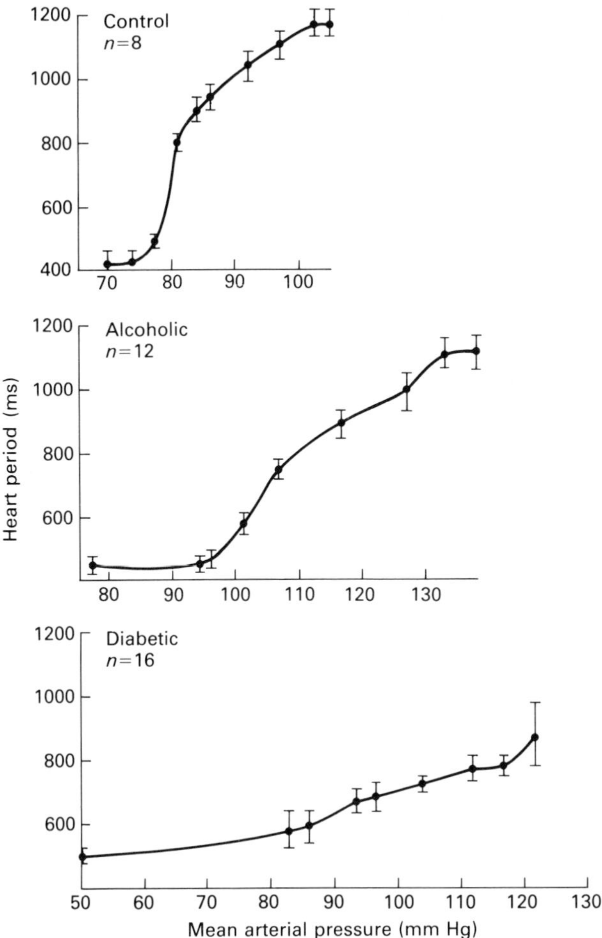

Fig. 34.4. Stimulus–response curves relating heart period to mean arterial pressure in control subjects and patients with diabetic and alcoholic neuropathy. (From McLeod (1980).)

Few pathological studies of the autonomic nervous system have been reported in alcoholic neuropathy. Appenzeller and Richardson (1966) found giant neurons in the sympathetic ganglia similar to those seen in diabetic neuropathy. Low *et al.* (1975*b*) found that the density and fibre diameter distribution of myelinated fibres in the splanchnic nerves of subjects with alcoholic neuropathy who had reduced myelinated fibre densities in the sural nerves did not differ significantly from those of controls and contrasted with the marked degenerative changes found in the splanchnic nerves of diabetics. Novak and Victor (1974) found active myelin degeneration in the paravertebral chain of one patient with

Wernicke's disease, hepatic encephalopathy, and severe peripheral neuropathy manifested by foot drop, wrist drop, and absent reflexes. These workers also found pathological evidence of active axonal degeneration of the vagus nerves in the same and one other case. We have recently demonstrated a significant reduction in the density of myelinated fibres in the distal parts of the vagus nerve at autopsy in chronic alcoholics (Guo *et al.* 1987).

Alcoholic neuropathy is a dying-back neuropathy identical to that of beriberi (Novak and Victor 1974). The most distal parts of the longest fibres in the vagus nerve are affected earliest and the shorter and more proximal myelinated fibres of the sympathetic system are not affected until later in the illness when the peripheral neuropathy is severe. The absence of postural hypotension and the relatively normal baroreflex function are consistent with a lack of pathology in the splanchnic nerves since postural hypotension is more likely to occur if the splanchnic outflow is involved. Disturbance of oesophageal motility in chronic alcoholics with peripheral neuropathy may be a manifestation of damage to the vagus nerve.

Malignancy

Impairment of sweating and postural hypotension may occur in association with the peripheral neuropathy of remote malignancies. In a patient with oat-cell carcinoma of the lung and pandysautonomia reported by Chiappa and Young (1973) there was no clinical or electrophysiological evidence of peripheral neuropathy, but, as well as severe orthostatic hypotension, there was an abnormal Valsalva response, impaired oesophageal and gastrointestinal motility, abnormal sweat and Schirmer tests, denervation supersensitivity to noradrenalin, and a flat cystometrogram. Autonomic dysfunction has also been described in association with carcinoma of the pancreas and lymphomas. Local hyperhidrosis and piloerection may result from direct irritation of nerves or roots by malignancies (Walsh *et al.* 1976).

Toxic causes

Vincristine

The vinca alkaloids are cytotoxic drugs used in the treatment of lymphoma, leukaemia, and some other malignancies. Vincristine, and occasionally vinblastine, cause peripheral neuropathy, the predominant pathological change in the peripheral nerve being axonal degeneration. Postural hypotension has been reported as a neurotoxic side-effect of vincristine and constipation, abdominal pain, paralytic ileus, urinary retention, and other bladder disturbances are well recognized complications. Published accounts of autonomic function studies in patients with vincristine-induced autonomic neuropathy are limited but have demonstrated abnormalities of postganglionic sympathetic efferent function and abnormal Valsalva responses in patients with postural hypotension. The sympathetic nerves and ganglia were normal in two cases in whom autopsy material was examined pathologically.

Autonomic dysfunction may develop within days of commencement of vincristine therapy. The mechanism of action is not clear, although there is some evidence in man and other animals that the primary site of damage is the unmyelinated noradrenergic fibres of the sympathetic nervous system. However the symptoms in man of constipation, paralytic ileus, and bladder disturbances indicate that parasympathetic fibres are also affected. Ultrastructurally, vinca alkaloids disrupt microtubules and cause an increase in the neurofilaments and the appearance of paracrystalline structures in axons. Unmyelinated fibres are more susceptible to the neurotoxin than myelinated fibres.

Heavy metal poisoning

There have been very few cases of heavy metal poisoning in which autonomic function has been adequately studied. In thallium poisoning, tachycardia and hypertension have been reported in association with peripheral neuropathy. In arsenical poisoning excessive sweating and impairment of sweating on the extremities have been described. Subacute or chronic inorganic mercury poisoning is the cause of acrodynia which occurs mainly in children and includes amongst its manifestations tachycardia, hypertension, and profuse sweating.

Organic solvents

Autonomic function has been shown to be disturbed in some workers exposed to organic solvents (Matikainen and Juntunen 1985).

Acrylamide

Excessive sweating was reported in association with the peripheral neuropathy resulting from industrial exposure to acrylamide in man.

Perhexiline maleate

Perhexiline maleate which is used in the treatment of angina pectoris may cause a peripheral neuropathy. Fraser *et al.* (1977) described three patients who developed autonomic neuropathy manifested by postural hypotension and an abnormal Valsalva ratio related to perhexiline maleate-induced neuropathy.

Connective tissue diseases

Rheumatoid arthritis

Impairment of sweating on the extremities is relatively common in rheumatoid arthritis and is probably related in most cases to damage of postganglionic sympathetic efferent fibres in the peripheral nerves. In addition, there may be vagal-nerve involvement since the heart-rate response to standing, to the Valsalva manoeuvre, and to respiration may be impaired particularly in patients with peripheral neuropathy. Rarely, autonomic neuropathy may be secondary to amyloidosis (McGill *et al.* 1986).

Systemic lupus erythematosus and mixed connective tissue diseases

Autonomic neuropathy has been reported as a complication of systemic lupus erythematosus and mixed connective tissue diseases (Gudesblatt *et al.* 1985; McCombe *et al.* 1987).

Leprosy

Cardiac denervation, postural hypotension, decreased sweating, and impaired response to the cold pressor test in the absence of other features of peripheral neuropathy have been described in patients with leprosy.

Chronic sensory neuropathy

Low *et al.* (1978) reported a unique patient with congenital sensory neuropathy in whom there was loss of pain but no other sensory modalities. Selective loss of small myelinated fibres with normal unmyelinated fibres was demonstrated on sural-nerve biopsy. Sweating was normal, but the Valsalva ratio was reduced, suggesting an abnormality of baroreceptor function resulting from involvement of cardiac autonomic nerves. Okajima *et al.* (1983) also reported autonomic neuropathy in association with a chronic sensory neuropathy.

EXPERIMENTAL AUTONOMIC NEUROPATHY

Autonomic disturbances have been extensively studied in animals with dying-back neuropathy induced by acrylamide (McLeod and Tuck 1987). Comparisons of the histological damage in the peripheral somatic, sympathetic, and parasympathetic nervous systems have demonstrated that the peripheral somatic nerves are damaged the most severely and the splanchnic nerves the least. The autonomic fibres are not greatly affected until the animals have developed a severe peripheral neuropathy; the vagus nerve is damaged to a greater extent than the splanchnic nerve. Vasomotor control of the mesenteric blood vessels and baroreflex control of heart rate and blood pressure is most severely affected when the peripheral neuropathy is advanced. In dogs, cardio-thoracic baroreceptors, oesophageal mechanoreceptors, pulmonary stretch receptors, and their innervating fibres are damaged before there are any overt clinical abnormalities (Chapter 10). These findings are relevant to the pathogenesis of autonomic dysfunction in alcoholic and other dying-back neuropathies.

The autonomic nervous system has also been studied in experimental allergic neuritis (EAN), the experimental model of the Guillain–Barré syndrome. The sympathetic and parasympathetic nervous systems are affected electrophysiologically and pathologically, and there is also some evidence that unmyelinated fibres may be damaged directly or indirectly in the splanchnic nerve (Tuck *et al.* 1981). These findings in EAN are relevant to the pathogenesis of autonomic dysfunction in the Guillain–Barré syndrome.

SUMMARY AND CONCLUSIONS

Disturbances of autonomic function are frequently present in patients with peripheral neuropathy. The autonomic nervous system is complex and may be damaged by disease in a variety of ways, giving rise to different clinical and pathological manifestations. Autonomic dysfunction is most likely to result from conditions such as primary amyloid and diabetes that affect the small myelinated and unmyelinated fibres in the baroreceptor afferents, the vagal innervation of the heart, and the sympathetic efferent fibres in the mesenteric vascular bed. Acute autonomic dysfunction can also occur in the Guillain–Barré syndrome in which there is segmental demyelination in the sympathetic and parasympathetic nerves; in vincristine neuropathy in which unmyelinated fibres may be preferentially damaged; and in acute prophyria in which the metabolic function of the autonomic nervous system may be disturbed.

REFERENCES

Appenzeller, O. and Richardson, E. P. (1966). The sympathetic chain in patients with diabetic and alcoholic polyneuropathy. *Neurology, Minneapolis* **16**, 1205–9.

Bird, T. D., Reenan, A. M., and Pfeifer, M. (1984). Autonomic nervous system function in genetic neuromuscular disorders. *Arch. Neurol., Chicago* **41**, 43–6.

Cable, W. J. L., Kolodny, E. H., and Adams, R. D. (1982). Fabry disease: impaired autonomic function. *Neurology, New York* **32**, 498–502.

Chiappa, K. H. and Young, R. R. (1973). A case of paracarcinomatous pandysautonomia. *Neurology, Minneapolis* **23**, 423.

Duncan, G., Johnson, R. H., Lambie, D. G., and Whiteside, E. A. (1980). Evidence of vagal neuropathy in chronic alcoholics. *Lancet* **ii**, 1053–6.

Dyck, P. J. and Lambert, E. H. (1968). Lower motor and primary sensory neuron disease with peroneal musclar atrophy. Part II. Neurologic, genetic and electrophysiologic findings in various neuronal degenerations. *Arch. Neurol. Chicago* **18**, 619–25.

Ewing, D. J. and Winney, R. (1975). Autonomic function in patients with chronic renal failure on intermittent haemodialysis. *Nephron* **15**, 424–9.

Fagius, J. and Wallin, G. (1983). Microneurographic evidence of excessive sympathetic outflow in the Guillain–Barré syndrome. *Brain* **106**, 589–600.

Fraser, D. M., Campbell, I. W., and Miller, H. C. (1977). Peripheral and autonomic neuropathy after treatment with perhexiline maleate. *Br. med. J.* **iii**, 675–6.

Gudesblatt, M., Goodman, A. D., Rubenstein, A. E., Bender, A. N., and Choi, H-SH. (1985). Autonomic neuropathy associated with autoimmune disease. *Neurology, New York* **35**, 261–4.

Guo, Y-P., McLeod, J. G., and Baverstock, J. (1987). Pathological changes in the vagus nerve in diabetics and chronic alcoholics. *J. Neurol. Neurosurg. Psychiat.* (In press.)

Jammes, J. L. (1972). The autonomic nervous system in peroneal muscular atrophy. *Arch. Neurol., Chicago* **27**, 213–20.

Krone, A., Reuther, P., and Fuhrmeister, U. (1983). Autonomic dysfunction in polyneuropathies: a report of 106 cases. *J. Neurol.* **230**, 111–21.

Low, P. A., Burke, W. J., and McLeod, J. G. (1978). Congenital sensory neuropathy with selective loss of small myelinated fibres. *Ann. Neurol.* **3**, 179–82.

Low, P. A., Dyck, P. J., Okazaki, H., Kyle, R., and Fealey, R. D. (1981). The splanchnic autonomic outflow in amyloid neuropathy and Tangier disease. *Neurology, New York* **31**, 461–3.

Low, P. A., Neumann, C., Dyck, P. J., Fealey, R. D., and Tuck, R. R. (1983). Evaluation of skin vasomotor reflexes by using laser Doppler velocimetry. *Mayo Clin. Proc.* **58**, 583–92.

Low, P. A., Walsh, J. C., Huang, C.-Y., and McLeod, J. G. (1975*a*). The sympathetic nervous system in diabetic neuropathy. A clinical and pathological study. *Brain* **98**, 341–56.

Low, P. A., Walsh, J. C., Huang, C.-Y., and McLeod, J. G. (1975*b*). The sympathetic nervous system in alcoholic neuropathy. A clinical and pathological study. *Brain* **98**, 357–64.

Matikainen, E. and Juntunen, J. (1985). Autonomic nervous system dysfunction in workers exposed to organic solvents. *J. Neurol. Neurosurg. Psychiat.* **48**, 1021–4.

McCombe, P. A. and McLeod, J. G. (1984). The peripheral neuropathy of vitamin B12 deficiency. *J. neurol. Sci.* **66**, 117–26.

McCombe, P. A., McLeod, J. G., Pollard, J. D., Guo, Y-P., and Ingall, T. J. (1987). Peripheral sensorimotor and autonomic neuropathy associated with systemic lupus erythematosus. *Brain* **110**, 533–49.

McGill, N. W., Tuck, R., and Hassall, J. E. (1986). Severe autonomic neuropathy in amyloidosis secondary to rheumatoid arthritis. *Aust. N.Z. J. Med.* **16**, 705–7.

McLeod, J. G. (1980). Autonomic nervous system. In *The physiology of peripheral nerve disease* (ed. A. J. Sumner), pp. 432–83. Saunders, Philadelphia.

McLeod, J. G. and Tuck, R. R. (1987). Disorders of the autonomic nervous system. *Ann. Neurol.* **21**, 419–31, 519–30.

Nies, A. S., Robertson, D., and Stone, W. J. (1979). Hemodialysis hypotension is not the result of uremic peripheral autonomic neuropathy. *J. lab. clin. Med.* **94**, 395–402.

Novak, D. J. and Victor, M. (1974). The vagus and sympathetic nerves in alcoholic neuropathy. *Arch. Neurol., Chicago* **30**, 273–84.

Oh, S. J. (1977). Botulism: electrophysiological studies. *Ann. Neurol.* **1**, 481–5.

Okajima, T., Yamamura, S., Hamada, K., Kawasaki, S., Ideta, T., Ueno, H., and Tokuomi, H. (1983). Chronic sensory and autonomic neuropathy. *Neurology, New York* **33**, 1061–4.

Stewart, P. M. and Hensely, W. J. (1981). An acute attack of variegate porphyria complicated by severe autonomic neuropathy. *Aust. NZ J. Med.* **11**, 82–3.

Tamura, N., Shimazu, K., Hienuki, M., Maruki, Y., Oiwa, K., Kim, H-T., Yamamoto, T., Omoto, K., and Hamaguchi, K. (1986). Sympathetic nervous function in motor neuron disease and spinocerebellar degeneration. *J. autonom. nerv. Syst.* (suppl.), 435–40.

Tuck, R. R. and McLeod, J. G. (1982). Autonomic dysfunction in Guillain–Barré syndrome. *J. Neurol. Neurosurg. Psychiat.* **44**, 983–90.

Tuck, R. R., Pollard, J. D., and McLeod, J. G. (1981). Autonomic neuropathy in experimental allergic neuritis: an electrophysiological and histological study. *Brain* **104**, 187–208.

Walsh, J. C., Low, P. A., and Allsop, J. L. (1976). Localized sympathetic overactivity: an uncommon complication of lung cancer. *J. Neurol. Neurosurg. Psychiat.* **39**, 93–5.

Yeung Laiwah, A. C., Macphee, G. J. A., Boye, P., Moore, M. R., and Goldberg, A. (1985). Autonomic neuropathy in acute intermittent porphyria. *J. Neurol. Neurosurg. Psychiat.* **48**, 1025–30.

Young, R. R., Asbury, A. K., Adams, R. D., and Corbett, J. L. (1969). Pure pandysautonomia with recovery. *Trans Am. neurol. Ass.* **94**, 355–7.

35. Acute and subacute autonomic neuropathies

Ramesh K. Khurana

INTRODUCTION

The peripheral autonomic nervous system is frequently affected in patients with somatic neuropathies. In contrast, isolated or predominant involvement of the autonomic nervous system, autonomic neuropathy, is uncommon. Autonomic neuropathies may be focal, multifocal, or generalized. Generalized autonomic neuropathies usually affect both sympathetic and parasympathetic fibres, but may predominantly affect one or the other component. Concomitant involvement of both components has been called pandysautonomia (Young *et al.* 1975). Autonomic neuropathies may be acute, subacute, or chronic in onset and progression. This chapter deals with acute and subacute autonomic neuropathies.

A clinical report consistent with acute autonomic neuropathy appeared in the literature in 1958. Barnett and Wagner described a 28-year-old male who acutely developed impotence, lower abdominal pain, diarrhoea, difficult and painful micturition, blurred near-vision, and orthostatic syncope. Dilated unreactive pupils, distended abdomen, and orthostatic hypotension were the only physical findings. Spinal fluid protein was 50 mg per cent. Autonomic tests demonstrated widespread sympathetic and parasympathetic dysfunction. Diarrhoea and urinary symptoms began to improve within 3 weeks. Young *et al.* (1969) provided a detailed account of a similar entity under the title, 'pure' pandysautonomia. Since these observations, several authors have added to the clinical spectrum of autonomic neuropathies (Anderson *et al.* 1972; Appenzeller and Kornfeld 1973; Bannister *et al.* 1986; Colan *et al.* 1980; Edelman *et al.* 1981; Estanol-Vidal *et al.* 1979; Fagius *et al.* 1983; Low *et al.* 1983).

CLINICAL FEATURES

Acute autonomic neuropathy affects previously healthy individuals of all ages and of either sex. There is generally no family history. The cases tend to be heterogeneous in terms of onset, evolution, autonomic defects, and recovery. Onset varies from a few days to a few months. It may start with non-specific symptoms of fatigue, lethargy, and headache (Low *et al.* 1983), or with autonomic symptoms such as blurred near-vision (Yee *et al.* 1976), vomiting (Thomashefsky *et al.* 1972), diarrhoea (Hopkins *et al.* 1974), and disturbed micturition. Occasionally, positive symptoms, e.g. profuse sweating, episodic piloerection, and hyper-salivation precede symptoms of autonomic hypoactivity (Hopkins *et al.* 1974). These symptoms may continue to evolve over a period of a few days to a few months. At the peak of the illness, symptoms involve multiple organs but to a variable degree. The patient is often disabled by cardiovascular, pupillary, gastrointestinal, and genitourinary symptoms. (Appenzeller and Kornfeld 1973; Okada *et al.* 1975; Young *et al.* 1975). Orthostatic lightheadedness and syncope, and blurred near-vision are the most prominent symptoms. Oral and gastrointestinal symptoms include pain in the parotid region, dry mouth, lack of appetite, nausea, vomiting, abdominal distension, abdominal colic, diarrhoea, constipation alternating with diarrhoea, and constipation unrelieved by laxatives. Genitourinary complaints consist of nocturnal polyuria, urinary hesitancy, urinary retention, and diminished to total loss of potency. Dry eyes, photophobia, nasal stuffiness, dryness of nasal passages, itching and peeling of skin, hypohidrosis or anhidrosis, cold intolerance, or heat intolerance are the other symptoms. The disease is usually monophasic and self-limiting. The occasional case may remit partially and relapse and may even be fatal (Estanol-Vidal *et al.* 1979; Fagius *et al.* 1983). Recovery may take several months, and may be complete but is usually incomplete.

Physical examination reveals tachycardia, orthostatic hypotension with fixed heart rate, dry and peeling skin, flushed skin, dry eyes, distended abdomen, distended urinary bladder, and absent bowel sounds. Neurological examination displays intact mental functions, extraocular movements, muscle strength, sensation, and co-ordination. Neurological abnormalitites usually seen are photophobia, dilated pupils unreactive to light or accommodation, unilateral or bilateral ptosis, diminished rectal tone, and absent bulbocavernosus reflex. The muscle stretch reflexes may be sluggish to absent (Appenzeller and Kornfeld 1973).

A subgroup of patients with autonomic neuropathy, age range 6–19 years, have 'pure' cholinergic dysautonomia (Anderson *et al.* 1972; Harik *et al.* 1977; Hopkins *et al.* 1981; Inamdar *et al.* 1982). It is of relatively acute onset and progression. Orthostatic hypotension is uncommon but tachycardia is a frequent manifestation.

Acute pandysautonomia was originally described as a 'pure' entity

(Young *et al.* 1969, 1975) with exclusive involvement of autonomic nerves. Description of subsequent cases indicates that autonomic nerves are predominantly, but not exclusively, affected. In a patient described by Young *et al.* (1975), absence of flare response to intradermal histamine seemed to indicate involvement of small dorsal-root ganglia neurons and their axons. Widespread dysautonomia which reversed with regression of oat-cell carcinoma of the lung, was reported in patients with electrophysiologically documented Lambert–Eaton myasthenic syndrome (Khurana *et al.* 1983; Mamdani *et al.* 1985). Colan and colleagues (1980) described a 9-year-old boy with pandysautonomia and loss of corneal reflexes, facial pain sensation, and gag reflex. He also had bilateral corneal ulceration, difficulty swallowing, frequent choking and regurgitation, and elevated cerebrospinal fluid protein. Sensory action potentials were absent. Another case of acute autonomic neuropathy with severe sensory deficit was reported by Fagius and associates (1983). Bannister and associates (1986) described a 45-year-old male with ulcerative colitis who developed progressive dysautonomia, neuropathy, and myelopathy. Abnormal electroencephalogram has been noted in some patients with acute and subacute dysautonomia (Anderson *et al.* 1972; Harik *et al.* 1977; Hopkins *et al.* 1974). These cases suggest that the criteria for the definition of this entity are arbitrary and that the spectrum of this entity ranges from pandysautonomia through predominantly cholinergic dysautonomia to dysautonomia together with other impairment of nervous system function at various levels of the neural axis.

PATHOGENESIS

In some cases of acute autonomic neuropathy no associated disease was found in spite of extensive work (Low *et al.* 1983; Thomashefsky *et al.* 1972; Young *et al.* 1975). Over the years, cases were reported in association with viral infections, malignancies, and connective tissue disorders. These associated diseases include infectious mononucleosis (Yahr and Frontera 1975), rubella (Bost *et al.* 1983), adenocarcinoma of the lung (Vasudevan *et al.* 1981), oat-cell carcinoma of the lung (Khurana *et al.* 1983; Mamdani *et al.* 1985), testicular malignancy (Fagius *et al.* 1983), Hodgkin's disease (Lieshout *et al.* 1986), and mixed connective-tissue disorder (Edelman *et al.* 1981). Amyloid deposits were noted on rectal biopsy in the case described by Wichser and associates (1972). Although direct viral invasion of peripheral autonomic ganglia or postganglionic neuronal elements has been speculated, most authors have suggested that the dysautonomia may be an acute immunological damage to peripheral fibres of the autonomic nervous system. The clinical features, course, and documented recovery, elevated cerebrospinal fluid protein without pleocytosis, association of dysautonomia with malignancy and mixed connective-tissue disease, and regeneration of unmyelinated fibres are consistent with this view. Appenzeller *et al.* (1965) produced a limited abnormality of vasomotor function in rabbits 6–8 days after the injection of sympathetic antigen with Freund's adjuvant. Ultrastructural studies of the sympathetic paravertebral chain, vasomotor nerves, and perivascular spaces showed no specific lesion (Becker *et al.* 1979). There were basophils in the perivascular tissues of the animals and antibody to the sympathetic antigen in sera of animals implicating immunological mechanisms. Fibre-size spectra of unmyelinated fibres in the paravertebral chain were shifted to the left suggesting regeneration of unmyelinated axons and four out of nine animals regained vasomotor function after 2 months. There was no immunofluorescence against neuronal components demonstrated. Whether this is an experimental model of acute autonomic neuropathy or just a thought-provoking experimental disorder in search of its human counterpart remains debatable.

PATHOLOGY

Pathological studies have been limited to biopsied material except in one case where the patient died of painless intestinal obstruction (Fagius *et al.* 1983). Biopsy of the colon in a single case demonstrated non-specific inflammation of the lamina propria (Hopkins *et al.* 1981). Skin biopsy in one patient with postganglionic cholinergic dysautonomia revealed positive immunofluorescence with IgG antibodies against cholinergic, possibly sudomotor, fibres (Harik *et al.* 1977). However, skin biopsy in another patient with a similar clinical presentation failed to demonstrate this finding (Inamdar *et al.* 1982).

Sural-nerve biopsy, performed at different times during the course of the disease, demonstrates variable pathology. Young *et al.* (1975) reported normal findings during the early symptomatic phase of the disease. Other authors described segmental demyelination and axonal degeneration (Colan *et al.* 1980; Estanol-Vidal *et al.* 1979). Low and colleagues (1983*b*) observed reduction of small myelinated and unmyelinated fibres, absent *in vitro* C-fibre potential, and an unmeasurable content of dopamine-β-hydroxylase. Morphometry of the sural nerve biopsied, 12 years after the onset, by Appenzeller and Kornfeld (1973) showed an increase of small unmyelinated fibres and multilamellated Schwann-cell processes. Neuropathological study in a single case revealed unilateral hippocampal necrosis and atrophy of dorsal columns (Estanol-Vidal *et al.* 1979). Dorsal-root ganglia displayed almost complete loss of neurons and increased collagen. Dorsal roots showed decreased myelinated fibres, increased collagen, and clusters of mononuclear inflammatory cells. Sciatic and femoral nerves also had a reduction in myelinated fibres. Intermediolateral-column neurons were normal. Study of the peripheral autonomic nervous system was unfortunately limited to the coeliac ganglion which was normal.

DIAGNOSIS

Diagnosis of acute and subacute autonomic neuropathy depends on the symptoms and signs of widespread autonomic involvement with relative sparing of the somatic nervous system. In addition to documenting autonomic dysfunction with special investigations, one should exclude other conditions which may mimic this syndrome. Botulinum A, B, and E toxins can produce partial cholinergic dysautonomia along with presynaptic neuromuscular dysfunction (Jenzer *et al.* 1975). Botulinum B may, however, produce cholinergic dysautonomia without muscle weakness in 20 per cent of cases. Symptoms of botulism include nausea, vomiting, blurred vision, dry mouth, constipation, abdominal cramps, disturbed micturition and sexual function, and orthostatic hypotension. The cases of botulism are usually not isolated, have a history of spoiled canned goods consumption, and are of rapid onset. Recovery is usually rapid and complete but abnormalities of Schirmer's test have been demonstrated 230 days after onset (Jenzer *et al.* 1975). Botulism should be excluded with appropriate toxicological studies. Atropine poisoning or Jimson-weed intoxication produces dose-related symptoms (Mikolich *et al.* 1975). Dryness of mouth occurs with a 0.5 mg dose, tachycardia with a 2 mg dose, and urinary retention beyond a 5 mg dose. These patients usually have altered states of consciousness, hallucinations, fever, decerebrate posture, hyperreflexia, postive Babinski sign, and electroencephalographic abnormalitites. Another rare entity is cholinergic dysautonomia following a box jellyfish sting which is acute in onset and quickly reversible (Chand and Selliah 1984). The patient may also show associated neurologic manifestations such as muscle weakness and central respiratory failure.

SPECIAL INVESTIGATIONS

Autonomic evaluation is necessary to make an appropriate diagnosis and to develop a reasonable plan of treatment (see Chapters 16, 17, 37, 38). Autonomic assessment is aimed at the following aspects: (1) to detect the presence of autonomic impairment; (2) to determine the involvement of various organs; (3) to assess the severity of autonomic dysfunction; (4) to apportion sympathetic and parasympathetic involvement of a particular organ; and (5) to localize the site of lesion in the peripheral autonomic nervous system. Various investigations are available for the assessment of autonomic function. These investigations are based on the following principles: (1) abnormalities of reflex responses mediated through autonomic pathways; (2) direct micro-electrode recordings of the sympathetic nerves; (3) altered pharmacological responses of the denervated target tissues; and (4) immunohistochemical changes in the tissues following denervation.

It is difficult to diagnose with certainty an afferent lesion in the presence of an efferent lesion or to localize a lesion in the preganglionic or postganglonic segment of the efferent pathway. Pharmacologic studies are based on the detection of denervation supersensitivity (Cannon's law), i.e. enhanced responsiveness of the effector cell to the neurotransmitter. Immunohistochemical techniques provide direct evidence of depletion of the neurotransmitter and presence of antibodies against the target tissues. Pharmacological and immunohistochemical studies provide perhaps the best evidence to localize the lesion. However, precise localization must be viewed as hypothetical on the basis of currently used tests for the assessment of autonomic function in humans.

TREATMENT

Symptom control is attempted until spontaneous recovery occurs. Paraneoplastic dysautonomia is an exception. Surgical resection of adenocarcinoma of the lung (Vasudevan *et al.* 1981) and chemotherapy of oat-cell carcinoma (Khurana *et al.* 1983; Mamdani *et al.* 1985) can cause regression of dysautonomia within a few days suggesting that treatment of the neoplasm rather than dysautonomia is a better alternative. Orthostatic hypotension is usually quite disabling. It may respond to a variety of treatments based upon the clinical and pharmacological assessment. Fludrocortisone acetate is the mainstay of treatment of orthostatic hypotension although other treatments may be more suitable in an individual patient. Corrective bifocal lenses relieve blurring of vision. Artificial tears and saliva provide relief in patients with dry eyes and dry mouth, respectively. Gastrointestinal and bladder dysfunction respond to bethanecol or carbachol treatment. These patients are hypersensitive to cholinomimetic drugs (Khurana *et al.* 1980). Bethanecol may have generalized rather than organ-specific effects and may cause problems initially. We have observed bronchorrhoea following administration of a small dose of bethanecol requiring atropine administration in a patient with paraneoplastic dysautonomia. Therefore, these patients should receive gradually increasing doses of these drugs as necessary.

REFERENCES

Anderson, O., Lindberg, J., Modigh, K., and Reske-Nielsen, E. (1972). Subacute dysautonomia with incomplete recovery. *Acta neurol. scand.* **48**, 510–19.

Appenzeller, O., Arnason, B. G., and Adams, R. D. (1965). Experimental autonomic neuropathy: an immunologically induced disorder of reflex vasomotor function. *J. Neurol. Neurosurg. Psychiat.* **28**, 510–15.

Appenzeller, O., and Kornfeld, M. (1973). Acute pandysautonomia. *Arch. Neurol.* **29**, 334–9.

Bannister, R., DaCosta, D. F., Hendry, W. G., Jacobs, J., and Mathias, C. J. (1986). Atrial demand pacing to protect against vagal overactivity in sympathetic autonomic neuropathy. *Brain* **109**, 345–56.

Barnett, A. J., and Wagner, G. R. (1958). Severe orthostatic hypotension: case report and description of response to sympathomimetic drugs. *Am. Heart. J.* **56**, 412–24.

Becker, W., Livett, B. G., and Appenzeller, O. (1979). Experimental autonomic neuropathy: ultrastructure and immunohistochemical study of a disorder of reflex vasomotor function. *J. autonom. nerv. Syst.* **1**, 53–67.

Bost, M., Rossignol, A.-M., Tachker, D., Batellier, H., and Jeannoel, P. (1983). Un cas de dysautonomie aigue reversible chez l'adolescent. *Pédiatrie* **38**, 29–36.

Chand, R. P. and Selliah, K. (1984). Reversible parasympathetic dysautonomia following stinging attributed to the box jellyfish (chironex fleckeri). *Aust. NZ J. Med.* **14**, 673–5.

Colan, R. V., Carter Snead, O., Oh, S. H., and Kashlan, B. (1980). Acute autonomic and sensory neuropathy. *Ann. Neurol.* **8**, 441–4.

Edelman, J., Gubbay, S. S., and Zilko, P. J. (1981). Acute pandysautonomia due to mixed connective tissue disease. *Aust. NZ J. Med.* **11**, 68–70.

Estanol-Vidal, B., Perez-Ortega, R., Vargas-Lugo, B., Chavez-Figarola, C., Viteri, M. S. D., and Loyo-Varela, M. (1979). Acute autonomic neuropathy. *Arch. invest. Med., Mexico* **10**, 53–64.

Fagius, J., Westerberg, C., and Olsson, Y. (1983). Acute pandysautonomia and severe sensory deficit with poor recovery. A clinical, neurophysiological and pathological case study. *J. Neurol. Neurosurg. Psychiat.* **46**, 725–33.

Harik, S. I., Ghandour, M. H., Farah, F. S., and Afifi, A. K. (1977). Postganglionic cholinergic dysautonomia. *Ann. Neurol,* **1**, 393–6.

Hopkins, A., Neville, B., and Bannister, R. (1974). Autonomic neuropathy of acute onset. *Lancet* **i**, 769–71.

Hopkins, I. J., Shield, L. K., and Harris, M. (1981). Subacute cholinergic dysautonomia in childhood. *Clin. exp. Neurol.* **17**, 147–51.

Inamdar, S., Easton, L. B., and Lester, G. (1982). Acquired postganglionic cholinergic dysautonomia: case report and review of the literature. *Pediatrics* **70**, 976–8.

Jenzer, G., Mumenthaler, M., Ludin, H. P., and Robert, F. (1975). Autonomic dysfunction in botulism B: a clinical report. *Neurology* **25**, 150–3.

Khurana, R. K., Koski, C. L., and Mayer, R. F. (1983). Dysautonomia in Eaton–Lambert syndrome. *Ann. Neurol.* **14**, 123.

Khurana, R. K., Nelson, E., Azzarelli, B., and Garcia, J. H. (1980). Shy–Drager syndrome: diagnosis and treatment of cholinergic dysfunction. *Neurology* **30**, 805–9.

Lieshout, J. J. V., Wieling, W., Montfrans, G. V., Settles, J. J., Speelman, J. D., Endert, E., and Karemaker, J. M. (1986). Acute dysautonomia associated with Hodgkin's disease. *J. Neurol. Neurosurg. Psychiat.* **49**, 830–2.

Low, P. A., Dyck, P. J., Lambert, E. H., Brimijoin, W. S., Trautmann, J. C., Malagelada, J. R., Fealey, R. D., and Barrett, D. M. (1983). Acute panautonomic neuropathy. *Ann. Neurol.* **13**, 412–17.

Mamdani, M. B., Walsh, R. L., Rubino, F. A., Brannegan, R. T., and Hwang, M. H. (1985). Autonomic dysfunction and Eaton–Lambert syndrome. *J. autonom. nerv. Syst.* **12**, 315–20.

Mikolich, J. R., Paulson, G. W., and Cross, C. J. (1975). Acute anticholinergic syndrome due to jimson seed ingestion, clinical and laboratory observation in six cases. *Ann. intern. Med.* **83**, 321–5.

Okada, F., Yamashita, I., and Suwa, N. (1975). Two cases of acute pandysautonomia. *Arch. Neurol.* **32**, 146–51.

Thomashefsky, A. J., Horwitz, S. J., and Feingold, M. H. (1972). Acute autonomic neuropathy. *Neurology, Minneapolis* **22**, 251–5.

Vasudevan, C. P., Suppiah, F., Udoshi, M. B., and Lusins, J. (1981). Reversible autonomic neuropathy and hypertrophic osteoarthropathy in a patient with bronchogenic carcinoma. *Chest* **79**, 479–81.

Wichser, J., Vijayan, N., and Dreyfus, P. M. (1972). Dysautonomia: its significance in neurologic disease. *Cal. Med.* **117**, 28–37.

Yahr, M. D. and Frontera, A. T. (1975). Acute autonomic neuropathy. *Arch. Neurol.* **32**, 132–3.

Yee, R. D., Trese, M., Zee, D. S., Kollarits, C. R., and Cogan, D. G. (1976). Ocular manifestations of acute pandysautonomia. *Am. J. Ophthalmol.* **81**, 740–4.

Young, R. R., Asbury, A. K., Adams, R. D., and Corbett, J. L. (1969). Pure pandysautonomia with recovery. *Trans. Am. neurol. Ass.* **94**, 355–7.

Young, R. R., Asbury, A. K., Corbett, J. L., and Adams, R. D. (1975). Pure pandysautonomia with recovery. Description and discussion of diagnostic criteria. *Brain* **98**, 613–36.

36. Clinical presentations of diabetic autonomic failure

Michael E. Edmonds and Peter J. Watkins

INTRODUCTION

Diabetic neuropathy is a common condition with highly characteristic features due to the early and extensive involvement of small nerve fibres. It is the commonest cause of autonomic neuropathy causing functional defects and symptoms in a wide variety of systems. The gastrointestinal tract, the genitourinary system, the heart, and blood vessels are all affected; there are abnormalities of sweating, pupillary defects, and a wide variety of metabolic disorders. Early small-fibre damage is manifested by impairment of vagally controlled heart-rate variability, while diminished peripheral sympathetic tone leads to increased blood flow which is detectable before there is clinical evidence of neuropathy (Archer *et al.* 1984). Diminished sweating is very common in diabetes (Low and Fealey 1987), and thermal sensation (a small-fibre modality) is lost before vibration sensation (a large-fibre modality) (Guy *et al.* 1985). Indeed, reduced thermal sensation is probably a very early marker of this and other neuropathies. Pain sensation has not been extensively assessed, but is abnormal in most diabetics with neuropathic ulcers and Charcot arthropathy.

The cause of the severe attack on small nerve fibres is not known, but there is now evidence that immunologically mediated damage could contribute to pathological changes of the autonomic nerves. Thus, at post-mortem, inflammatory cellular infiltrations of lymphocytes, macrophages, and occasionally plasma cells were found, particularly related to autonomic nerve bundles and ganglia, in or around bundles of unmyelinated nerve fibres and in the superior cervical sympathetic ganglion (Duchen *et al.* 1980). Our observation (Guy *et al.* 1984*b*) that iritis commonly occurs in severe autonomic neuropathy (14 of 47 patients under 40 years old), though not confirmed, lends further weight to this hypothesis, and we have also shown that immune complexes may be increased in these patients (Gilbey *et al.* 1986). The idea that antibodies to exogenous insulin might interfere with the action of nerve growth factor with which it has structural similarities was raised by Bennett (1984): nerve growth factor is required in animals for growth and survival of sympathetic nerves, and also accumulates in the denervated iris. The idea merits further study.

This chapter describes the clinical consequences of the autonomic defects which occur in diabetes.

BLOOD FLOW IN THE NEUROPATHIC FOOT

Peripheral neuropathy in the foot leads to both somatic and autonomic damage. Small-fibre loss may predominate leading to loss of pain and thermal sensation before light touch and vibration senses are blunted (Guy *et al.* 1985). Small-fibre neuropathy may produce a pseudo-syringomyelic picture with a distal-length related sensory loss mainly affecting pain and temperature sensation. Small-fibre loss also leads to sympathetic denervation which is characteristic of diabetic neuropathy (Watkins and Edmonds 1983). A peripheral sympathetic defect has been demonstrated by direct measurement of sympathetic activity in postganglionic C fibres in the diabetic neuropathic limb (Fagius 1982). Sympathetic nerve endings to small arterioles in the diabetic limb are entirely absent or are found at significantly greater distance from effector sites compared with controls. Recent studies of the circulation in the neuropathic foot have shown that blood flow is increased with arteriovenous shunting, and that the peripheral arteries are dilated and stiff. These abnormalities may be responsible (in part) for the pathogenesis of the neuropathic complications of the diabetic foot, and may also be important in acute, painful neuropathy.

Autonomic denervation may be responsible for abnormalities in blood flow. Doppler studies have shown that there is increased velocity of forward flow in dilated peripheral arteries. Venous occlusion plethysmography has demonstrated increased peripheral blood flow (Archer *et al.* 1984) (Fig. 36.1). Measurements of the big toe and midfoot have shown high blood flows, on average five times above normal, in diabetic patients with peripheral neuropathy. These recordings have confirmed earlier observations demonstrating a fixed increased resting blood flow in patients with severe neuropathy. Spontaneous variations in resting flow which are secondary to sympathetic activity are considerably reduced in the neuropathic diabetic foot. All these observations were made in the supine patient. However, high blood flows and overperfusion have also been demonstrated in the dependent foot. In normal subjects standing causes precapillary vasoconstriction in the foot, limiting the increment in

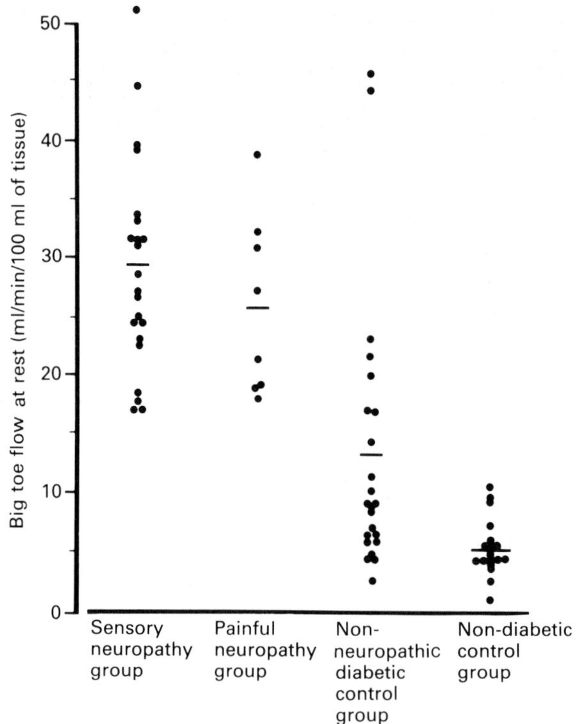

Fig. 36.1. Blood flow measured by plethysmography in the hallux of diabetics with severe sensory neuropathy, severe painful neuropathy, non-neuropathic diabetic controls, and normal controls. (Taken from Archer *et al.* (1984) by kind permission of the editor of *Diabetologia.*)

capillary pressure and reducing blood flow (Tooke 1986). This veni-arteriolar response is dependent upon a sympathetic axon reflex. Laser doppler flowmetry which measures superficial microvascular flow, has shown that in the neuropathic foot the percentage fall in skin blood flow on dependency is less than normal. This suggests that postural control of blood flow is disturbed in patients with diabetic neuropathy, and this abnormality is compatible with loss of sympathetic vascular tone. Increase in blood flow is associated with arteriovenous shunting in the neuropathic limb resulting in prominent turgid veins over the dorsum of the foot and lower part of the calf in the recumbent position (Ward *et al.* 1983). Furthermore, evidence derived from Doppler sonography, microsphere partitioning, and foot venous blood sampling supports the concept of arteriovenous shunting. In the neuropathic limb the arterial walls are stiff probably as a result of medial wall calcification (Fig. 36.2), and sympathetic neuropathy may be an important aetiological factor. Recently, calcification has been reported following sympathectomy.

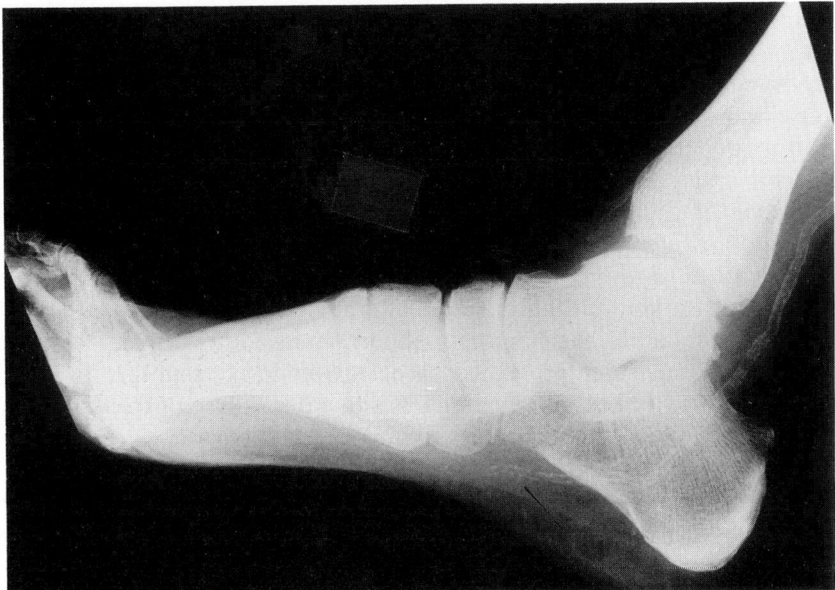

Fig. 36.2. Medial calcification in the arteries of a young severely neuropathic insulin-dependent diabetic.

Eleven of 13 patients who underwent unilateral sympathectomy developed medial calcification on the operative side having had normal radiographs before the procedure. Bilateral sympathectomy was carried out on seven patients, all of whom showed calcification on both sides later

Autonomic neuropathy may be responsible for two other abnormalities in the foot, namely disordered thermal regulation and disturbances of sweating (see p. 000). Increased blood flow leads to reaised skin temperature in the resting neuropathic limb (Ward *et al.* 1983). In a recent study, mean skin temperature was 33.5°C in neuropathic feet compared with 25.8°C in control subjects (Archer *et al.* 1984). However, vasoconstriction in response to local cold is often prolonged. A disturbed autonomic balance with unopposed sympathetic nervous activity may be responsible for such vasospasm; alternatively, a sympathetic denervation hypersensitivity may be the cause.

Degenervation of postganglionic unmyelinated sudomotor axons leads to a reduction in sweating. Quantitative tests of sweat function have been developed using pilocarpine stimulation or acetylcholine electrophoresis; these have confirmed the close relationship between sweating deficiency and loss of pain perception.

Abnormalities in blood flow, thermoregulation, and sweating which follow from autonomic neuropathy may be responsible for the complications of the neuropathic foot.

Several studies have now shown that there is greater autonomic impairment in diabetics with neuropathic ulceration compared to those with neuropathy but no ulceration (Edmonds *et al.* 1986). Rigid dilated arteries and shunting lead to a rapid increase of flow with short-circuiting of capillaries and distal ischaemia. They also lead to raised venular pressure and venous distension. Indeed, in one animal study, arteriovenous shunting was a necessary requirement for neuropathic ulceration (Borkowski 1973). Autonomic neuropathy also predisposes to ulceration by other mechanisms. Abnormal responses to temperature changes, in particular prolonged vasoconstriction on exposure to cold, could be harmful. Loss of sweating leads to a dry skin with thick plaques of hard callus which readily crack. This can lead to fissuring of the skin and eventual ulceration.

Although less frequent, the Charcot joint can be a devastating complication of the neuropathic foot. Circulatory changes can lead to abnormalities in bone structure (Fig. 36.3). In the experimental animal increased blood flow leads to rarefaction and demineralization of bone, and in the human there is a reduction in bony cortical thickness rendering the foot susceptible to even minor trauma. Nevertheless, somatic neuropathy is also a necessary prerequisite, patients with Charcot arthropathy having absent flare response after axon reflex stimulation, indicating degeneration of unmyelinated nociceptive fibres. The combination of somatic and autonomic neuropathy permits abnormal mechanical stress to occur resulting in fracture and finally bone and joint disorganization.

Peripheral oedema, sometimes of considerable severity and resistance to treatment, is a rare feature of some cases of diabetic neuropathy. It may be related to overperfusion, especially in the dependent position, together with arteriovenous shunting, raised venous pressure, and venous distension. The use of sympathometic agents by stimulating vasoconstriction may be expected to reduce this form of oedema. We have shown that ephedrine is of value in treating neuropathic oedema (Edmonds *et al.* 1983). It results in a rapid decrease of weight, a reduction in peripheral diastolic flow, and an increase in sodium excretion, all associated with diminution of oedema. The effect of ephedrine is, however, complex and, as well as its peripheral effects, it may have central effects on the control of sodium and water homeostasis.

High peripheral blood flow and increased warmth have been observed in the acutely painful neuropathic limb (Archer *et al.* 1984). Reduction of this blood flow either by sympathetic stimuli or by inflation by a sphygmomanometer cuff, was associated with a reduction in pain. This

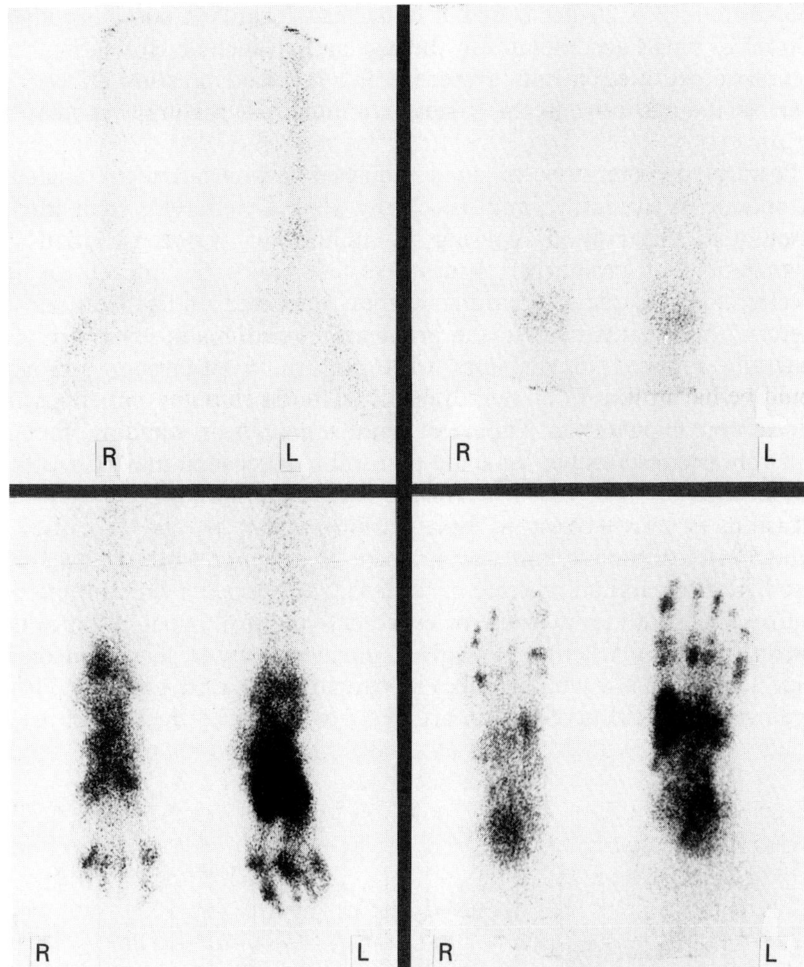

Fig. 36.3. Isotope uptake in the feet of a normal subject (top pair) and a patient with severe diabetic neuropathy (bottom pair), indicating the greatly incresed bone blood flow which occurs in diabetic neuropathy.

finding could explain the observation that this pain could be diminished by cooling the feet (Ward *et al.* 1983) and therapeutic reduction of blood flow may be a possible treatment for painful diabetic neuropathy.

POSTURAL HYPOTENSION

Maintenance of blood pressure on standing depends on afferent impulses from baroreceptors (namely in the carotid sinus and aortic arch) and on efferent sympathetic impulses to the heart and blood vessels. In normal people there is a 20 per cent fall in cardiac output on standing; about 700 ml of blood accumulates in the legs and splanchnic circulation, but compensatory mechanisms prevent a fall in blood pressure. If one or more of the pathways in this system are impaired, postural hypotension results.

Postural hypotension is an established complication of diabetic autonomic neuropathy, and is chiefly due to efferent sympathetic vasomotor denervation causing a failure of vasoconstriction in splanchnic and peripheral tissues (Hilsted 1982). Failure of cardiac acceleration and reduced cardiac output (exhibited under the stress of exercise) both contribute to the problems. Noradrenalin levels are also generally reduced in diabetics with postural hypotension, although occasionally an excess of noradrenalin is found in some patients with low-volume hypotension. Failure of renin responses on standing, though probably not responsible for acute postural hypotension, may (Christlieb and Bratten 1974) or may not (Hilsted 1982) be abnormal.

Insulin is now known to have cardiovascular effects. It causes a reduction of plasma volume, an increase of peripheral blood flow from vasodilatation, and an increase of heart rate. In patients with autonomic neuropathy, insulin may cause or exacerbate postural hypotension to the point of fainting whether it is given intravenously or subcutanteously (Fig. 36.4). It has a similar effect in sympathectomized patients. These cardiovascular effects of insulin are likely to be due to the insulin itself,

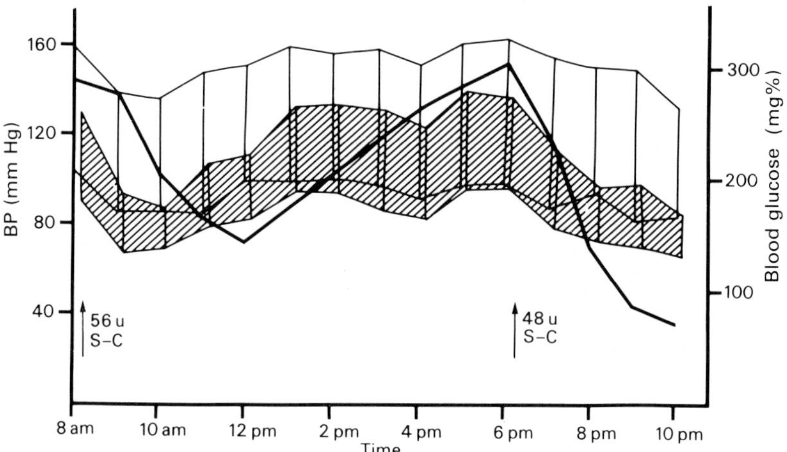

Fig. 36.4. Diurnal variation of lying and standing blood pressures in a 48-year-old man with severe autonomic neuropathy. Insulin was given subcutaneously (S–C) at times shown by the vertical arrows. The unhatched area shows supine blood pressure, the hatched area the standing blood pressure, and the continuous line the blood glucose.

and not changes of blood glucose, and in other types of postural hypotension the insulinaemia following a meal can be sufficient to exacerbate the hypotension.

Postural hypotension (a fall of systolic pressure of more than 30 mm Hg) occurs in diabetics with advanced neuropathy although symptoms are infrequent and were noted in only 23 of 73 autonomic neuropathy patients described by Ewing and Clarke (1986) and eight of 125 neuropathy patients examined by Rundles (1945). Disabling hypotension, when systolic pressure falls below 70 mm Hg, is rare. Both hypotension and its symptoms vary spontaneously to a remarkable degree. The explanation for this is unclear, although insulin itself may be partly responsible by exacerbating the condition, and fluid retention (for example from cardiac failure) may ameliorate it.

Treatment of postural hypotension

Few diabetics develop symptoms sufficiently severe to need treatment. When they do, it is first essential to stop any drugs which exacerbate hypotension, notably diuretics, tranquillizers, and antidepressants. Simple treatments should always be tried and include raising the head of the bed and full-length elastic stockings, but the benefits are slight. Complicated anti-g suits may be helpful but are too cumbersome to be acceptable. Measures which increase plasma volume are the most effective although oedema is a troublesome side-effect which often renders treatment unacceptable. A high salt intake or fludrocortisone sometimes in high doses (up to 0.4 mg daily) can, however, be effective. The use of an orally active adrenergic agonist, midodrine, can help; it has an exclusively peripheral pressor effect on arterial and venous capacitance vessels. We found that it improved both standing blood pressure and symptoms in two of three patients severely affected by postural hypotension.

Many other treatments have been suggested: their effectiveness is inconsistent, some regimes are hazardous, and supine hypertension is a common sequel. These treatments include β-blockers with partial agonist activity, such as pindolol and xamoterol, and the use of ergotamine, vasopressin, caffeine, non-steroidal inflammatory drugs, clonidine, and metoclopramide (Chapter 32).

SWEATING ABNORMALITIES

Defective sweating in diabetic neuropathy was described many years ago. There is renewed interest in this field brought about by development of new techniques. Measurement of sweating in the periphery is one of the few quantitative methods for assessing sympathetic nerve function. Loss of sweating may be of particular importance in the development of neuropathic foot lesions, and this represents another area of recent investigation.

There are four methods for studying sweat responses (Low and Fealey 1987). The thermoregulatory sweat test involves whole-body testing and sweating is detected by application of alizarin red powder: this method assesses peripheral sympathetic function (pre-plus postganglionic). The quantitative sudomotor axon reflex test stimulates sweating by iontophoresis of acetylcholine, and assesses postganglionic sympathetic function by the axon reflex. Direct stimulation of sweat glands by iontophoresis of pilocarpine and recording by counting sweat droplets on a silastic imprint assesses postganglionic sweat gland denervation. Finally, the dermal sweat glands are normally activated by a sympathetic discharge, and this provides the galvanic skin response. This is a biphasic charge of electric potential that can be recorded from the skin using electrocardiogram electrodes. The quantitative sudomotor axon reflex test is probably the most sensitive of these four tests.

The commonest sweating deficit is in the feet in the classical stocking distribution. There is a close correlation with other autonomic defects, especially with postural hypotension, but also with cardiac vagal denervation, although the cardiovascular autonomic function tests tend to be abnormal before there is evidence of peripheral sweating loss. There is some relationship between loss of sweating and diminished pain sensation, and with absence of sympathetic activity obtained by direct microneurographic nerve recordings (Fagius 1982). Abnormal responses may be found in cases of painful neuropathy, and patients with truncal mononeuropathies may have patchy sweating defects. These tests all confirm the widespread small nerve-fibre damage which occurs in diabetic neuropathy.

Loss of sweating in neuropathic feet may act as a prelude to the dry, cracked skin which offers a portal of entry for sepsis. Feet with neuropathic ulcers do not however always show an absence of sweating, and in recent work as many as 25 per cent of these feet, and 64 per cent of those with Charcot arthropathy, retained the ability to sweat as demonstrated by the axon reflex test. The role of sympathetic failure in the genesis of diabetic foot lesions may need some reappraisal though our own studies have shown that cardiovascular reflexes are always abnormal in these patients (Edmonds *et al.* 1986).

Gustatory sweating is a highly characteristic and not uncommon symptom of diabetic autonomic neuropathy (Fig. 36.5). Sweating begins minutes after starting to chew tasty food, especially cheese. It starts on the forehead, and spreads to involve the face, scalp, and neck, and sometimes the shoulders and upper part of the chest, compelling patients to keep a towel at the dinner table. Distribution of the sweating is in the

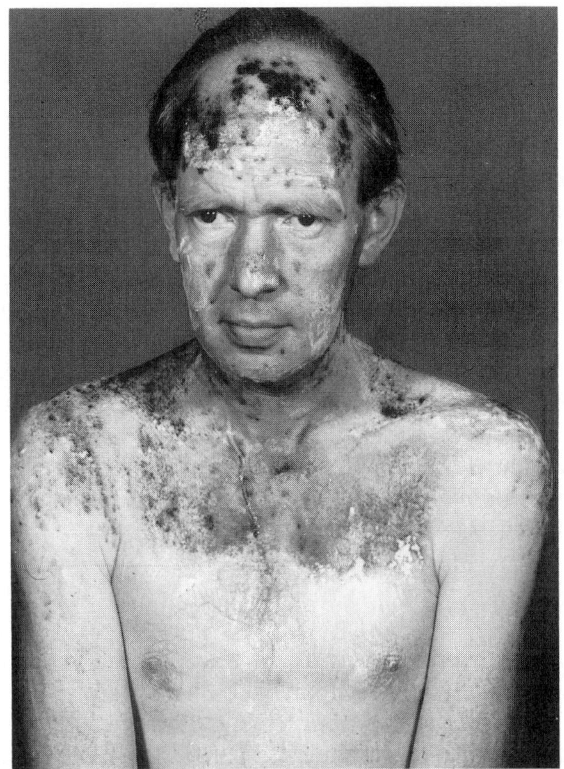

Fig. 36.5. Severe facial and shoulder sweating (gustatory sweating) seen a few minutes after eating cheese. The area of sweating is clearly delineated by the application of quinizarin powder which turns blue when moist.

territory of the superior cervical ganglion. It may be of sudden onset; its cause is unknown, although aberrant nerve regeneration has been suggested. It is occasionally sufficiently severe to need treatment: anticholinergic drugs are highly effective though side-effects may limit their use. Poldine methylsulphate (*Nacton*) is the best agent, and propantheline bromide (*Pro-banthine*) can also be used. They are given half an hour before meals, but may also be effective if given before single meals at social occasions.

DIABETIC DIARRHOEA

Diarrhoea is a very disagreeable symptom of autonomic neuropathy. Abdominal rumbling and discomfort precede attacks of watery diarrhoea, without pain or bleeding, and usually without malabsorption. Faecal incontinence is common, especially at night, when exacerbations seem to be worse. Symptoms last from a few hours to a few days and then remit, with normal bowel action or even constipation (sometimes induced by treatment) in between attacks. Constipation is not in our view otherwise a particular problem experienced by neuropathic diabetics.

The cause of diabetic diarrhoea is not known, and there have been few recent advances. Abnormalities of gut motility, decreased gut transit time, bacterial overgrowth, and bile salt malabsorption have all been described (Chapter 14).

The diagnosis of diabetic diarrhoea must be established by confirming the presence of autonomic neuropathy, and excluding other causes of diarrhoea.

Tetracycline offers effective treatment in approximately half the patients, and is given in one or two doses of 250 mg at the onset of an attack which is abruptly aborted. If this fails, one must try all the usual antidiarrhoea remedies, notably codeine phosphate, lomotil, or loperamide (*Imodium*). The use of clonidine has also been described (Fedorak *et al.* 1985).

GASTROPARESIS

Vomiting from gastroparesis is a rare complication of autonomic neuropathy. It is usually intermittent, and only rarely so persistent that surgery may be needed. Gastroparesis is characterized by a gastric splash, and radiologically by large food residues, absent peristalsis, a failure to empty the stomach, and a patulous pylorus. Failure to advance a jejunal biopsy capsule beyond the pylorus is also a feature.

Gastroparesis is most probably due to vagal degeneration. Several post-mortem studies have demonstrated loss of myelinated fibres in the vagus nerve, but only recently, loss of unmyelinated fibres has been shown in a vagus nerve removed at laparotomy from a patient with intractable vomiting from gastroparesis (Guy *et al.* 1984*a*). Subtotal smooth-muscle cell atrophy in the muscularis propria of the stomach has been described in these patients, associated with transformed, smooth-muscle cells undergoing a form of necrobiosis appearing as highly distinctive, homogeneous, round, eosinophilic bodies (Moscoso *et al.* 1986).

Gastric motility and emptying studies are generally difficult to perform, and yield variable results. Liquids, solids, and indigestible solids are emptied by the stomach at different rates, and by different mechanisms (Minami and McCallum 1984). Radioisotope studies in diabetics with autonomic neuropathy have variously shown normal solid emptying, impairment of the usual differentiation between solid and liquid emptying, abnormal solid but normal liquid emptying, and abnormal solid and liquid emptying (DePonti *et al.* 1987). Abnormal liquid emptying probably represents advanced disease; it can be assessed with relative simplicity by a new technique measuring epigastric impedance (Gilbey and Watkins 1987) (Fig. 36.6). This technique seems to be a reliable diagnostic tool, and distinguishes those with vomiting from gastroparesis from the many patients with severe autonomic neuropathy who have normal gastric liquid emptying (Fig. 36.7).

Dopamine antagonists (metoclopramide and domperidone) enhance gastric tone and emptying. They may accelerate gastric emptying in

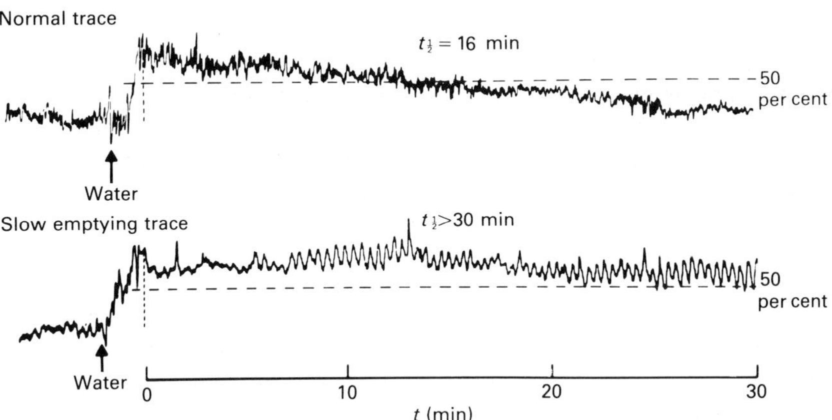

Fig. 36.6. Gastric emptying measured by epigastric impedance, showing normal emptying (above) and grossly delayed emptying in gastroparesis (below). $t_{1/2}$ is the time taken for impedance to return to 50 per cent of maximum deflection.

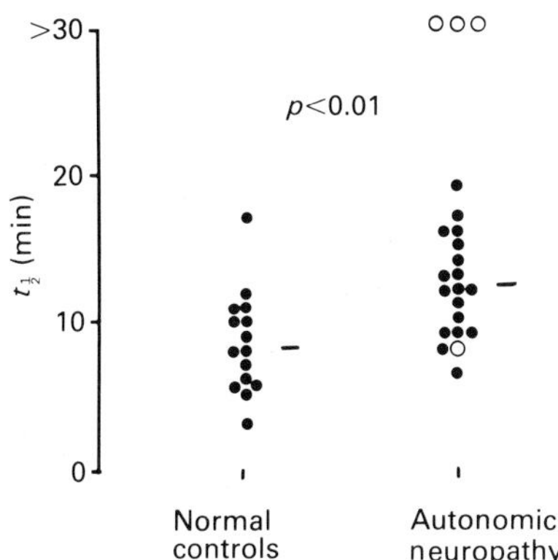

Fig. 36.7. Gastric emptying times in normal subjects (left) and those with severe autonomic neuropathy (right). The technique distinguishes those with vomiting (O) due to gastroparesis from other causes. Not all diabetics with autonomic neuropathy show a delay in gastric emptying. (Taken from Gilbey and Watkins (1987) by kind permission of the editor of *Diabetic Medicine*.)

diabetic autonomic neuropathy occasionally with considerable effect. They form the mainstay of treatment during vomiting bouts. Rarely, when vomiting becomes persistent, a drainage operation is needed. There are few reports of the procedure, and it may fail. We reported two cases, only one of which succeeded (Guy *et al.* 1984*a*). Roux-en-Y gastrectomy is recommended, together with vagotomy and antrectomy, to minimize biliary reflux and stomal ulceration.

OESOPHAGUS

Abnormal oesophageal motility has been described in diabetic autonomic neuropathy although there are no convincing clinical manifestations of this. The subject was reviewed by Ewing and Clarke (1986). Recent studies by Maddern *et al.* (1985) describe relief of heartburn and dysphagia by domperidone, noting however no improvement in solid emptying.

GALL BLADDER

Enlargement of the gall bladder, probably due to poor contraction, may be a feature of diabetes related to autonomic neuropathy. Studies by ultrasonography have not confirmed the enlargement of the gall bladder, but do suggest impaired muscular contraction. There are no known clinical effects from this.

NEUROGENIC BLADDER

Autonomic neuropathy affecting the sacral nerves causes bladder dysfunction. Bladder-function tests are commonly abnormal in neuropathic diabetics but symptoms from neurogenic bladder in diabetes are relatively rare, usually occurring in diabetics who already have advanced complications. Most patients with neurogenic bladder are also impotent.

Impairment of bladder function is chiefly the result of detrusor-muscle afferent sensory abnormalities, while pudendal innervation of perineal and periurethral striated muscle is usually unaffected in diabetic neuropathy. Afferent damage results in impaired sensation of bladder filling, and leads to detrusor areflexia: thus, the bladder pressure during cystometrography fails to increase as the bladder is filled. In advanced cases bladder emptying is reduced because of impaired detrusor activity and possibly failure of the internal sphincter to open adequately. Measurements of urine flow show that the peak flow rate is reduced and that duration of flow is increased.

There are no symptoms in the early stages, but later patients experience hesitancy during micturition, develop the need to strain, a feeble stream, and a tendency to dribble. Micturition is sometimes in short interrupted spurts which results from straining. Patients may be aware of lengthening intervals between micturition, and also experience a sensation of inadequate bladder emptying. Gradually residual urine volume increases and, in severe cases, gross bladder retention occurs with abdominal swelling, and sometimes overflow incontinence as well. Bladder capacity may exceed 1 litre.

Diagnosis of neurogenic bladder is usually simple because patients have obvious and severe neuropathy. It is, however, important to exclude bladder-neck obstruction, and especially prostatic obstruction in men. Cystoscopy is therefore needed, and intravenous pyelography too may be helpful: rarely, diabetic neurogenic bladder causes hydroureter and hydronephrosis. Ultrasound examination provides a simple measurement of bladder emptying, but more sophisticated bladder function tests are sometimes needed. These include cystograms, cystometrography, and urine flow-rate measurements.

The principles of treatment are to compensate for deficient bladder sensation and thus prevent the development of a high residual urine volume. For those diabetics who have few symptoms of cystopathy, education is important and may suffice. In particular, the patient should be told to void every three hours during the daytime. Straining may be required, and the Crede manoeuvre can increase the efficiency of bladder emptying. With more severe symptoms, more active measures are needed. Cholinergic drugs are used to increase intravesical pressure, and maintain a small bladder capacity. Bethanecol is the best availble drug, although side-effects of sweating, salivation, and tachycardia can be a nuisance. Administration of prazosin may help by reducing urethral resistance. If it is ineffective alone, catheterization with regular clamping and release can help to overcome the problem. Surgery is sometimes needed. Careful bladder-neck resection, even in women, provides very effective relief in the more severe cases by lowering the propulsive force needed to empty the bladder, In the most disabled patients, long-term catheterization is the only solution to the problem.

The most serious consequence of urinary retention is the development of urinary-tract infections which are severe or even fatal. Diabetic cystopathy sometimes occurs in the presence of advanced nephropathy, and then infections may accelerate the decline of renal function. If the residual bladder volume is very large, transplantation is usually contraindicated because postoperative sepsis is almost inevitable.

IMPOTENCE

Autonomic neuropathy is still considered to be the main aetiological factor in diabetic impotence (Chapter 13). It is due to erectile failure resulting from damage to both parasympathetic and sympathetic innervation of the corpora cavernosa. VIPergic nerves are also important in the vasodilatation of erection and the concentration of vasoactive inhibitive polypeptide (VIP) is low in the penile corpora in diabetics with autonomic neuropathy. Failure to achieve erection may also be the result of a concomitant sensory deficit in the dorsal nerve of the penis. The onset of neuropathic impotence is always gradual, progressing slowly over months, but complete erectile failure is usually present within 2 years of the onset of symptoms. This history contrasts with psychogenic impotence which begins suddenly and in which nocturnal erections are present.

Impotence may also be due to vascular occlusion of the branches of the internal pudendal artery. Furthermore, in rare cases, erectile failure may be caused by the Gluteal Steal syndrome.

The diagnosis of neuropathic impotence in diabetics is difficult. However, the quantitation of erectile function has been improved recently by several techniques, especially by the measurement of continuous nocturnal penile tumescence and rigidity by recording of circumferential penile expansion, and concurrent rigidity during sleep. Absence of tumescence and rigidity over 3 successive nights is a strong indication for an organic cause of impotence. Vasculogenic impotence can be confirmed by a measurement of penile blood pressure, and by comparing it with a brachial systolic pressure, thereby achieving a penile brachial index. When the ratio of brachial-to-penile pressure is 0.75 or less, a diagnosis of penile vascular disease can be strongly considered. Autonomic function tests give some guidance to the presence of autonomic neuropathy, but they do not establish conclusively in an individual whether it is the cause of the impotence. A neuropathic cause can be more exactly defined by electrophysiological testing of reflex sexual pathways. Conduction velocity is reduced in the dorsal nerve of the penis in diabetic impotent patients, and the latency of the bulbocavernosus reflex is prolonged.

The rational treatment of diabetic impotence depends on a careful history, in particular to evaluate any psychological component. If this factor is present, then the patient and his partner may be helped by appropriate discussion and advice. For younger patients, penile implants, either rigid or inflatable, have been of value. In vasculogenic impotence, arterial disease is often distal, and arterial reconstruction is only useful in those with major arterial diseases.

RESPIRATORY RESPONSES AND ARRESTS

Sudden cardiorespiratory arrests have been well described in diabetes with autonomic neuropathy. In most of these episodes, there was some interference with respiration either by anaesthesia, drugs, or bronchopneumonia. These observations have led to further investigation of the respiratory system of diabetics with autonomic neuropathy; first, the control of ventilation in response to hypoxia and hypercapnoea; second, the pattern of respiration during sleep; and third, the bronchial reactivity to chemical and physical agents.

The integrity of the ventilatory responses in autonomic neuropathy has been studied by measuring response to hypoxia and hypercapnoea in diabetics with and without neuropathy. The results of these are conflicting. Normal increased ventilatory responses to transient hypoxia during excercise and to progressive hypoxia have been reported, implying that peripheral chemoreceptors and their afferent nerves are intact in diabetic autonomic neuropathy. Although Williams *et al.* (1984) studied diabetics as a whole, up to 25 per cent had abnormal response to hypoxia, and these patients also had evidence of defective autonomic innervation from pupillary studies. Similarly, Monserrat *et al.* (1985) found a defective response to hypoxia in autonomic neuropathy. The results regarding responses to hypercapnoea have also been conflicting; both normal ventilatory and reduced responses have been detected (Ewing and Clark 1986). Thus the true importance of abnormal ventilatory responses as a cause of respiratory arrest has yet to be established.

In 1981, Guilleminault *et al.* reported four insulin-dependent diabetics with apnoeic episodes during sleep. These apnoeic episodes occurred not only during rapid-eye-movement sleep when they are a normal event, but also during non-rapid eye movement when they are definitely pathological. In the same year Rees *et al.* (1981) reported three further diabetics with autonomic neuropathy who also had sleep apnoea. However, two of these patients were older than any of the control group, and the incidence of sleep apnoea in normal subjects is known to rise with increasing age.

In recent studies of unselected diabetic patients, five of 12 insulin-dependent diabetic patients had abnormal breathing patterns, and four of these had evidence of autonomic neuropathy. Interestingly, the heart-rate adaptation to the apnoeic episodes was also abnormal in these patients. However, when well-matched groups of diabetics with and without autonomic neuropathy were studied, the number of apnoeic episodes per night was not significantly different in the two groups. It was concluded that diabetic patients with severe autonomic neuropathy have normal breathing patterns, and oxygenation during sleep, and that it is unlikely that sleep apnoea is a cause of respiratory arrest and sudden death in patients with autonomic neuropathy (Catterall *et al.* 1984).

The third area of study has assessed the integrity of respiratory reflexes which affect bronchomotor tone. Airways tone is mainly under vagal control, and it is reduced in diabetics with autonomic neuropathy. Administration of ipratropium to normal subjects blocks efferent vagal tone in the airways, causing marked bronchal dilatation. This response is, however, reduced in diabetics with autonomic neuropathy, indicating that the patient has reduced airways tone. Furthermore, diabetics with autonomic neuropathy have a diminished bronchial reactivity to cold air (Heaton *et al.* 1984). To determine whether this defect was due to a neurodeficit or an abnormality of bronchial smooth muscle, reactivity to inhaled histamine, which has a direct effect on bronchial smooth muscle, was studied in diabetics with and without autonomic neuropathy. There was no difference in reactivity; thus, failure of autonomic-neuropathy patients to respond to cold-air inhalation is due to vagal impairment. Furthermore, these patients also have an impaired cough reflex as demonstrated by high cough threshold to inhalation of citric acid (Fig. 36.8).

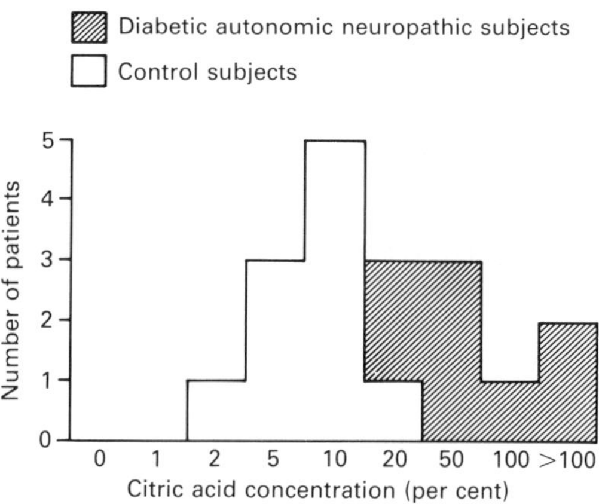

Fig. 36.8. Cough responses to inhaled citric acid in normal subjects and diabetics with severe autonomic neuropathy. The response may be impaired or even absent in autonomic neuropathy.

Respiratory arrests in diabetics with autonomic neuropathy continue to be reported as do sudden deaths. Control of ventilation may contribute to these events although it is unlikely that sleep apnoea causes unexpected deaths in diabetics with autonomic deficit. Respiratory protective reflexes, including the cough reflex, are definitely impaired.

HYPOGLYCAEMIA: EFFECTS OF NEUROPATHY AND β-BLOCKADE

Hypoglycaemia is a powerful stimulus of autonomic function, both sympathetic and parasympathetic. Autonomic stimulation accounts for at least some of the clinical symptoms which alert patients to the need for sugar. Loss of these early warning symptoms is common amongst diabetics, who may suddenly lose consciousness when they become hypoglycaemic. It probably occurs in as many as one in 10 insulin-treated diabetics within a year, and may affect patients of almost any age or duration, with or without diabetic complications. Autonomic neuropathy has been blamed as the cause of this failure to respond to hypoglycaemia. However, it is unlikely that autonomic neuropathy alone is responsible: patients experiencing this problem may or may not be affected by autonomic neuropathy, and it occurs inconsistently at different times in the same patient. Among 28 of our own severe autonomic neuropathy patients, 19 retained normal warning symptoms, three thought they were diminished, and only six had lost them altogether. Abnormalities of metabolic and endocrine responses to hypoglycaemia in patients with neuropathy might provide some clues to these problems.

Glucagon

Pancreatic islets receive a rich autonomic innervation and it is well established that neural influences modulate the release of glucagon and insulin. Hypoglycaemia is a powerful stimulus of glucagon release which is a major source of the changes necessary for rapid recovery from hypoglycaemia. Early studies described defective glucagon release in diabetics with autonomic neuropathy, but more recently this has been refuted. Thus, glucagon responses to hypoglycaemia in tetraplegics are normal and not reduced by atropine, indicating independence of autonomic innervation (Frier 1986) (Fig. 36.9). There is indeed a defect of hypoglycaemia-induced glucagon release in long-term diabetics, but this is very variable, and independent of autonomic neuropathy.

Catecholamines

Adrenalin release occurs rapidly, within 20 to 30 minutes, following hypoglycaemia, and together with glucagon is one of the major counter-regulatory hormones responsible for recovery from hypoglycaemia. The response is mediated by sympathetic nerves. There is evidence for a diminished response in autonomic neuropathy, although this also occurs in diabetics of long duration without detectable neuropathy (Frier 1986).

Tetraplegic subjects (i.e. sympathectomized by cord transection) lose both their awareness of hypoglycaemics, and their adrenalin responses to it. Adrenalin release may be of major importance with regard to awareness of hypoglycaemics, and its failure could be an important cause for the loss of warning. The reasons why the adrenalin response may fail in diabetics are not clear.

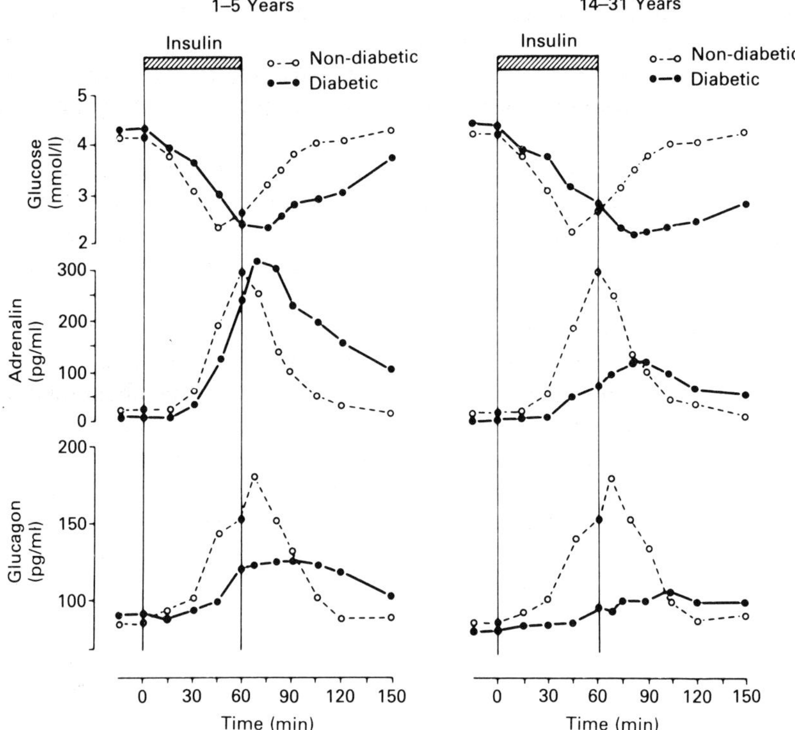

Fig. 36.9. Mean responses of blood glucose, plasma adrenalin, and glucagon in groups of non-diabetic and insulin-dependent diabetic subjects (durations shown above each graph) following intravenous infusions of insulin to induce hypoglycaemia. (Reproduced by kind permission of Frier (1986) and the editor of *Diabetic Medicine.*)

Noradrenalin also increases in response to hypoglycaemia but does not play an important role in recovery from hypoglycaemia.

Pancreatic polypeptide

Hypoglycaemia reliably stimulates the release of pancreatic polypeptide; this is blocked by atropine indicating that this is mediated by parasympathetic nerves. The response is defective or absent in diabetics with established autonomic neuropathy and this response is now considered to be a useful test for the integrity of the autonomic innervation of the pancreatic islets.

BLOOD-PRESSURE CHANGES

Insulin administration and hypoglycaemia cause major changes of blood pressure, which differ from normal in neuropathic patients and those on

β-blockers. Insulin administration to sympathectomized or severe neuropathy patients causes a decrease of blood pressure and even severe hypotension when upright. This hypotensive effect of insulin may account for occasional black-outs in neuropathic patients previously attributed to hypoglycaemia. In normal subjects taking β-blocking drugs, hypertension occurs during hypoglycaemia (increase of systolic and diastolic pressures) in contrast to the normal response, which is an increase of systolic but a decrease of diastolic pressure. It is unlikely that the hypertensive effect of hypoglycaemia in diabetics on β-blocking drugs has serious consequences.

In conclusion, unconsciousness from hypoglycaemia is a distressingly common problem in insulin-treated diabetics. It is, however, very unlikely that autonomic neuropathy is responsible for this phenomenon. Failure of adrenalin release may be important in this regard, but is not solely due to autonomic failure. Frier (1986) has described various defects of hypothalamic (β-endorphin) and pituitary secretions (ACTH, growth hormone, prolactin) which could indicate a role for the central nervous system. Finally, insulin-induced hypotension in neuropathic diabetics may occasionally cause a black-out which could be confused with hypoglycaemia.

REFERENCES

Archer, A. G., Roberts, V. C., and Watkins, P. J. (1984). Blood flow patterns in painful diabetic neuropathy. *Diabetologia* **27**, 563–7.

Bennett, T. (1984). Diabetic autonomic neuropathy and iritis. *Br. med. J.* **289**, 1231.

Borkowski, M. (1973). An experimental study on the role of arteriovenous anastomoses in the pathogenesis of trophic ulcer. *Arch. Immunol. Ther. exp.* **21**, 363–75.

Catterall, J. R., Claverly, P. M. A., Ewing, D. J., Shapiro, C. M., Clarke, B. F., and Douglas, N. J. (1984). Breathing, sleep and diabetic autonomic neuropathy. *Diabetes* **33**, 1025–7.

Christlieb, A. R. and Bratten, J. T. (1974). Decreased response of plasma renin activity to orthostasis in diabetic patients with orthostatic hypotension. *Diabetes* **23**, 835–40.

DePonti, F., Fealey, R. D., and Malagelada, J.-R. (1987). Gastrointestinal syndromes due to diabetes mellitus. In *Diabetic neuropathy* (ed. P. J. Dyck, P. K. Thomas, A. K. Asbury, A. I. Winegrad, and D. Porte Jr), pp. 155–61. W. B. Saunders, Philadelphia.

Duchen, L. W., Anjorin, A., Watkins, P. J., and MacKay, J. D. (1980). Pathology of autonomic neuropathy in diabetes mellitus. *Ann. intern. Med.* **92**, 301–3.

Edmonds, M. E., Archer, A. G., and Watkins, P. J. (1983). Ephedrine: a new treatment for diabetic neuropathic oedema. *Lancet* **i**, 548–51.

Edmonds, M. E., Nicolaides, K. H., and Watkins, P. J. (1986). Autonomic neuropathy in diabetic foot ulceration. *Diabetic Med.* **3**, 56–9.

Ewing, D. J. and Clarke, B. F. (1986). Autonomic neuropathy: its diagnosis and prognosis. In *Clinics in endocrinology and metabolism* (ed. P. J. Watkins), pp. 855–88. W. B. Saunders, London.

Fagius, J. (1982). Microneurographic findings in diabetic polyneuropathy with special reference to sympathetic nerve activity. *Diabetologia* **23**, 415–520.

Fedorak, R. N., Field, M., and Chang, E. B. (1985). Treatment of diabetic diarrhoea with clonidine. *Ann. intern. Med.* **102**, 197–9.

Frier, B. M. (1986). Hypoglycaemia and diabetes. *Diabetic Med.* **3**, 513–25.

Gilbey, S. G., Guy, R. J. C., Jones, H., Vergani, D., and Watkins, P. J. (1986). Diabetes and autonomic neuropathy: an immunological association? *Diabetic Med.* **3**, 241–5.

Gilbey, S. G. and Watkins, P. J. (1987). Measurement by epigastric impedance of gastric emptying in diabetic autonomic neuropathy. *Diabetic Med.* **4**, 122–6.

Guilleminault, C., Briskin, J. G., Greenfield, M. S., and Silvestri, R. (1981). The impact of autonomic nervous system dysfunction on breathing during sleep. *Sleep* **4**, 263–78.

Guy, R. J. C., Clark, C. A., Malcolm, P. N., and Watkins, P. J. (1985). Evaluation of thermal and vibration sensation in diabetic neuropathy. *Diabetologia* **28**, 131–7.

Guy, R. J. C., Dawson, J. L., Garrett, J. R., Laws, J. W., Thomas, P. K., Sharma, A. K., and Watkins, P. J. (1984*a*). Diabetic gastroparesis from autonomic neuropathy: surgical considerations and changes in vagus nerve morphology. *J. Neurol. Neurosurg. Psychiat.* **47**, 686–91.

Guy, R. J. C., Richards, F., Edmonds, M. E., and Watkins, P. J. (1984*b*). Diabetic autonomic neuropathy and iritis: an association suggesting an immunological cause. *Br. med. J.* **189**, 343–5.

Heaton, R. W., Guy, R. J. C., Gray, B. J., Watkins, P. J., and Costello, J. F. (1984). Diminished bronchial reactivity in cold air in diabetic patients with autonomic neuropathy. *Br. med. J.* **189**, 149–51.

Hilsted, J. (1982). Pathophysiology in diabetic autonomic neuropathy: cardiovascular, hormonal and metabolic studies. *Diabetes* **31**, 730–7.

Low, P. A. and Fealey, R. D. D. (1987). Sudomotor neuropathy. In *Diabetic neuropathy* (ed. P. J. Dyck, P. K. Thomas, A. K. Asbury, A. I. Winegrad, D. Porte, Jr), pp. 140–5. W. B. Saunders, Philadelphia.

Maddern, G. J., Horowitz, M., and Jamieson, G. G. (1985). The effect of domperidone on oesophageal emptying in diabetic autonomic neuropathy. *Br. J. clin. Pharmacol.* **19**, 441–4.

Minami, H. and McCallum, R. W. (1984). The physiology and pathophysiology of gastric emptying in humans. *Gastroenterology* **86**, 1592–610.

Monserrat, J. M., Cochrane, G. M., Wolf, C., Picado, C., Roca, J., and Agusti-Vidal, A. (1985). Ventilatory control in diabetes mellitus. *Eur. J. resp. Dis.* **67**, 112–17.

Moscos, G. J., Driver, M., and Guy, R. J. S. (1986). A form of necrobiosis and atrophy of smooth muscle in diabetic gastric autonomic neuropathy. *Path. Res. Pract.* **181**, 188–94.

Rees, P. J., Prior, J. C., Cochrane, G. M., and Clarke, T. J. H. (1981). Sleep apnoea in diabetic patients with autonomic neuropathy. *J. R. Soc. Med.* **74**, 192–5.

Rundles, R. W. (1945). Diabetic neuropathy: a general review with a report of 125 cases. *Medicine, Baltimore* **24**, 111–60.

Tooke, J. E. (1986). Microvascular haemodynamics in diabetes mellitus. *Clin. Sci.* **70**, 119–25.

Ward, J. D., Simms, J. M., Knight, G., Boulton, A. J. M., and Sandler, D. A. (1983). Venous distension in the diabetic neuropathic foot (physical sign of arteriovenous shunting). *J. R. Soc. Med.* **76**, 1011–14.

Watkins, P. J. and Edmonds, M. E. (1983). Sympathetic nerve failure in diabetes. *Diabetologia* **25**, 73–7.

Williams, J. G., Morris, A. I., Hayter, R. C., and Ogilvie, C. M. (1984). Respiratory responses of diabetics to hypoxia, hypercapnia and exercise. *Thorax* **39**, 529–34.

37. Cardiovascular pathophysiology in diabetes mellitus: a reappraisal

Terence Bennett and Sheila M. Gardiner

INTRODUCTION

Although many papers on diabetic autonomic neuropathy have been published since the appearance of the first edition of this book, our basic understanding of the problem in human patients has improved little. In the case of clinical investigations in Nottingham the relative lack of forward movement has been due to the increasing conviction that measurements made under less than strictly controlled conditions could only serve to confuse rather than to enlighten. As a result, recent time has been spent devising experimental protocols that might provide more reliable data. However, such cogitation has also served to highlight the multifaceted nature of the problem and (for these writers at least) has led to a point where, although the questions to be asked are clearer, the solutions require an experimental approach that may be unethical and/or very difficult to achieve in patients with diabetes mellitus. Notwithstanding this dilemma, the following comments are made in the hope that colleagues will find them of interest and, possibly, helpful.

WHAT IS NORMAL?

One of the main questions that must tax any investigator can be considered under the subheading 'conditions under which the measurement is made'. Intuitively, most of us feel that these conditions should be controlled. Indeed, in work with animals great trouble is taken to ensure that, as far as possible, individuals are of the same sex, genotypically homogeneous, eating the same food, exposed to the same housing conditions, studied at the same time of day using the same experimental protocol, etc. When it comes to the study of normal human subjects, many of us confine our studies to the same time of day, on fasted subjects, of the same sex, under the same environmental conditions. Evidence that such caution is justified comes from recent studies of the influence of factors such as starvation or exercise on cardiovascular reflexes. Following a 48-h fast Bennett *et al.* (1984*a*) found that normal male subjects showed a reduction in diastolic blood pressure and forearm vascular resistance when they were supine. Furthermore, they showed abnormal baroreflex responses to lower body subatmospheric pressure or to standing. While 48-h starvation may seem an unlikely stress in regard to normal subjects, it may be highly relevant to the acute metabolic disturbances experienced by patients with diabetes mellitus (see below). Perhaps a more frequently encountered, and difficult to control, variable is the amount of exercise a subject has taken. In both normotensive and hypertensive subjects, moderate levels of exercise produce persistent (8 h or more) effects on cardiovascular reflexes. Although this intervention lowers systemic arterial blood pressure, it is accompanied by signs of resetting and sensitization of cardiac and vascular reflexes (Bennett *et al.* 1984*b*). While there is some evidence this might be due to central opioidergic influences on sympathetic efferent outflow, more work needs to be done, since Floras *et al.* (1986) found muscle sympathetic efferent activity was *suppressed* 60 min after exercise, whereas Bennett *et al.* (1984*b*) observed forearm vascular resistance was *elevated* at this time. The greater effects of exercise on cardiovascular reflexes in hypertensive patients is noteworthy in the context of the frequent occurrence in diabetic patients of elevated systemic arterial blood pressures. There have been no studies of the influence of exercise on cardiovascular reflexes in diabetic patients, although exercise may be an important factor in treatment of diabetes mellitus.

It is surprising how few investigators consider environmental temperature an important variable in studies of cardiovascular reflexes. In the light of the fact that patients with diabetes mellitus may show substantial abnormalities of thermoregulatory reflexes (Scott *et al.* 1987), the need to carry out studies under thermally controlled conditions is now undeniable. Furthermore, it would be of great value if all laboratories reported data at agreed thermoneutral temperatures.

Examination of the literature gives the impression that there are currently available large data bases for normal responses to a variety of manoeuvres, that take into account age and sex. However, most of these data have been collected under uncontrolled conditions, and they often refer only to the simplest of measurements. None of us have yet taken the trouble to establish normal ranges for a spectrum of cardiovascular reflexes, in the same normal subjects, assessing the responses under controlled conditions through time. Of course, the latter point raises the spectre of reproducibility. Even controlling all known variables as tightly as possible, one not infrequently encounters big differences in experimental results obtained from homogeneous groups of animals at different times. (One is willing to accept these as seasonal differences in rats, but wonders where such seasonal differences are to be seen in man.) Other important factors bearing upon the question of reproducibility in studies in man are those of habituation and tachyphylaxis (in many animal studies this does not arise because the animals are investigated once only). Taking insulin-induced hypoglycaemia as an example of a substantial challenge that should elicit reproducible responses in the same individual, it is notable that in one normal subject (T.B.) there has been a marked diminution in the subjective effects elicited by this stimulus repeated many times over a period of years. In this context it is of interest that recent observations indicate current metabolic status may influence hypoglycaemic awareness in normal subjects and this clearly could have profound implications for the interpretation of abnormalities of responsiveness in patients with diabetes mellitus.

All these various areas cry out to be studied, especially since longitudinal investigations of the therapeutic efficacy of diverse drugs are being carried out now in patients with diabetes mellitus, in spite of the fact that many of the results will be uninterpretable, or physiologically meaningless. (An example of the latter problem is seen in a recent study in which active drug treatment produced a statistically significant increase of 0.7 ± 0.24 m/s in peroneal motor nerve conduction velocity in a group of diabetic patients, against a background of the two 'normal' groups in the study having values of 46.5 ± 3.9 and 49.1 ± 2.4 m/s for this variable.)

WHAT IS ABNORMAL?

In the light of the above comments it is worthwhile running through the particular problems that may arise in trying to assess what is abnormal when studying cardiovascular reflexes in patients with diabetes mellitus. It is clear that those variables one tries to control for in normal subjects may be more important in patients. For example, it is not necessarily true that an overnight-fasted (or fed) diabetic patient has normal fluid and electrolyte balance or, if studied under something other than thermoneutral conditions, would be in a comparable state to a normal subject. However, the biggest problem arises with those variables, such as glucose and insulin 'status', that one knows will be abnormal. All of us in the past (and many of us still) have been guilty of studying diabetic patients under conditions in which metabolic variables must have been changing throughout the experimental protocol. It is possible to avoid this problem by admitting the patient to hospital the night before the study and controlling plasma glucose by continuously adjusting the rate of intravenous administration of glucose and insulin until the study is finished the next morning (Scott *et al.* 1987). However, this does not obviate the important consideration: how long before the study should one attempt such control to distinguish between disorders attributable to acute or chronic metabolic abnormalities? This and many other questions remain unanswered, including that to do with the possibility of prolonged administration of insulin influencing insulin sensitivity and all that goes with it. The other side of the coin is related to the reasons for making the measurements (see below). From a clinical point of view it is important to know what the patient's cardiovascular status is under everyday circumstances. It may be, then, that all measurements should be carried out under both laboratory and field conditions, the former serving as objective assessments that can be compared from time to time, the latter being indices of clinical progression. A systematic comparison of these two sets of data might throw up some interesting results.

WHAT MEASUREMENTS TO MAKE?

In the early days of a new area of study, workers are prone to stick with the measurements that are easy to make and/or those with which they are familiar. With the passage of time, some people come to appreciate that the nuances of the problem under study need subtler approaches. Progress depends on reconsideration of fixed views and development of new techniques. However, the latter also must be examined critically since they are often of the 'hi-tech' variety and, apart from anything else, the more technically difficult the measurements, the greater the inclination of the more enthusiastic devotees to make them under less than rigorous conditions. It is a truism that more data are obtained the more measurements one makes, but too few investigators consider what the measurements mean. Certainly there is the tacit assumption, on the part of many, that the measurement means the same thing under all conditions. If one takes the example of sinus arrhythmia, it is clear one can quantitate it precisely, but it does not follow that reduction in sinus arrhythmia is due to the same thing under all conditions. Strictly speaking, in order to make any meaningful statement it is necessary to be able to quantitate all components of the system—afferent input, central transmission, efferent output, and effector responsiveness (which includes membrane receptor number and affinity and all those events that represent 'post-receptor coupling'). The latter assertion is not too far-fetched since there is much evidence for marked changes in myocardial receptors in animals with experimentally induced mellitus, yet this possibility has not been investigated in diabetic patients.

At present, then, while all the 'easy' measurements are routinely made, it is not obvious to us what useful information they provide, except where they signal clinical intervention, e.g. postural hypotension or, possibly, tachycardia. Given the multifactorial nature of many of the disturbances it is clearly quite unjustifiable to extrapolate from one system to another (e.g. reduced sinus arrhythmia does not provide evidence of an organic lesion underlying diabetic impotence). It is, therefore, incumbent upon those who routinely assess autonomic function to consider why they do it, given that the simple repetition of a procedure tells one nothing about the mechanisms involved, or the nature of the longitudinal changes, especially if the measurements are made under uncontrolled conditions.

The following sections are written with the express intention of highlighting areas that would benefit from increased research effort.

DIABETIC AUTONOMIC DYSFUNCTION

Diabetic autonomic dysfunction may result from afferent, central, or efferent 'disorders' (these disorders may be due to anything from frank neuronal degeneration through to acute neuronal dysfunction attributable to metabolic disturbance, for example). It is possible, indeed likely, that a combination of disorders may be present, but for convenience the problems will be considered individually. Except where stated, the studies quoted have not been done under controlled conditions of the sort described above.

Afferent disorders

The cause(s) of these (as with all other neuronal disorders in diabetes mellitus) is unresolved. Factors such as neuronal hypoxia, impaired axonal transport, and membrane dysfunction are being mooted.

It is not routinely possible to assess cardiovascular afferent integrity independent of other mechanisms in man, and the relevant physiological experiments have not been done in experimental animals. However, one study bearing on this point is that of Fagius *et al.* (1985) who examined the responses of normal subjects to anaesthesia of the glossopharyngeal and vagal nerves (to achieve cessation of afferent inflow independent of manipulation of sensory terminals). This manoeuvre induced hypertension and tachycardia, associated with intense muscle sympathetic activity—signs similar to those seen in the Guillain–Barré syndrome. Although hypertension and tachycardia are common in diabetes mellitus, they are not associated with increased muscle sympathetic activity, and it has been suggested this might argue against an afferent disorder (Fagius 1985). However, if selective afferent dysfunctions develop, other afferent or central processes may readjust, or other dysfunctions may occur concurrently. An example that may be analogous to the changes in the former category is that of baroreceptor deafferentation or cardiac denervation which do not produce sustained elevations in systemic arterial blood pressure or vasopressin release in experimental animals.

There have been no studies involving electrical stimulation of the carotid-sinus nerve or examining responses to carotid-sinus suction in diabetic patients, but these would not provide information about afferent function independent of central or efferent mechanisms.

There is some evidence for a relatively selective impairment of afferent input from peripheral chemoreceptors in patients with diabetes mellitus, since hypoxic ventilatory drive may be abnormal when hypercapnic drive is not. However, it is difficult to control for the relative strengths of these two stimuli. Other afferent systems, such as thermoreceptors, that may influence cardiovascular function have been shown to be defective in diabetics, but not in a systematic way that excluded the possibility of impaired central mechanisms.

One way of investigating the integrity of afferent systems (although not strictly 'cardiovascular') independently of central processes would be to challenge with a chemical stimulus that produced an axon reflex. Afferent fibres in the skin when stimulated with capsaicin release neuropeptides (including substance P and calcitonin gene-related peptide (CGRP)) and there is an accompanying 'flare'. It has been shown that diabetic patients may have an impaired microvascular hyperaemic response to skin trauma (Rayman *et al.* 1986), and it is possible that this is due to loss of capsaicin-sensitive afferent fibres (Aronin *et al.* 1984). However, in rats made diabetic with streptozotocin, diminished capsaicin-mediated plasma extravasation is not associated with reduced skin content of substance P. Thus, the phenomenon may be complicated by changes in microvascular permeability which also occur in diabetic patients (Tooke 1986). In passing, it is noteworthy that those afferent fibres sensitive to capsaicin are dependent on nerve growth factor, and hence may be impaired by insulin antibodies. Furthermore, in experimental animals, treatment with capsaicin produces changes in cardiovascular control mechanisms remarkably similar to those seen in diabetic animals (Bennett and Gardiner 1985; Hebden *et al.* 1987). Finally, capsaicin is a particularly potent stimulus for eliciting 'gustatory sweating' and the latter may occur in response to abnormal stimuli in diabetic patients.

Central disorders

It is not routinely possible non-invasively to monitor central events (such as evoked potentials) associated with processing of cardiovascular information in man, and we know of no data in animals. However, there is electrophysiological evidence that central pathways subserving auditory function may be abnormal in diabetic patients (e.g. Eckberg *et al.* 1986), but further controlled studies are required. Eckberg *et al.* (1986) cited some of our earlier data in support of the proposition that there may be reversible abnormalities in the central 'setting' of cardiovascular mechanisms, but these possibilities have not been investigated systematically.

As alluded to above, major questions regarding hypothalamic glucose sensitivity and other possibilities, such as the involvement of insulin and/or glucagon and/or vasopressin in disorders of central cardiovascular regulation in diabetes mellitus, have barely been thought about, let alone studied.

Efferent disorders

Neuronal dysfunction

While, theoretically, it might be possible to gain some information regarding preganglionic efferent activity by monitoring the changes in postganglionic muscle or skin sympathetic activity (Fagius 1985) in response to edrophonium, this has not yet been done. At a more peripheral level, as mentioned above, there have been few systematic comparative studies of effector responses (however assessed—see below) to different manoeuvres under different conditions. This is partly to do with the nature of the measurement, since, generally, those activities directed towards understanding pathophysiological processes are more invasive than 'bedside tests'. However, the understandable inclination to keep invasive measurements to a minimum probably accounts for the current confusion regarding the relations between peripheral blood flow, muscle sympathetic activity, and catecholamine release (as indices of sympathetic efferent activity). In this context, peripheral blood flow usually means that through the forearm *or* calf (but see Scott *et al.* 1987). However, there is evidence for differential blood flow responses in these two limbs following a particular stimulus (see Chapter 5) which is an intriguing observation, since baroreceptor-mediated modulation of muscle symapthetic activity is directed equally to the two limbs (Victor *et al.* 1986). Furthermore, there is a linear relationship between forearm venous plasma noradrenalin concentrations and muscle sympathetic activity in the leg during drug-induced changes in blood pressure. However, the physiological meaning of this impressive correlation needs some reconsideration. First, the drugs used to elicit changes in muscle sympathetic activity (secondary to changes in systemic arterial pressure) may themselves affect perfusion in the forearm and leg (possibly differentially) and hence may influence catecholamine extraction at those sites

(Chang *et al.* 1986). Second, the differential flow changes in the two limbs in response to a specific stimulus (see above) would be likely to lead to differential changes in venous plasma catecholamine concentrations at those sites. The relationship between leg and forearm venous plasma catecholamines in response to specific stimuli has yet to be delineated. Nevertheless, there is the important observation that the flow changes (reflecting the summation of all the various inputs) may be different in the two limbs. If the changes in sympathetic efferent outflow *are* the same in the arm and leg in response to any particular manoeuvre then it is possible that differences in the distribution of postjunctional receptor types and/or release of local vasodilator substances may account for the differential flow responses.

The fact that forearm venous catecholamine concentration seems to be a good index of sympathetic efferent outflow to the forearm vascular beds (Grassi *et al.* 1985) also needs to be examined critically. Catecholamines in antecubital vein plasma may arrive there from the arterial inflow and/or from the forearm. Measurement of arterial and venous concentrations simultaneously with blood flow would permit calculation of a 'spillover' rate (Chang *et al.* 1986), but this does not take account of the bidirectional flux of catecholamines that may be occurring. For example, if the forearm removed all the inflowing noradrenalin, but release of noradrenalin in the forearm (subserving vasomotor tone) added a similar amount, the apparent spillover rate would be zero (Jie 1986), and one might infer there was no noradrenergic 'tone'. The proper calculation of regional noradrenalin release rate requires the simultaneous measurement of noradrenalin extraction by the tissue, ideally using radiolabelled noradrenalin. However, administering the latter by constant infusion produces problems with recirculation, while bolus administration requires assumptions to be made regarding the disposition of the radiolabelled marker in the non-steady state. Furthermore, it is now apparent that estimation of extraction by use of trace amounts of ^{3}H-noradrenalin may not give a complete answer since it is possible that the effluent radioactivity may not all be associated with noradrenalin (Howes *et al.* 1986). The definitive experiment, i.e. simultaneous measurement of forearm and calf flows, muscle sympathetic activity, and regional noradrenalin release rates at rest and following physiological manoeuvres that load or unload arterial and/or cardiopulmonary baroreceptors, has yet to be done!

In the light of the problems mentioned above, the recent observations of Eckberg *et al.* (1986) are of interest. These investigators studied 10 unselected, young, adult, insulin-dependent, diabetic patients with no symptoms or signs of autonomic neuropathy, and compared them with 12 age-matched non-diabetic subjects. Eckberg *et al.* measured forearm venous plasma noradrenalin levels and R–R interval variability under resting conditions, and during changes of arterial blood pressure elicited by infusions of nitroprusside or phenylephrine. The latter manoeuvres produced complex changes in forearm plasma noradrenalin levels in the non-diabetic subjects, but had little effect on the group mean values in the diabetic patients. However, there were marked interindividual differences in the latter. Nevertheless, Eckberg *et al.* (1986) felt their results in diabetic patients signified 'profound disturbances of sympathetic control' with 'no credible evidence that sympathetic outflow was modulated by changes of arterial pressure'. Several points need to be made here: (1) since the patients were asymptomatic, it would have to be argued that the abnormality detected by Eckberg *et al.* was confined to the forearm (and, possibly, other vascular beds not involved in orthostatic reflexes); (2) patients similar to those in the studies by Eckberg *et al.* show competent forearm vasoconstriction in response to manoeuvres such as lower-body subatmospheric pressure. Hence, antecubital venous plasma noradrenalin levels in such subjects may not reflect end-organ responses. It is possible there are abnormalities of postjunctional adrenoceptors (see below) or endothelial cell function in the diabetic forearm that may influence any relation between vasoconstriction and venous noradrenalin concentration, but it is not unlikely that a different answer to that arrived at by Eckberg *et al.* (1986) would be obtained if the definitive experiment described above was carried out in his patients with diabetes mellitus.

The earlier findings indicating disorders of catecholamine biosynthesis in diabetic patients with impaired cardiovascular control (Hoeldtke and Cilmi 1984) also need to be re-examined in the light of the more sophisticated approaches described above. However, it is of interest that postural hypotension in some diabetic patients is *not* associated with signs of a hyperdopaminergic state (Hoeldtke and Cilmi 1984), since the vasodilator effects of dopamine have been thought to explain the effectiveness of treatment with metoclopramide in diabetic postural hypotension (see below).

One (of the many) complications of cardiovascular studies in man (or animals) is to do with the different receptor sites that the catecholamines may act upon to influence regional flows. Jie and his colleagues (Jie 1986) carried out elegant investigations examining the effects of local arterial infusions of agonists and antagonists on forearm blood flow. In normal subjects, in this vascular bed, there appear to be postjunctional α_1- and α_2-adrenoceptors that are capable of mediating vasoconstriction. The marked hyperaemia seen with yohimbine (an α_2-antagonist) would seem to indicate an important contribution of the postjunctional α_2-adrenoceptors to the maintenance of resting vascular tone, but the fact that this response is markedly inhibited by β-adrenoceptor antagonism indicates that it might be due to active vasodilatation. A similar phenomenon occurs in conscious rats (Gardiner and Bennett 1987*b*) and cautions against simplistic explanations. The important experiment of assessing the forearm vascular responses to release of endogenous noradrenalin in the presence of an antagonist of the vasodilator β_2-adrenoceptors and delineating the influences of selective α_1- and α_2-adrenoceptor antagonists on these responses remains to be done, as does the experiment demonstrating a role of dopamine receptors in peripheral vascular control. Needless to say, these are even more virginal territories as far as diabetic patients are concerned. However, they are likely to be fecund fields, judging by the abnormalities of cardiovascular reactivity seen in animals with experimental diabetes mellitus.

Given the current uncertainty about the physiological role (if any) of pre- or postjunctional vascular α_2-adrenoceptors in normal man, and the lack of any evidence that adrenoceptors on non-vascular tissues are 'models' of vascular adrenoceptors, one can only be entertained by the gazelle-like conceptual leaps involved in getting from the finding of decreased α_2-adrenoceptors on platelet membranes to the occurrence of orthostatic hypotension in patients with diabetes mellitus (Abrahm *et al.* 1986).

Hormonal dysfunction: vasopressin

A role for vasopressin (ADH) in cardiovascular regulation has been widely debated (e.g. Bennett and Gardiner 1986; Gardiner and Bennett 1987*a*) and in the context of diabetes mellitus ADH takes on an intriguing aspect since its release is normally influenced by extracellular fluid osmolality (which may be abnormal in diabetic patients) and ADH may exert important influences on hepatic metabolism and haemostasis. A particularly nice point in regard to the osmoreceptor control of ADH release in diabetic patients is to do with the possibility that glucose could act as a stimulus for thirst and vasopressin release if its normal lack of effectiveness in this regard was due to an insulin-dependent uptake into osmoreceptor cells (Zerbe *et al.* 1985). Although infusion of hypertonic glucose did not stimulate ADH release in either normal subjects or diabetic patients, Zerbe *et al.* (1985) pointed out the latter were not insulin-deficient at the time of the measurements. Indeed, it has been shown (Vokes *et al.* 1987) that acute insulin deficiency increases ADH secretion by sensitizing the osmoreceptor stimulation to hyperglycaemia in patients with insulin-dependent diabetes mellitus. It is noteworthy that infusion of hypertonic saline induced similar rises in plasma ADH in both groups (although diabetic patients had consistently higher levels of plasma ADH (Zerbe *et al.* 1985)), since only in the normal subjects did infusion of hypertonic saline cause an increase in blood pressure. Thus these results do not fit readily into the dogma regarding ADH and baroreflex mechanisms (see Bennett and Gardiner, 1986). However, a greater responsiveness of ADH release to orthostatic stimuli in diabetic patients without postural hypotension (Zerbe *et al.* 1985) and a greater postural fall in blood pressure in diabetic patients showing diminished ADH release (Zerbe *et al.* 1983; Grimaldi *et al.* 1985), indicates the hormone may play an overt role in cardiovascular regulation when other systems are impaired, but, presumably, only if vascular sensitivity to ADH is not diminished. This proposition is supported by the finding that antagonism of V_1-receptors for ADH exacerbates diabetic postural hypotension (Ribeiro *et al.* 1987). The finding that ADH release in response to haemodynamic stimuli can be impaired when that to osmotic stimuli is not may provide evidence of selective baroreceptor afferent dysfunction (Zerbe *et al.* 1983).

In summary, there is a little direct information regarding the cardiovascular influences of ADH in patients with diabetes mellitus, but it may be we know more than we know we know! For example, based on the proposition that excessive dopamine secretion could, by dint of its vasodilator action, cause orthostatic hypotension, it was found that treatment with metoclopramide (a dopamine antagonist) facilitated vasoconstriction, and hence opposed diabetic orthostatic hypotension (Bessa *et al.* 1984). However, we suggest the action of metoclopramide may have been due to augmented ADH release, since (although there have been no studies in diabetic patients) the drug stimulates basal release of ADH in normal subjects. The cardiovascular sequelae of possible interactions between metoclopramide and other ADH-releasing mechanisms (insulin, hypoglycaemia, neuroglycopenia) in normal subjects and diabetic patients await investigation.

Hormonal dysfunction: other hormones

Lack of space prevents us doing justice to the possible cardiovascular consequences of disorders of the renin–angiotensin–aldosterone system and atrial natriuretic peptides, bradykinin, eicosanoids, and the sequelae of insulin administration. But we would predict many of these factors will be found to have overlapping and interactive influences on various processes, including cardiovascular function. Indeed, we are seeing, already, evidence that inhibition of angiotensin-converting enzyme may improve renal perfusion and insulin sensitivity. However, it is feasible that the concurrent interference with metabolism of bradykinin could exacerbate postural hypotension in patients with impaired cardiovascular regulation (Miyamori *et al.* 1986). The ability of insulin to influence cardiovascular mechanisms has taken on a new dimension recently with the finding that diabetic patients with hypotension may show profound exacerbation of their abnormalities when exposed to lower-body subatmospheric pressure during a euglycaemic, hyperinsulinaemic clamp.

REFERENCES

Abrahm, D. R., Hollingsworth, P. J., Smith, C. B., Jim, L., Zucker, L. B., Sobotka, P. A., and Vinik, A. I. (1986). Decreased α_2-adrenergic receptors on platelet membranes from diabetic patients with autonomic neuropathy and postural hypotension. *J. clin. Endocrinol. Metab.* **63**, 906–12.

Aronin, N., Leeman, S. E., and Clements, R. S. (1984). Substance P deficiency in peripheral and cutaneous nerves of diabetics with polyneuropathy. *Clin. Res.* **32**, 388A.

Bennett, T. and Gardiner, S. M. (1985). Neonatal capsaicin treatment impairs vasopressin-mediated blood pressure recovery following acute hypotension. *Br. J. Pharmacol.* **81**, 341–5.

Bennett, T. and Gardiner, S. M. (1986). Influence of exogenous vasopressin on baroreflex mechanisms. *Clin. Sci.* **70**, 307–15.

Bennett, T., Macdonald, I. A., and Sainsbury, R. (1984*a*). The influence of acute starvation on the cardiovascular responses to lower body subatmospheric pressure or to standing in man. *Clin. Sci.* **66**, 141–6.

Bennett, T., Wilcox, R. G., and Macdonald, I. A. (1984*b*). Post-exercise reduction in blood pressure in hypertensive men is not due to acute impairment of baroreflex function. *Clin. Sci.* **67**, 97–103.

Bessa, A. M., Zanella, T., Saragoca, M. A., Mulinari, R. A., Czepielewski, M., Ribeiro, A. B., and Ramos, O. L. (1984). Acute hemodynamic and humoral effects of metoclopramide on blood pressure control improvement in subjects with diabetic orthostatic hypotension. *Clin. Pharmacol. Ther.* **36**, 738–44.

Chang, P. C., van der Krogt, J. A., Vermey, P., and van Brummelen, P. (1986). Norepinephrine removal and release in the forearm of healthy subjects. *Hypertension* **8**, 801–9.

Eckberg, D. L., Harkins, S. W., Fritsch, J. M., Musgrave, G. E., and Gardner, D. F. (1986). Baroreflex control of plasma norepinephrine and heart period in healthy subjects and diabetic patients. *J. clin. Invest.* **78**, 366–74.

Fagius, J. (1985). Autonomic neurophysiology in long-term diabetes. *Clin. Physiol.* **5** (Suppl. 5), 74–8.

Fagius, J., Wallin, B. G., Sundlof, G., Nerhed, C., and Englesson, S. (1985). Sympathetic outflow in man after anaesthesia of the glossopharyngeal and vagus nerves. *Brain* **108**, 423–38.

Floras, J. S., Aylward, P. E., Sinkey, C., and Mark, A. L. (1986). Post-exercise decreases in blood pressure are accompanied by decreases in muscle sympathetic nerve activity. *Clin. Res.* **34**, 708A.

Gardiner, S. M. and Bennett, T. (1987*a*). Influence of endogenous vasopressin on baroreflex mechanisms. *Brain Res. Rev.* **11**, 317–34.

Gardiner, S. M. and Bennett, T. (1987*b*). Influence of β-adrenoceptor antagonism on the cardiovascular responses to α-adrenoceptor antagonism in conscious, unrestrained, Long Evans and Brattleboro rats. *Br. J. Pharmacol.* (In press).

Grassi, G., Gavazzi, C., Cesura, A. M., Picotti, G. B., and Mancia, G. (1985). Changes in plasma catecholamines in response to reflex modulation of sympathetic vasoconstrictor tone by cardiopulmonary receptors. *Clin. Sci.* **68**, 503–10.

Grimaldi, A., Pruszczynski, W., Thervet, F., and Ardaillou, R. (1985). Antidiuretic hormone response to volume depletion in diabetic patients with cardiac autonomic dysfunction. *Clin. Sci.* **68**, 545–52.

Hebden, R. A., Bennett, T., and Gardiner, S. M. (1987). Abnormal blood pressure recovery during ganglion blockade in diabetic rats. *Am. J. Physiol.* **252**, R102–R108.

Hoeldtke, R. D. and Cilmi, K. M. (1984). Norepinephrine secretion and production in diabetic autonomic neuropathy. *J. clin. Endocrinol. Metab.* **59**, 249–52.

Howes, L. G., MacGilchrist, A., Hawksby, C., Sumner, D., and Reid, J. L. (1986). An improved approach for the determination of plasma [^{3}H]-noradrenaline kinetics using high-performance liquid chromatography. *Clin. Sci.* **71**, 211–15.

Jie, K. (1986). Characterization and (patho)-physiology of vascular α-adrenoceptors: studies in the forearm. MD thesis, Leiden.

Miyamori, I., Takeda, Y., Koshida, Ikeda, M., Yasuhara, S., Nagai, K., Morise, T., Takimoto, H., and Takeda, R. (1986). Role of bradykinin for orthostatic hypotension in diabetes mellitus. *Exp. clin. Endocrinol.* **87**, 169–75.

Rayman, G., Williams, S. A., Spencer, P. D., Smaje, L. H., Wise, P. H., and Tooke, J. E. (1986). Impaired microvascular hyperaemic response to minor skin trauma in type I diabetes. *Br. med. J.* **292**, 1295–8.

Ribeiro, A. B., Saadi, C. I., Zanella, T., Mulinari, R. A., Kohlmann, O., and Gavras, H. (1987). Vasopressin maintains blood pressure in diabetic orthostatic hypotension. *Hypertension* **9**, 557 (Abstract 137).

Scott, A. R., Bennett, T., and Macdonald, I. A. (1987). Diabetes mellitus and thermoregulation. *Can. J. Physiol. Pharmacol.* **65**, 1365–76.

Tooke, J. E. (1986). Microvascular haemodynamics in diabetes mellitus. *Clin. Sci.* **70**, 119–25.

Victor, R. G., Leimbach, W. L., Kempf, J., and Mark, A. L. (1986). Unloading of cardiopulmonary baroreflex markedly increases muscle sympathetic outflow to the leg in humans. *Fed. Proc.* **45**, 156 (Abstract 11).

Vokes, T. P., Aycinena, P. R., and Robertson, G. L. (1987). Effect of insulin on osmoregulation of vasopressin. *Am. J. Physiol.* **252**, E538–E548.

Zerbe, R. L., Henry, D. P., and Robertson, G. L. (1983). Vasopressin response to orthostatic hypotension. *Am. J. Med.* **74**, 265–71.

Zerbe, R. L., Vinicor, F., and Robertson, G. L. (1985). Regulation of plasma vasopressin in insulin-dependent diabetes mellitus. *Am. J. Physiol.* **249**, E317–E325.

38. Recent advances in the non-invasive investigation of diabetic autonomic neuropathy

David J. Ewing

INTRODUCTION

Clinical investigation into diabetic autonomic neuropathy has advanced considerably during the past 5 years. Non-invasive cardiovascular reflex tests are increasingly being applied to give an objective assessment of autonomic involvement. Testing techniques have been refined, normal ranges for results extended, and new approaches utilized. Increasingly, too, by using these tests as markers for autonomic damage, abnormalities in other body systems are being uncovered, and treatment of diabetic neuropathy objectively assessed. Tests of autonomic function other than those based on cardiovascular reflexes are also being developed and adding to current knowledge of the underlying pathophysiology of diabetic autonomic neuropathy. With these advances, of course, some areas of controversy and incomplete understanding have emerged. Standardization of testing and measurement of abnormality is still far from complete, and interpretation of some findings is contentious.

The purpose of this chapter is to update information on cardiovascular reflex testing in the light of recent studies both in normal and diabetic subjects. In addition, it will chart progress in non-invasive investigation of cardiovascular autonomic abnormalities in diabetes, and outline studies in other body systems, particularly those utilizing non-invasive investigative techniques. For further and more extensive references to studies mentioned in this chapter, readers are directed to two recent reviews (Ewing 1984; Ewing and Clarke 1986).

BEDSIDE CARDIOVASCULAR REFLEX TESTS

Five simple non-invasive tests using cardiovascular reflexes are now widely accepted for routine diagnostic use in the assessment of autonomic neuropathy. Three, the responses to the Valsalva manoeuvre, deep breathing, and standing up, are based on the measurement of heart-rate changes, while the other two, the responses to standing up and sustained handgrip depend on blood-pressure measurements. Other cardiovascular tests that have been utilized include the heart-rate responses to atropine and propranolol, testing the baroreflex arc, and the cold pressor test, but none appears as reliable in distinguishing normal from abnormal, or as easily performed.

Normal ranges

During the past 7 years there have been reports from over 30 groups giving normal ranges for these five tests. Table 38.1 details 10 recent articles with large numbers of normal subjects. A problem with such studies is that of standardization, both of the techniques and the indices used to describe the results. The lying-to-standing heart-rate and blood-pressure responses were carried out similarly in most studies, as was sustained handgrip. However, with both the Valsalva manoeuvre and the heart-rate response to deep breathing, slightly different techniques were employed in the different studies. Of the six accounts of normal Valsalva responses, four were conducted sitting and two lying down. In five, blowing was held for 15 seconds and in one for only 10 seconds. With tests of heart-rate variation during breathing there have been several different combinations, with subjects lying or sitting, breathing quietly or breathing deeply, and taking a single or repeated deep breaths.

The measurements used to assess the responses have also differed. There have been no disagreements about measurements of systolic blood pressure to assess postural hypotension, or diastolic blood pressure to assess sustained handgrip, or about the Valsalva ratio. However, the lying-to-standing heart-rate response has been assessed both by the 30:15 ratio and by the maximum:minimum heart-rate ratio, although, in practice, the two ratios are almost identical. Other studies, however, have used the rise in heart rate on standing, instead of the rebound bradycardia. The heart-rate response to breathing has yielded the most varied measurements. Some groups have used the maximum:minimum heart-rate response, others the expiration to inspiration ratio (E:I ratio), and yet others the coefficient of variation or standard deviation (SD) of the heart rate.

One further factor in the establishment of normal ranges has been the relation between results and the ages of the normal subjects. Heart-rate variation, however measured, declines with increasing age (Fig. 38.1). Most authors have also found that the lying-to-standing heart-rate response is related to age, whereas there have been differing views about

Table 38.1. Some recent large series of cardiovascular reflex tests in normal subjects: different techniques and measurements

Study	*Number of subjects*	*Test*						
		Valsalva manoeuvre		*Heart-rate (HR) variation*		*Lying-to-standing heart-rate measurement*	*Postural blood-pressure (BP) measurement*	*Sustained handgrip measurement*
		Technique	*Measurement*	*Technique*	*Measurements*			
Smith (1982)	174	—	—	Lying single breath	E:I ratio	—	—	—
Wieling *et al.* (1982)	133	—	—	Lying deep breathing	Max–min HR	HR rise	—	—
Smith (1984)	150	Lying 10 s	Valsalva ratio	—	—	—	—	—
Ewing *et al.* (1985)	139	Sitting 15 s	Valsalva ratio	Sitting deep breathing	Max–min HR	30:15 ratio	Systolic BP fall	Diastolic BP rise
Masaoka *et al.* (1985)	143	—	—	Sitting deep breathing	Max–min HR	—	—	—
Oikawa *et al.* (1985)	162	—	—	Lying quiet breathing Lying deep breathing	Max–min HR SD	HR rise	—	—
Clark and Mapstone (1986)	85	Sitting 15 s	Valsalva ratio	Sitting deep breathing	Max–min HR	30:15 ratio	Systolic BP fall	—
Gautschy *et al.* (1986)	120	Sitting 15 s	Valsalva ratio	Sitting deep breathing	E:I: ratio SD	30:15 ratio	Systolic BP fall	Diastolic BP rise
O'Brien *et al.* (1986*a*)	310	Lying 15 s	Valsalva ratio	Lying single breath Lying quiet breathing	Max–min HR E:I ratio SD	Max–min ratio	—	—
Vita *et al.* (1986)	66	Sitting 15 s	Valsalva ratio	Lying quiet breathing Sitting deep breathing	SD Max–min HR	30:15 ratio	Systolic BP fall	Diastolic BP rise

SD, standard deviation of the heart rate

the effect of age on the Valsalva manoeuvre and the postural fall in blood pressure. The sustained handgrip response is related more to the strength of contraction rather than to age *per se.*

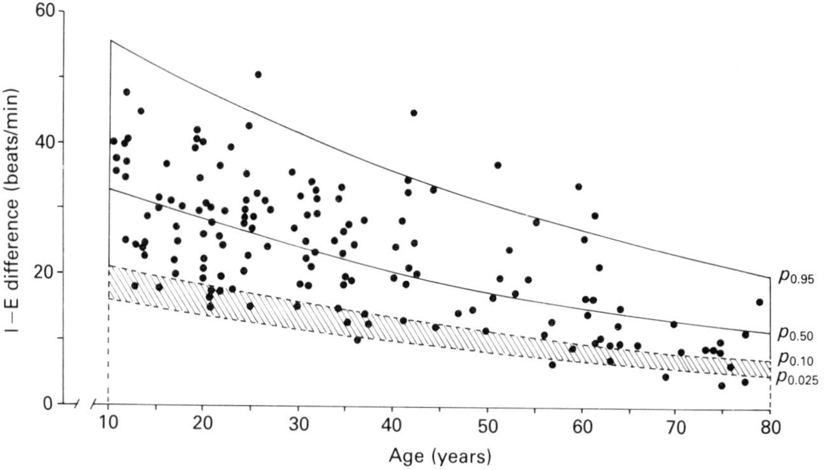

Fig. 38.1. Heart-rate variation during deep breathing (I—E difference) in relation to age in 133 normal subjects, recorded in the lying position. The hatching indicates the area of uncertainty: values below it are abnormal, and values above normal. (Modified from Wieling *et al.* (1982) and Dambrink and Wieling (1987).)

In view of these discrepancies it is difficult to compare different normal values. From a practical point of view, however, it would seem desirable to try and achieve more standardization of the tests, both in their techniques and in the actual measurements used for assessment. While, of course, there is no absolute right or wrong method for performing the tests or calculating the results, the following is a brief account of how the five tests can be performed simply, based on our experience over some years.

Simple non-invasive tests

Heart-rate response to the Valsalva manoeuvre

This test is performed by asking the subject to sit quietly and then blow into a mouthpiece attached to an aneroid pressure gauge at a pressure of 40 mm Hg and to hold the pressure for 15 seconds. The ratio of the longest R–R interval shortly after the manoeuvre (within about 20 beats) to the shortest R–R interval during the manoeuvre is then measured. The result is expressed as the Valsalva ratio which is taken as the mean ratio from three successive Valsalva manoeuvres.

Heart-rate response to standing up

The subject is asked to lie quietly on a couch and then to stand up unaided as quickly as practicable. The characteristic heart-rate response can be expressed by the 30:15 ratio which is the ratio of the longest R–R interval around the thirtieth beat after standing up to the shortest R–R interval around the fifteenth beat.

Heart-rate response to deep breathing

The patient sits quietly and then breathes deeply and evenly at 6 breaths per minute (5 seconds in and 5 seconds out). The maximum–minimum heart rate during each 10-second breathing cycle is measured and the mean of the differences during three successive breathing cycles gives the 'maximum–minimum heart rate'.

Blood-pressure response to standing up

This test is performed by measuring the blood pressure while the subject is lying down, and again 1 minute after standing up. The difference in systolic blood pressure is taken as the measure of postural blood-pressure change.

Blood-pressure response to sustained handgrip

Handgrip is maintained at 30 per cent of the maximum voluntary contraction up to a maximum of 5 minutes, using a handgrip dynamometer, and the blood pressure measured each minute. The difference between the diastolic blood pressure just before release of handgrip and before starting is taken as the measure of response.

Assessment of cardiovascular autonomic damage

Assessment of cardiovascular autonomic nerve damage can be made from the combined results of these five tests, which we have employed over several years in a large number of normal (Fig. 38.2), diabetic, and other subjects (Ewing *et al.* 1985). Table 38.2 gives the normal and abnormal values we use in Edinburgh for routine clinical and diagnostic purposes. It might be argued that because clinical measurements such as these are not done under tightly controlled conditions, the results obtained are invalid (see Chapter 37). However, in clinical practice, provided test conditions are standardized as much as practicable, factors such as the time of testing, relation to meals and exercise, temperature of the laboratory, etc. appear to have little effect on the actual results

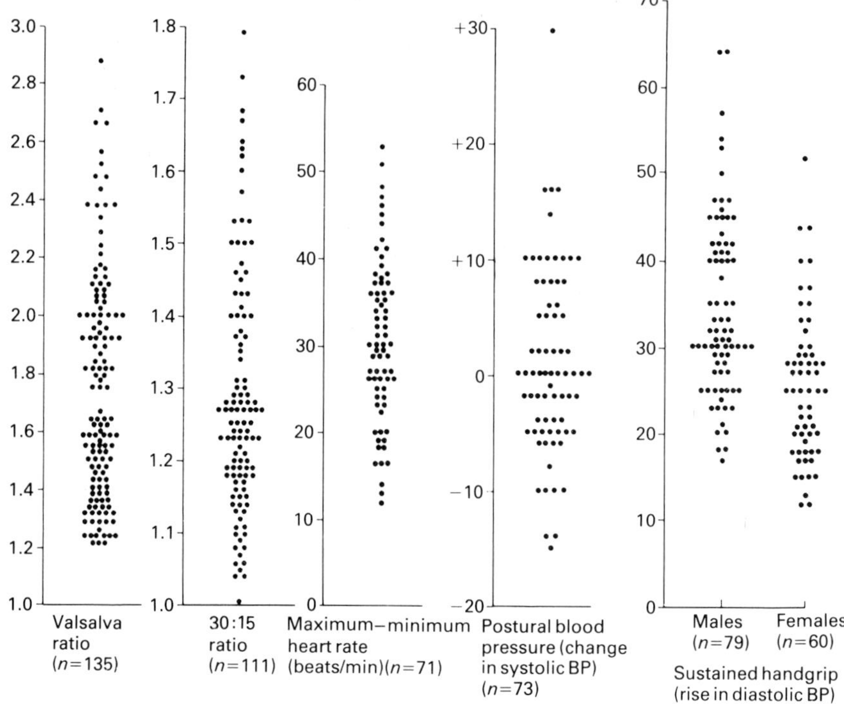

Fig. 38.2. Individual responses to five cardiovascular reflex tests in normal subjects aged 16–69 years. (From Ewing *et al.* (1985).)

Table 38.2. Normal and abnormal values for simple bedside cardiovascular reflex tests

Test	*Normal*	*Borderline*	*Abnormal*
Valsalva manoeuvre (Valsalva ratio)	1.21 or more	—	1.20 or less
Heart-rate variation (Maximum–minimum heart rate)	15 beats/min or more	11–14 beats/min	10 beats/min or less
Heart-rate response to standing (30:15 ratio)	1.04 or more	1.01–1.03	1.00 or less
Blood pressure response to standing (postural fall in systolic BP)	10 mm Hg or less	11–29 mm Hg	30 mm Hg or more
Sustained handgrip (increase in diastolic BP)	16 mm Hg or more	11–15 mm Hg	10 mm Hg or less

obtained. In addition, the tests have proved of considerable diagnostic use in relating autonomic abnormalities to symptoms and prognosis. Figures for repeatability are available for each of the tests (Ewing *et al.* 1985). Although these are less than perfect, it must be remembered that a borderline area of uncertainty exists between normal and abnormal. The figures quoted do not take age into account. More stringent criteria should be applied in research studies, allowing for age, particularly when one of the heart-rate variation tests is used.

Autonomic neuropathy can be classified according to the severity of damage into one of five groups:

1. Normal: all five tests normal or one borderline.
2. Early involvement: one of the three heart-rate tests abnormal or two borderline.
3. Definite involvement: two or more of the heart-rate tests abnormal.
4. Severe involvement: two or more of the heart-rate tests abnormal, plus one or both of the blood-pressure tests abnormal or both borderline.
5. Atypical pattern: any other combination of abnormal tests (in the study quoted above only 6 per cent of patients tested were 'atypical').

An alternative to this classification of severity is to give each individual test a score of 0, 1, or 2 depending on whether they are respectively normal, borderline, or abnormal. An overall 'autonomic test score' of 0–10 can then be obtained. Although increasing scores of 0–10 correlate closely with grades of severity given above, scoring of the tests in this way allows the 'atypical' pattern to be given an actual numerical value. This battery of cardiovascular tests can be performed very easily in the clinic situation with only minimal equipment. All that is needed are a sphygmomanometer, an ECG machine, an aneroid pressure gauge attached to a mouthpiece by a rigid or flexible tube, and a handgrip dynamometer. With practice a planned sequence of tests can be performed within 15–20 minutes.

Measurement and calculation of the various ratios can be done in two ways. Before the advent of microcomputer systems, and still useful when tests are only occasionally performed, all that is required is a ruler and an ECG strip. Nowadays, however, a number of computer programs have been written which measure the R–R interval automatically, calculate the required ratios, and group the results. Several systems have been described, incorporating measurements of heart rate. In Edinburgh, a system now in routine use based on the five tests described above can operate with a BBC or IBM pc or compatible microcomputer. It has the advantages of allowing blood-pressure measurements to be entered and automatically classifying the results.

Although it was stated in the previous edition that heart-rate responses are indicative of cardiac parasympathetic integrity, while blood-pressure changes are only abnormal with more extensive and widespread 'extra cardiac' sympathetic damage, it has become increasingly apparent that the autonomic pathways involved in these reflexes are extremely complex and encompass both parasympathetic and sympathetic fibres to a greater or lesser extent. While a division into parasympathetic and sympathetic tests is clinically convenient, this does not strictly reflect all the complex underlying physiological mechanisms. Of the five tests, most observers now agree that the heart-rate response to deep breathing is mediated almost exclusively by cardiac parasympathetic pathways. Both the Valsalva manoeuvre and the lying-to-standing heart-rate response rely to some extent on the integrity of sympathetic as well as parasympathetic pathways (see Chapter 17). While postural blood-pressure control is predominantly dependent on intact peripheral sympathetic vasoconstriction, other factors such as blood volume may also contribute. Some recent evidence has suggested that the degree of orthostatic hypotension is partly related to the degree of parasympathetic baroreflex dysfunction (Olshan *et al.* 1983). The blood-pressure response to sustained handgrip appears to be predominantly mediated by sympathetic pathways.

The classification proposed here for cardiovascular autonomic neuropathy avoids labelling the reflex pathways as either precisely parasympathetic or sympathetic as it seems more logical to define autonomic involvement merely as early, definite, or severe. One trap for the unwary is to use a single cardiovascular-reflex test for assessment of autonomic damage (usually the heart-rate response to deep breathing) as this is misleading. It presumes that autonomic neuropathy is 'all or nothing' and does not allow for a range of nerve damage from minimal to extremely extensive.

SOME NEWER APPROACHES TO CARDIOVASCULAR REFLEX FUNCTION

Immediate heart-rate response to lying down

When a normal subject lies down there is a small but consistent immediate rise in heart rate over 3 or 4 beats, followed by a fall in heart rate to below the standing level over the next 25 to 30 beats. This pattern of response is altered by atropine, which abolishes the initial shortening of the R–R interval over the first 10 beats. Thereafter slow but steady lengthening of the R–R interval occurs. With additional propranolol the later part of the response is further attenuated. Propranolol alone does not affect the response (Fig. 38.3). This suggests that the first part of the heart-rate response to lying down (over the first

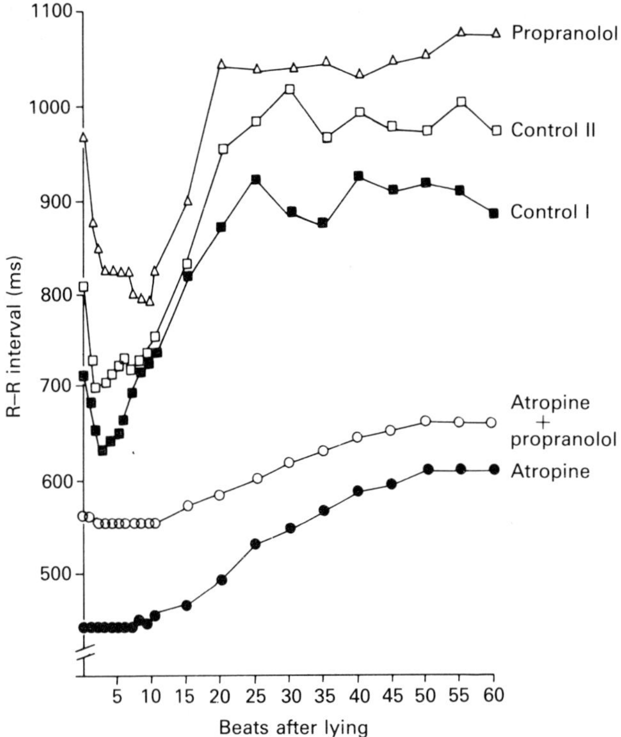

Fig. 38.3. Immediate heart-rate response to lying down before and after cardiac autonomic blockade in eight young normal subjects: group mean R–R interval measurements (ms) before and during the first 60 beats after lying down. (From Bellavere and Ewing (1982).)

10 beats) is under cardiac parasympathetic control, while the later part comes more under sympathetic control (Bellavere and Ewing 1982). This response has been adapted as a further possible test for cardiac parasympathetic damage in diabetics. The standing to lying ratio (S:L ratio) is the ratio of the longest R–R interval during the 5 beats before lying down to the shortest R–R interval during the 10 beats after lying down. Results in diabetics with different degrees of autonomic damage are shown in Fig. 38.4, and suggest that this could be a way of detecting early cardiac parasympathetic damage (Rodrigues and Ewing 1983). In a further study the later part of the response has been suggested as a marker of sympathetic damage (Bellavere *et al.* 1987). Further investigations are awaited to see whether or not this test will be useful clinically.

Heart-rate response to coughing

Coughing produces rapid intrathoracic pressure fluctuations, with

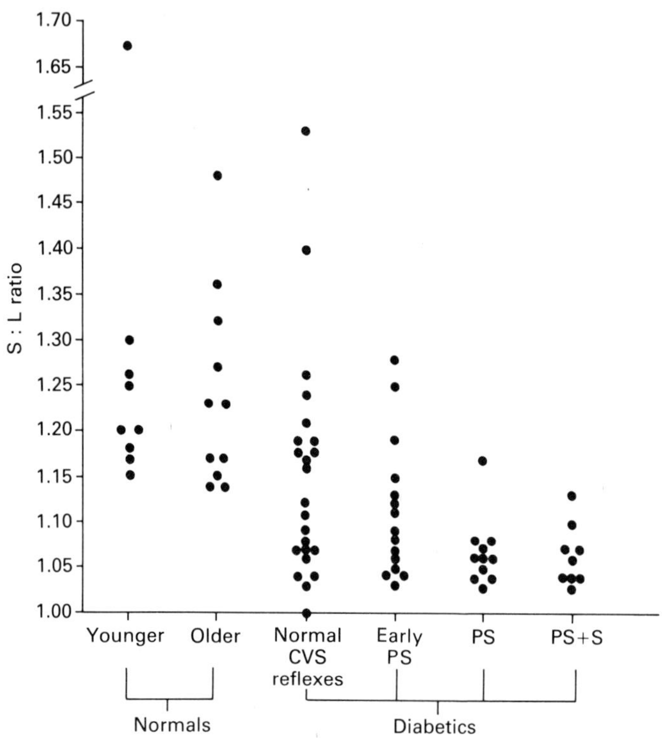

Fig. 38.4. Standing-to-lying heart-rate ratios (S:L ratio) in 20 normal subjects and 58 diabetics with different degrees of autonomic damage (CVS, cardiovascular; PS, parasympathetic; S, sympathetic). (From Rodrigues and Ewing (1983).)

consequent haemodynamic and cardiovascular reflex effects. Normally a brief cough produces an immediate shortening of R–R interval (or increase in heart rate) reaching a peak in 2–3 seconds, and is followed by R–R interval lengthening back to the resting value over the next 18–20 seconds. The cardiac acceleration is abolished by atropine, but not propranolol, showing that it is dependent on cardiac parasympathetic pathways (Cardone *et al.* 1987). Diabetics with autonomic neuropathy have a response similar to normal subjects after autonomic blockade, unlike diabetics with intact cardiovascular reflexes (Fig. 38.5). It is possible that this manoeuvre could be adopted as a further simple test of cardiac parasympathetic function.

Complex analyses of heart-rate variation

Heart-rate variability has been analysed by several groups using complex spectral analysis techniques. While these approaches may have relevance in the theoretical understanding of the basis of heart-rate variability

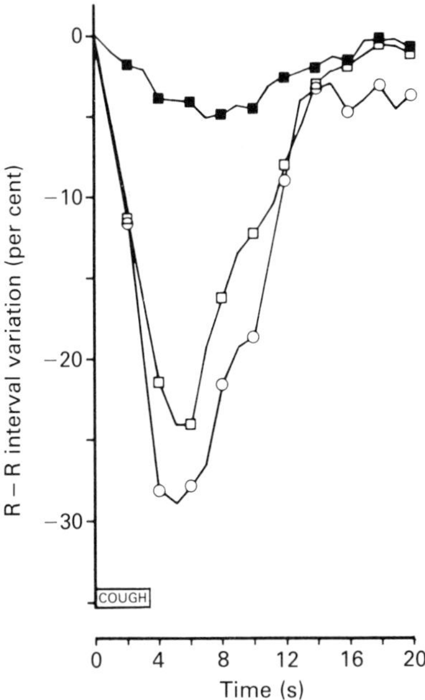

Fig. 38.5. Instantaneous heart-rate response to coughing in (○) six normal subjects, (□) six diabetics without, and (■) six with autonomic neuropathy: group mean R–R interval variation (per cent) from baseline during the first 20 seconds. (From Cardone *et al.* (1987).)

they probably have no advantage over simpler measures of heart-rate variation for day-to-day clinical use.

Longer term assessment of heart-rate variation

A new approach to assessment of autonomic function has recently been developed using 24-hour ECG recordings of heart rate and assessing heart-rate variability continuously (Ewing *et al.* 1984). The method allows an 'on-line' assessment of autonomic function from minute to minute and hour to hour. In normal subjects, in addition to the well recognized sinus arrhythmia, there are large numbers of frequent but irregular larger changes in beat-by-beat heart rate. If a lower cut-off point of 50 ms is adopted for changes between successive R–R intervals, then in normal subjects about 200 'step counts' per hour can be recorded during the day and about 400 per hour at night. In diabetics with cardiac parasympathetic damage, and in cardiac transplant patients, these 'step counts' in heart rate are almost entirely abolished (Fig. 38.6). This method has proved a very sensitive way of detecting early cardiac parasympathetic function, and shows abnormalities more often than conventional cardiovascular reflex tests as about half the

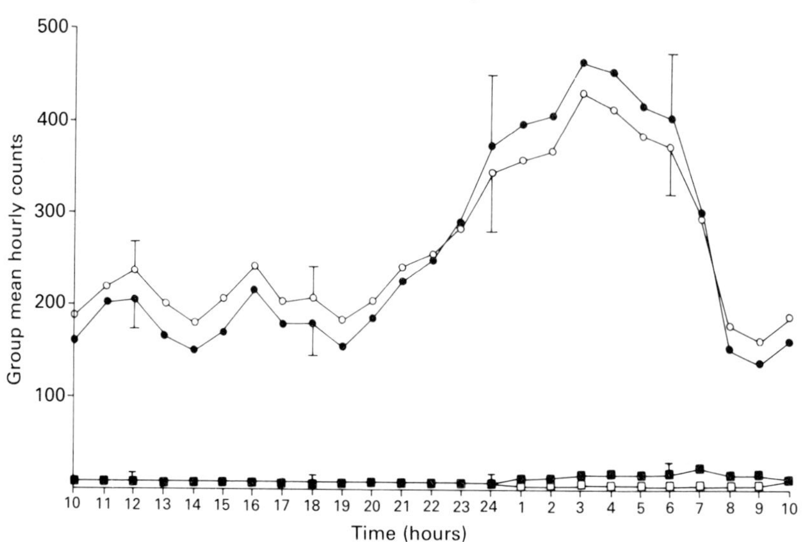

Fig. 38.6. Group mean hourly R–R interval step counts in (○, positive; ●, negative) 25 normal subjects; (■) 12 diabetics with cardiac parasympathetic damage; and (□) six cardiac transplant patients. Bars represent ±SEM. (From Ewing *et al.* (1984).)

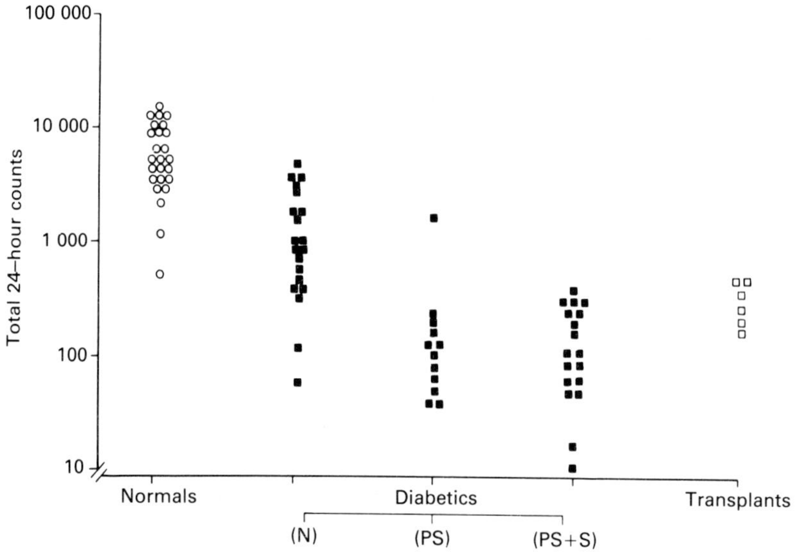

Fig. 38.7. Total number of R–R interval step counts accumulated over the whole 24-hour period in (○) 25 normal subjects; (■) 50 diabetics; and (□) six cardiac transplant patients. The diabetics were grouped into 20 with normal cardiovascular reflexes (N), 12 with cardiac parasympathetic damage (PS), and 18 with parasympathetic and additional sympathetic abnormalities (PS+S).

diabetics with normal cardiovascular reflexes, nevertheless, had abnormally low 'step counts' (Fig. 38.7). The potential for this method has not yet been fully developed but it is likely that subtle variations of cardiac parasympathetic activity in response not only to specific manoeuvres but also to normal everyday events can be examined, and very early damage to cardiac parasympathetic nerves detected, both in diabetics and in other disorders.

CARDIOVASCULAR AUTONOMIC ABNORMALITIES IN DIABETICS

Prevalence of abnormalities

Two large studies have recently reported the prevalence of abnormal cardiovascular autonomic function in diabetics. O'Brien and colleagues (1986*b*) found abnormal heart-rate variation tests in 17 per cent of over 500 unselected insulin-dependent diabetics. The frequency of abnormalities was greatest in diabetics aged 40–49 years and those with diabetes of 20 or more years duration. They also found a drop in systolic blood pressure of 20 mm Hg or more in 10 per cent, although only half had abnormal heart-rate variation. In a second study 700 individuals were selected as a representative sample of surviving diabetics first diagnosed between 1939 and 1965. Orthostatic hypotension, defined as a fall of 25 mm Hg or more in systolic blood pressure, was observed in approximately 12 per cent, with the highest prevalence in older diabetics, and young diabetics with long duration of diabetes (Krolewski *et al.* 1985). In other studies, 31 per cent of teen-age diabetic subjects and 15 per cent of diabetic children had abnormal cardiovascular reflexes. Several studies have confirmed that autonomic function tests may be abnormal without autonomic symptoms, and that autonomic damage can be detected within the first 2 years after diagnosis of diabetes, again without symptoms (see Ewing and Clarke 1986).

Sequence of abnormalities

The sequence of cardiovascular reflex abnormalities in diabetics is now becoming clearer. Autonomic damage is not simply present or absent but can be anywhere on a spectrum from minimal to severe. Cardiac parasympathetic function may be impaired without sympathetic damage, but not the reverse, whereas detectable sympathetic lesions were found in one study only in longstanding diabetic subjects with extensive cardiac vagal damage. In individuals followed prospectively the heart rate first increased and later decreased, suggesting that cardiac vagal fibres are affected before cardiac sympathetic fibres.

Cardiovascular tests deteriorate with time. In a large group of diabetic patients heart-rate tests were abnormal more commonly and earlier than blood-pressure tests. When tests were repeated, three-quarters were unchanged, one-quarter deteriorated, but only a very few improved (Ewing *et al.* 1985). Early parasympathetic involvement may, however, be more apparent than real as heart-rate tests are much more sensitive than blood-pressure tests and therefore more likely to be abnormal. There is increasing evidence that deranged sympathetic function elsewhere can be found even in mild autonomic neuropathy with for example, abnormal noradrenalin responses to exercise and arterial pressure changes, and impaired iris sympathetic function. Within the heart, however, it is likely that cardiac parasympathetic fibres are involved more extensively and earlier than cardiovascular sympathetic nerves, possibly because they are longer and therefore more liable to damage. Computer simulation models of random nerve damage where longer fibres were affected first also support this view (see Ewing 1984; Ewing and Clarke 1986).

Baroreflex damage

Two recent studies (Olshan *et al.* 1983; Eckberg *et al.* 1986) have looked at baroreflex function in diabetics using amyl nitrite inhalation and phenylephrine infusions. Both showed abnormalities of baroreflex control in diabetic patients with and without autonomic symptoms, signifying defects of both parasympathetic and sympathetic innervation.

Relation to somatic neuropathy

As peripheral nerves contain both autonomic (small) and somatic (large) fibres, associations between autonomic and somatic neuropathy have inevitably been reported. Studies have included autonomic-function tests in subjects with symptomatic peripheral neuropathy, nerve electrophysiology in symptomatic autonomic neuropathy, or both somatic and autonomic function in asymptomatic patients. Recently, this relationship has been re-examined in diabetic subjects with different presentations of clinical neuropathy, and in untreated non-insulin dependent diabetic subjects. These studies support the view that a diffuse, generalized, and symmetrical involvement of peripheral nerves can be detected, although different fibre types may be involved in varying proportions with different clinical presentations (see Ewing and Clarke 1986).

24-hour heart-rate monitoring

Several studies have now looked at 24-hour ambulatory ECG monitoring in diabetics. In one, 64 diabetics with varying severity of autonomic damage were analysed. The frequency of arrhythmias was no higher than in normal subjects. The diabetics had higher mean hourly heart rates, and, with increasing autonomic damage, there was reduction in diurnal heart-rate variation. The mean waking and sleeping heart rates were higher in the diabetics. The maximum heart rates achieved were not significantly different, but the minimum heart rates were significantly higher in the diabetics. These previously unrecognized abnormal 24-hour heart-rate patterns provide further evidence of damage to the autonomic mechanisms controlling heart rate in diabetes mellitus (see Ewing 1984). Two further studies have now confirmed these findings (Rubler *et al.* 1985; Valensi *et al.* 1985). Our own study also showed that only one subject had a persistent heart rate above 90 beats per minute throughout the 24 hours, despite the previously reported clinical descriptions of 'persistent tachycardia' as a well-recognized feature of diabetic autonomic neuropathy. A second clinical suggestion of the 'fixed heart rate' was also uncommon. Despite considerable autonomic involvement in one-third of the diabetics, only one subject had a relatively 'fixed' heart rate. Even this patient had a variation between maximum and minimum heart rates of 16 beats/min over the 24-hour recording period.

Recently, we studied a further group of diabetics with severe cardiovascular autonomic abnormalities who were given single oral doses of three different β-adrenoceptor-blocking drugs (Reid *et al.* 1987). Although they were in theory 'medically' denervated, heart rates were still altered during the 24-hour recordings in proportion to the degree of partial agonist activity of each drug. These surprisingly normal heart-rate responses suggest that the concept of 'cardiac denervation' requires some modification. Diabetics who have abnormal cardiovascular reflex responses to the usual conventional reflex tests may not necessarily be completely denervated, as more severe stresses may provoke some changes in heart rate.

Relationship between cardiac neural damage and cardiac function

Work on the cardiovascular effects of autonomic neuropathy in diabetics has concentrated mainly on damage to the cardiac nerve supply to the heart. Little attention has been paid to the effect either of poor cardiac function on heart-rate and blood-pressure responses to autonomic stimuli, or to the possible effects of abnormal autonomic innervation on cardiac function itself. It has been well recognized for many years that subjects with cardiac failure have abnormal responses to the Valsalva manoeuvre, and care has therefore been taken in most studies to exclude subjects with clinical cardiac failure. Whether, however, there are more subtle interplays between neural supply and haemodynamic changes is only now beginning to be appreciated. Diabetics with postural hypotension may have some myocardial contractility impairment, possibly caused either by diabetic cardiopathy or by cardiac sympathetic nerve damage (see Ewing 1984). Recently Kahn and colleagues (1986*a*) confirmed this observation and suggested that diminished heart-rate and blood-pressure alterations during exercise could reflect deranged parasympathetic and sympathetic control of the sinoatrial node and vascular resistance beds.

Radionuclide ventriculography studies have shown depressed left ventricular diastolic filling and left ventricular performance on exercise in diabetics with autonomic neuropathy which was not found in those without (Zola *et al.* 1986; Kahn *et al.* 1986*b*). The authors suggested that the depressed myocardial performance could not be entirely explained by microvascular disease and that the effect on left ventricular function might be a direct result of damaged autonomic innervation to the heart. They also postulated that diminished cardiac catecholamine responsiveness might play a part. These studies have not yet been confirmed by other groups, but if substantiated may lead to further understanding of autonomic nervous control of normal and abnormal cardiac function.

INVOLVEMENT OF OTHER SYSTEMS

Respiratory studies

Recent respiratory investigations in diabetics with autonomic neuropathy have focused on three areas: ventilatory control, respiratory reflexes, and breathing abnormalities during sleep (see Ewing and Clarke 1986). Differing results have been found in studies on the control of breathing. Ventilatory responses to both transient and progressive hypoxia have been found to be both normal and abnormal. Similarly, responses to hypercapnia have also produced conflicting results. Different conclusions have therefore been reached about whether there is damage to peripheral chemoreceptor or central ventilatory control mechanisms in diabetic autonomic neuropathy. In a recent case report, it was suggested that both mechanisms might be involved. Impaired bronchomotor function has been described, with diminished bronchodilatation following inhalation of ipratropium bromide (an atropine-like drug) found in one study, and no fall in specific airways conduction after a provocation test with cold air in a second study. Reports of breathing patterns during sleep have been in conflict. The earliest two studies suggested that breathing abnormalities were common during sleep in diabetic autonomic neuropathy, although the authors did not take account of normal variability or age. In another study abnormal sleep-related breathing patterns were described in approximately one-quarter of a mixed group of diabetic patients. By contrast, a carefully controlled study concluded that diabetic patients with severe autonomic neuropathy had normal breathing patterns and oxygenation during sleep. Further studies are clearly needed to resolve these various discrepancies.

Pupillary abnormalities

Pupillary abnormalities in diabetics are reviewed in detail in Chapter 22. Two simple bedside techniques to assess autonomic pupil function have recently been described. The first measures the diameter of the dark-adapted pupil using a polaroid photograph of the eye taken by electronic flash. When standardized against the outer diameter of the iris, the dark adapted pupil diameter provides a quantitative estimate of sympathetic innervation (Smith and Dewhirst 1986). The second technique, measurement of pupil cycle time (PCT), depends on the observation that regular oscillations of the pupil can be induced with a slit lamp beam in normal subjects and timed with a stop watch (Martyn and Ewing 1986). Pharmacological testing confirms that PCT is a sensitive measure of parasympathetic dysfunction and in diabetics with autonomic neuropathy, it is considerably prolonged (Fig. 38.8). These techniques provide two additional simple methods of testing autonomic reflexes independent of cardiovascular pathways.

Sudomotor and skin tests

Two recent new tests of local sweating have been suggested. Low and colleagues (1983) have described a sophisticated quantitative sudomotor axon reflex test (Q-SART) in which local sweating is stimulated by acetylcholine iontophoresis. Kennedy *et al.* (1984) used a different approach, counting the number of imprints that sweat drops make in a soft silastic impression material after stimulation of local sweating with pilocarpine iontophoresis. These two approaches allow local sympathetic sweat production to be measured quantitatively. Low *et al.* (1986) used their Q-SART test to compare distal sympathetic function with vagal function in diabetic neuropathy. They found abnormal Q-SART tests in the foot and abnormal heart-rate variation in roughly equal proportions and much more frequently than either orthostatic hypotension or sweating abnormalities in the arm (Fig. 38.9). This suggests that abnormalities of distal sympathetic function occur early in the natural history of diabetic autonomic neuropathy, and, in view of the findings in the arms, lend further support to the view that longer fibres are damaged before shorter fibres.

Another skin-testing technique was described by Hoffmann *et al.* (1982) who measured the skin flare response to intradermal histamine

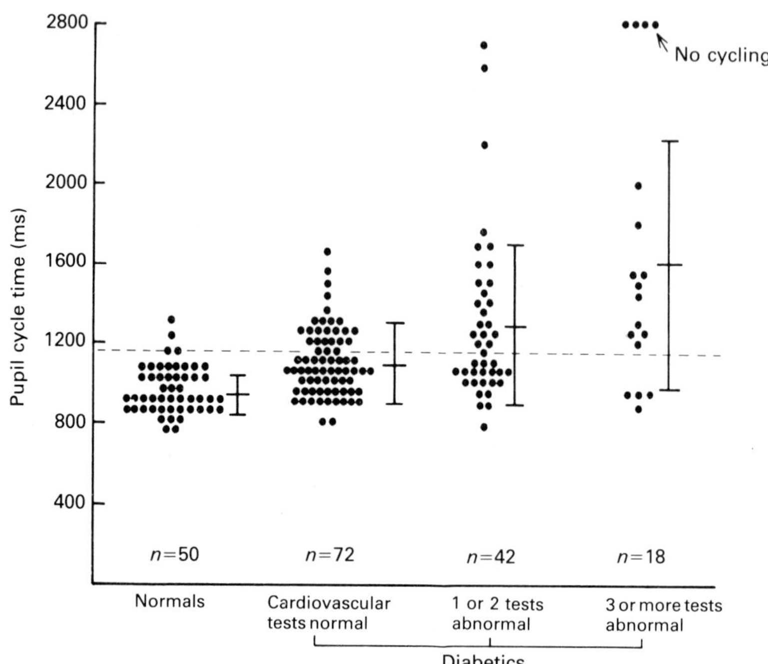

Fig. 38.8. Pupil cycle times in normal subjects and diabetics. The diabetics are grouped according to the numbers of abnormal results found on cardiovascular reflex testing. Group mean ±SD are indicated. The upper limit of normal is shown by the dotted line. (From Martyn and Ewing (1986).)

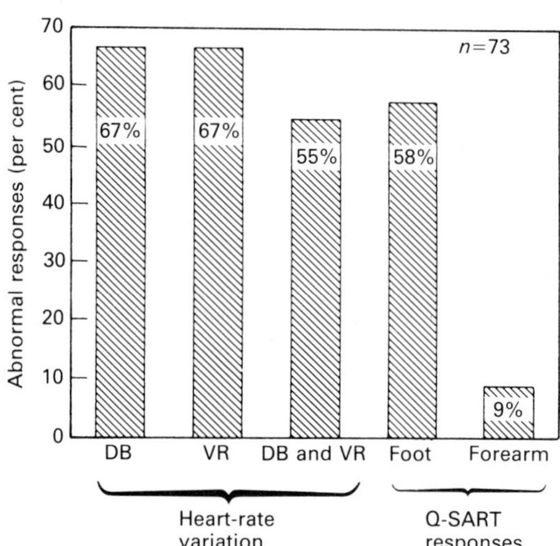

Fig. 38.9. Percentage frequency of abnormal heart-rate variation tests (heart-rate responses to deep breathing (DB) and the Valsalva manoeuvre (VR)) and Q-SART responses (in the foot and forearm) in 73 patients with diabetic neuropathy. (From Low *et al.* (1986).)

before and after the addition of noradrenalin or terbutaline (adrenoceptor agonists) in normal subjects and diabetics with and without autonomic neuropathy. Diabetics with autonomic neuropathy showed no change in the skin response after noradrenalin in contrast to the other subjects, thus suggesting a defect at the distal adrenoceptor level in these patients. The authors proposed that this could be used as a simple additional test for identifying patients with autonomic neuropathy.

Gastrointestinal function

While not strictly 'non-invasive', gastrointestinal findings in diabetics with autonomic neuropathy are included here for completeness.

Oesophagus

Oesophageal function can be assessed by cineradiography, manometry, or scintiscanning. Scintiscanning techniques measuring both solid and liquid transit times may show abnormalities in diabetic autonomic neuropathy. Multi-peaked oesophageal pressure waves were recently found in most diabetics studied with neuropathy, in only a few without neuropathy, and rarely in non-diabetics referred with suspected oesophageal disease. These abnormal motility patterns confirm previous reports that diabetics with autonomic neuropathy frequently have diminished or disordered oesophageal peristalsis and delayed oesophageal emptying (see Ewing and Clarke 1986).

Stomach

Isotopic gastric scanning techniques have confirmed that liquid emptying is normal but solid emptying is delayed in diabetics with other evidence of autonomic neuropathy. Impaired gastric accommodation to distension has also been reported, and vagally mediated gastric acid secretion in response to sham feeding is reduced. An enhanced gastrin response in diabetics with abnormal cardiovascular reflexes has also been shown (see Ewing and Clarke 1986).

Small and large intestine

Abnormalities of proximal small intestinal motility involving both parasympathetic and sympathetic innervation have been described in diabetics with gastric autonomic problems, including decreased intestinal transit times and absence of interdigestive migrating motor complexes (see Ewing and Clarke 1986).

Neuroendocrine abnormalities

A number of recent studies have examined the role of gastrointestinal hormones and catecholamines in diabetic autonomic neuropathy (see Ewing and Clarke 1986). Pancreatic polypeptide (PP) release from the pancreatic islets is partly under parasympathetic control, and in diabetics with cardiac vagal abnormalities the PP responses to exercise, hypoglycaemia, sham feeding, and a meal are significantly reduced. Little is known about the exact neural mediation of somatostatin release but vagal pathways may be involved. The regulation of glucagon secretion is controversial but may be partly under autonomic control. Both somatostatin and glucagon responses to hypoglycaemia have been shown to be reduced in diabetic autonomic neuropathy. Gastric inhibitory peptide secretion after a meal is diminished in diabetics with autonomic damage, although its impaired secretion may, in fact, be secondary to delayed gastric emptying rather than direct neural damage. Motilin may play a key role in regulating gastric motility and intestinal transit. It is probably modulated primarily by vagal fibres, and its release is also abnormal in these diabetics. High fasting and postprandial gastrin levels have been reported in diabetics with autonomic damage, although gastrin secretion is probably mediated by other factors in addition to autonomic mechanisms. An enhanced gastrin response may occur because of loss of normal vagal inhibition of the gastrin-secreting cells. Autonomic modulation therefore influences the secretion of these polypeptides, which in turn may regulate in part gastrointestinal motility, and digestion and absorption of nutrients. Abnormalities of these gastrointestinal hormones may also contribute to the clinical sequelae of delayed gastric emptying, diarrhoea, and constipation.

Catecholamine responses are abnormal in diabetic subjects with autonomic neuropathy. Noradrenalin responses are blunted during standing, exercise, and edrophonium administration, but not with hypoglycaemia (although this has recently been disputed). One group have distinguished a 'hypoadrenergic' pattern with diminished noradrenalin levels due to sympathetic damage from a 'hyperadrenergic' pattern resulting from a diminished intravascular volume. Another group of workers looked at catecholamine kinetics and showed that noradrenalin production and turnover were reduced in autonomic neuropathy. Plasma adrenalin responses are blunted by hypoglycaemia, but hydroxylation of dopamine seems to be normal.

Renal involvement

Two studies of renal function in diabetics with autonomic neuropathy found that renal haemodynamics may be deranged in diabetics with autonomic neuropathy and suggested that autonomic neuropathy may affect the kidney independently from microvascular changes (Lilja *et al.* 1985; Winocour *et al.* 1986).

Sudden deaths in diabetics

In three large series where there was prospective follow-up of diabetics with autonomic neuropathy, some sudden and unexpected deaths were described, for which no cause could be found (see Ewing and Clarke 1986). Four possible explanations have been put forward, none of which is entirely convincing. Diabetics with damaged autonomic pathways might not respond normally to hypoxia, and this could lead to cardio-respiratory arrests under certain conditions, such as chest infections or surgery. However, as mentioned above (p. 682), the evidence relating to hypoxic responses in diabetics is far from conclusive. Second, cardiac arrhythmias might be the cause of these sudden deaths. Diabetics do not, however, have more arrhythmias during 24-hour ECG monitoring than normal subjects. Sleep apnoea has also been proposed as a mechanism, but we found normal breathing patterns during sleep in diabetics with autonomic neuropathy. The fourth possibility is that of some as yet unknown homeostatic mechanism or reflex that fails to function under certain conditions, and which may lead to unexpected death.

CONCLUSION

The place of non-invasive cardiovascular reflex tests is now firmly established for the objective bedside or out-patient assessment of diabetic autonomic neuropathy. There are, however, some controversies about how exactly the tests should be performed, and what measurements should be made to determine the integrity of responses. Newer non-invasive tests, such as the standing-to-lying and cough tests, have recently been proposed, and new ways are being developed to look at autonomic damage over longer periods using 24-hour heart-rate recordings.

Over the past 5 years, too, further insight has been gained into the consequences of cardiovascular autonomic damage in diabetes, its natural history, and relation to somatic neuropathy. Although not always clinically evident, it is also becoming apparent that disordered autonomic function can be detected throughout the body, if techniques are sensitive enough. The effect of autonomic damage on the function of different organs is only just beginning to be appreciated in diabetics. While there have been many recent advances in the assessment and understanding of diabetic autonomic neuropathy and its pathophysiology, many further areas still wait to be explored.

REFERENCES

Bellavere, F., Cardone, C., Ferri, M., Guarini, L., Piccoli, A., and Fedele, D. (1987). Standing to lying heart rate variations. A new simple test in the diagnosis of diabetic autonomic neuropathy. *Diabetic Med.* **4**, 41–3.

Bellavere, F. and Ewing, D. J. (1982). Autonomic control of the immediate heart rate response to lying down. *Clin. Sci.* **62**, 57–64.

Cardone, C., Bellavere, F., Ferri, M., and Fedele, D. (1987). Autonomic mechanisms in the heart rate response to coughing. *Clin. Sci.* **72**, 55–60.

Clark, C. V. and Mapstone, R. (1986). Age-adjusted normal tolerance limits for cardiovascular autonomic function assessment in the elderly. *Age Ageing* **15**, 221–9.

Dambrink, J. H. A. and Wieling, W. (1987). Circulatory response to postural change in healthy male subjects in relation to age. *Clin. Sci.* **72**, 335–41.

Eckberg, D. L., Harkins, S. W., Fritsch, J. M., Musgrave, G. E., and Gardner, D. F. (1986). Baroreflex control of plasma norepinephrine and heart period in healthy subjects and diabetic patients. *J. clin. Invest.* **78**, 366–74.

Ewing, D. J. (1984). Cardiac autonomic neuropathy. In *Diabetes and heart disease* (ed. R. J. Jarrett), pp. 99–132. Elsevier Biomedical Press, Amsterdam.

Ewing, D. J. and Clarke, B. F. (1986). Diabetic autonomic neuropathy: present insights and future prospects. *Diabetes Care* **9**, 648–65.

Ewing, D. J., Martyn, C. N., Young, R. J., and Clarke, B. F. (1985). The value of cardiovascular autonomic function tests: 10 years experience in diabetes. *Diabetes Care* **8**, 491–8.

Ewing, D. J., Neilson, J. M. M., and Travis, P. (1984). New method for assessing cardiac parasympathetic activity using 24 hour electrocardiograms. *Br. Heart. J.* **52**, 396–402.

Gautschy, B., Weidmann, P., and Gnadinger, M. P. (1986). Autonomic function tests as related to age and gender in normal man. *Klin. Wochenschr.* **64**, 499–505.

Hoffman, A., Conen, D., Leibundgut, U., and Berger, W. (1982). A skin test for autonomic neuropathy. *Eur. Neurol.* **21**, 29–33.

Kahn, J. K., Zola, B., Juni, J. E., and Vinik, A. I. (1986*a*). Decreased exercise heart rate and blood pressure response in diabetic subjects with cardiac autonomic neuropathy. *Diabetes Care* **9**, 389–94.

Kahn, J. K., Zola, B., Juni, J. E., and Vinik, A. I. (1986*b*). Radionuclide assessment of left ventricular diastolic filling in diabetes mellitus with and without cardiac autonomic neuropathy. *J. Am. Coll. Cardiol.* **7**, 1303–9.

Kennedy, W. R., Sakuda, M., Sutherland, D., and Goetz, F. C. (1984). The sweating deficiency in diabetes mellitus: methods of quantitation and clinical correlation. *Neurology, Cleveland* **34**, 758–63.

Krolewski, A. S., Warram, J. H., Cupples, A., Gorman, G. K., Szabo, A. J., and Christlieb, A. R. (1985). Hypertension, orthostatic hypotension and the microvascular complications of diabetes. *J. chron. Dis.* **38**, 319–26.

Lilja, B., Nosslin, B., Bergstrom, B., Sundkvist, G. (1985). Glomerular filtration rate, autonomic nerve function and orthostatic blood pressure in patients with diabetes mellitus. *Diabetes Res.* **2**, 179–81.

Low, P. A., Caskey, P. E., Tuck, R. R., Fealey, R. D., and Dyck, P. J. (1983). Quantitative sudomotor axon reflex test in normal and neuropathic subjects. *Ann. Neurol.* **14**, 573–80.

Low, P. A., Zimmerman, B. R., and Dyck, P. J. (1986). Comparison of distal sympathetic with vagal function in diabetic neuropathy. *Muscle Nerve* **9**, 592–6.

Martyn, C. N. and Ewing, D. J. (1986). Pupil cycle time: a simple way of measuring an autonomic reflex. *J. Neurol. Neurosurg. Psychiat.* **49**, 771–4.

Masaoka, S., Lev-Ran, A., Hill, L. R., Vakil, G. and Hon, E. H. G. (1985). Heart rate variability in diabetes: relationship to age and duration of the disease. *Diabetes Care* **8**, 64–8.

O'Brien, I. A. D., O'Hare, P., and Corrall, R. J. M. (1986*a*). Heart rate variability in healthy subjects: effects of age and the derivation of normal ranges for tests of autonomic function. *Br. Heart. J.* **55**, 348–54.

O'Brien, I. A. D., O'Hare, J. P., Lewin, I. G., and Corrall, R. J. M. (1986*b*). The prevalence of autonomic neuropathy in insulin-dependent diabetes mellitus: a controlled study based on heart rate variability. *Quart. J. Med.* **61**, 957–67.

Oikawa, N., Umetsu, M., Toyota, T., and Goto, Y. (1985). Quantitative evaluation of diabetic autonomic neuropathy by using heart rate variations—determination of the normal range for the diagnosis of autonomic neuropathy. *Tohoku J. exp. Med.* **145**, 233–41.

Olshan, A. R., O'Connor, D. T., Cohen, I. M., Mitas, J. A., and Stone, R. A. (1983). Baroreflex dysfunction in patients with adult-onset diabetes and hypertension. *Am. J. Med.* **74**, 233–42.

Reid, W., Ewing, D. J., Harry, D. J., Smith, H. J., Neilson, J. M. M., and Clarke, B. F. (1987). Effects of β-adrenoceptor blockade on heart rate and physiological tremor in diabetics with autonomic neuropathy. A comparative study of epanolol, atenolol and pindolol. *Br. J. clin. Pharmacol.* **23**, 383–9.

Rodrigues, E. A. and Ewing, D. J. (1983). Immediate heart rate response to lying down: simple test for parasympathetic damage in diabetes. *Br. med. J.* **287**, 800.

Rubler, S., Chu, D. A. and Bruzzone, C. L. (1985). Blood pressure and heart rate responses during 24-hour ambulatory monitoring and exercise in men with diabetes mellitus. *Am. J. Cardiol.* **55**, 801–6.

Smith, S. A. (1982). Reduced sinus arrhythmia in diabetic autonomic neuropathy: diagnostic value of an age-related normal range. *Br. med. J.* **285**, 1599–601.

Smith, S. A. (1984). Diagnostic value of the Valsalva Ratio reduction in diabetic autonomic neuropathy: use of an age-related normal range. *Diabetic Med.* **1**, 295–7.

Smith, S. A. and Dewhirst, R. R. (1986). A simple diagnostic test for pupillary abnormality in diabetic autonomic neuropathy. *Diabetic Med.* **3**, 38–41.

Valensi, P., Attali, J. R., Sachs, R.-N., Palsky, D., Lanfranchi, J., and Sebaoun, J. (1985). Abnormalities of 24 hour continuous electrocardiographic monitoring in diabetes mellitus: involvement of cardiac autonomic neuropathy and/or insulin treatment. *Diabet. Metab* **11**, 337–42.

Vita, G., Princi, P., Calabro, R., Toscano, A., Manna, L., and Messina, C. (1986). Cardiovascular reflex tests: assessment of age-adjusted normal range. *J. neurol. Sci.* **75**, 263–74.

Wieling, W., Van Brederode, J. F. M., De Rijk, L. G., Borst, C., and Dunning, A. J. (1982). Reflex control of heart rate in normal subjects in relation to age: a data base for cardiac vagal neuropathy. *Diabetologia* **22**, 163–6.

Winocour, P. H., Dhar, H., and Anderson, D. C. (1986). The relationship between autonomic neuropathy and urinary sodium and albumin excretion in insulin-treated diabetics. *Diabet. Med.* **3**, 436–40.

Zola, B., Kahn, J. K., Juni, J. E. and Vinik, A. I. (1986). Abnormal cardiac function in diabetic patients with autonomic neuropathy in the absence of ischemic heart disease. *J. clin. Endocrinol. Metab.* **63**, 208–14.

39. Autonomic failure in alcoholics

Ralph H. Johnson

INTRODUCTION

Common experience and frequent printed references in plays, novels, or newspapers to human problems related to alcohol indicate that its acute effects on autonomic nervous system function are well known. Shakespeare's comment in *Macbeth* that alcohol, 'provokes the desire but it takes away the performance' points to the development of sexual impotence. Newspaper reports of drunks found by the roadside dead after a cold night would suggest interference with thermoregulatory mechanisms. Nevertheless, the effects of chronic alcohol ingestion upon autonomic pathways have not attracted as much research as the equivalent defects that occur in diabetes mellitus (Johnson *et al.* 1984) even though clinicians are aware that impotence is a common complaint in chronic alcoholics and that sudden death is not uncommon in them. This chapter describes the features of autonomic failure which occur in alcoholics and shows, in the second part of the chapter, that autonomic dysfunction involving the heart has a clear relationship with increased mortality. In our patients in whom autonomic function tests were abnormal the mortality rate beyond a further 6 years is significantly increased and is three times the expected rate of an age-matched population. Dysfunction of the sympathetic nervous system is considered first, followed by a description of parasympathetic nervous dysfunction.

SYMPATHETIC NERVOUS SYSTEM FAILURE

Blood-pressure regulation

The acute affects of alcohol on autonomic function are generally related to the changes consequent on peripheral vasodilatation although blood pressure is largely unaffected. Both hypertension and orthostatic hypotension may, however, occur with alcohol. The latter problem is only occasional but can be the result of an acute toxic effect of alcohol, due to sympathetic damage or as a consequence of several pathophysiological changes during withdrawal. These are discussed in the following sections.

Hypertension

It is probable that there is a causative association between regular, moderate, or heavy alcohol consumption and raised blood pressure (Potter and Beevers 1984). This may account for 30 per cent of hypertension in affluent countries. Hypertension while imbibing and also additional symptoms of sympathetic overactivity (tremor, sweating, and tachycardia) during alcohol withdrawal, are related to increased concentrations of circulating catecholamines. There is debate about the causation of arterial hypertension in chronic alcoholics (Johnson *et al.* 1987). Discussion of this problem, however, is outside the scope of this chapter which is concerned with features of autonomic failure in alcoholics.

Orthostatic hypotension: acute effect of alcohol

Excess alcohol in both non-alcoholics and alcoholics may cause autonomic failure with orthostatic hypotension due to a toxic effect of alcohol lasting days or weaks. Sympathetic failure in both situations was explained by a block of baroreceptors on the afferent side of the reflex arc (Barraclough and Sharpey-Schafer 1963). In alcoholics in whom orthostatic hypotension is found as an acute toxic response to excess alcohol, recovery is usual with abstinence and treatment with vitamins and a normal diet (Barraclough and Sharpey-Schafer 1963) (Fig. 39.1).

Orthostatic hypotension: due to sympathetic damage

Although in alcoholics, in whom orthostatic hypotension develops as an acute response to excess alcohol, recovery generally occurs, there may be impairment of sympathetic outflow at central or peripheral levels as a cause of orthostatic hypotension in this group (Victor *et al.* 1971). When Wernicke's encephalopathy and chronic liver disease develop, alcoholics are particularly prone to develop orthostatic hypotension (Bernardi *et al.* 1982). In Wernicke's encephalopathy pathological changes may occur in the brainstem, as discussed later. There is evidence in a small proportion of chronic alcoholics, particulary those with a polyneuropathy, of efferent sympathetic dysfunction including absence of normal sympathetic vasoconstriction (Jensen *et al.* 1984). Abnormal ganglion cells and degeneration in sympathetic nerves have also been reported, implying efferent sympathetic dysfunction (Appenzeller and Richardson 1966; Appenzeller and Ogin, 1974). Another pathological study of patients with alcoholic neuropathy, however, failed to reveal significant degeneration in splanchnic nerves (Low *et al.* 1975). These authors did

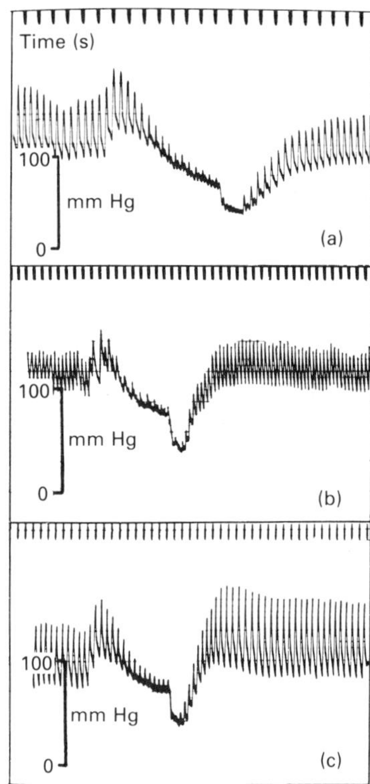

Fig. 39.1. The arterial blood pressure with Valsalva's manoeuvre in a patient with chronic alcoholism admitted with orthostatic hypotension. (a) On admission, syncope occurred at the end of the period of raised intrathoracic pressure. (b) 1 month and (c) 2 months, after treatment with vitamins and a normal diet. Some recovery of circulatory reflexes is shown by the beginnings of an overshoot in (b), while in (c) the response is normal; after treatment, symptoms of orthostatic hypotension recovered. (Taken with permission from Barraclough and Sharpey-Schafer (1963).)

not find any evidence of orthostatic hypotension in their alcoholic patients and concluded, 'The absence of significant disturbance of blood pressure control correlates well with the absence of pathology in the greater splanchnic nerve'. The divergence in these observations indicates considerable differences in the susceptibility of individual alcoholics to the effects of alcohol. It is, therefore, apparent that the frequency of orthostatic hypotension varies in alcoholic groups and is probably related to the severity of the disorder and to whether complications, including neurological damage, have developed.

Orthostatic hypotension: during withdrawal

There are several possible explanations for orthostatic hypotension:

1 There may be reduced numbers of α-adrenergic receptors as a response to previously increased sympathetic nervous activity.

2 Catecholamine secretion may be reduced.
3 β-adrenoceptor vasodilatation may occur.
4 Hypovolaemia may occur during withdrawal, although raised blood volumes are usual.
5 Thiamine is frequently administered to alcoholics during withdrawal and this causes peripheral vasodilatation which could result in hypotension. Hypotension can however occur without thiamine being administered.

The most likely causes of orthostatic hypotension are sympathetic nervous system dysfunction (1 and 2 above) and hypovolaemia either separately or together.

Evidence for sympathetic dysfunction during withdrawal includes the observation of altered plasma catecholamine responses to change of posture (Fig. 39.2). Similar findings were obtained during abstinence for the whole period studied (up to 7 weeks) (Eisenhofer *et al.* 1985). In this study we confirmed that alcohol withdrawal is associated with increased sympathetic activity as reflected by raised supine and standing plasma concentrations of catecholamines. After 2–7 weeks of abstinence from alcohol, plasma noradrenalin concentrations may be higher than controls. Despite increased sympathetic nervous responses to standing, alcoholics during withdrawal have impaired blood-pressure control (Fig. 39.3), and some exhibit orthostatic hypotension. A likely explanation for this which we are currently exploring is depressed α-receptor activity consequent upon excess catecholamine levels during alcohol excess. Orthostatic hypotension may also be observed in alcoholics after continued abstinence. The falls in one group of six patients after abstinence for 4–6 weeks were from 143/83 mm Hg to 84/55 mm Hg (means) (Eisenhofer *et al.* 1985). In some of these there is a total failure of reflex noradrenalin release in response to standing and this probably contributes to orthostatic hypotension. Absence of a significant postural increase in plasma noradrenalin probably implies that the sympathetic failure is postganglionic. De Marchi and Cecchin (1986) confirmed the occurrence of orthostatic hypotension as an occasional finding. In their series, however, very few patients suffered from orthostatic hypotension; only two patients of 60 had orthostatic hypotension during withdrawal. One of these patients still exhibited a fall in blood pressure after 8 weeks of abstinence. The frequency of orthostatic symptoms in different groups therefore differs widely, and is probably dependent upon the severity of their alcoholism.

Temperature regulation

Not all the mechanisms involved in theremoregulation are specifically autonomic. For example, shivering depends upon somatic nerves to muscle and an important aspect of human thermoregulation is conscious

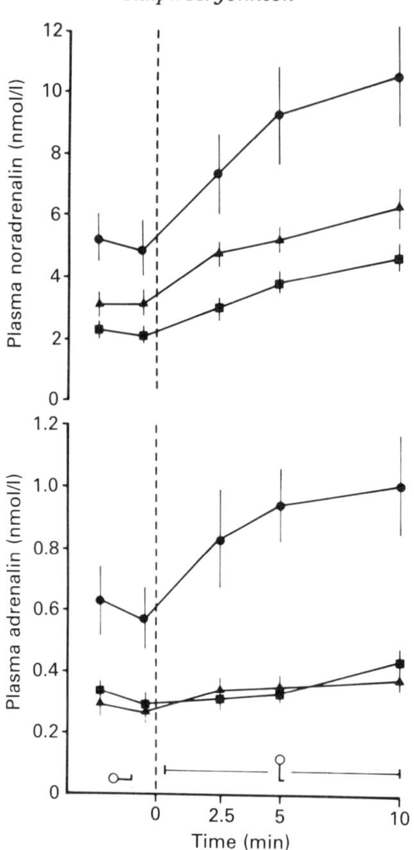

Fig. 39.2. Plasma catecholamine concentrations (mean ±SEM) in the supine position (○⊣) and in response to standing (♀) in (●) 10 withdrawing alcoholics, (▲) 10 abstinent alcoholics without orthostatic hypotension, and (■) 10 control subjects. Withdrawing alcoholics had supine and standing noradrenalin and adrenalin concentrations which were significantly ($p < 0.05$) higher than abstinent alcoholics or control subjects. Abstinent alcoholics had supine noradrenalin concentrations which were significantly ($p < 0.05$) higher than control subjects. Plasma adrenalin concentrations 10 min after standing were significantly ($p < 0.01$) higher than supine concentrations in all groups. (Taken with permission from Eisenhofer *et al.* (1985).)

appreciation of temperature change by which clothing and other features of external thermoregulation are controlled. However, human thermoregulation is so dependent on sympathetic function via the control of vasomotor tone and sweating, that any disorder affecting the sympathetic system and its major thermoregulatory control centres in the hypothalamus can put an individual at great risk of wide fluctuations in body temperature which may become dangerous for survival (Johnson and Spalding 1974). It is convenient in discussing

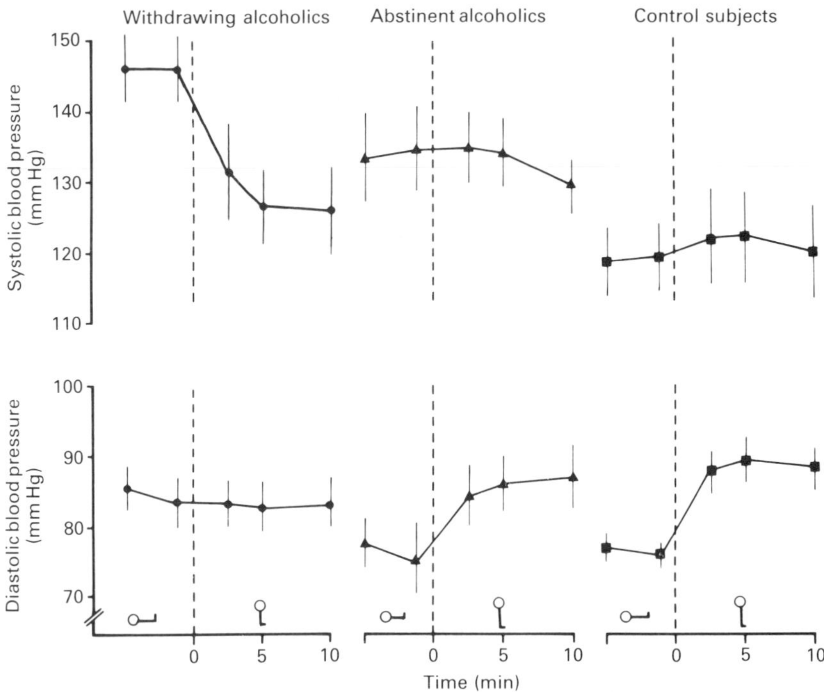

Fig. 39.3. Observations on the same subjects as in Fig. 39.2. Systolic and diastolic blood pressure (mean ±SEM) in the supine position (○⏌) and in response to standing (⚲) in (●) 10 withdrawing alcoholics, (▲) 10 abstinent alcoholics, and (■) 10 control subjects. Withdrawing alcoholics had significantly ($p > 0.02$) higher supine systolic and diastolic blood pressures than control subjects. Withdrawing alcoholics showed impaired systolic and diastolic blood-pressure responses to standing which were significantly ($p < 0.05$) different from the responses of abstinent alcoholics or control subjects even though catecholamine concentrations were higher (Fig. 39.2). (Taken with permission from Eisenhofer *et al.* (1985).)

thermoregulatory dysfunction due to alcohol to discuss, first, the risk of hypothermia occurring and, second, to describe disorders of sweating, vasoconstriction, and vasodilatation.

Liability to hypothermia

Acutely, alcohol causes peripheral vasodilatation. This may be hazardous in situations where the subject is exposed to cold, for example, when somebody becomes intoxicated to the point of impairment of their level of consciousness so that they become chilled in a cold environment. Accidental hypothermia is also common in alcoholic populations. In this group increased heat loss because of vasodilatation in the skin related to high blood alcohols will be contributory but there is also the possibility of major dysfunction of thermoregulatory controlling mechanisms in the hypothalamus. A review of patients admitted with accidental hypothermia over a 10-year period to a New York hospital indicated that by far the majority were alcoholic male 'derelicts', drunk at the time of admission, who were found by police in the street. No information was given about levels of blood alcohol (Weyman *et al.* 1974). This description, incidentally, underlines some reasons why clinical physiological research has been limited in this group: they are not always pleasant or easy to deal with and their habits make them difficult to follow up. The peripheral effects of alcohol coupled with impairment of normal thermoregulatory mechanisms due to a central depressant effect of alcohol and/or pathological damage to the hypothalamus result in inhibition of shivering and inappropriate vasodilatation of central origin. There is evidence that neuropeptides including vasopressin, are involved in the development of tolerance to the hypothermic effects of alcohol (Pittman *et al.* 1982). Vasopressin-deficient rats become very liable to develop hypothermia. Since ethanol inhibits vasopressin release (Eisenhofer and Johnson 1982), it is possible that ethanol induces suceptibility to hypothermia through reduced vasopressin concentrations.

Thermolability is particularly likely in alcoholism complicated by Wernicke's encephalopathy (Lipton *et al.* 1978). Indeed, one of Wernicke's original patients suffered from hypothermia (1881–3). The syndrome of Wernicke's encephalopathy, which is due to thiamine deficiency, consists of disturbances of consciousness and memory, abnormalities of eye movement, ataxia, and often polyneuropathy. Lack of discomfort to thermal stress may also contribute to hypothermia in patients with Wernicke's encephalopathy (Lipton *et al.* 1978). In Wernicke's encephalopathy there may be small petecheal haemorrhages occurring in the hypothalamus, the brainstem, and the corpora mammalaria (Harper 1979). In chronic alcoholism, hypothermia may therefore be a result of structural damage to the hypothalamus (Hunter 1976; Victor *et al.* 1971). Hypothermia may frequently be missed unless expressly looked for and, since Wernicke's encephalopathy responds dramatically to thiamine, it is a condition which it is important to diagnose. It has been shown that improvement in thermoregulatory functions also occurs after treatment with thiamine (Lipton *et al.* 1978) (Fig. 39.4).

Sweating

Chronic alcoholics with peripheral neuropathy may be noted to have hands and feet that are dry and the skin of their feet and legs may be hairless and shiny. Sweating loss usually has a 'glove and stocking' distribution, suggesting involvement of postganglionic sympathetic nerves. The condition appears to be common, all subjects in one series having absent or reduced distal sweating (Low *et al.* 1975). A

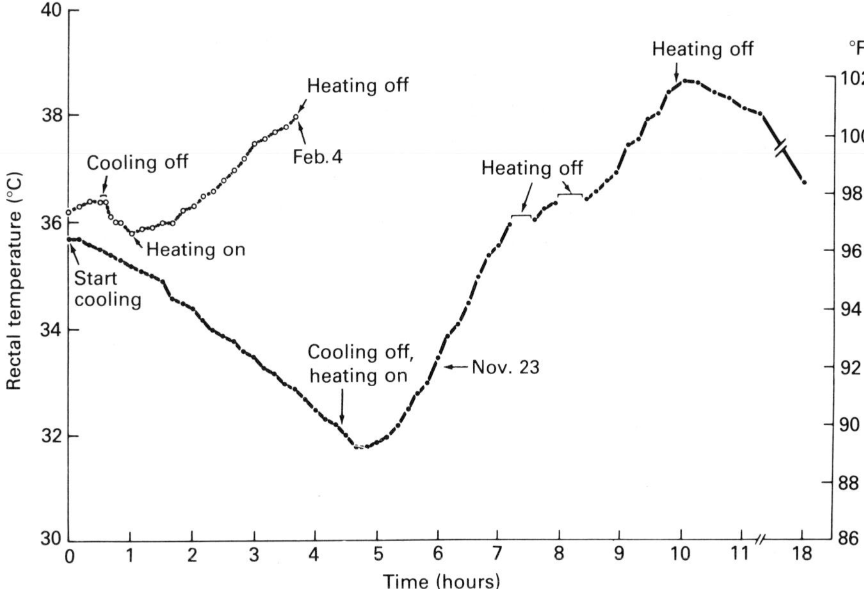

Fig. 39.4. Changes in rectal temperature in a 53-year-old alcoholic man during cooling and warming. Nov. 23: prior to treatment with thiamine. He tolerated cooling and warming easily without feeling 'too hot or too cold' and without shivering while being cooled or sweating while being warmed. Feb. 4 (73 days later): after treatment, he shivered while his skin was cooled and his rectal temperature rose. He sweated while being warmed. Both procedures were stopped because his tolerance of them was reduced compared with the first investigation. In both he was conscious and speaking throughout. (Taken with permission from Lipton *et al.* (1978).)

consequence of loss of sweating might be reduced fluid loss and thermal instability with hyperthermia being a likely complication.

Surprisingly, Zazgornik and his co-workers (1972) reported that chronic alcoholics have a higher loss of fluid during heat stress compared with control subjects. This could be due to the development of 'compensatory sweating', a phenomenon that has been observed in diabetics with partial loss of sympathetic function causing incomplete anhidrosis.

Diabetic patients sweated more profusely in those areas in which normal sweating is retained (Goodman 1966). We, therefore, studied whether alcoholics have increased or decreased susceptibility to thermal stress (Robinson *et al.* 1985). A group of alcoholics were compared with control subjects during a period of 30 minutes in a sauna. There was a marked reduction in sweat rates over the forearm in the alcoholics compared with the sweat rates in control subjects. Weight losses were significantly greater in the control subjects whereas central temperatures (oral) were higher in the alcoholic subjects (Fig. 39.5). There was, therefore, no evidence of compensatory sweating. In one of the alcoholic patients central temperature rose over $2\frac{1}{2}$°C higher than the highest temperature obtained in the control subjects. It is, therefore, apparent that alcoholics have major impairment of thermoregulation for responding to a thermal load; discomfort in hot environments and even accidental hyperthermia are therefore possible.

Vasomotor control

As already described, acute ingestion of alcohol is usually considered to have a dilatory effect on blood vessels. Generally, however, blood pressure and cardiac output remain unchanged and therefore vasodilatation in skin must be accompanied by vasoconstriction in other vascular beds. There is evidence of vasoconstriction in muscle (Fewings *et al.* 1966). This may be an active mechanism involving sympathetic nerves. The vasodilatory effect is probably related to a direct effect of alcohol on blood vessels (Johnson and Robinson 1987).

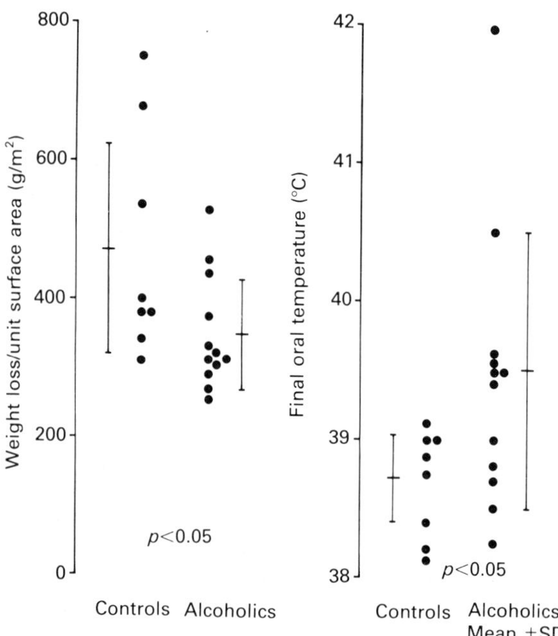

Fig. 39.5. Final weight losses (g/m^2) and oral temperatures (°C) after heat exposure in a sauna in age- and weight-matched male alcoholics (12 subjects) and controls (8 subjects). The alcoholics had significantly lower weight losses ($p < 0.05$) and significantly higher ($p < 0.05$) final oral temperatures than the control subjects. The patient with the highest temperature did not complain of any discomfort during investigation. (Taken with permission from Robinson *et al.* (1985).)

PARASYMPATHETIC NERVOUS SYSTEM FAILURE

Is parasympathetic function, through the cranial outflow (third, seventh, ninth, and tenth cranial nerves) or the sacral outflow, largely spared in chronic alcoholics as has been suggested (Low *et al.* 1975)? If there is dysfunction, can this involve an individual nerve trunk or are other parts of the parasympathetic system also likely to be affected?

Studies of vagal nerve function in chronic alcoholics are described first as these were the starting points for this series of studies in my laboratory.

Vagus nerve (tenth nerve) to the heart

Hoarseness of the voice and difficulty in swallowing are among the symptoms which may develop as a result of nervous system damage. Recognition of these clinical symptoms, now known to be due to damage to the vagus nerve, occurred in clinical accounts about 100 years ago. In 1885 a description was given in the *American Journal of Medical Science* of a man of 28 who was a severe alcoholic. In addition to developing a progressive peripheral neuropathy in the 4 months before he died, he could only speak in a whisper in the week or so prior to his death. A similar case was also described in London the same year. Dejerine was one of those who studied alcoholic pathology and in 1887 he reported studies showing abnormalities of the vagus nerve. In 1893 two patients were described who had evidence of vagal nerve damage which in one was so severe that he had 'a feeble and husky' voice. Nevertheless, it was not until 1974 that Novak and Victor, who also reviewed previous case reports, gave greater prominence to these symptoms. These authors described four patients with alcoholic neuropathy in whom dysphonia and dysphagia were prominent clinical features. They drew attention to the similarity with beriberi, in which vagus-nerve damage is well described. They considered that the voice and swallowing problems were due to varying degrees of degeneration of the vagus nerves. The degeneration was similar to that occurring in peripheral sensory and motor nerves. One of the four patients also had degeneration of nerves in sympathetic trunks and had clinical symptoms of hypothermia and hypotension due to sympathetic dysfunction. Parasympathetic dysfunction however, has not been commonly recognized in alcoholic neuropathy. A 1975 report by Low *et al.* gave details of studies of autonomic function in 12 subjects with alcoholic neuropathy. Details of sympathetic function found in this investigation have already been noted. Parasympathetic function was studied by observing heart rate at rest, during and after the Valsalva manoeuvre, and during drug infusion (phenylephrine). Although two patients had abnormal Valsalva ratios and one had a heart-rate response to raising the blood pressure which was 'well below . . . the control range', the authors concluded that 'quantitative assessment of baroreceptor function was . . . within the control range'. Pathological changes in the sympathetic nervous system were studied but no post-mortem observations were made of the vagus nerves in these patients.

It appeared that one possible explanation for the lack of clear evidence of parasympathetic failure in Low and his colleagues' study is that in their series of alcoholics there was only a minor degree of general neurological disability. It was apparent from Novak and Victor's post-mortem studies that their patients with vagus-nerve damage suffered from severe polyneuropathy. We therefore studied a group of chronic alcoholic patients with varying degrees of alcohol-related peripheral and central neurological damage. Some of the patients had severe neurological deficits (Duncan *et al.* 1980). Without reference to autonomic dysfunction, the patients were divided into two groups according to the severity of their neurological symptoms and signs. Studies were also carried out of their autonomic function. None of these alcoholics had orthostatic hypotension, but those with the greatest degree of peripheral and central nervous damage were more likely to have abnormal heart-rate responses to Valsalva manoeuvre, deep breathing, change of posture, baroreceptor stimulation by means of neck suction, and intravenous atropine. Our results, therefore, indicated that chronic damage to the vagus as a feature of alcoholic polyneuropathy, can be determined clinically, although it had largely been unrecognized previously except in the post-motem report by Novak and Victor (1974). Details of the tests of heart-rate change used in this investigation follow. A continuous electrocardiogram was taken in each test.

1. Standing. After lying for 15 minutes the subjects were rapidly tipped so that the patients stood. The 30:15 ratio was calculated as the ratio of the R–R interval at beat 30 after standing (approximate time of longest interval) to the R–R interval at beat 15 after standing (approximate time of shortest interval). The ratio was considered abnormal below 1.04.

2. Valsalva manoeuvre. This was performed with an expiratory pressure of 40 mm of water for 10 seconds and the 'Valsalva ratio' was calculated as the ratio of the longest R–R interval after the manoeuvre to the shortest R–R interval during the manoeuvre (Levin 1966). The ratio was considered abnormal below 1.50 (Fig. 39.6).

3. Deep breathing. While supine the subject breathed deeply at the rate of 6 breaths per minute and the heart-rate change with breathing was then calculated as the difference between the average maximum heart rate during deep expiration and the average minimum heart rate

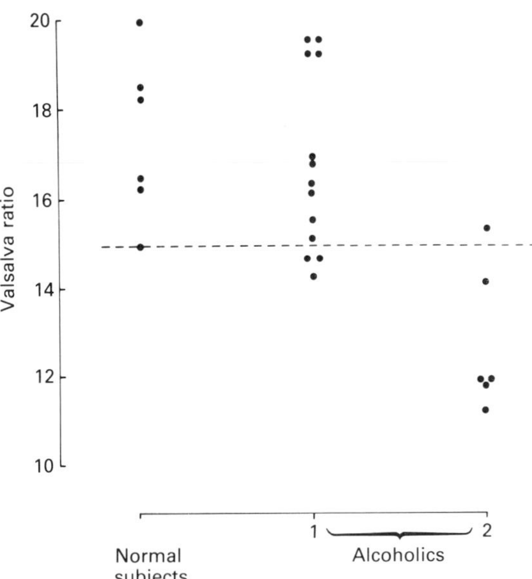

Fig. 39.6. Valsalva ratio in normal subjects and alcoholics with little or no evidence of neurological damage (group 1) and alcoholics with evidence of neurological damage (group 2). Normal range ⩾1.50. (Taken with permission from Duncan *et al.* (1980).) The greater depression in Valsalva ratio in alcoholics with neurological damage indicates that they also suffer from parasympathetic (vagal) damage.

during deep inspiration. A heart-rate increase below 15 beats/min was considered abnormal.

4. Atropine test. Atropine (1.8 mg) was administered intravenously at a rate of 0.6 mg/min with an interval of 1 min between successive 0.6 mg doses. The heart rate reached a maximum in 10–15 min and the maximum change from resting values was then calculated. An increase in heart rate below 30 beats/min was considered abnormal (Fig. 39.7).

5. Baroreceptor stimulation. Negative pressure was applied to the subject's neck using a lead cuff moulded to the neck (Eckberg *et al.* 1975). The negative pressure was applied at a suction pressure of −50 mm Hg and R–R interval was recorded throughout the procedure. An increase in R–R interval of less than 80 ms was considered abnormal (Fig. 39.8).

Other studies have subsequently confirmed that heavy drinkers may show depressed reflex heart-rate responses (Melgaard and Somnier 1981; Johnston *et al.* 1983). One study reported beat-to-beat variation of resting heart rate and the other study reported heart-rate change on taking a deep breath.

Parasympathetic dysfunction could be clinically important as vagal

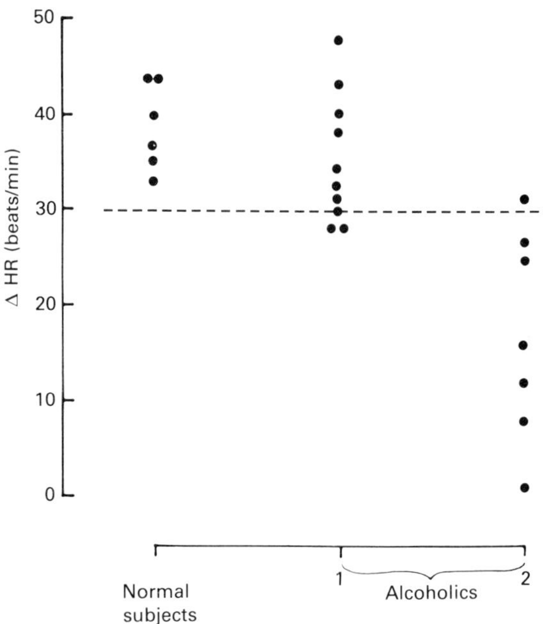

Fig. 39.7. Heart-rate response to atropine (1.8 mg i.v.) in normal subjects and group 1 (with little or no evidence of general neurological damage) and group 2 (with major evidence of neurological damage) alcoholic patients. Normal range ⩾ 30 beats/min. (Taken with permission from Duncan *et al.* (1980).) The heart-rate response to atropine is reduced in alcoholics with a greater degree of peripheral and central nervous damage suggesting that there is also chronic damage to the vagus nerve.

neuropathy may contribute to poor exercise tolerance. Patients with autonomic neuropathy due to diabetes mellitus have been found to have a smaller change in heart rate and lower tolerable workloads than controls when doing exercise (Hilsted *et al.* 1982). In general, once autonomic tests in diabetics become abnormal, they remained abnormal. Symptoms of autonomic neuropathy, particularly orthostatic hypotension, gastric symptoms, and hypoglycaemic unawareness, together with abnormal autonomic function tests, carried a poor prognosis in these patients.

The mortality in patients with diabetes mellitus with evidence of autonomic neuropathy was 44 per cent after $2\frac{1}{2}$ years and 56 per cent after 5 years (Ewing *et al.* 1980). Half of the deaths in those with abnormal tests were due to renal failure, but, in the remainder, including some in whom death was sudden or unexpected, autonomic failure could be contributory either directly or indirectly. Cerebrovascular accidents could have been due to a fall in cerebral blood flow associated with abnormal cardiovascular reflexes. The relationship of autonomic dysfunction to 'sudden' death is discussed later.

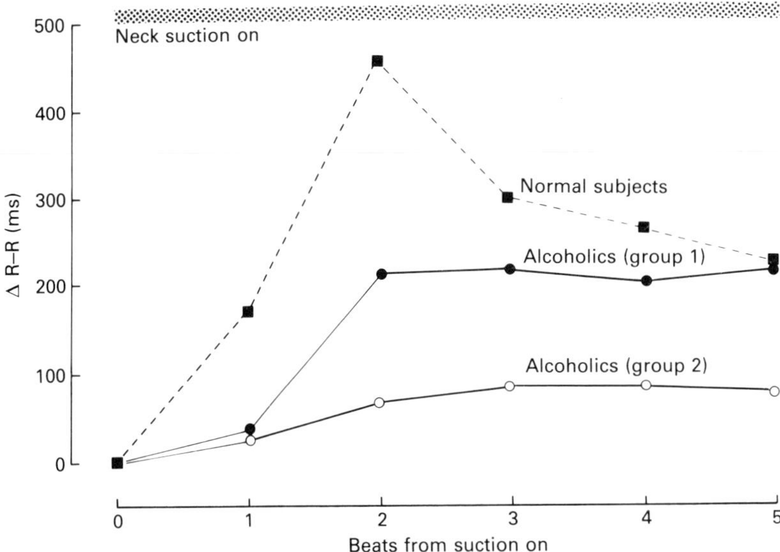

Fig. 39.8. Increases in heart rate during the first five beats after onset of neck suction. Means of results for six normal subjects, nine alcoholics with little or no evidence of neurological damage (group 1), and seven alcoholics with evidence of neurological damage (group 2). (Taken with permission from Duncan *et al.* (1980).) The depressed heart-rate response in alcoholics with neurological deficit indicates that they also suffer from parasympathetic (vagal) damage.

The situation in alcoholics might be somewhat different. Although alcoholics may show extensive evidence of a polyneuropathy they do not, in general, have orthostatic hypotension and will not, therefore, have complications related to it, as may diabetics. Alcoholism, moreover, is reversible and, therefore, particularly if patients become abstinent, the prognosis might not be as bad. We, therefore, investigated a group of alcoholic patients immediately following withdrawal before and after abstinence for 27 months. There was significant improvement in autonomic function in the total patient group and only two subjects eventually had abnormal test results compared with the original six who had had evidence of vagal neuropathy (Tan *et al.* 1984*b*). Vagal neuropathy in alcoholics may therefore be reversible with abstinence. One explanation could be improved nutrition.

In a further study we have prospectively followed alcoholics for up to 6–7 years to observe whether abnormal autonomic function is associated with an altered survival rate (Johnson and Robinson 1988). Figure 39.9 indicates that parasympathetic dysfunction in alcoholism has a highly significant association with increased mortality. Details of the major tests used are given in Table 39.1. The tests most likely to show an abnormality in borderline autonomic neuropathy were the 30:15 ratio on standing and

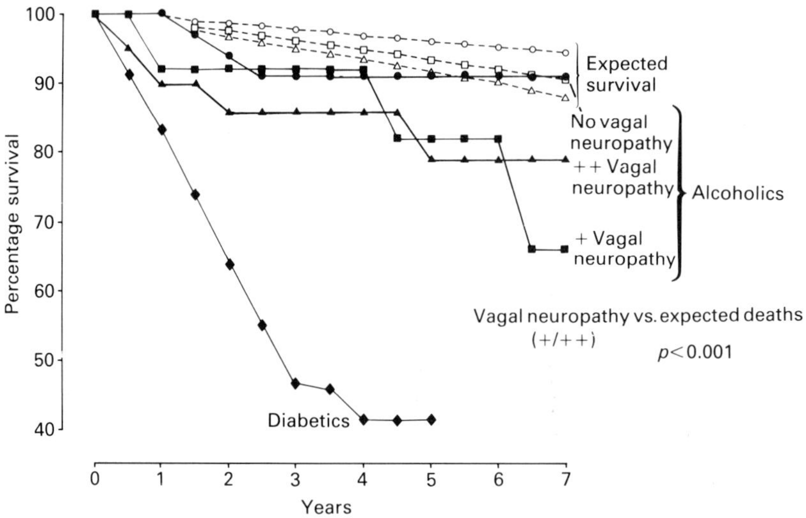

Fig. 39.9. Seven-year survival curves for alcoholics upon whom autonomic function tests were carried out. (●) 32 alcoholics had no evidence of parasympathetic neuropathy, (■) 25 alcoholics had only one abnormal test, and (▲) 22 alcoholics had two or more abnormal tests (Johnson and Robinson 1988). Expected survival curves for the general New Zealand population are shown by broken lines with age matching for each group (open symbols). Survival curves for a diabetic population with autonomic neuropathy are also shown (◆, from Ewing *et al.* 1980). The survival rate of alcoholics was significantly decreased in the patients who had evidence of parasympathetic neuropathy ($p < 0.001$).

the heart-rate response to deep breathing. There was a very marked overrepresentation beyond what would be expected in deaths from cardiovascular and respiratory causes and this was highly significant in our series. Sudden death or death from exposure were also recorded in several patients. It should be noted that prognosis is poor even if only one test result is abnormal. We have not distinguished the outcome according to whether our patients have continued to drink or become abstinent. In the latter situation, as already discussed, improvement in test results may occur (Tan *et al.* 1984*b*). The finding of such a grave prognosis with borderline results may therefore have considerable clinical significance. We have previously studied mortality in an alcoholic population in New Zealand and the death rate we have found in a large group of alcoholics was in keeping with the overall mortality rate in this study (Lambie *et al.* 1983).

Parasympathetic damage is, therefore, an indicator of a reduced chance of survival beyond 6 years. What, however, is the relationship of the autonomic failure to the death rate? Is it indirect—autonomic failure being a concomitant of widespread pathology due to alcohol or does the autonomic dysfunction have a direct causal relationship? As noted

Table 39.1. The tests of parasympathetic function used in a series of 79 alcoholics whose survival was studied prospectively (see Fig. 39.9). The most sensitive tests in patients who showed borderline results were the heart-rate changes on standing and with deep breathing. A Valsalva ratio of ⩾1.20 has been used as the lower level of normal (Ewing *et al.* 1973)

Test	*Technique*	*Measurement*	*Normal value*	*Abnormal results in alcoholics (per cent)*		
				Nil ($n = 32$)	*1 abnormal test* ($n = 25$)	*2 abnormal tests* ($n = 22$)
Standing 30:15 ratio	Rapid standing	R–R interval 30th beat after standing / R–R interval 15th beat after standing	⩾1.04	0	48	86
Valsalva ratio	Valsalva's manoeuvre for 10 s at 40 cm water pressure	Longest R–R interval after manoeuvre / Shortest R–R during manoeuvre	⩾1.20	0	8	52
Breathing—Deep breathing	Six slow breaths/min	Fast heart rate – slowest heart rate	+ 15 beats/min	0	40	91
Atropine	1.8 mg i.v. Slow infusion over 5 min with 1 min intervals between each 0.6 mg	Increase in heart rate	⩾ 30 beats/min	0	4	81

above, Ewing and his colleagues considered that up to 50 per cent of the diabetic deaths might be attributable to autonomic disorder. In alcoholics prolonged syncope and failure of cerebral perfusion leading to stroke are unlikely as orthostatic hypotension is rare. There is a possibility however, that alcoholic cardiomyopathy may be related to autonomic dysfunction. Patients with cardiomyopathy had impairment of parasympathetic function (Amorim *et al.* 1981; Amorim and Olsen 1982). Vagal neuropathy may also contribute to hyponatraemia and altered blood volumes in alcoholic cirrhosis (Decaux *et al.* 1986).

Another contributory cause of sudden death may be disordered respiration. The cause for the increase in mortality in diabetics is unknown, but the possibility exists that cardiorespiratory arrests are common. These have been reported in a series of diabetic patients and it was argued that, as there was no evidence of myocardial infarction, cardiac arrhythmia, or hypoglcyaemia and as several patients had evidence of interference with respiration, it was likely that the cardiorespiratory arrests were due to defective respiratory reflexes (Page and Watkins 1978). There is also a possibility that patients with an autonomic neuropathy may have a diminished hypoxic drive to ventilation.

Disordered breathing, with periods of apnoea probably central in origin, has been observed in subjects with autonomic neuropathy associated with multiple system atrophy with autonomic failure, or familial dysautonomia (Guilleminault *et al.* 1981). We therefore studied respiration during sleep in alcoholic patients compared with controls. The alcoholic patients had an increased number of episodes of central and of obstructive apnoea and also of hypopnoea compared with controls. There was a significant correlation between the frequency of central apnoea or hypopnoea and clinical evidence of central nervous system damage. There was also a significant association between vagal neuropathy and hypopnoea (Tan *et al.* 1985). We have also found that alcoholics who were still drinking had more episodes of apnoea when their blood alcohol levels were raised after withdrawal. This is in keeping with the observation that in normal subjects acute ingestion of alcohol increases the incidence of abnormal respiratory events (Taasen *et al.* 1981).

There are several possible explanations for the occurrence of sleep apnoea in alcoholic patients. One is that vagal neuropathy could have a role. It may be related to damage to afferent vagal fibres from the lungs interfering with respiratory reflexes during sleep. Vagal neuropathy in our studies however, has been associated with other signs of nervous system damage and, in any case, not all of the patients had a vagal neuropathy. A relationship between vagal neuropathy and all abnormal respiratory events during sleep could not be confirmed. Another explanation is that there is central nervous system damage affecting the brainstem and pons. Central nervous system damage, as already discussed, has been found pathologically in chronic alcoholics. There is, however, no evidence of altered chemosensitivity either peripherally or centrally, as an explanation of abnormal respiratory events in these patients during sleep (Lambie *et al.* 1987). Indeed, brainstem pathology could be a consequence, rather than a cause, of apnoea and hypopnoea. On the other hand, the explanation of obstructive apnoea in alcoholics could be vagal damage causing laryngeal paresis. This is consistent with the vocal and swallowing defects, which as noted initially in this section, may occur in alcoholics. The possibility of this explanation has been identified in autonomic failure due to multiple system atrophy (Guindi *et al.* 1981).

Vagus nerve (tenth nerve) to the alimentary system

Mobility may be impaired in the lower two-thirds of the oesophagus in patients who have alcoholism severe enough to cause a peripheral neuropathy (Winship *et al.* 1968). Nausea and vomiting are common complaints in chronic alcoholics and these upper gastrointestinal symptoms could be related to gastric motor dysfunction. In diabetes mellitus abnormal oesophageal and stomach motility are common and delayed stomach emptying is probably related to vagal denervation (Guy *et al.* 1984). Gastric secretion of acid, induced by insulin hypoglycaemia, is also reduced in some diabetics, suggesting vagal damage. This may explain the infrequency of duodenal ulcer in diabetics. A study has been carried out to make similar observations on gastric motility in alcoholism (Keshavarzian *et al.* 1986). There was no difference however, in the gastric emptying time of alcoholics compared with normal controls. It was suggested that the upper gastrointestinal complaints could therefore be due to chronic gastritis as this is more common in alcoholics than in non-alcoholic subjects (Atkinson and Hosking 1983). It is noteworthy, however, that in this study the patients were free of any evidence of a clinical peripheral neuropathy. Our previous observations have indicated that parasympathetic abnormalities are more common when other evidence of neurological damage is also present. This problem, together with studies of acid secretion, therefore requires further investigation in alcoholics.

In keeping, however, with normal observations about gastric motility we have observed that glucagon is not affected in alcoholics with damage to the vagus nerves innervating the heart (Tan *et al.* 1983). There is conflicting evidence about whether glucagon release is dependent upon vagus nerve function and our results may therefore be interpreted as supporting those authors who consider this nervous influence to be insignificant. It could be, however, that the nerve supply to the alpha cells of the pancreas, which secrete glucagon, is not affected in chronic alcoholics or that the vagal neuropathy is incomplete, with sufficient innervation to still allow stimulation of glucagon.

Oculomotor nerve (third nerve) to the pupil

Parasympathetic denervation hypersensitivity of the iris has been found in three-quarters of diabetics diagnosed within the preceding 2 years (Sigsbee *et al.* 1974). A study was therefore carried out to determine the sensitivity of irises in the eyes of alcoholics to metacholine (Myers *et al.* 1979). It was found that the same proportion of alcoholics and control subjects had an iris constriction of 1 mm or more. However, 60 per cent of the alcoholic patients had no evidence of peripheral neuropathy and none had orthostatic hypotension, alteration of the heart-rate response to Valsalva's manoeuvre, dysphonia, or dysphagia. In view of our finding of vagal neuropathy in alcoholics, particularly those with central or peripheral nerve damage, it appeared likely that the patients who had been studied were not as severely affected by alcohol as many available to us. We therefore repeated the investigation but, in addition, obtained a permanent photographic record by studying pupillary dilatation to 2 per cent methacholine in an ambient light using a studio flash unit with 1/60th second exposure (Tan *et al.* 1984*c*). It was then possible to measure the changes in pupillary diameter without any knowledge of the patient's condition. In addition, four of the vagal function tests previously described were carried out. Our observations indicated that resting pupillary diameters were greater in those alcoholics who had evidence of cardiac vagal neuropathy (Fig. 39.10). Their responses to methacholine were also greater than in control subjects or alcoholics without vagal neuropathy (Fig. 39.11). Our findings therefore implied that lesions occur in the parasympathetic supply to the pupil and that there is congruence of parasympathetic abnormality between the oculomotor and the vagus nerves. In some patients there is no increased sensitivity to methacholine which might be because the lesions in these patients are preganglionic. There is however, some evidence that there is no difference in the methacholine response between pre- and post-ganglionic third-nerve lesions (Ponsford *et al.* 1982). Alcoholism can also affect the pupils' response to light, there being a greater degree of constriction during light exposure in non-alcoholics than in alcoholics (Rubin *et al.* 1977).

Sacral outflow: sexual function

Erectile impotence is a common complaint in alcoholics. There are several possible abnormalities which can contribute to it with varying degrees of importance in individual patients. Endocrine dysfunction

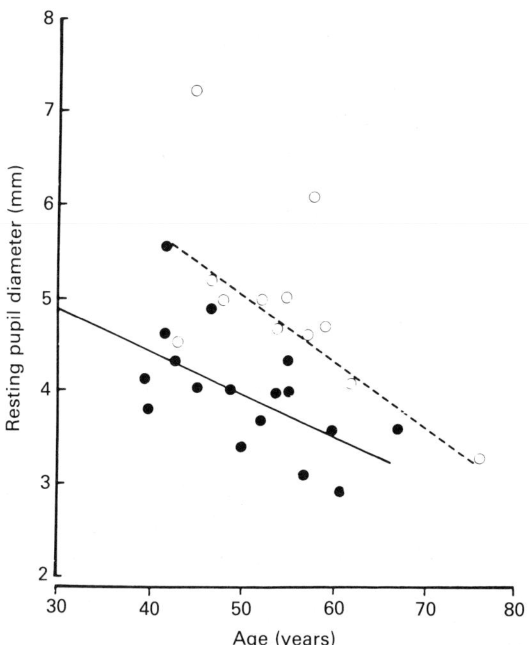

Fig. 39.10. Correlation between resting pupil size and age in chronic alcoholics: (●) group 1, without vagal neuropathy and solid line ($r=0.64$, $p<0.005$); (○) group 2, with vagal neuropathy and dashed line ($r=0.61$, $p<0.01$). (Taken with permission from Tan *et al.* (1984*c*).) The resting pupillary diameters were larger in the chronic alcoholics with vagal neuropathy suggesting that there is also a lesion in the parasympathetic supply to the pupil.

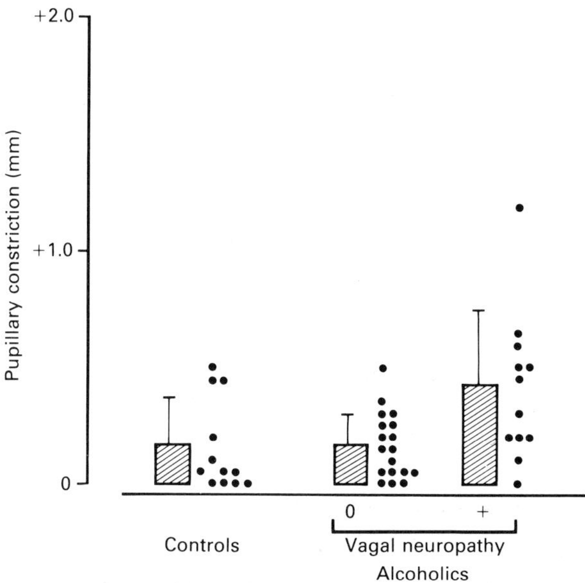

Fig. 39.11. Pupillary constriction after 2 per cent methacholine. Horizontal bars indicate mean values. Responses in alcoholics with vagal neuropathy were significantly greater than in normal controls ($p<0.05$) or in alcoholics without vagal neuropathy ($p<0.05$). (Taken with permission from Tan *et al.* (1984*c*).)

occurs in many chronic alcoholics resulting in symptoms such as hypogonadism and gynaecomastia. Feminizing hormones, including oestrogens, follicle-stimulating hormone (FSH), and luteinizing hormone (LH) are frequently raised, although testosterone levels are usually normal. Psychogenic factors could be important, and have been shown to contribute to the impotence of a large proportion of diabetics (Hosking *et al.* 1979). It has also been suggested that in some diabetics impairment of nocturnal erection is due to a neuropathy at sacral levels (Karacan 1980). We therefore examined whether impotence occurs in alcoholics in relation to widespread evidence of nervous system damage, particularly whether it is associated with dysfunction of vagal parasympathetic fibres to the heart (Tan *et al.* 1984*a*).

Half of the subjects studied had normal penile erections and their impotence was therefore pyschogenic. In the others, however, nocturnal erections were either diminished or absent. All these subjects had raised FSH and LH concentrations with the exception of one patient who had only raised FSH. They also had more evidence of neurological damage than the patients who had normal penile erection. Two of this group had evidence of parasympathetic nervous system dysfunction affecting the heart and in one of these it appeared clear that the major degree of parasympathetic damage which was found was more significant than

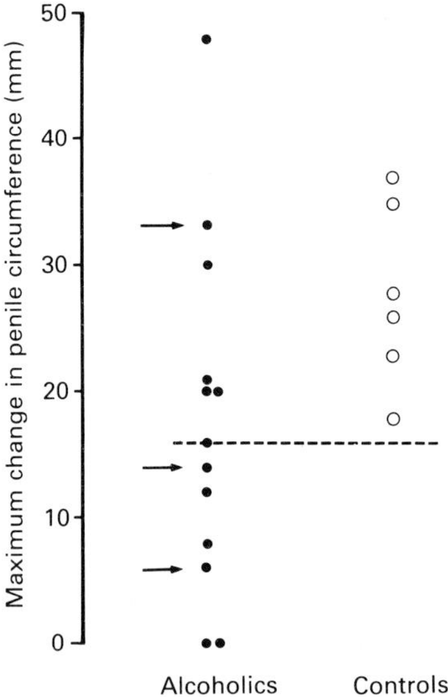

Fig. 39.12. Maximum change in penile circumference during sleep for (●) 13 alcoholic patients and (○) six age-matched controls. The probable lower limit of the normal range is shown by the interrupted line. The three patients who had vagal neuropathy are shown by the arrows. (Taken with permission from Tan *et al.* (1984*a*).)

very minor endocrine abnormalities. This presupposes that there is a degree of concordance, as was found between ocular parasympathetic dysfunction and that of the heart, between that of the sacral outflow and that of the heart. Such concordance is not however absolute as one patient with a vagal neuropathy affecting the heart had normal penile erections (Fig. 39.12).

It has already been noted that parasympathetic dysfunction of the heart may improve during long-term withdrawal from alcohol. It is, therefore, possible that organic impotence, due to dysfunction of the parasympathetic nerves in the sacral outflow subserving erection, may also improve with abstinence. It would be of value to study this in order to be able to give clear advice when counselling alcoholics about sexual function.

REFERENCES

Amorim, D. S., Dargie, H. J., Heer, K., Brown, M., Jenner, D., Olsen, E. G. J., Richardson, P., and Goodwin, J. F. (1981). Is there autonomic impairment in congestive (dilated) cardiomyopathy? *Lancet* **i**, 525–7.

Amorim, D. S. and Olsen, E. G. J. (1982). Assessment of heart neurons in dilated (congestive) cardiomyopathy. *Br. Heart J.* **47**, 11–18.

Appenzeller, O. and Ogin, G. (1974). Myelinated fibres in human paravertebral sympathetic chain: white rami communicantes in alcoholic and diabetic patients. *J. Neurol. Neurosurg. Psychiat.* **37**, 1155–61.

Appenzeller, O. and Richardson, E. P. Jr. (1966). The sympathetic chain in patients with diabetic and alcoholic polyneuropathy. *Neurology* **16**, 1205–7.

Atkinson, M. and Hosking, D. J. (1983). Gastrointestinal complications of diabetes mellitus. *Clin. Gastroenterol.* **12**, 633–50.

Barraclough, M. A. and Sharpey-Schafer, E. P. (1963). Hypotension from absent circulatory reflexes: effects of alcohol, barbiturates, psychotherapeutic drugs and other mechanisms. *Lancet* **ii**, 1121–6.

Bernardi, M., Trevisani, F., Santini, C., Ligabue, A., Capelli, M., and Gasparrini, G. (1982). Impairment of blood pressure control in patients with liver cirrhosis during tilting: study on adrenergic and renin–angiotensin systems. *Digestion* **25**, 124–30.

Decaux, G., Cauchie, P., Soupart, A., Kruger, M., and Delwiche, F. (1986). Role of vagal neuropathy in the hyponatraemia of alcoholic cirrhosis. *Br. med. J.* **293**, 1534–6.

De Marchi, S. and Cecchin, E. (1986). Are orthostatic hypotension and impaired blood pressure control common features of the alcohol withdrawal syndrome? *Clin. Sci.* **70**, 213–14.

Duncan, G., Johnson, R. H., Lambie, D. G., and Whiteside, E. A. (1980). Evidence of vagal neuropathy in chronic alcoholics. *Lancet* **ii**, 1053–7.

Eckberg, D. L., Cavanagh, M. S., Mark, A. L., and Abboud, F. M. (1975). A simplified neck suction device for activation of carotid baroreceptors. *J. lab. clin. Med.* **85**, 167–73.

Eisenhofer, G. and Johnson, R. H. (1982). Effect of ethanol ingestion on plasma vasopressin and water balance in humans. *Am. J. Physiol.* **242,** R522–R527.

Eisenhofer, G., Whiteside, E. A., and Johnson, R. H. (1985). Plasma catecholamine responses to change of posture in alcoholics during withdrawal and after continued abstinence from alcohol. *Clin. Sci.* **68,** 71–8.

Ewing, D. J., Campbell, I. W., Burt, A. A., and Clarke, B. F. (1973). Vascular reflexes in diabetic autonomic neuropathy. *Lancet* **ii,** 1354–6.

Ewing, D. J., Campbell, I. W., and Clarke, B. F. (1980). The natural history of diabetic autonomic neuropathy. *Quart. J. Med.* **49,** 95–108.

Fewings, J. D., Hanna, M. J. D., Walsh, J. A., and Whelan, R. F. (1966). The effects of ethyl alcohol on the blood vessels of the hand and forearm in man. *Br. J. Pharmacol. Chemother.* **27,** 93–106.

Goodman, J. I. (1966). Diabetic anhidrosis. *Am. J. Med.* **41,** 831–5.

Guilleminault, C., Briskin, J. G., Greenfield, M. S., and Silvestri, R. (1981). The impact of autonomic nervous system dysfunction on breathing during sleep. *Sleep* **14,** 263–78.

Guindi, G. M., Bannister, R., Gibson, W. P. R., and Payne, J. K. (1981). Laryngeal electromyography in multiple system atrophy with autonomic failure. *J. Neurol. Neurosurg. Psychiat.* **44,** 49–53.

Guy, R. J. C., Dawson, J. L., Garrett, J. R., Laws, J. W., Thomas, P. K., Sharma, A. K., and Watkins, P. J. (1984). Diabetic gastroparesis from autonomic neuropathy: surgical considerations and changes in vagus nerve morphology. *J. Neurol. Neurosurg. Psychiat.* **47,** 686–91.

Harper, C. (1979). Wernicke's encephalopathy: a more common disease than realised. *J. Neurol. Neurosurg. Psychiat.* **42,** 226–31.

Hilsted, J., Galbo, H., Christensen, N. J., Parving, H. H., and Benn, J. (1982). Haemodynamic changes during graded exercise in patients with diabetic autonomic neuropathy. *Diabetologia* **22,** 318–23.

Hosking, D. J., Bennet, T., Hampton, J. R., Evans, D. F., Clark, A. J., and Robertson, G. (1979). Diabetic impotence studies of nocturnal erection during REM sleep. *Br. med. J.* **2,** 1394–6.

Hunter, J. M. (1976). Hypothermia and Wernicke's encephalopathy. *Br. med. J.* **2,** 563–4.

Jensen, K., Andersen, K., Smith, T., Henricksen, O., and Melgaard, B. (1984). Sympathetic vasoconstrictor nerve function in alcoholic neuropathy. *Clin. Physiol.* **4,** 253–63.

Johnson, R. H., Lambie, D. G., and Eisenhofer, G. (1987). The effects of acute and chronic ingestion of ethanol on the autonomic nervous system. *Drug Alcohol Dependence* **18,** 319–28.

Johnson, R. H., Lambie, D. G., and Spalding, J. M. K. (1984). *Neurocardiology: the interrelationships between dysfunction in the nervous and cardiovascular systems.* W. B. Saunders, London.

Johnson, R. H. and Robinson, B. J. (1987). Local autonomic failure affecting a limb. *J. Neurol. Neurosurg. Psychiat.* **50,** 738–42.

Johnson, R. H. and Robinson, B. J. (1988). Mortality in alcoholics with autonomic neuropathy. *J. Neurol. Neurosurg. Psychiat.* (In press.)

Johnson, R. H. and Spalding, J. M. K. (1974). *Disorders of the autonomic nervous system.* Blackwell, Oxford.

Johnston, L. C., Patel, S., Vankineni, P., and Kramer, N. (1983). Deficient slowing of the heart among very heavy social drinkers. *J. Stud. Alcohol.* **44**, 505–14.

Karacan, I. (1980). Diagnosis of erectile impotence in diabetes mellitus. *Ann. intern. Med.* **92**, 334–7.

Keshavarzian, A., Iber, F. L., Greer, R., and Wobblelon, J. (1986). Gastric emptying of solid meal in male chronic alcoholics. *Alcoholism* **10**, 432–5.

Lambie, D. G., Tan, E. T. H., and Johnson, R. H. (1987). Respiratory responsiveness in alcoholic patients after withdrawal. *Alcoholism* **11**, 49–51.

Lambie, D. G., Whiteside, E. A., Bell, J., and Johnson, R. H. (1983). Mortality associated with alcoholism in New Zealand. *NZ med. J.* **96**, 199–202.

Levin, A. B. (1966). A simple test of cardiac function based upon the heart rate changes induced by the Valsalva manoeuvre. *Am. J. Cardiol.* **18**, 90–9.

Lipton, J. M., Payne, H., Garza, H. R., and Rosenberg, R. N. (1978). Thermolability in Wernicke's encephalopathy. *Arch. Neurol.* **35**, 750–3.

Low, P. A., Walsh, J. C., Huang, C. Y., and McLeod, J. G. (1975). The sympathetic nervous system in alcoholic neuropathy: a clinical and pathological study. *Brain* **98**, 357–64.

Melgaard, B. and Somnier, F. (1981). Cardiac neuropathy in chronic alcoholics. *Clin. Neurol. Neurosurg.* **83–4**, 219–24.

Myers, W., Willis, K., and Reeves, A. (1979). Absence of parasympathetic denervation of the iris in alcoholics. *J. Neurol. Neurosurg. Psychiat.* **42**, 1018–19.

Novak, D. J. and Victor, M. (1974). The vagus and sympathetic nerves in alcoholic polyneuropathy. *Arch. Neurol.* **30**, 273–84.

Page, M. McB. and Watkins, P. J. (1978). Cardiorespiratory arrest and diabetic autonomic neuropathy. *Lancet* **i**, 14–16.

Pittman, Q. J., Rogers, J., and Bloom, F. E. (1982). Arginine vasopressin deficient Brattleboro rats fail to develop tolerance to the hypothermic effects of alcohol. *Regulatory Peptides* **4**, 33–41.

Ponsford, J. R., Bannister, R., and Paul, E. A. (1982). Methacholine pupillary responses in third nerve palsy and Adie's syndrome. *Brain* **105**, 583–97.

Potter, J. F. and Beevers, D. G. (1984). Pressor effect of alcohol in hypertension. *Lancet* **i**, 119–22.

Robinson, B. J., Johnson, R. H., Lambie, D. G., and Whiteside, E. A. (1985). Thermoregulatory responses in alcoholism. *Austral. Alcohol Drug Rev.* **4**, 157–9.

Rubin, L. S., Gottheil, E., Roberts, A., Alterman, A. I., and Holstine, J. (1977). Effect of stress on autonomic reactivity in alcoholics pupillometric studies. *J. Stud. Alcohol.* **38**, 2036–48.

Sigsbee, B., Torkeson, R., Kadis, G., Wright, J. W., and Reeves, A. G. (1974). Parasympathetic denervation of the iris in diabetes mellitus. *J. Neurol. Neurosurg. Psychiat.* **37**, 1031–4.

Taasan, V. C., Block, A. J., Boysen, P. G., and Wynne, J. W. (1981). Alcohol increases sleep apnea and oxygen desaturation in asymptomatic men. *Am. J. Med.* **71**, 240–5.

Tan, E. T. H., Johnson, R. H., Lambie, D. G., Vijayasenan, M. E., and Whiteside, E. A. (1984*a*). Erectile impotence in chronic alcoholics. *Alcoholism* **8**, 297–301.

Tan, E. T. H., Johnson, R. H., Lambie, D. G., and Whiteside, E. A. (1984*b*). Alcoholic vagal neuropathy: recovery following prolonged abstinence. *J. Neurol. Neurosurg. Psychiat.* **47**, 1335–7.

Tan, E. T. H., Lambie, D. G., Johnson, R. H., Robinson, B. J., and Whiteside, E. A.

(1985). Sleep apnoea in alcoholic patients after withdrawal. *Clin. Sci.* **69**, 655–61.

Tan, E. T. H., Lambie, D. G., Johnson, R. H., and Whiteside, E. A. (1983). Release of glucagon in male alcoholics with vagal neuropathy. *Alcoholism* **7**, 416–19.

Tan, E. T. H., Lambie, D. G., Johnson, R. H., and Whiteside, E. A. (1984*c*). Parasympathetic denervation of the iris in alcoholics with vagal neuropathy. *J. Neurol. Neurosurg. Psychiat.* **47**, 61–4.

Victor, M., Adams, R. D., and Collins, G. H. (1971). *The Wernicke–Kersakoff syndrome.* Blackwell, Oxford.

Wernicke, C. (1881–3). *Lehrbuch der Gehirnkrankheiter für Aertze und Studierende*, Vol. 2, p. 229. Fisher, Berlin.

Weyman, A. E., Greenbaum, D. M., and Grace, W. J. (1974). Accidental hypothermia in an alcoholic population. *Am. J. Med.* **56**, 13–21.

Winship, D. H., Caflisch, C. R., Zboralske, F. F., and Hogan, W. J. (1968). Deterioration of oesophageal peristalsis in patients with alcoholic neuropathy. *Gastroenterology* **55**, 173–8.

Zazgornik, J., Irsigler, K., Kline, E., and Kryspin-Exner, K. (1972). The eccrine sweat-gland function of chronic alcoholics. *Nutrition Metab.* **14**, 307–12.

40. Autonomic neuropathy in porphyria

Abel Gorchein

INTRODUCTION

The acute hepatic porphyrias are rare hereditary disorders of haem synthesis characterized principally by acute attacks of abdominal pain, autonomic dysfunction, motor neuropathy, and neuropsychiatric manifestations. The most severe attacks may progress rapidly to quadriplegia with bulbar and respiratory paralysis while some individuals may have only abdominal pain recurring over many years. The severity of the pain often simulates an abdominal emergency. A recent comprehensive review is that by Kappas *et al.* (1983). In each of the acute porphyrias, acute intermittent porphyria (AIP), variegate porphyria (VP), and hereditary coproporphyria (HC), deficiency of a single enzyme of the haem biosynthetic pathway is inherited as an autosomal dominant characteristic (Fig. 40.1).

The activity of the first, and normally rate-limiting enzyme of the haem pathway, δ-aminolaevulinate synthetase (ALA-S) undergoes a compensatory increase, and in attacks, precursors up to the particular enzyme 'block' are produced in increased amounts. Thus in all these conditions δ-aminolaevulinic acid (ALA) and porphobilinogen (PBG) are both excreted in increased amounts in the urine. In addition, in HC and VP, coproporphyrin and protoporphyrin are increased and may cause cutaneous photosensitivity. A more recently described and extremely rare acute porphyria is due to deficiency of ALA-dehydratase (PBG-synthetase). It has similar clinical manifestations to AIP and has an excess of ALA in the urine, but not of PBG. Other disorders of porphyrin metabolism (Fig. 40.1) are not associated with excessive excretion of ALA and PGB, and do not have neurological manifestations.

The levels of ALA and PBG are much increased during attacks, but the precise relationship of the disturbance in the haem pathway and the excessive production of these precursors to the development of neurological manifestations is unclear. Even the most severely affected

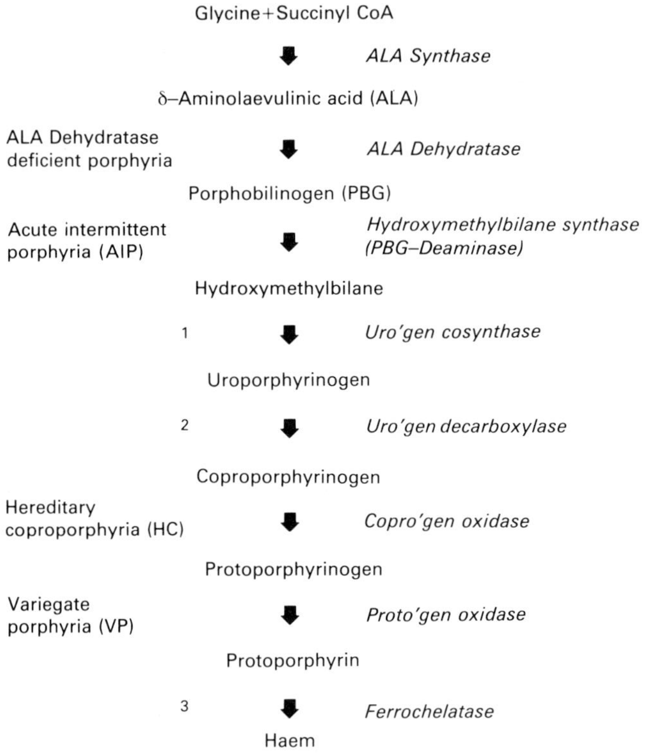

Porphyria	Pathway	Enzyme
	Glycine+Succinyl CoA	
	↓	*ALA Synthase*
	δ–Aminolaevulinic acid (ALA)	
ALA Dehydratase deficient porphyria	↓	*ALA Dehydratase*
	Porphobilinogen (PBG)	
Acute intermittent porphyria (AIP)	↓	*Hydroxymethylbilane synthase (PBG–Deaminase)*
	Hydroxymethylbilane	
1	↓	*Uro'gen cosynthase*
	Uroporphyrinogen	
2	↓	*Uro'gen decarboxylase*
	Coproporphyrinogen	
Hereditary coproporphyria (HC)	↓	*Copro'gen oxidase*
	Protoporphyrinogen	
Variegate porphyria (VP)	↓	*Proto'gen oxidase*
	Protoporphyrin	
3	↓	*Ferrochelatase*
	Haem	

Fig. 40.1. The haem biosynthetic pathway. The acute porphyrias are listed on the left with their enzyme deficiency on the right. The 'non-acute' porphyrias are indicated by numbers opposite their corresponding enzyme defects. 1. Congenital porphyria. 2. Cutaneous hepatic porphyria (porphyria cutanea tarda). 3. Erythropoeitic protoporphyria.

individuals may, however, with appropriate management recover from seemingly catastrophic neurological deficit.

NEUROPATHOLOGY

Nearly all the clinical manifestations of acute intermittent porphyria can be attributed to widespread neurological dysfunction (Goldberg 1959). Peripheral neuropathy has been studied in some detail and a brief account of the results will be given since these are likely to be relevant to the pathology of the autonomic nervous system, which can only rarely be subjected to electrodiagnostic investigation. It is now generally agreed that peripheral neuropathy is due to a primary axonal disorder which may be followed by 'dying-back' degeneration, and secondary demyelination. Motor fibres are principally affected with definite but lesser sensory changes. The pattern of involvement does not preferentially involve the longest fibres, so that proximal muscle weakness may in fact precede more distal involvement. The reasons for this distribution are not clear, but the larger size of the motor units of the proximal muscles has been suggested as a factor increasing their vulnerability to a possible metabolic derangement. These earlier conclusions, summarized by Ridley (1969), have generally been supported by electrodiagnostic studies (see Bonkowski and Schady 1982 for a review) and by more recent histopathological studies (Thorner *et al.* 1981; Yamada *et al.* 1984). Thus nerve conduction velocities are not slowed to the levels observed in demyelinating lesions and unmyelinated, as well as myelinated fibres, were found to show morphological features of axonopathy.

Electromyography supports histological observations of extensive degeneration of motor fibres within affected skeletal muscle with the general demonstration of spontaneous fibrillation, poor recruitment of motor unit action potentials, and polyphasia and giant units. These changes indicate distal axonal degeneration and reinnervation by collateral sprouting.

A feature commented on by a number of authors is the non-synchronous nature of the nerve lesions apparent from both post-mortem and electromyographic studies. Regenerating nerve fibres together with areas of dying-back degeneration can be detected, consistent with recurrent exacerbations and remissions of attacks.

In addition, Mustajoki and Seppalainen (1975) found slowing of nerve conduction velocities of the slower motor fibres of the ulnar nerve and slower sensory conduction of ulnar and median nerves in latent porphyrics (genetic carriers with no clinical attacks), which would indicate ‘subclinical’ neuropathy.

AUTONOMIC NEUROPATHY

A number of the most prominent clinical features of the acute porphyrias (Table 40.1) can be attributed to autonomic neuropathy with effects on the gastrointestinal system, and on cardiovascular function. Other manifestations include disorders of sweating and loss of sphincter control.

The high incidence of some of these manifestations, particularly abdominal pain and tachycardia, may indicate a particular susceptibility of the autonomic nerves to disturbed function in porphyria (Goldberg 1959; Ridley *et al.* 1968). Thus, abdominal pain and tachycardia almost invariably precede muscle weakness due to somatic nerve dysfunction and may be the only clinical abnormalities in some attacks. Autonomic dysfunction can recover and the cessation of tachycardia has been

Table 40.1. Clinical features of acute porphyria attributable to autonomic neuropathy

Gastrointestinal	Abdominal pain Nausea, vomiting Constipation Diarrhoea (rare)
Cardiovascular	Sinus tachycardia Hypertension Hypotension (rarer)
Others	Disorders of sweating: hyperhydrosis, patchy anhydrosis Bladder sphincter disturbance: retention of urine

considered an early indication of remission (Waldenström 1957; Ridley *et al.* 1968).

Fewer studies are available of the pathology of autonomic nerve tissue in porphyria compared with somatic nerves, but these strongly support the belief that extensive involvement of the autonomic nervous system is the basis for clinical disease. Thus lesions of the vagus, including axonal degeneration and demyelination, and chromatolysis of dorsal nuclei, and of the sympathetic chain, have been reported (Gibson and Goldberg 1956; Yamada *et al.* 1984), and also chromatolysis and diverse abnormalities in splanchnic motor cells of the lateral horns, and in cells of the coeliac ganglion.

Despite these findings, specific and objective clinical evidence of autonomic nerve dysfunction is often lacking, particularly in relation to abdominal pain. Clinical studies of cardiovascular autonomic function and of gastrointestinal motility have more recently been applied, however, and may eventually provide a fuller understanding of the autonomic disturbances in porphyria. These studies will now be reviewed in the context of the earlier observations.

GASTROINTESTINAL TRACT

Early observations radiologically and at laparotomy supported the belief that the abdominal pain of the porphyric attack was due to incoordinated contractions and dilatation of bowel segments (Berlin and Cotton 1950). The severe vomiting, constipation, or diarrhoea could thus also be accounted for. Precise information about the pathophysiology of the gut in this condition has, however, remained fragmentary despite increasing interest in the study of motor activity as an index of control mechanisms (e.g. Wingate 1981), and relationships between the enteric nervous system and the large number of regulatory peptides in both gut mucosa and enteric nerves.

Studies on gastrointestinal motility and circulating gut peptides

Proximal gastrointestinal motility was studied in three patients with acute intermittent porphyria, and levels of circulating gut peptides were also measured (Gorchein *et al.* 1982; and unpublished results). Patients 1 and 2 both had severe paralytic manifestations, requiring assisted ventilation and intensive care and were studied for periods of up to 72 h using a triple-lumen perfused tube system with attached transducers.

Patient 1 was the most severely affected and was studied twice. At the time of the first study he had required total parenteral nutrition for 7 months. A number of attempts to provide nutrition through a naso-gastric tube had failed because of apparent lack of absorption of even isotonic solutions of nutrients, which resulted in haemoconcentration, hypotension, abdominal distention, and diarrhoea. He thus appeared to have 'total gut failure'. Clinical evidence of improvement of somatic neurological function, as well as an increase in bowel sounds and the ability to occasionally eat and retain small meals prompted the second study 2 months after the first.

In patient 2 nutrition was maintained by continuous infusion of *Isocal* and carbohydrate supplements through a fine-bore nasogastric tube. Attacks of abdominal pain requiring pethidine for their alleviation continued but with decreasing frequency and spontaneous respiration returned after 3 months. Restoration of other peripheral neurological function continued steadily, but after 6 months nasogastric-tube feeding was still required to supplement the oral intake.

Patient 3 had suffered from abdominal pain and AIP-related psychiatric disorder for at least 10 years but had never had any paresis. He was studied using two ingested tethered pressure-sensitive radio-telemetric capsules.

Patterns of abnormal motility

All the studies showed deviations from the pattern of periodic fasting activity found in healthy controls.

Patient 1. The first study showed no motor activity in either antrum or small intestine for the first 90 min. Then strong antral contractions at a frequency of 3/min were observed which continued for the subsequent 55 h, after which the frequency of antral contractions varied between 3/min, and a tachygastric rhythm of 10/min. The duodenum appeared to be completely atonic throughout. Neither the gastric contractions nor duodenal atony were modified by oral beef broth, perfusion of the duodenum with nutrient solution, or even intraluminal instillation of neostigmine. In the second study carried out 2 months later, no evidence of gastric motor activity was seen but in contrast, bursts of propagated motor activity indistinguishable from normal migrating complexes (MCs) occurred throughout the study, and their frequency was increased compared with those in healthy controls (Table 40.2). Oral feeding did not induce the characteristic postprandial response, which is replacement of the fasted pattern with irregular contractile activity, and did not lengthen the inter-MC interval. The response to a small dose (0.5 mg) of locally instilled neostigmine was now marked, with the onset of borborygmi and contractile activity.

Table 40.2. Incidence of motor complexes during fasting

Patient number	1	1	2	3	Controls*
Study number	1	2	3	4	—
Study time (h)	72	60	24	48	—
Number of MCs	0	70	12	57	—
Number of intervals	0	66	7	51	193
Intervals (min)					
(1) Range	—	9/135	30/308	24/96	10/380
(2) Mean	—	48	56	49	110
(3) Median	—	42	51	42	90

* Thompson *et al.* (1980).

Patient 2 showed a median inter-MC interval during fasting reduced by nearly half when compared to healthy controls (Table 40.2). Feeding either orally or enterically resulted in only incomplete inhibition of periodic activity, the overall median interval remaining similar to that of (fasting) healthy controls, although the patient was fed for more than half the study. In addition, prolonged and vigorous irregular contractile activity was found in the jejunum but not in the antrum. No clear correlation of these events was found with episodes of abdominal pain and borborygmi.

Patient 3 had frequent MC-like episodes which appeared to suppress after a meal, but returned relatively rapidly. Several episodes of abdominal pain occurred during the study but did not correlate with the records of motility.

Peptides

In patient 1 no detectable motilin immunoreactivity was demonstrable at the time he had 'total gut failure'. Subsequently, the level of motilin came within the normal range (Table 40.3), coincident with the return of periodic activity. The values of other peptides studied in this patient, and in the two others (Table 40.3) did not provide evidence of definable abnormalities.

The disturbed period of fasting motor activity found in all three

Table 40.3. Plasma peptide levels in acute intermittent porphyria

Patient	*Date of sample*		*Level (pmol/l)*				
			Motilin	*VIP*	*PP*	*Gastrin*	*Glucagon*
1	5.1.81	1400	ND	2	212	11	17
	15.1.81	0900	ND	2	200	27	5
	29.1.81	0935*	ND	2	350	31	22
	19.3.81	1000	22	8	240	6	22
	27.3.81	1000*	29	8	410	6	35
	30.3.81	0900*	24	14	300	5	5
2	14.4.81	0930	39	8	30	10	87
	28.4.81	1000	88	3	30	12	21
	23.6.81	0930*	140	3	119	72	16
3	17.11.81	0850	7	2	18	8	5
	17.11.81	0910*	44	2	94	25	11
Normal values			3–300	2–21	10–200	2–30	5–40

* Postprandial samples.
ND, not detected.

patients, with the MCs more closely spaced, had not previously been described in man, but is similar to the pattern induced in dogs in which segments of small intestine have been subjected to various degrees of denervation (Sarr and Kelly 1981). In addition, in three out of the four studies, there was impairment of the normal response to food.

From the clinical state at the time of the first study in patient 1, it seems clear that nerve damage was then maximal. The findings could therefore be accounted for in the following way: (1) the continual activity of the distal stomach suggests that the fundamental gastric motor activity is myogenic, but normally suppressed and modulated into a pattern by extrinsic and humoral factors; (2) the complete duodenal atony suggests that, in contrast to the stomach, intestinal motor activity required neural activation; (3) the lack of response of the duodenum to neostigmine suggested that the damage also extended to involve the enteric nervous system. Support for these interpretations was provided by the results of the second study, when returning neural control suppressed automatic gastric motor activity and reimposed some periodic motor activity in the small intestine although at an abnormal frequency.

The complete absence of plasma motilin immunoreactivity in a human subject was also a novel finding. The association of MCs with plasma motilin is well established and it is generally considered that motilin exerts its effects after release from mucosal endocrine cells in response to chemical stimulation. Study 1 suggests that release of motilin may in fact depend on neural integrity. Some neural control returned between the two studies. The relatively normal concentrations of the other peptides, however, suggests that AIP does not impair the release of gut mucosal peptides as a general phenomenon. The unique observation of total lack of motilin spanning a period of about 4 weeks during which there was no periodic activity (Patient 1, Study 1), supports its role in the initiation, but not in the timing of MCs, since no such abnormalities of motilin levels were found in the other studies, where increased frequency of MCs was observed.

The interpretation of the studies on individual very-ill patients raises difficulties in terms of the specificity of the observations in relation to the porphyria. It is, however, notable that patient 1 acted to some extent as his own control in terms of severe debility, intermittent positive-pressure respiration, and total parenteral nutrition between the two studies and it is on this common background that the differences were found. Additionally, patient 3 was ambulant, not debilitated, and not receiving total parenteral nutrition, but he also showed the reduced MC interval pattern and abnormal suppression by feeding. It seems reasonable to conclude that AIP induces a characteristic disturbance of gut motor activity, that this is due to autonomic and/or enteric nerve damage, and that this damage can recover.

Relation of gut motility to abdominal pain

Neither in the least severely affected subject (patient 3), who had no somatic paralysis but complained of recurrent severe abdominal pain, nor in the more severely affected patient 2, was it possible to correlate exacerbations of abdominal pain with episodic increase in upper gut motility. It is possible that the pain originated from a site in the gut not probed by the pressure transducers; alternatively, it may be that pain is not principally related to gut motility. Autonomic disturbance of the gall bladder and bile ducts, pancreatic ducts, or ureters could be responsible by mechanisms analogous to those postulated for the gastrointestinal tract. There is no evidence that the pain results from direct pharmacological effects of haem precursors on gut or vascular smooth muscle. Wehrmacher (1952) reported relief of pain after sympathetic blockade by drugs acting at ganglia or adrenergic nerve endings, or by procaine-induced splanchnic block. Pain relief by chlorpromazine (Melby *et al.* 1956) was also attributed to its adrenolytic effect. These observations support the role of the autonomic nervous system in the generation of pain, but give no indication of a particular mechanism. The cause of the abdominal pain cannot therefore be considered to be understood.

CARDIOVASCULAR SYSTEM

Tachycardia

Already referred to as a prominent early sign of the porphyric attack, sinus tachycardia is generally attributed to autonomic cardioneuropathy

(Ridley *et al.* 1968). Vagal damage would allow unopposed action of the sympathetic cardioaccelerator nerves.

Tests of autonomic function

More recently, non-invasive and simple bedside tests, originally developed and applied for assessment of autonomic function in diabetes (see Chapter 38), have been used in subjects with acute porphyrias in attempts to obtain a more precise assessment of their autonomic function. These have included determination of the Valsalva 'ratio' of the longest R–R interval, after the manoeuvre, to the shortest during its performance, the immediate response of the heart rate to standing (30:15 ratio), and the beat-to-beat heart-rate variation during deep breathing, to test parasympathetic function. The extent of elevation of blood pressure by isometric exercise (sustained handgrip) has been used as a test of sympathetic function. Detection of postural hypotension indicates damage to the baroreflex arc, but does not indicate its site.

Patients in acute attacks

In patients tested during acute attacks it has generally been possible to demonstrate objective abnormalities, consistent with their clinical presentation. Thus Stewart and Hensley (1981) reported a patient in an acute attack of variegate porphyria who presented with abdominal pain and aching legs and 4 days later developed a fixed tachycardia and severe postural hypotension 'to the point of syncope'. She was found to have no reflex bradycardia following the Valsalva manoeuvre (ratio was 1.0), and the heart period range and mean gain values were consistent with impaired baroreceptor function. There was no evidence of denervation hypersensitivity to phenylephrine. The pain improved and no clinical features of autonomic neuropathy remained after 14 days, but it is not stated whether the autonomic function tests had also returned to normal.

Using the immediate heart-rate response to standing (30:15 ratio), Gupta *et al.* (1983*a*) found all seven of their patients with AIP in attack to be abnormal, consistent with the clinical finding of tachycardia in all, and hypertension in six. The Valsalva ratio was, however, abnormal in only five of these (Gupta *et al.* 1983*b*). These results were confirmed and extended by Yeung Laiwah *et al.* (1985) in a group of eight patients with AIP in attacks who were found to have abnormal beat-to-beat variation in heart rate in response to deep breathing, in addition to abnormal Valsalva ratio and immediate heart-rate response to standing (30:15 ratio). These patients also had a grossly impaired rise in blood pressure following a modified sustained handgrip test. The greatest differences from the normal were with the 30:15 ratio and the blood-pressure response to sustained handgrip. Despite these abnormalities, however, the patients could not be shown to have significant postural hypotension. Six of these eight patients were retested during remission, at least 6 months later, when the tests showed a marked improvement.

Subjects in remission and with latent porphyria

Application of these tests to porphyric patients in remission (subjects with at least one previous attack but with no current acute symptoms) and with latent porphyria (genetic carriers with no clinical attacks) provided less consistent results. Thus, while each group of workers could demonstrate abnormalities in their asymptomatic or latent subjects with either the test of immediate heart-rate response to standing (30:15 ratio; Gupta *et al.* 1983*a*) or the Valsalva ratio (Yeung Laiwah *et al.* 1985), neither could demonstrate abnormalities with both tests. In addition, the magnitude of the differences from normal were generally very small with very few subjects unequivocally abnormal and nearly all in the 'overlap' range with the controls (Fig. 40.2).

Further experience with these types of tests may clarify this matter,

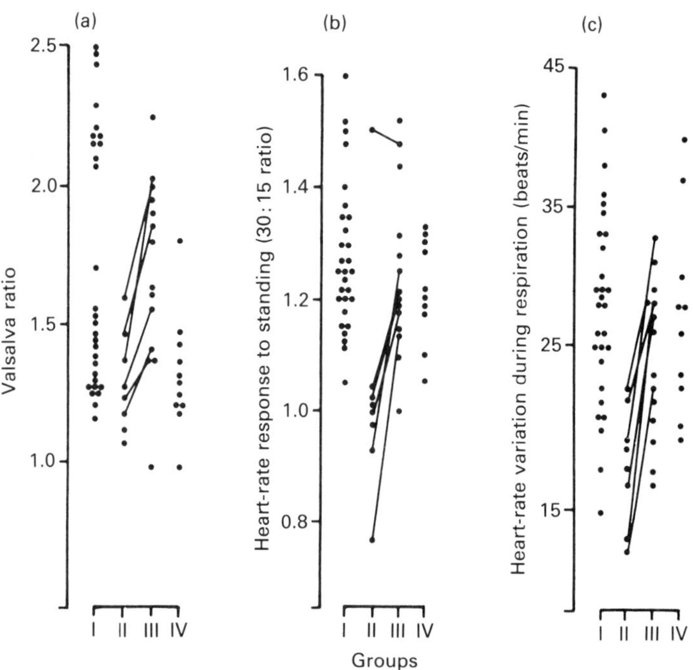

Fig. 40.2. Results of (a) Valsalva manoeuvre; (b) 30:15 ratio; and (c) heart-rate variation during respiration in different groups: (I) young normal subjects; (II) acute intermittent porphyria in acute attack; (III) acute intermittent porphyria in remission; and (IV) latent acute intermittent porphyria. Each line represents individual patients tested during an acute attack and during remission. (Taken with permission from Yeung Laiwah *et al.* (1985).)

but it would seem from the results available so far that these essentially 'clinical' tests may not be sufficiently sensitive to detect physiological abnormalities in porphyrics who are not in acute attacks.

Thus it seems highly likely, but is not unequivocally established, that subclinical autonomic neuropathy occurs in latent porphyrics, in addition to the abnormalities previously reported in their somatic peripheral nervous system (Mustajoki and Seppalainen 1975).

The demonstration of neurological defects in latent porphyrics has important implications in relation to aetiological factors. Unequivocal demonstration of neuropathy, with normal levels of ALA and PBG, would strongly favour the view that these metabolites are not directly involved as neurotoxic agents.

Hypertension

During porphyric attacks, hypertension is commonly found, but orthostatic hypotension has also been described (Shirger *et al.* 1962; Stewart and Hensley 1981). A likely mechanism for the hypertension is 'deafferentation' of carotid and aortic baroceptors by damage to the glossopharyngeal and vagus nerves, their nuclei, or central connections. Such lesions interrupt the normally continuous inhibitory control on the medullary vasomotor centres and lead to activation of the sympathetic outflow. The central connections of the baroceptor reflex are now well described (e.g. Palkovits 1980). This mechanism has long been proposed to explain hypertension in acute poliomyelitis and the Guillain–Barré syndrome. It is supported, in porphyria specifically, by the post-mortem demonstration of damage to the vagus and glossopharyngeal nerves (Baker and Watson 1945; Gibson and Goldberg 1956), and by a detailed study of a patient developing an acute attack of porphyria (Kezdi 1954). In the presence of hypertension and tachycardia, digital pressure on the carotid sinus failed to decrease the pulse rate or lower the blood pressure, and blocking the carotid-sinus nerve by local injection of procaine did not lead to their further elevation. As the patient's symptoms of glossopharyngeal and vagal paralysis improved, the blood pressure decreased, and there was also a return of responsiveness of the carotid sinus to digital pressure which now caused a slowing of the pulse.

Increased urinary excretion of catecholamines has been reported in acute attacks of porphyria with hypertension by Schley *et al.* (1970*b*) and confirmed by others. The levels reached may be of the order found in phaeochromocytoma. It seems likely that this also reflects the increased peripheral sympathetic activity brought about by reduced afferent input. Similar elevations of catecholamines have been reported in Guillain–Barré polyneuritis (e.g. Ventura *et al.* 1986). Beal *et al.* (1977) found that ALA and PBG inhibited uptake of catecholamines by platelets from six porphyric subjects (three in remission and three latent) but not from normal controls, and suggested that this could in part explain the raised catecholamine levels in the porphyric attack. Their proposal that the basis of their findings was a fundamental difference in membrane receptors or uptake systems of porphyric as opposed to normal subjects does not appear to have been extended.

Chronic hypertension and renal function in porphyria

Although the hypertension commonly found during acute attacks generally subsides in remission, it is now clear that AIP additionally predisposes to chronic hypertension. In a study extending over 20 years, Beattie and Goldberg (1976) found that about half the survivors of 38 patients who had had an acute attack of porphyria in early adulthood had diastolic pressures exceeding 100 mm Hg, and of the six deaths, four were due to hypertension-related causes. A highly significant association was also reported (Yeung Laiwah *et al.* 1983) between AIP and 'early-onset' (before age 65) chronic renal failure. Thus in a retrospective survey of 65 patients with AIP in remission, six were found with chronic renal failure due to end-stage renal disease and associated hypertension. Information is not available, however, on the aetiological relationship between the development of hypertension and renal failure since, at the time sustained hypertension was diagnosed, their patients already had established renal damage. In the absence of evidence for any other causes they concluded that porphyria-induced hypertension was the most important factor in the aetiology of the chronic renal failure, and this was supported by the finding that renal function in their two living patients remained stable following control of their blood pressure.

It is, however, well recognized also (Stein and Tschudy 1970; Schley *et al.* 1970*a*,*b*) that renal functional impairment occurs during porphyric attacks. Its nature is not well-defined and interpretation may be complicated by the presence of prerenal factors including loss of fluid and electrolytes due to vomiting and disturbed gastrointestinal function and, more rarely, by inappropriate secretion of antidiuretic hormone (ADH). Although tubular damage may be found in subjects who die in acute attacks, it is not established that this is the basis of the more commonly found renal defect, which is generally considered to be minor and transient, although there is evidence also that it may persist (Schley *et al.* 1970*a*).

Hypertension in porphyria: a role for the renal nerves?

Recognition of disturbed baroreflex control in porphyria (see above) has probably resulted in disregard of the possible direct involvement of the renal nerves in the aetiology of the hypertension. Their importance in the regulation of body fluids and cardiovascular homeostasis is becoming increasingly recognized (Katholi 1983) and it would seem likely also that they are damaged as part of the extensive neuropathy of the porphyric attack.

It is particularly difficult to study this relationship because of the relative rarity of appropriate patients and also because of the primary needs of their immediate clinical care during attacks. In these circumstances, single-case, anecdotal reports may be justified on the grounds that they may provide insights not otherwise available, as illustrated by the following case (Gorchein and Peart, unpublished).

Case report

The patient, now 51 years old, had a life-threatening attack of AIP at the age of 23. Following severe abdominal pain she rapidly became tetraplegic and required artificial ventilation. Some milder attacks of pain occurred over the following year but neurological recovery continued and was nearly complete 2 years later. She was left with bilateral weakness of wrist extension.

Slight impairment of renal function of undetermined nature, with the blood urea raised to 60–80 mg %, in apparent disproportion to the creatinine (0.9–1.1 mg %) was recorded. The blood pressure which had been high during the attack returned to normal (105/80 mm Hg), but increased with her first and only pregnancy in 1964 from 130/84 at 14 weeks to 160/100–110 mm Hg at 33 weeks. An intravenous pyelogram several months after delivery was normal. No further clinical attacks of porphyria occurred but the urinary excretion of ALA (15–30 mg/24 h) and PBG (35–55 mg/24 h) have always remained grossly elevated. Blood pressure remained high following the pregnancy and an upward trend was noted 8 years ago and treatment was deemed necessary.

At this time, the patient indicated that for many years most of her urine output had been at night. In-patient studies confirmed this (Fig. 40.3(a)) with night:day volume ratios between 1.8:1 and 2.5:1. There was also a marked nocturnal natriuresis. Differences in the night:day excretion of creatinine were small, indicating that simple differences in glomerular filtration could not account for the obervations. Slight differences only were noted with K^+ excretion, and also with the excretion of ALA, consistent with its renal handling being similar to that of creatinine (Gorchein and Webber 1987), and with PBG. When the patient was kept supine during the day, both the volume of urine and Na^+ excretion markedly increased (Fig. 40.3(a)) indicating that the abnormalities were dependent on posture rather than on alterations of circadian rhythms. Blood-pressure measurements at 6-h intervals during these studies showed a small and inconsistent postural drop but there was no marked increase in supine blood pressure. Normal levels of

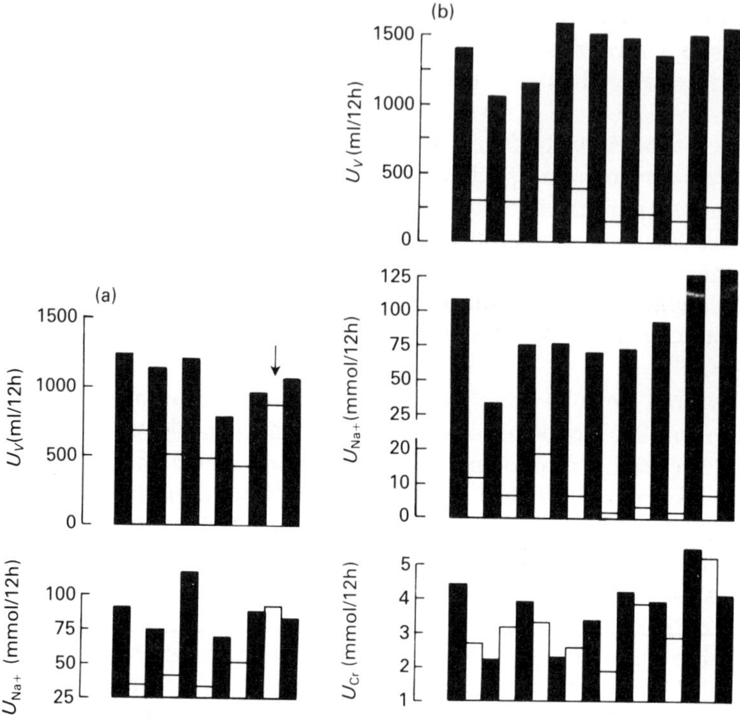

Fig. 40.3. Night and day urine volumes and sodium excretion in a porphyric subject. Consecutive 12-h urine collections are shown for two studies done 8 months apart: Night (20.00–08.00 h) in black, and day (08.00–20.00 h) in white. The arrow in panel (a) indicates a 12-h period of recumbency during the day. The creatinine excretion for the later study (panel (b)) is also shown.

plasma noradrenalin and plasma renin activity were demonstrated in response to change from the supine to erect posture and also following a period of ambulation. Thus, despite the slight postural falls in blood pressure, no evidence was obtained of gross abnormalities of sympathetic response to changes in posture. The differences in her night:day urine ratios were even more pronounced (Fig. 40.3(b)) in a further pretreatment study 8 months later. Little urine or Na^+ was excreted during the day, but creatinine excretion was not significantly different between night and day (Wilcoxon matched-pairs rank test).

Blood pressure was then maintained between 140/90 and 150/100 mm Hg with a small dose of bethanidine (10 mg twice daily) with a slight asymptomatic postural drop.

Renal function has remained stable over the last 6–7 years with serum creatinine raised at 140 μmol/l and creatinine clearance approximately 35 ml/min.

Tests of autonomic function were done late in 1986 after temporarily stopping the bethanidine, but autonomic neuropathy could not be demonstrated.

Retrospective examination of fluid charts available from 1961 and 1964 when the blood pressure was normal showed qualitatively similar but less pronounced abnormalities in the night:day ratios of urine volumes. It seems likely therefore that longstanding, primarily renal abnormalities are responsible for the abnormal night:day urine ratios and the development of hypertension, which then caused additional renal damage.

It is suggested that damage to renal nerves occurred as part of the autonomic neuropathy of the porphyric attack, and that this involved the neural control of tubular sodium transport. This can be modulated independently of changes in overall sympathetic output to the kidneys and thus of vasoconstriction or other renal haemodynamic changes (DiBona 1985).

Since, however, increased tubular Na^+ reabsorption is associated with increase in efferent sympathetic activity, it would seem necessary to speculate that the neural lesion selectively involves the afferent pathway and that this normally exerts inhibitory control on sympathetic efferent activity mediating tubular Na^+ reabsorption. Thus renal deafferentation would result in the increased tubular Na^+ reabsorption observed in the upright position. Diuresis and natriuresis when supine would occur because there would be reduction in centrally-mediated sympathetic outflow to the kidneys from changes in baroreceptor activity (with recovery of neural function following the acute attack) and, probably with more importance, effects arising from reabsorption of Na^+ and water into the vascular compartment leading to volume expansion and its consequences (e.g. release of atrial natriuretic peptide, changes in activity of the renin–angiotensin system, and in ADH).

In summary, it is proposed that attacks of porphyria may cause renal afferent neuropathy resulting in impaired Na^+ excretion by the kidney. This is then responsible for the development of the sustained hypertension commonly found in long-term survivors of acute porphyric attacks. Prospective studies after acute porphyric attacks should be directed to determine whether a renal abnormality in Na^+ handling can be confirmed. Examination of this possibility may be relevant also to our understanding of the wider problem of the aetiology of essential hypertension, in which defective Na^+ excretion by the kidney may be an important primary determinant (Haddy and Pamnani 1985).

CONCLUSIONS

Autonomic neuropathy is a major feature of attacks of the acute porphyrias and can account for clinically obvious disturbance of gastrointestinal and cardiovascular function. It seems probable also that other disorders of autonomic function occur, which are not as readily assessed but may lead to long-term effects such as altered renal function and sustained hypertension. Methodological limitations make it difficult to determine with certainty whether disturbed autonomic function is a feature of latent porphyria.

In contrast to the explosive increase in recent years in information about the molecular genetics of these diseases (e.g. Nordmann 1986), fundamental clinical questions remain unanswered, including the cause of the abdominal pain and of the neuropathy itself. The apparently widening gap between knowledge of nuclear events and their relation to neurological deficiency should, however, sustain the exciting challenge of future investigation.

REFERENCES

Baker, A. B. and Watson, C. J. (1945). The central nervous system in porphyria. *J. Neuropathol. exp. Neurol.* **4**, 68–76.

Beal, M. F., Atuk, N. O., Westfall, T. C., and Turner, S. M. (1977). Catecholamine uptake, accumulation and release in acute porphyria. *J. clin. Invest.* **60**, 1141–8.

Beattie, A. D. and Goldberg, A. (1976). Acute intermittent porphyria: natural history and prognosis. In *Porphyrias in human diseases* (ed. M. Doss), pp. 245–50. Karger, Basel

Berlin, L. and Cotton, R. (1950). Gastro-intestinal manifestations of porphyria. *Am. J. digest. Dis.* **17**, 110–14.

Bonkowski, H. L. and Schady, W. (1982). Neurologic manifestations of acute porphyria. *Sem. liver Dis.* **2**, 108–24.

Di Bona, G. F. (1985). The kidney in the pathogenesis of hypertension: The role of renal nerves. In *Hypertension and the kidney* (ed. J. G. Porush), pp. A27–A31. Grune and Stratton, Orlando, Florida.

Gibson, J. B. and Goldberg, A. (1956). The neuropathology of acute porphyria. *J. Pathol. Bacteriol.* **71**, 495–509.

Goldberg, A. (1959). Acute intermittent porphyria—a study of 50 cases. *Quart. J. Med.* (New ser.) **28**, 183–209.

Gorchein, A., Valori, R. M., Wingate, D. L., and Bloom, S. R. (1982). Abnormal proximal gut motility in acute intermittent porphyria (AIP): a neuropathic model. *Gastroenterology* **5**, 1070.

Gorchein, A. and Webber, R. (1987). δ-Aminolaevulinic acid in plasma, cerebrospinal fluid, saliva and erythrocytes: studies in normal, uraemic and porphyric subjects. *Clin. Sci.* **72**, 103–12.

Gupta, G. L., Saksena, H. C., and Gupta, B. D. (1983*a*). Cardiac dysautonomia in acute intermittent porphyria. *Ind. J. med. Res.* **78**, 253–6.

Gupta, G. L., Saksena, H. C., and Gupta, B. D. (1983*b*). Autonomic neuropathy and hypertension in acute intermittent porphyria. *J. Ass. Physcns, India* **31**, 259.

Haddy, F. J. and Pamnani, M. B. (1985). The kidney in the pathogenesis of hypertension: The role of sodium. In *Hypertension and the kidney* (ed. J. G. Porush), pp. A5–A13. Grune and Stratton, Orlando, Florida.

Kappas, A., Sassa, S., and Anderson, K. E. (1983). In *The metabolic basis of inherited disease*, 5th edn. (ed. J. B. Stanbury, J. B. Wyngaarden, D. S. Fredrickson, J. L. Goldstein, and M. S. Brown), pp. 1301–84. McGraw-Hill, New York.

Katholi, R. (1983). Renal nerves in the pathogenesis of hypertension in experimental animals and humans. *Am. J. Physiol.* **245**, F1–F14.

Kezdi, P. (1954). Neurogenic hypertension in man in porphyria. *Arch. intern. Med.* **4**, 122–30.

Melby, J. C., Street, J. P., and Watson, C. J. (1956). Chlorpromazine in the treatment of porphyria. *J. Am. med. Ass.* **162**, 174–8.

Mustajoki, P. and Seppalainen, A. M. (1975). Neuropathy in latent hereditary hepatic porphyria. *Br. med. J.* **2**, 310–12.

Nordmann, Y. (Ed.) (1986). *Porphyrins and porphyrias* (Proceedings Second International Congress on Porphyrins and Porphyrias, Paris, 1985). Inserm/John Libby Eurotext, London.

Palkovits, M. (1980). The anatomy of central cardiovascular neurones. In *Central adrenaline neurons* (ed. K. Fuxe, M. Goldstein, T. Hökfelt, and B. Hökfelt), pp. 3–17, Pergamon Press, Oxford.

Ridley, A. (1969). The neuropathy of acute intermittent porphyria. *Quart. J. Med.* **38**, 307–33.

Ridley, A., Hierons, R., and Cavanagh, J. B. (1968). Tachycardia and the neuropathy of porphyria. *Lancet* **ii**, 708–10.

Sarr, M. G. and Kelly, K. A. (1981). Myoelectric activity of the autotransplanted canine jejunoileum. *Gastroenterology* **81**, 303–10.

Shirger, A., Martin, W. J., Goldstein, N. P., and Huizenga, K. A. (1962). Orthostatic hypotension in association with acute exacerbations of porphyria. *Proc. Mayo Clin.* **37**, 7–11.

Schley, G., Bock, K. D., Desbusmann, E. R., Hocevar, V., Merguet, P., Paar, D., and Rausch-Stroomann, J-G. (1970*a*). Untersuchungen über die Nierenfunktion bei der akuten intermittierenden Porphyrie. *Klin. Wschr.* **48**, 616–23.

Schley, G., Bock, K. D., Hocevar, V., Merguet, P., Rausch-Strooman, J-G., Schröder, E., and Schümann, H. J. (1970*b*). Hochdruck und Tachykardie bei der akuten intermittierenden Porphyrie. *Klin. Wschr.* **48**, 36–42.

Stein, J. A. and Tschudy, D. P. (1970). Acute intermittent porphyria—a clinical and biochemical study of 46 patients. *Medicine* **49**, 1–16.

Stewart, P. M. and Hensley, W. J. (1981). An acute attack of variegate porphyria complicated by severe autonomic neuropathy. *Aust. NZ J. Med.* **11**, 82–3.

Thompson, D. G., Wingate, D. L., Archer, L., Benson, M. J., Green, W. J., and Hardy, R. J. (1980). Normal patterns of human upper small bowel motor activity recorded by prolonged radiotelemetry. *Gut* **21**, 500–6.

Thorner, P. S., Bilbao, J. M., Sima, A. A. F., and Briggs, S. (1981). Porphyric neuropathy: an ultrastructural and quantitative case study. *Can. J. neurol. Sci.* **8**, 281–7.

Ventura, H. O., Messerli, F. H., and Barron, R. E. (1986). Norepinephrine-induced hypertension in Guillain–Barré syndrome. *J. Hypertension* **4**, 265–7.

Waldenström, J. (1957). The porphyrias as inborn errors of metabolism. *Am. J. Med.*

22, 758–73.

Wehrmacher, W. H. (1952). New symptomatic treatment for acute intermittent porphyria. *Arch. intern. Med.* **89**, 111–14.

Wingate, D. L. (1981). Backwards and forwards with the migrating complex. *Dig. Dis. Sci.* **26**, 641–66.

Yamada, M., Kondo, M., Tanaka, M., Okeda, R., Hatakeyama, S., Fukui, T., and Tsukagoshi, H. (1984). An autopsy case of acute porphyria with a decrease of both uroporphyrinogen I synthetase and ferrochelatase activities. *Acta Neuropathol., Berlin* **64**, 6–11.

Yeung Laiwah, A. A. C., MacPhee, G. J. A., Boyle, P., Moore, M. R., and Goldberg, A. (1985). Autonomic neuropathy in acute intermittent porphyria. *J. Neurol. Neurosurg. Psychiat.* **48**, 1025–30.

Yeung Laiwah, A. A. C., Mactier, R., McColl, K. E. L., Moore, M. R., and Goldberg, A. (1983). Early-onset chronic renal failure as a complication of acute intermittent porphyria. *Quart. J. Med.* **52**, 92–8.

41. Pain and the sympathetic system

Peter W. Nathan

THE SYNDROMES

Most doctors feel confused about the sympathetic system and painful states. After they have read this chapter, they will, no doubt, still be confused but, I hope, at a higher level.

The sympathetic system was labelled sympathetic by Galen because its function is to harmonize the parts of the body. In the group of cases considered here, there is disharmony. The feature they have in common is that the disharmony is relieved or even cured by sympathetic blocks. This large group of rare cases is called algodystrophy or reflex sympathetic dystrophy. Other features commonly found in these cases are these: the pain is persistent; it is described as burning; it is usually severe; and in most cases there are also other pains, such as aching and sudden shoots of pain. Typically, there is a particular kind of hypersensitivity. This includes hyperpathia: here, there is a slight delay in feeling a stimulus, a pointed stimulus feels less pointed and more diffuse than normal, and the stimulus causes a dreaded penetrating burning pain and is followed by a painful aftersensation. There is allodynia or pain felt with a stimulus that does not cause pain in normal tissues. Often in these patients even blowing on the skin causes pain. There is an abnormal sensitivity to warmth and cold: not only do thermal stimuli appear excessively warm or cold but there is also a lowering of threshold so that stimuli within a neutral range in normal people cause sensations of warm or cold. Usually the tissues beneath the skin are tender to pressure. The patient commonly protects the affected part of his body from stimulation, even by himself. He avoids moving the limb and when he is persuaded to do so, his efforts are feeble. This symptom is commoner in the upper than the lower limb. The condition spreads; if it starts peripherally it spreads to the central nervous system and if it starts in the central nervous system it spreads to the periphery. Occasionally, though rarely, the state spreads into a whole forequarter or hindquarter of the body.

In these cases, the limb is often cold, the skin becomes smooth and shiny, the pulps of the fingers atrophy and the fingers become tapered, and there is decalcification of the bones. The vascular changes do not occur in most of the cases. They are usually attributed to the algodystrophy, but it is possible that they are at least partly due to disuse of the limb. For disuse alone in an upper limb can cause atrophy. This is seen in some patients with catatonia who stand all day without moving and with their arms hanging by their sides. More rarely it occurs in hysteria, where the patient is convinced she cannot use the limb and does not do so. There is no evidence that these features occur more in causalgia and other cases of reflex sympathetic dystrophy than in complete lesions of peripheral nerves without the painful syndrome.

Coming within the category of algodystrophy are several groups of pathological conditions. The cases fall easily into two categories, those starting in the peripheral and those starting in the central nervous system. The cases starting in the periphery include cases of amputation, painful hypersensitive scars, and causalgia, mainly occurring with partial lesions of the median nerve and thus after Colles fractures and in the carpal tunnel syndrome, often following surgery.

Of the cases that originate in the periphery, there is a separate group in which abnormal vascular irrigation is the main element of the syndrome. This occurs after neural damage such as injury to the median nerve or following fractures without any damage to a peripheral nerve. When this condition is severe, there can be such decalcification of the bone that it is said to cut like cheese. This group includes cases of Sudeck's atrophy. Associated with the radiological appearances of the bone are atrophic changes in the skin, connective tissues, and musculature.

Whether the peripheral blood flow is increased or decreased, the pain and hypersensitivity are usually relieved by sympathetic blocks, particularly by regional guanethidine. Sometimes, though rarely, this condition can be cured by reducing the abnormal vascular supply. Two cases were reported by Foix *et al.* (1919) of causalgia cured by ligating the radial artery in one case and the posterior tibial artery in the other. One should, but does not, keep such cases in mind.

In some patients with reflex sympathetic dystrophy, Blumberg (1985) found that the normal constriction of cutaneous blood vessels to noxious stimulation no longer occurred. There was either no response or else cutaneous vasodilatation.

Leriche (1937) thought that the outgrowing axons in a neuroma formed the first afferent link in a vasomotor reflex. He suggested that the next link was constriction of the blood vessels, and that that caused 'une véritable maladie nouvelle'. This condition was shown up by decreased temperature, cyanosis, oedema, trophic disturbances, and pains. However, he was fully aware that vasoconstriction did not cause pain. He noted that in some cases there was decreased, and occasionally, increased tone of the muscles outside of the territory 'legitimately paralysed'. One must point out that neuromata form on all peripheral nerves divided or partially divided by trauma, and yet the painful cases under discussion are quite rare. Leriche (1930) also recorded cases in which the abnormal state originated from the supposedly inert peripheral cord of a severed nerve. Not only did local anaesthetic injected into this divided peripheral cord temporarily remove the pain and abnormal vascular state but electrical stimulation at operation also induced severe pain and local vasoconstriction. This is due to occasional anastamoses with neighbouring nerves.

In the predominantly vascular cases, the central nervous system can also play a part in the development of the condition. For instance, as in other examples of algodystrophy, Sudeck's atrophy with associated pathological changes may spread to the opposite limb. The central lesions giving rise to algodystrophy include the lesions of multiple sclerosis and lesions in or near the thalamus, causing the thalamic syndrome; and the shoulder–hand syndrome has been recorded as a transient effect of migraine, where the vascular disturbance is affecting the cerebral cortex.

Only certain pains are sympathetically maintained. A nice example of this selection is a case recorded by Schott (1986). The patient had an infarct of the right parietal cortex followed by severe burning pain down the left side of the body and extreme hypersensitivity. When he came into hospital he also had a painful bunion on the left little toe. 'A regional intravenous guanethidine infusion in his left leg abolished all the causalgic pain in his left side, except for the pain in his toe.'

When, in sympathetically maintained pains, the lesion is in the central nervous system, the particular pain of algodystrophy depends on events in the periphery. For, in these central cases also, sympathetic blocks or local anaesthetic blocks of the somatic nerves remove the pain.

Although the relief by sympathectomy is so striking that this component of these conditions is usually taken to be the outstanding and characteristic feature, in clinical practice one's experience is that more cases are not relieved by sympathetic blocks than are. Further, we have all seen cases of chronic pain without hyperpathia and allodynia in which the pain was relieved by sympathetic blocks. Nevertheless, in view of the remarkable removal of extreme sensitivity and burning pain produced by blocking the sympathetic innervation of the region and the momentary increase in pain produced by any sort of stress which activates the sympathetic system, it is probable that sympathetic postganglionic fibres are necessary to cause this kind of extreme cutaneous and deep hypersensitivity. But this is so only when there is already a state of hyperpathia with allodynia; for in the normal patient sympathetic stimulation or giving noradrenalin or adrenalin has no effect on sensation.

One hypothesis might well be that in all of these states, central and peripheral, the sympathetic regulatory function of the limbs has gone wrong, and that the absence of sympathetic control affects not only the thermal regulation and the vascularity of the limbs but also the sensitivity of mechanoreceptors.

DO SYMPATHETIC NERVES CONTROL THE SENSITIVITY OF RECEPTORS?

For many years physiologists have been producing contradictory evidence of the effects of sympathetic nerves on mechanoreceptors. There is evidence that many mechanoreceptors in frogs and the cat are accompanied by at least one sympathetic nerve fibre, and that this has some effect on their function. Tournay (1921, 1927, 1931, 1939), who thought that the sympathetic system regulated sensibility, concluded from unsatisfactory experiments in the cat and the rabbit that the influence of the sympathetic system became clear after its removal. He believed that sympathectomy increased sensibility and that normally the sympathetic system damped it down.

Dusser de Barenne (1931) produced better evidence. After unilateral extirpation of the sympathetic chain in the cat's abdomen, he found ipsilateral 'hyperaesthesia for tactile excitation and a very definite hyperalgesia for painful excitation of the skin'. It was unrelated to the skin temperature. It was still present 8 weeks later when the animals were killed. It occurred in six out of eight animals. But Van Petten *et al.* (1983) looked for such hyperaesthesia in the sympathectomized cat: none of their six cats showed any evidence of permanent change in cutaneous sensibility.

Cutaneous hypersensitivity has been reported immediately after sympathectomy; it is usually attributed to some damage to the somatic nerves during the operation. It is not usually recorded, though Brown and Adson (1929) did report it. 'Following thoracic ganglionectomy, cutaneous hyperaesthesia was noted in some degree in every case. Soreness of the muscles, nerve trunks and large arteries of the arm was brought out by mild palpation.' It diminished within a fortnight and was gone in 4 to 5 weeks. They accepted the explanation that it was due to damage to the somatic nerves. But perhaps it was not. Livingston (1935, p. 179) reported a personal communication of Donal Sheehan. Sheehan said he found a slightly lowered threshold for touch in all of 15 patients having had sympathectomy; but it was insufficient to call it hyperaesthesia. But thousands of sympathectomies have been carried out for Raynaud's syndrome, for occlusive vascular states of the lower limb, and for hyperhidrosis, and no changes in sensibility have been observed. Hyperaesthesia is not reckoned to be a complication of this operation.

Further, in cases of phaeochromocytomata, there is a large amount of circulating noradrenalin which reaches the receptors; there is no change in cutaneous sensibility. The same applies to hypothyroidism with diminished sympathetic activity and hyperthyroidism with excessive activity.

The evidence on the effects of sympathetic stimulation on mechanoreceptors in mammals will now be briefly reviewed. In some classes of mechanoreceptors, sympathetic stimulation can raise the threshold to mechanical stimulation; it can decrease their firing rate and stop spontaneous firing of these receptors. This decrease in responsiveness might be seen as complementary to the reported hypersensitivity following sympathectomy. But in other mechanoreceptors it may increase the resting discharge without causing change in threshold. The effect of stimulation on intra-oral mechanoreceptors of the cat was examined by Cash and Linden (1982). Stimulation of the cervical trunk affected about a half of these mechanoreceptors and had no effect on the others. The threshold of the receptors was raised, and spontaneous activity was removed. Also in the cat, Pierce and Roberts (1981) examined the effect of sympathetic stimulation on G-hairs (guard hairs: rapidly adapting units with low thresholds for hair movement and conduction velocities in the A-beta range) and on type II mechanoreceptors ('responsive to skin compression and stretch . . . responsive to movements of the joints in humans'). These mechanoreceptors were of two types: (1) excited by stretch parallel to the long axis of the receptor; (2) excited by stretch perpendicular to the long axis of the leg. Sympathetic stimulation raised the threshold of the guard hair receptors to 2.2 times their previous value; and a third of the more slowly adapting guard hair receptors showed sympathetically induced spontaneous activity. Of the type II mechanoreceptors, the (1) receptors were unaffected by sympathetic stimulation and the (2) receptors had an increased resting discharge but no change in mechanical sensitivity. Roberts and Levitt (1982) examined the effect of sympathetic stimulation on the D hair afferents. These receptors became less sensitive: the intensity of repetitive mechanical stimulation had to be increased during repetitive sympathetic stimulation in order to maintain the response to stimulation. Roberts *et al.* (1985) went on to examine the effect of sympathetic stimulation on Type I slowly adapting mechanoreceptors. It had 'predominantly excitatory effects'. In some units, there was an increase in any existing discharge and in silent units, a discharge was induced. In some units there was 'a reduction in the threshold for mechanical activation'. Roberts and Elardo (1985*a*, *b*) found that the effect of sympathetic stimulation on A-delta nociceptors was to 'induce firing in a small population of A mechanoheat receptors', but only after 'they had been sensitized by noxious heating of their receptive fields'. The effect of stimulating the sympathetic trunk on C fibre mechanoreceptors of the cat's skin was to induce repetitive discharge. The activation of these receptors by the sympathetic system and the fact that they were activated at the low rate of 2-Hz stimulation made the authors question whether these afferents were used to report external events. Those working on man with intraneural recordings have not found these non-myelinated mechanoreceptors.

Barasi and Lynn (1983) demonstrated that non-myelinated mechanoreceptors in the rabbit were excited at the onset of sympathetic stimulation. Sympathetic stimulation produced no change in the responsiveness of A-delta mechanoreceptor units to pressure. C polymodal nociceptors showed no effect from sympathetic stimulation when tested with pressure stimuli. Barassi and Lynn's conclusion from all the experiments was that the effects of sympathetic stimulation were only small; they thought it unlikely that causalgia could be due to sympathetic effects on nociceptors. Shea and Perl (1985) found that stimulation of the sympathetic trunk in the rabbit had no effect on cutaneous polymodal nociceptors (C fibres). The absence of any effect from stimulating sympathetic nerves on C fibre nociceptors fits in well with Robert's (1986) finding that sympathetic stimulation of the periphery causes rapid firing of the wide-dynamic-range neurons of the posterior horns but not of the nociceptor-specific neurons.

In man, Hallin and Wiesenfeld-Hallin (1983) recorded sympathetic activity in the peripheral nerves of seven normal subjects. They 'observed that changes in spontaneous ongoing activity of the Pacinian corpuscle afferents were closely associated with decrease or increase in skin' sympathetic discharge; this afferent discharge was very marked when the subjects did mental arithmetic.

Thus, we see that the physiological evidence is inconsistent. The effects of sympathetic stimulation vary from increasing the activity of these receptors and increasing their sensitivity to reducing this activity and raising their threshold.

The data on the effects of cutting out the sympathetic supply of a region and of stimulating the sympathetic supply to receptors are shown in an abbreviated form in Tables 41.1 and 41.2.

That hyperpathia and allodynia are not due to impulses in peripheral C fibres nor in A-delta fibres is shown by the fact that they are caused by the lightest of stimuli; such stimuli do not excite fibres within the delta and C fibre range. Further, when only C fibres are conducting after 25 min or more of ischaemia produced by a sphygmomanometer cuff, the extreme sensitivity has long disappeared. That this abnormal sensitivity depends above all on the large mechanoreceptive fibres is

Table 41.1. Data on sympathectomy

Author	*Date*	*Species*	*Effect of sympathectomy*
Tournay	1921 1927 1931 1939	Dog	Reflex effects from chronic ulcer only on sympathectomized side. Noxious and cold stimuli caused nocifensor reactions only on sympathectomized side.
Dusser de Barenne	1931	Cat	Hyperaesthesia and hyperalgesia.
Brown and Adson	1929	Man	Hyperaesthesia; soreness of deep tissues.
Sheehan (reported on p. 179 of Livingston 1935)	1935	Man	Lowered threshold for touch.

Table 41.2. Data on stimulating sympathetic supply of receptors

Author	*Date*	*Species*	*Effect of sympathetic stimulation*
Cash and Linden	1982	Cat	Effects were on a half the population of periodontal mechanoreceptors; no effects on other half: stopped spontaneous firing; decreased firing rate to a controlled pressure; raised threshold.
Pierce and Roberts	1981	Cat	On rapidly adapting units activated by hair movements; raised threshold. If no piloerection occurs on type II mechanoreceptors, increased resting discharge but no change in threshold.
Roberts and Levitt	1982	Cat	On D-hair receptors; raised threshold.
Roberts *et al.*	1985	Cat	Type I slowly adapting mechanoreceptors: excitatory effects; sometimes increased resting discharge; some showed reduction in threshold.
Roberts and Elardo	1985*a*	Cat	On A-delta nociceptors: firing induced in units with high mechanical thresholds but only after sensitization of field by noxious heat.
Roberts and Elardo	1985*b*	Cat	On non-myelinated mechanoreceptors: repetitive discharge induced.
Barasi and Lynn	1983	Rabbit	On A-delta mechanoreceptors: no effect; On non-myelinated mechanoreceptors: at first, excitatory effect: after 1 min depressing effect; on non-myelinated polymodal nociceptors: no effect.
Shea and Pearl	1985	Rabbit	On non-myelinated polymodal nociceptors: no effect.
Hallin and Weisenfeld-Hallin	1983	man	Pacinian corpuscles: excitatory.

indicated by the fact that only these fibres have a low enough threshold to be activated by the minimal contact that causes sensation—admittedly a painful sensation—in these states. This fact probably means that an input in these large fibres arriving at neurons of the spinal cord that also receive a noxious input is necessary to cause pain and allodynia. Roberts (1986) proposed that this occurs at the convergent or wide-dynamic range neurons of the posterior horns. From there impulses pass to higher centres in the spinothalamic and spinoreticular tracts.

In man, Francini *et al.* (1979) and Procacci *et al.* (1979) produced evidence that, in every case of reflex sympathetic dystrophy, skin potential responses and cutaneous sensory thresholds differed in the pathological limb from the contralateral limb; moreover they were abnormal also in the contralateral limb. After sympathetic blocks, the total pattern became normal. Their work indicates that the sensory thresholds are under the control of sympathetic efferents. They concluded that the sympathetic blocks 'provide a re-setting of the sensory thresholds and of the reflexes to another steady state similar to that observed in normal subjects'.

Two points may be emphasized. First, the sensory threshold is abnormal in the two contralateral limbs; thus, the harmonizing function of the sympathetic control is disturbed. Second, when the sympathetic supply is removed not in the presence of this condition, one does not see any changes in sensibility or somatic sensation.

EXPERIMENTALLY INDUCED REFLEX SYMPATHETIC DYSTROPHY

Sympathetic nerves affect capillary permeability. Engel (1941) showed in rabbits, cats, and dogs that sympathetic activity increases and sympathectomy decreases capillary permeability. After sympathectomy, 'in spite of marked vaso-dilatation, dye excretion was considerably reduced on the sympathectomised side'. He considered that these changes in permeability 'would counteract or balance the effect of vasomotor changes'.

Thorban (1962) believed that he induced reflex limb dystrophy in the rabbit. To do so, he had to induce a fracture plus a partial peripheral-nerve lesion. He could not induce it with a complete nerve lesion nor with a fracture without a nerve lesion. Microscopic examination of the capillaries showed that they were dilated and packed full of blood, and that eventually there was oedema of the soft tissues and endarteritis obliterans. However, one cannot immediately relate these findings to the state occurring in man. For in clinical medicine, these states are rare. Nearly all peripheral-nerve lesions occur without a concomitant reflex dystrophy; and reflex dystrophy can accompany fractures without any peripheral-nerve involvement, partial or complete.

Krediet (1964) and Folkerts *et al.* (1969) were also able to induce this condition in the rabbit but not in the dog or rat. They produced it by injecting phenol either into the stellate ganglion or into the hypogastric plexus. This is surprising because one treats these conditions in man by the injection of phenol into the chain or ganglia. These investigators showed that there was a greatly abnormal increase in the number of capillaries and that this increase in the region of the motor end-plates caused them to degenerate. They also examined muscle fibres and muscle end-plates in the biceps brachialis of a patient with reflex sympathetic dystrophy and found degenerated muscle fibres and motor end-plates.

The findings in the human patient carry more weight than those obtained in the rabbit. But there is other experimental work showing that the sympathetic control of blood vessels can become abnormal after a peripheral-nerve lesion. Blumberg and Jänig (1981, 1983) induced a neuroma in a cat's peripheral nerve and then examined the sympathetic control of the blood vessels of the limb. In many animals the reflex responses of cutaneous blood vessels of the entire limb had become abnormal. Instead of sudden noxious stimulation inhibiting the cutaneous vasoconstrictor neurons, it either excited them or it had no effect on the cutaneous blood vessels. Furthermore, the cutaneous vasoconstrictor neurons now responded to baroreceptors, whereas normally only the muscular vasoconstrictor neurons respond to this pulsatile stimulation.

REGIONAL INTRAVENOUS GUANETHIDINE IN MAN

The introduction by Hannington-Kiff (1974) of the regional intravenous injection of guanethidine gave us an easily repeatable therapy for painful sympathetically maintained states and it also introduced some new problems. We will now consider these.

As blocks of the sympathetic ganglia and chain by local anaesthetics remove or even cure algodystrophy, it appears likely that guanethidine acts by depleting the noradrenalin content of the sympathetic fibres. However, evidence obtained during this form of treatment has shown that guanethidine does not act therapeutically in this way. There is little correlation between the relief of pain and any blocking of sympathetic function by guanethidine. For instance, Fig. 41.1 shows the excitation of the arrectores pili distal to the occluding cuff following the injection of guanethidine. This appears within minutes of the injection and lasts up to a few hours. Apart from the first 4 or 5 minutes after the injection of

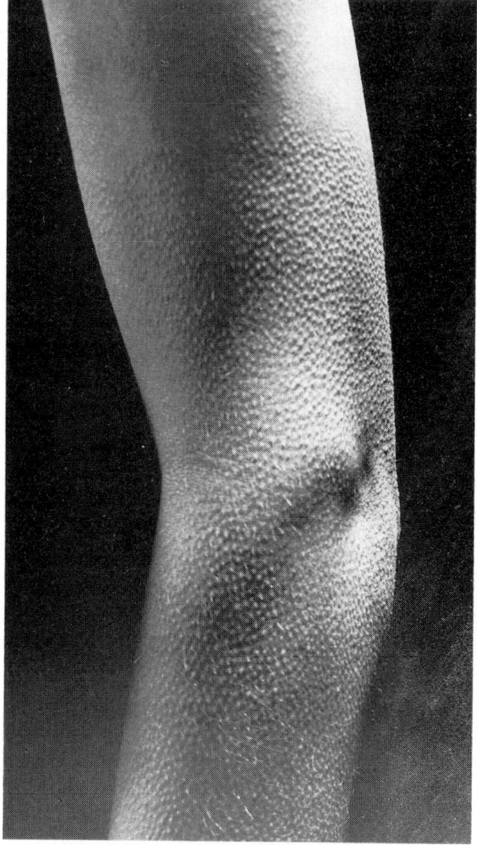

Fig. 41.1. Piloerection in man following the infusion of guanethidine. (From Loh *et al.* (1980).)

guanethidine, the painful state and hyperpathia are removed. And yet this stimulation of the arrectores pili is evidence of the local presence of noradrenalin, presumably in abnormally high concentration.

In the series of cases reported by Loh *et al.* (1980), guanethidine did not remove all sympathetic activity from the treated limb. In only one of 50 or more regional injections was the reactivity of the digital blood vessels completely removed; in all others the block was partial. The reactivity of these vessels to a simple mathematics test was always similar to that of the vessels of the contralateral limb, but it was less.

Although the relief of pain almost always occurred within 20 min of the injection, the cutaneous vasodilatation was often not immediate and in many cases came on only after 8 hours. Furthermore, the lack of relationship between relief of pain and onset of vasodilatation was strikingly demonstrated in two patients in whom pain and hyperpathia returned during the period of vasodilatation; a second infusion of guanethidine given during this period had the same therapeutic effect as the first, the relief of pain and hyperpathia lasting between 12 and 36 hours. In one patient we gave a regional block with guanethidine, knowing that she already had had a sympathectomy to the lower limbs. At the time of the injection, there was full cutaneous vasodilatation. Nevertheless, the reginal guanethidine relieved the pain for 48 hours. One may ask if these infusions work because they cause prolonged vasodilation, and not because they block other sympathetic control. But this question cannot be answered. For the block of all sympathetic functions comes on at the same time, and at that time the pain and hyperpathia are removed.

Finally, there is an important investigation of the effects of guanethidine and reserpine given as regional blocks to normal subjects (McKain *et al.* 1983). Reserpine did not cause vasodilatation. Guanethidine did so, and it lasted up to 3 days. We found the same in our patients. They concluded that reserpine does not induce sympathetic blocking and that 'intravenous regional guanethidine produces not sympathetic block but selective peripheral vasodilatation. . . . It may be preferable to sympathetic block or surgical sympathectomy'. One must note, however, that other methods of causing vasodilatation do not help cases of reflex sympathetic dystrophy and they may make the pain worse. And cases of causalgia and reflex sympathetic dystrophy occur in hot countries where there is always full vasodilatation of the digital vessels.

The most surprising therapeutic effect of guanethidine is in cases of limb dystrophy with Sudeck's atrophy. Guanethidine which causes vasodilatation frequently cures the condition, and does so with greater probability and more effectively than sympathetic blocks of the chain and ganglia.

We must conclude that we do not know why guanethidine is effective in cases of reflex sympathetic dystrophy. Its effect does not come from blocking the sympathetic control of blood vessels, nor is it related to piloerection. It is unlikely to be effective due to any sympathetic influence on mechanoreceptors.

TWO HYPOTHESES

Two hypotheses have been put forward to account for these pathological states. Blumberg and Jänig (1981, 1983, 1985) proposed that, following the lesions of peripheral nerves, many afferent nerve fibres, both myelinated and non-myelinated, show continuous activity. This causes an abnormal state in the local region of the spinal cord, and that results in abnormal activity in sympathetic vasomotor and sudomotor neurons. They propose that this abnormal sympathetic discharge affects the local afferent nerve fibres and thus prolongs the pathological process as a vicious circle. Roberts (1986) proposed that nociceptor input due to trauma has sensitized wide-dynamic range neurons of the posterior horns so that they discharge on receiving a mechanoreceptive input. 'Chronic sympathetically maintained pains are mediated by activity in low-threshold myelinated mechanoreceptors . . . this afferent activity results from sympathetic efferent actions upon their receptors or upon afferent fibres ending in a neuroma . . . these afferent fibres evoke sufficient activity in sensitized spinal wide-dynamic range neurons to produce a painful sensation.' These two hypotheses may account for the different conditions that may be relieved by sympathetic blocks. The first may be held to explain the abnormal vascular state of these conditions and the second to explain the burning pain and the allodynia.

TREATMENT

We do not stimulate the sympathetic system; we block it. Loh and Nathan (1978) showed that the kinds of cases that are likely to benefit from blocks are those with hyperpathia. In all these cases, either blocks of the sympathetic ganglia and/or chain or the regional infusion of guanethidine into the limb should be tried. For the upper limb, the kind of block which should be used depends on the kind of block of which the doctor has the greatest experience. For the lower limb, guanethidine infusion is easier to do, does not need to be done in the department of radiology with an image intensifier, and is less unpleasant for the patient. In a minority of cases, several blocks or infusions may be needed to cure the condition. Immediately after the block, the patient should use the limb. It is good for this to be done under the eye of a physiotherapist, who can rub and stimulate the skin that is no longer tender and encourage the patient to feel objects and various textures, using active touch.

In most cases, blocks need to be repeated; one is then faced with the question whether they should be made permanent by the injection of sclerosing solutions or by surgery. This is not an easy question to answer. Repeated blocks may be more therapeutic than extirpation of parts of the sympathetic chain and ganglia. There are also complications from injecting local anaesthetic into the ganglia and chain, others from injecting phenol or alcohol, and others from surgery. Surgery or the injection of sclerosing solutions should never be carried out without some preceding blocks with local anaesthetic solutions or with guanethidine. Surgery for the removal of the stellate ganglion causes a permanent Horner's syndrome; this may also occur when the operation is done to divide the sympathetic fibres to the upper limb. Cousins *et al.* (1979) compared in a series of 386 patients the results of injecting the lumbar chain with 100 per cent alcohol, 6 per cent phenol in water, and 10 per cent phenol in Conray contrast medium. All three solutions produced equally satisfactory results; the Conray solution produced more complete anhidrosis provided that under X-ray control it was seen to cover the L 3,3 and 4 vertebral bodies. The results were as good as those obtained by open surgery.

Surprisingly, it was shown by Loh *et al.* (1981) that, when hyperpathia and extreme cutaneous sensitivity so typical of causalgia occur with central lesions, the same sympathetic blocks to the periphery are worth trying. When they are effective, they remove some of the pain, all the hyperpathia, and most of the abnormal posture and dystonic movements of the thalamic syndrome. Again, although illogical, one finds that not all the peripheral nerves of the affected region have to have their sympathetic nerve supply blocked. For instance, a painful hyperpathic state of the whole of the upper limb can be alleviated by the infusion of guanethidine into the tissues below the elbow.

One should not consider that blocks of the sympathetic system have failed until one has tried them several times. In practice, this hardly applies to blocking the chain for the lower limb as this procedure is not simple, takes more time, and tends to be painful. With regard to the infusions, if they are helpful, then two or three a week for 1 or 2 weeks are likely to be better than merely one or two. If the beneficial effects last for many months or a year or more and then pass off, the patient should have one or two blocks repeated.

The dose of guanethidine that we use at the National Hospital for Nervous Diseases, London is 20 mg. It is given in 40 ml of fluid. The solution is made up as follows. Ten ml of 1 per cent lignocaine is added to 20 mg of guanethidine. This solution is then made up to 40 ml with normal saline.

Occasionally, the local infusion of guanethidine does not help but the injection of local anaesthetic into the sympathetic ganglion improves the condition; occasionally it is the other way round.

Patients can learn to block the sympathetic supply to the periphery of their limbs by biofeedback (Blacker 1980); this can alleviate causalgia.

Apart from, and in addition to, blockage of the sympathetic system, all the usual methods of dealing with chronic pain are worth trying. These include cold sprays, cold packs, either wet or dry, and transcutaneous nerve stimulation. This stimulation is worth trying on the side opposite to the lesion if it cannot be tolerated or is inneffective in the painful, hyperpathic area.

REFERENCES

Barasi, S. and Lynn, B. (1983). Effects of sympathetic stimulation on mechanoreceptor and nociceptor afferent units with small myelinated (A-delta) and unmyelinated (C) axons innervating the rabbit pinna. *J. Physiol. London* **341**, 51P.

Blacker, H. M. (1980). Volitional sympathetic control. *Anesth. Analg.* **59**, 785–8.

Blumberg, H. (1985). Einfluss akuter and chronischer Schmerzen auf das sympathische Nervensystem des Menschen. *Der Anaestheth.* **34**, 2–3.

Blumberg, H. and Jänig, W. (1981). Neurophysiological analysis of efferent sympathetic and afferent fibres in skin nerves with experimentally produced neuromata. In *Phantom and stump pain* (ed. J. Siegfried and M. Zimmerman) pp. 15–31. Springer Verlag, Berlin.

Blumberg, H. and Jänig, W. (1983). Changes of reflexes in vasoconstrictor neurons supplying the cat hindlimb following chronic nerve lesions: a model for studying mechanisms of reflex sympathetic dystrophy. *J. auton. nerv. Syst.* **7**, 399–411.

Blumberg, H. and Jänig, W. (1985). Reflex patterns in postganglionic vasoconstrictor neurons following chronic nerve lesion. *J. auton. nerv. Syst.* **14**, 157–80.

Brown, G. F. and Adson, A. W. (1929). Physiological effects of thoracic and lumbar sympathetic ganglionectomy or section of the trunk. *Arch. Neurol. Psychiat., Chicago* **22**, 322–57.

Cash, R. M. and Linden, R. W. A. (1982). Effects of sympathetic nerve stimulation in intra-oral mechanoreceptor activity in the cat. *J. Physiol., London* **329**, 451–63.

Cousins, M. J., Reeve, T. S., Glynn, C. J., Walsh, J. A., and Cherry, D. A. (1979). Neurolytic lumbar sympathetic blockade: duration of denervation and relief of rest pain. *Anaesth. intens. Care* **7**, 121–35.

Dusser de Barenne, J. G. (1931). L'influence du système nerveux autonome sur la sensibilité de la peau. *J. de Psychol.* **28**, 177–82.

Engel, D. (1941). The influence of the sympathetic nervous system on capillary permeability. *J. Physiol., London* **99**, 161–81.

Foix, C., Mouchet, and Rimette (1919). Sur une variété de causalgie aisément curable par une ligature artérielle. *Rev. neurol.* **26**, 141–3.

Folkerts, J. F., Wiertz-Hoessels, E. L. M. J., Krediet, P., and Sneep, A. J. (1969). Reflex sympathetic dystrophy. A clinical, histological, histochemical and experimental study. *Conf. neurol.* **31**, 145–75.

Francini, F., Zoppi, M., Mareca, N., and Procacci, P. (1979). Skin potential and emg changes induced by cutaneous electrical stimulation. 1. Normal man in arousing and non-arousing environment. *Appl. Neurophysiol.* **42**, 113–24.

Hallin, R. G. and Wiesenfeld-Hallin, Z. (1983). Does sympathetic activity modify afferent inflow at the receptor level in man? *J. auton. nerv. Syst.* **7**, 391–7.

Hannington-Kiff, J. (1974). Intravenous regional sympathetic block with guanethidine. *Lancet* **i**, 1019–20.

Krediet, P. (1964). Experimental post-traumatic dystrophy in the rabbit. *Nature* 538–9.

Leriche, R. (1930). Du role du bout périphérique d'un nerf sectionné dans la génèse de certains syndromes douloureux. *Presse Méd.* **38** (i), 777–9.

Leriche, R. (1937). *Chirurgie de la douleur.* Masson, Paris.

Livingston, W. K. (1935). *The clinical aspects of visceral neurology with special reference to the surgery of the sympathetic nervous system.* Charles C. Thomas,

Springfield, Illinois.

Loh, L. and Nathan, P. W. (1978). Painful peripheral states and sympathetic blocks. *J. Neurol. Neurosurg. Psychiat.* **41**, 664–71.

Loh, L., Nathan, P. W., and Schott, G. D. (1981). Pain due to lesions of central nervous system removed by sympathetic block. *Brit. med. J.* **282**, 1026–8.

Loh, L., Nathan, P. W., Schott, G. D., and Wilson, P. G. (1980). Effects of regional guanethidine infusion in certain painful states. *J. Neurol. Neurosurg. Psychiat.* **43**, 446–51.

McKain, C., Urban, B. J., and Goldner, J. L. (1983). The effects of intravenous regional guanethidine and reserpine. *J. Bone Jt. Surg.* **65A**, 808–11.

Pierce, J. and Roberts, W. J. (1981). Sympatheticaly induced changes in the responses of guard hair and Type II receptors in the cat. *J. Physiol., London* **314**, 411–28.

Procacci, P., Francini, F., Maresca, M., and Zoppi, M. (1979). Skin potential and emg changes induced by cutaneous electrical stimulation. II Subjects with reflex sympathetic dystrophies. *Appl. Neurophysiol.* **42**, 125–34.

Roberts, W. J. (1986). A hypothesis on the physiological basis for causalgia and related pains. *Pain* **24**, 297–311.

Roberts, W. J. and Elardo, S. M. (1985*a*). Sympathetic activation of A-delta nociceptors. *Somatosens. Res.* **3**, 33–44.

Roberts, W. J. and Elardo, S. M. (1985*b*). Sympathetic activation of unmyelinated mechanoreceptors in cat skin. *Brain Res.* **339**, 123–5.

Roberts, W. J., Elardo, S. M., and King, K. A. (1985). Sympathetically induced changes in the responses of slowly-adapting type I receptors in cat skin. *Somatosens. Res.* **2**, 223–36.

Roberts, W. J. and Levitt, G. R. (1982). Histochemical evidence for sympathetic innervation of hair receptor afferents in cat skin. *J. comp. Neurol.* **210**, 204–9.

Schott, G. D. (1986). Mechanisms of causalgia and related clinical conditions: the role of the central and of the sympathetic nervous systems. *Brain* **109**, 717–38.

Shea, V. K. and Perl, E. R. (1985). Failure of sympathetic stimulation to affect the responsiveness of rabbit polymodal nociceptors. *J. Neurophysiol.* **54**, 513–19.

Thorban, W. (1962). Klinische und experimentelle Untersuchungen zur Ätiologie und Pathogenese der postraumatischen Sudeckschen Gliedmassendystrophie. *Acta Neuroveg.* **25**, 1–62.

Tournay, A. (1921). Influence de sympathetique sur la sensibilité: effets de la résection du sympathique sur le reliquat de sensibilité d'un membre dont les nerfs ont été sectionnés en presque totalité. *Comptes Rend. Acad. Sci.* 939–42.

Tournay, A. (1927). Recherches expérimentales sur les effets sensitifs des perturbations sympathiques. *Rev. neurol.* **II**, 622–32.

Tournay, A. (1931). Nouvelles remarques et recherches expérimentales sur les effets sensitifs des perturbations sympathiques. *Rev. neurol.* **I**, 413–35.

Tournay, A. (1939). Remarques neurologiques sur des perturbations du système végétatif avec réflexions explicatives selon la neurophysiologie actuelle. Troisième Congrès Neurol. Internat.

Van Petten, C., Roberts, W. J., and Rhodes, D. L. (1983). Behavioural test of tolerance for aversive mechanical stimuli in sympathectomised cats. *Pain* **15**, 177–89.

42. Autonomic control of sweat glands and disorders of sweating

K. J. Collins

INTRODUCTION

Three main types of exocrine gland are found in human skin—eccrine, apocrine, and sebaceous; the apocrine and sebaceous glands are associated as a unit with hair follicles (epitrichial glands) while the eccrine glands are not associated with hairs (atrichial glands). Earlier distinctions between epitrichial and atrichial glands on the basis of necrobiosis, a process in which cells of the epitrichial glands lose some structural integrity during secretion, have, in the course of investigations by electron microscopy, been found not to show such clear-cut histological differences as was originally claimed. The ultrastructure of the three types of gland have now been investigated in some detail (Hashimoto 1978) and recent major advances in elucidating their secretory function have come from the use of micropuncture techniques and studies on the isolated gland *in vitro* (Sato 1977).

In the human, eccrine glands totalling more than two million are found over the whole body surface and subserve a primary thermoregulatory function. Apocrine glands are mostly concentrated in axillary, pubic, circumanal, ceruminal, and circumareolar areas. Little is known of the physiological function of apocrine sweat in humans though the secretion is thought to subserve a vestigial sexual (attractant) role. Eccrine and apocrine glands are innervated by the sympathetic nervous system and their function can be profoundly affected by failure of autonomic nervous control. No motor innervation has been demonstrated in human sebaceous glands which appear to be solely under hormonal control.

SECRETORY FUNCTION

Eccrine glands

Two functional types of eccrine glands are recognized in human skin—those on the general body surface which are concerned with temperature regulation and respond in accord with the intensity of afferent thermal stimulation, and those on the palms and soles and other areas such as the forehead which respond to mental, emotional, and sensory stimuli. Palmar and plantar glands are usually the first to react to emotional stimulation and are the only ones to do so if the stimulus is weak (Kuno 1956). In the case of extreme mental excitement, fear, or violent sensory stimulation, there is often a profuse and sudden outbreak of sweat on the general body surface (cold sweat) as well as on the normal 'emotional' sweating areas. Palmar and plantar glands do not normally react to thermal stimulation unless the heating is sufficiently intense to cause emotional sweating. Thus there appears to be a degree of overlap in the central control and functional activity of the 'thermal' and 'emotional' eccrine glands.

In conditions of high heat stress an acclimatized man is capable of sustaining a sweat rate of at least 1 litre per hour for some hours. Complete evaporation of 1 litre of sweat will eliminate 675 W of thermal power. The salient feature of sweat secreted on to the skin surface is that it is hypotonic compared to extracellular fluid, with sodium and chloride ions accounting for about 90 per cent of its osmotic activity. The secretory process involves two stages: the formation of an isotonic precursor fluid in the secretory coil and the reabsorption of sodium in the sweat-gland duct. The use of cryoscopic techniques, micropuncture techniques, and isolated glands have verified that precursor sweat secreted into the coil is isotonic with respect to interstitial periglandular fluid (Sato 1977). The sodium chloride concentration of sweat secreted on to the skin surface is usually in the range 0.1 to 0.4 g/dl (17–68 mM) and this concentration will vary according to the rate of sweating, the level of skin temperature, dietary intake of salt, adrenocortical hormone activity, sweat suppression (hidromeiosis, see p. 761), and the state of heat acclimatization, all of which are factors shown to alter the composition of sweat.

Apocrine glands

In a few species apocrine sweating is accredited with a specific thermoregulatory function, the best known example of which is in the horse where failure of apocrine sweat secretion leads to a condition of 'dry-coat' which bears a resemblance to the anhidrosis and heat intolerance associated with eccrine sweat-gland failure in man. In some animals, apocrine glands located in special sites such as in the perianal or inguinal areas are regarded as scent glands which come into activity with phases of the sexual cycle. In the human, apocrine glands do not appear to have either a definite thermoregulatory or sexual function, though they do not develop fully until puberty and are said to involute after the menopause. Cyclic activity of the glands in relation to the human menstrual cycle has not been established. Shelley and Hurley (1953) claim that the human apocrine secretion is odourless and that odour only develops as the result of bacterial contamination. As in many other species, emotional stimuli can evoke a rapid discharge of the human apocrine glands, but if the secretion is odourless when it is newly discharged it is difficult to attribute to it a sexual role. Qualitatively, Shelley and Hurley (1953) found that uncontaminated axillary sweat collected directly from follicle openings was milky in appearance and contained protein, reducing sugar, and ammonia. The range of electrolyte concentration is not clearly documented though the evidence is that it is hypotonic like eccrine sweat (Weiner and Hellman 1960).

CENTRAL NERVOUS CONTROL AND INNERVATION

Eccrine glands

In experimental animals it has been established that local heating of the pre-optic hypothalamic area (heat loss centre) induces generalized sweating, vasodilatation, and polypnoea, whereas local cooling of this area causes vasoconstriction and thermogenesis. A heat-gain centre in the posterior hypothalamus with cross-inhibition to the pre-optic area has also been described. In the control of sweating, the temperature of blood reaching the hypothalamus cannot be the only drive, although such a system has been proposed (Benzinger 1959). There is abundant evidence that cutaneous temperatures also influence sweat rate (Kerslake 1972, pp. 142–5); for example, an intense heat stimulus applied to a limb can elicit generalized sweating within minutes, before deep body temperature begins to increase. The stimulation of sweating by internal temperature and afferent information from skin thermoreceptors is augmented by the local skin temperature in a multiplicative fashion with a Q_{10} of approximately 3. Thus, when mean skin temperature and core temperature remain unchanged, an increase in local skin temperature of 10°C will increase local sweat-gland activity by about threefold.

Efferent nerve fibres originating from the hypothalamic preoptic area descend through the brainstem and spinal tract and transmit to the sympathetic sudomotor system. Nerves surrounding the eccrine glands are composed of non-myelinated class-C fibres which react strongly in tests for cholinesterase. The postganglionic sudomotor nerves are cholinergic as demonstrated by the classical studies of Dale and Feldberg (1934). These fibres branch repeatedly in the skin and are distributed to the secretory coil of the gland as well as to the coiled portion of the duct. Free endings of the peripheral sympathetic nerves in relation to the secretory cells have rarely, if ever, been visualized. Instead, there is a dense network of very fine fibres, described by Hillarp (1959) as a 'ground plexus' in the vicinity of the glands. Individual fibres exhibit a series of varicosities strung out along their length and these probably represent the presynaptic terminal endings from which transmission is effected *en passage* (Fig. 42.1). Each effector cell is therefore probably innervated by many fibres arising from different sudomotor neurons and each fibre innervates many effector cells. Acetylcholine is released at the sympathetic terminals in close proximity to the eccrine sweat-gland capsule from whence it reaches the gland through the basal lamina and interstitial channels (Fig. 42.1). The infolded basal cytomembranes of the secretory cells become depolarized, sodium ions and interstitial fluid derived from dilated blood vessels flow into the cell, and the secretory process is initiated.

Uno and Montagna (1975) also demonstrated a loose network of catecholamine-containing nerves around the eccrine glands of the monkey paw. This observation has revived the longstanding theory of a dual adrenergic and cholinergic innervation which was first proposed when catecholamines were found to have some secretory effect on the eccrine sweat glands. The demonstration of adrenergic nerves in the monkey paw innervation may simply be a species-specific difference, but, nevertheless, human eccrine glands do respond weakly to local infusion of catecholamines. In a more recent histofluorescent study of human eccrine glands from the skin of the back and the chest, Uno (1977) described numerous cholinergic and a few adrenergic terminals around the secretory cells.

In animal studies, developmental changes have been described in the properties of cholinergic sympathetic neurons. The developing sweat gland in the footpads of rodents appear to be innervated by noradrenergic axons that lose their store of endogenous catecholamines but not their capacity for uptake and storage (on exposure to exogenous catecholamine) as they elaborate an axonal plexus in the maturing glands (Landis and Keefe 1983). The hypothesis is put forward that cholinergic sympathetic neurons appear to undergo a transition from noradrenergic to cholinergic function during development *in vivo* similar to that described previously in cell cultures.

Denervation hypersensitivity

The human eccrine neuroglandular unit has often been singled out as a possible exception to Cannon's rule of hypersensitivity following postganglionic denervation. The response to acetylcholine is reported to gradually diminish after denervation (Coon and Rothman 1941). In contrast, the eccrine sweat glands of the cat (or monkey) paw are found

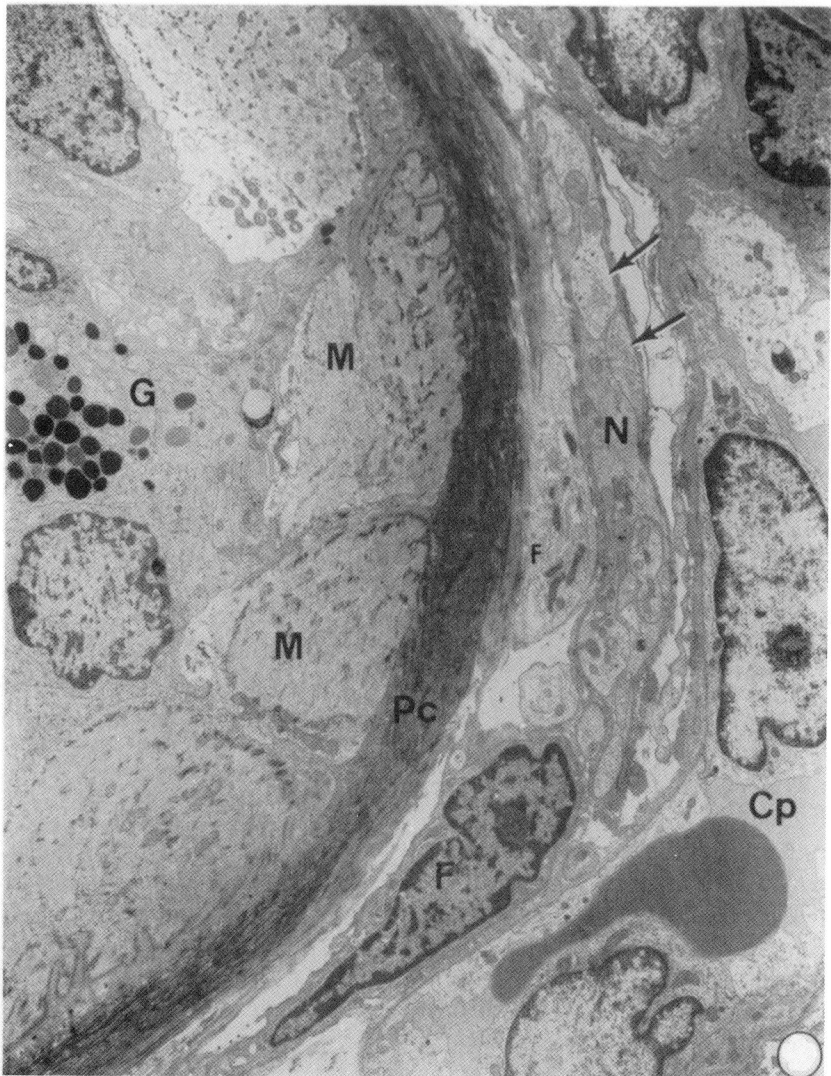

Fig. 42.1. Electron micrograph of the periglandular tissue of an eccrine sweat gland. M, myoepithelial cells with myofilaments; G, secretory cell; Pc, periglandular collagenous tissue; F, fibrocyte; Cp, capillary; N, cholinergic terminal nerve containing agranular vesicles (arrowed). (From Uno (1977).)

to become hypersensitive to acetylcholine for several weeks after postganglionic denervation (Reas and Trendelenburg 1967), reduced sensitivity during the first two postoperative days being followed by hypersensitivity from the fourth postoperative day onward. Although it is not clear whether the difference is species-specific or due to different experimental conditions, the timing in these investigations is often inconsistent. Coon and Rothman's studies were performed 1–2 years after denervation while in the cat's paw experiments tests were made from 1 day to several weeks after denervation. One other factor that may influence interpretation is the trophic changes which have been described in human skin following sympathectomy and which may affect the ability to detect sweat responses on the skin surface.

Apocrine glands

Uno (1977) observed adrenergic fibres occurring sporadically in the connective tissue of the human axilla. None formed a dense network around the glands but the evidence favoured a few adrenergic fibres innervating the apocrine secretory coil. Cholinergic terminals were also found to be present around both secretory coil and ducts. It was concluded that the eccrine and apocrine glands of humans were innervated by predominantly cholinergic fibres with a few adrenergic fibres also. To some extent this arrangement of the neural network with cholinergic dominance in a dual innervation corresponds to the pharmacological responsiveness of the two types of sweat gland, both of which appear to respond to cholinergic and adrenergic agents, the former being a stronger stimulant to secretion (Sato 1980). This view, however, is challenged by Robertshaw (1974) who maintains that apocrine glands of all species are more responsive to catecholamines and are more easily stimulated by adrenalin than noradrenalin or acetylcholine.

PHARMACOLOGY OF SWEATING

Eccrine glands

The fundamental cholinergic nature of the sympathetic innervation of the eccrine glands has been established from early classic experiments. Parasympathomimetics such as the naturally occurring alkaloid pilocarpine are potent sudorific agents while 0.5 mg atropine sulphate administered intravenously in man is sufficient to inhibit thermal sweating within 2 or 3 minutes (Craig and Cummings 1965). Human eccrine glands have, however, long been known to respond to intradermally administered catecholamines and also to intraarterial though not intravenous infusion of adrenalin (Foster and Weiner 1970). The question, therefore, has been raised whether spontaneous sweating in thermogenic areas in patients with phaeochromocytoma may be at least partly due to the direct stimulation of the glands by circulating adrenalin. This suggestion was discounted by Foster and Weiner (1970) who observed that the quantity of intraarterial adrenalin required to stimulate sweating is rather high and by Prout and Wardle (1969) who abolished sweating in phaeochromocytoma with hyoscine. Local adrenalin-induced sweating is quantitatively only about 10 per cent of that produced by parasympathomimetics. It is blocked by priscol and dibenamine but not by atropine which suggests specific adrenergic receptors in the glands. The use of specific α- and β-adrenergic blockers have not completely clarified the problem. α-blockers such as phentolamine and guanethidine have been shown to inhibit adrenalin-induced sweating, but these substances are also reported to possess anticholinergic properties (Foster and Weiner 1970).

The question remains as to the possible role of the adrenergic component. One possibility is that the myoepithelial cells of the gland receive an adrenergic innervation (Robertshaw 1974). It has, however, been demonstrated that in the isolated eccrine gland the myoepithelial cells contract in response to cholinergic stimuli and not to α- or β-adrenergic agents (Sato 1977). One further observation from the laboratory of Sato may be of significance. Both adrenalin and the β-adrenergic agonist isoproterenol significantly enhance the amount of glucose metabolized via the pentose cycle and this is inhibited by propanolol. It has been suggested that the control of glandular growth, including hypertrophy, and morphological changes in the glands during secretory activity may be a role subserved by the β-adrenergic component. To draw an analogy with the salivary glands, the parotid and submaxillary glands have a dual innervation and can be shown to hypertrophy with increased nuclear division as the result of treatment with β-adrenergic agents. The sublingual gland which lacks an adrenergic innervation is unaffected (Seifert 1967). The fact remains that adrenergic blocking agents do not inhibit thermoregulatory or emotional eccrine sweating although complete inhibition is obtained by atropine.

Nicotine injected intradermally was used by Coon and Rothman (1941) to demonstrate a local reflex sweat response similar to the well-known axon reflex flare of the Lewis triple response. The response can be produced in the human and in the cat's paw by local injections of nicotine and acetylcholine but not by methacholine (acetyl-β-methylcholine), and it is blocked by high concentrations of nicotine and by hexamethonium and curare (Collins and Weiner 1961). In their response to these substances the neureoglandular units resemble sensory receptor responses producing axon reflexes in the skin and mesentery. The cutaneous network of sympathetic nerves appear to furnish the pathways for the sweating axon reflex, but there is no evidence that this local response is concerned with normal thermogenic sweating. Sweat reactions sometimes observed in the periphery of ulcers, whitlows, or in other local inflammatory skin conditions may be due to stimulation of the axon reflex pathways.

Second messengers in cholinergic neurons

In studies of the cholinergic and adrenergic mechanisms of eccrine sweat secretion (Sato 1977) it was demonstrated that both cholinergic and α-adrenergic sweating *in vitro* are absolutely dependent on extracellular calcium whereas β-adrenergic sweating is not. The role of cAMP has been established as an intracellular mediator of some hormones and β-adrenergic agonists in a variety of tissues. This appears to hold also for isoprenaline-induced β-adrenergic sweating.

It has generally been assumed that one neuron produces and releases only one transmitter ('Dale's principle') but much recent research has shown the coexistence of two putative transmitters, e.g. peptides and classical transmitters in one neuron (Hökfelt *et al.* 1980). Such neurons were first observed in the lumbosacral sympathetic ganglia which contain one of the best defined cholinergic neuron populations (which are acetylcholinesterase- and cholineacetylase-rich) and involved in the regulation of the sweat glands. These neurons also contain vasoactive intestinal polypeptide (VIP). A dense network of VIP-immunoreactive fibres has been identified around the sweat glands of the cat foot pad. Both varicose and thin immunoreactive fibres were observed close to the sweat-gland ducts and acini. These sweat-gland nerve terminals are also acetylcholinesterase-rich. A hypothesis has therefore been put forward to explain the regulation of sweat secretion (Lundberg *et al.* 1979). It is suggested that acetylcholine produces secretion by an action on the secretory cells and this effect is atropine-sensitive. Concomitantly, there is a local vasodilatation which occurs on stimulation of the post-ganglionic nerves which is atropine-resistant. It may be postulated that there are two effects, with secretion and vasodilatation in exocrine glands being induced by acetylcholine and VIP, respectively, and released from the same nerve terminals synergistically (Fig. 42.2).

In view of the similarity between sudomotor and cutaneous vasomotor responses to changes in metabolic rate or external environment it is attractive to suppose that these efferent systems may be linked. This was proposed earlier by Fox and Hilton (1958) who demonstrated that sweat contains the vasoactive peptide bradykinin which, by analogy with other exocrine glands, might be expected to increase blood flow in the neighbourhood of an active gland. VIP has a well-established vasodilatory effect but it may also influence blood circulation and capillary permeability indirectly by activation of a kinin system.

Apocrine glands

Hurley and Shelley (1960) proposed that, as human axillary apocrine glands can be made to expel their preformed sweat by intradermal or intravenous injections of adrenalin and not by parasypathomimetics nor

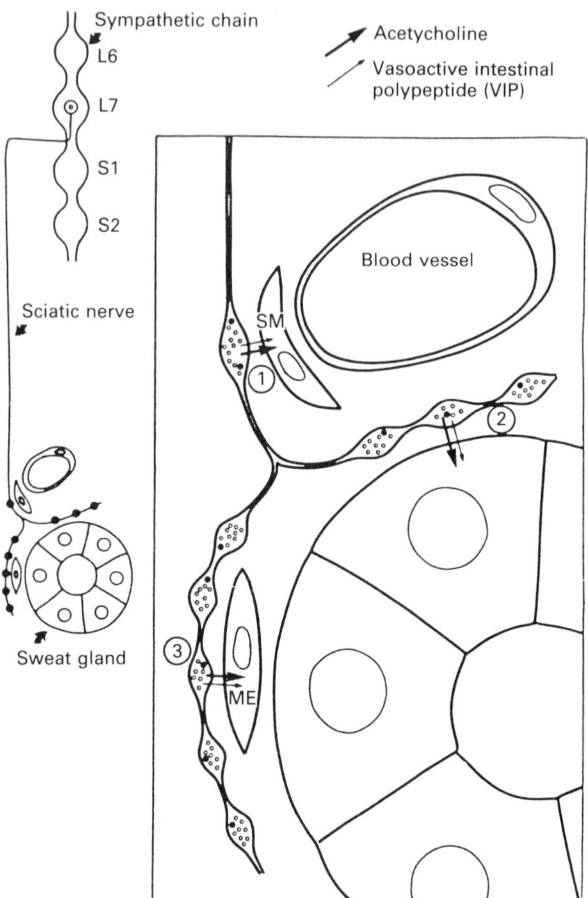

Fig. 42.2. Postulated neuronal mechanisms involved in the control of sweat secretion in the cat paw. The secretomotor neurons are cholinergic but also contain a VIP-like peptide. The nerve terminals may hypothetically influence sweat secretion by an action on several sites. Acetylcholine and VIP may act on (1) smooth muscle (SM) cells around arterioles and/or on capillaries, (2) directly on the gland cells, or (3) indirectly on the gland cells via an action on the myoepithelial (ME) cells. (From Lundberg *et al.* (1979).)

when blocked by atropine, a predominantly adrenergic control system was involved. However, Aoki (1962) was able to stimulate apocrine secretion by acetylcholine. The parasympathomimetics caused profuse eccrine sweating also in the axilla, but in some subjects this was only slight and apocrine secretion could be easily identified. Robertshaw (1974) believed that this is of minor importance since apocrine sweating was only produced with a high concentration of acetylcholine and the amount produced was very small.

The apocrine gland has a well-developed myoepithelium and the secreting tubule has a large luminal space in which to retain preformed sweat. In the isolated apocrine gland, the myoepithelium contracts in response to α-adrenergic stimulation (phenylephrine) but not to β-adrenergic stimulation (isoproterenol) (Sato 1980). However, α-adrenergic stimulation was found to be the least effective stimulant of apocrine secretion. Acetylcholine in the physiological range of concentration did not produce myoepithelial contraction though higher concentrations did. The possibility therefore exists that secretory cell function and myoepithelial contraction may be dissociated pharmacologically (Sato 1980) with cholinergic and β-adrenergic elements controlling secretion and α-adrenergic stimulation controlling myoepithelial function.

DISORDERS OF SWEATING

Sweating disorders may take the form of an increase in sweat production above normal for a given stimulus (hyperhidrosis), a reduction below normal (hypohidrosis), or a complete absence of sweating (anhidrosis). Each of these conditions may be localized or generalized. With regard to apocrine sweating the glands have been implicated in the pathogenesis of four clinical conditions: apocrine bromhidrosis, apocrine chromidrosis, Fox–Fordyce disease, and hidroadenitis suppurativa. The involvement of the autonomic system in the aetiology of these conditions is not known. The role of the autonomic nervous system in disorders of the eccrine glands and eccrine sweating has received considerably more attention and the following discussion will focus on changes in the neural control, effector function, and morphological changes in the skin which have a bearing on functional disturbances.

Increased sweat secretion

An increased sweat volume for a given thermal stimulus is the normal physiological response to the effect of repeated exposures to environmental heat. This is part of the well-known adaptive response to hot climates described as acclimatization. Much of the improvement in sweat response stems from a training effect of the sweat glands themselves as was demonstrated in a series of experiments to show the effect of independently varying the central and peripheral drive to sweating during acclimatization (Collins *et al.* 1965). It may be shown that, in the absence of central thermoregulatory drive, it is possible to train sweat glands by repeated daily treatment with acetylcholine and to induce an improvement in sweat output similar to that achieved by acclimatization (Fig. 42.3). The possibility that there are also adaptive changes taking

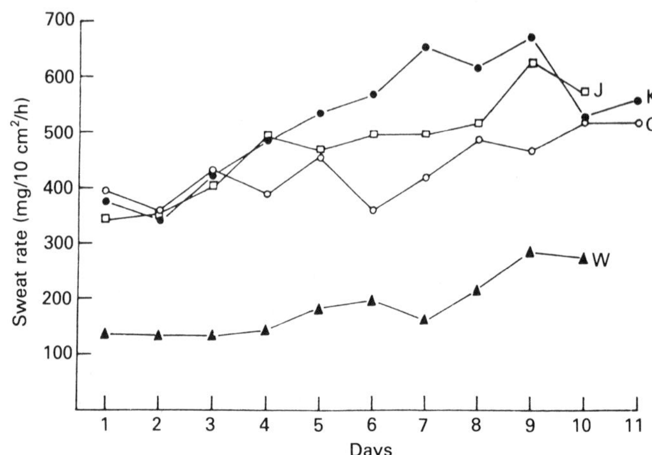

Fig. 42.3. Sweat responses measured on the forearm of four subjects showing the improvement in sweating capacity induced by daily intradermal injections of methacholine. (From Collins *et al.* (1965).)

place in the central nervous control during acclimatization cannot be discounted, however.

Excessive generalized sweating is sometimes reported as a syptom of central nervous disturbances and irritative lesions of the hypothalamus. Large volumes of sweat may be produced also by administration of parasympathomimetics or cholinesterase inhibitors. An increase in metabolic rate in thyrotoxicosis is sometimes associated with abnormal sweating and an alteration in hypothalamic activity is thought to produce the night sweats of tuberculosis, lymphomas, and brucellosis. Increased sweating has been described with phaeochromocytoma, carcinoid syndrome, acromegaly, diabetes mellitus, hyperpituitarism, and gout. The excess sweating in many of these conditions can be inhibited by anticholinergic agents.

Palmar, plantar, and axillary hyperhidrosis

Excessive sweat production on the emotional sweating areas, sometimes described as essential hyperhidrosis, appears to be produced by an exaggerated central drive to the eccrine glands. Though usually restricted to the palms, soles, and axillae, it sometimes may occur over the general body surface in areas normally reacting only to thermal stimulation (Allen *et al.* 1974). In the axillae, though in the presence of high-density and well-developed apocrine glands, hyperhidrosis has been considered to be due to intense activity of the eccrine glands. However, in view of the profuse nature of the apocrine secretion demonstrated in isolated human axillary glands, it appears likely that apocrine secretion contributes substantially in axillary hyperhidrosis.

The use of anticholinergic agents such as atropine, scopolamine, and probanthine has for long been a popular form of treatment. Their local or systemic administration may, however, produce unacceptable side-effects such as dry mouth, blurred vision, and urinary retention. The few attempts made to use anti-adrenergic agents in the treatment of hyperhidrosis have, not surprisingly, met with little success. In the axilla, surgical excision of the well-localized hyperhidrotic area is effective, and transaxillary symphathectomy may be used for suppression of both palmar and axillary hyperhidrosis (Ellis 1979).

Hyperhidrosis is a self-limiting condition though it may last for many years. Topical sweat suppressants are commonly used for treatment especially in mild to moderately severe cases. Methenamine, believed to act by slow release of formaldehyde, has been used successfully even in patients with known formaldehyde sensitivity. Aluminium salts which block the sweat duct in the stratum corneum by protein precipitation are also effective. Shelley and Hurley (1975) claim that complete control of axillary hyperhidrosis can be achieved by a careful regime involving: (1) local application of 20 per cent aluminium chloride hexahydrate in anhydrous ethyl alcohol; (2) application when the axillary glands are inactive; and (3) covering the area for 6 to 8 hours with impermeable film after application.

Decreased sweat secretion without morphological changes in the skin

Neurological disorders

Emotional sweating on the palmar and plantar areas is under control from the cerebral cortex and bursts of sweating occur on these areas in anticipation of contact with objects. Cortical lesions can abolish the emotional sweating response. Thermal sweating over the general body surface may, however, remain intact if lesions are above the level of the hypothalamus. Lesions in the hypothalamic area, e.g. as the result of trauma or surgical operations on the floor of the third ventricle, can produce anhidrosis and intolerance to heat and cold.

Transection of the cord results in an anhidrosis below the level of transection by interfering with sympathetic nervous pathways, but sweating on contralateral surfaces can be elicited by spinal reflexes, for example in response to local heating. The success of surgical sympathectomy is often tested by the demonstration of anhidrosis in sympathectomized areas. Hemihidrosis on one side of the face occurs in Horner's syndrome induced by tumours or lesions in the area of the cervical sympathetic chain.

Patients with diabetic neuropathy often show evidence of anhidrosis over the lower extremities or trunk, but other distributions are not uncommon. There may be compensatory hyperhidrosis of the face and neck in such patients and drenching nocturnal sweats independent of hypoglycaemia are sometimes reported. Another unusual feature of diabetic neuropathy is the occurrence of severe facial sweating at mealtimes. The distribution of gustatory sweating is within the area supplied by sympathetic fibres from the superior cervical ganglia.

Segmental or unilateral loss of sweating has been described with orthostatic hypotension and sexual impotence due to degeneration of sympathetic neurons especially in the intermediolateral spinal columns. This is usually found in middle-aged males where autonomic failure may be associated with other primary neuronal degenerations such as that found in olivopontocerebellar atrophy, parkinsonism, and motor neuron disease.

Anhidrosis has been reported in alcoholic polyneuritis and Wernicke's encephalopathy. It may occur in alcoholic patients without postural hypotension and is evidence of the involvement of postganglionic sympathetic fibres of the limbs, which alone is not sufficient to cause loss of baroreflexes or postural hypotension. Hypohidrosis and anhidrosis, especially in the lower extremities, are often noted in patients with postural hypotension.

Impairment of sweating and of vasodilatation is often described in tetraplegics who may become vulnerable to the effects of environmental heat and to hyperpyrexia in infections. Involvement of the peripheral nerves in leprosy similarly results in anhidrotic areas. Impaired sweating is a consequence of the involvement of the autonomic nervous system in the Guillain–Barré syndrome and in the Holmes–Adie syndrome.

Heat-stroke

The thermoregulatory system is capable of maintaining a high rate of sweating in hot, dry environments in the face of significant dehydration. Leithead and Pallister (1960) found that sweat rates tended to diminish progressively with dehydration, and, reviewing the literature on this vexed question, considered that the weight of evidence favoured the view that there was some decrease in thermal sweating in water depletion. Water- and salt-deficiency heat exhaustion or extreme heat exposure may lead to heat-stroke which is characterized by hyperpyrexia (41°C deep body temperature or more), central nervous system disturbances leading to convulsions, delirium, and coma, and anhidrosis. Anhidrosis with a hot, dry skin is often present but it cannot be claimed that it is pathognomic of heat-stroke. At autopsy, destructive lesions in the hypothalamus have been described which represent a disturbance in the control of sweating at the highest level of autonomic control.

Decreased sweat secretion with morphological changes in the skin

Hidromeiosis

This term is used to describe a particular type of reduction in sweating associated with sustained wetting of the skin in warm ambient temperatures. Formerly, this phenomenon was considered to represent a 'sweat-gland fatigue', implying exhaustion and metabolic changes in the glands. It has been shown that it is possible to inhibit sweating over the body surface by hydrating the stratum corneum through direct wetting, by local tape occlusion, or by enclosing a limb in an impermeable armbag (Fig. 42.4). By suppressing sweat-gland activity in a local area of the enclosed arm by atropine it was possible to show that hidromeiosis did not occur in the atropinized area. This suggested that hidromeiosis

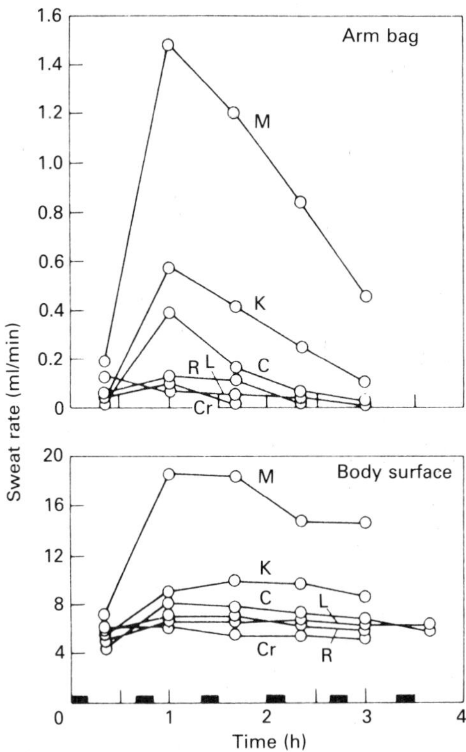

Fig. 42.4. Sweat rates from the arm and hand enclosed in an arm bag to show hidromeiosis, and from the general body surface. Six subjects (identified by letters) performed a work and rest routine in a hot environment. Blocks on the abscissa indicate work periods. After the first hour there is a decline in sweat rate from the arm, while general sweat production falls only slightly. (From Collins and Weiner (1962).)

occurs only in regions which are actively sweating. The phenomenon was analysed by Kerslake (1972) who concluded that epidermal hydration in the presence of active sweating leads to blockage of sweat ducts (hidromeiosis) and that there was no conclusive evidence for the existence of glandular fatigue as the result of continuous osmotic work or failure of the neuroglandular junction. Suppression of sweating which occurs most readily in hot humid environments with excessive skin wetting may lead to heat exhaustion and heat-stroke.

Prickly heat (miliaria rubra) carries a similar aetiology to hidromeiosis though the condition is less readily reversible. It is one of the most common skin problems encountered in hot climates and may sometimes lead to anhidrotic heat exhaustion. Like hidromeiosis, the reduction in sweating is associated with sustained wetting of the skin, but excessive hydration of the epidermis is not sufficient in itself to cause the syndrome. Prickly heat occurs in some susceptible individuals, in whom the cause is not known, though it is observed that a number of different types of injury to the epidermis may cause sweat-duct blocking and, consequently, the trapping of sweat in the ducts.

A number of skin diseases may be associated with hypohidrosis or anhidrosis without involvement of the sudomotor nerves. Hereditary ectodermal dysplasia is characterized by absence, hypoplasia, or markedly decreased numbers of sweat, sebaceous, and mucous glands. In some forms of icthyosis the sweat glands are hypoplastic or absent and reduced sweating is noticeable in skin areas affected by scleroderma, erythroderma, exfoliative dermatitis, and other atrophic skin disorders.

Effects of ageing

It has frequently been reported that there is a reduction in the number of active eccrine sweat glands and a reduced secretory output per gland in old age. This has been ascribed to intrinsic degenerative changes in the glands and to a change in the sensitivity to cholinergic stimulation. Thermoregulatory impairment due to diminished or absent sweating is considered to be one of the factors responsible for the greater incidence of heat illness which occurs during heat waves in cities outside the tropics, predominantly affecting the elderly population. Most of the increased mortality in the elderly is probably due to increased cardiovascular strain imposed by the heat, but the impairment of sweating must be considered to be an aggravating factor. Investigations of the eccrine-sweat response in the aged by thermal stimulation and by local injections of parasympathomimetics have shown marked age-related reductions in sweat-gland activity (Fig. 42.5) (Foster *et al.* 1976). The evidence for failure of autonomic control of sweating with age has been discussed (Collins and Exton-Smith 1981) and found to be inconclusive. At least part of the phenomenon of decreased sweating with age may be

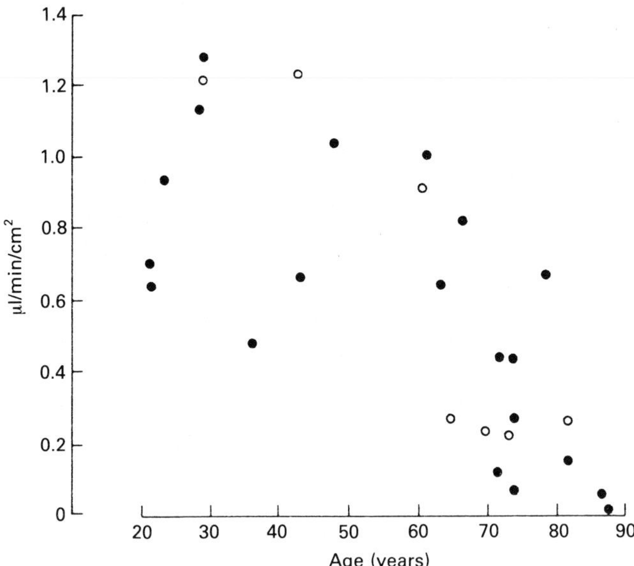

Fig. 42.5. Variations in maximum sweating response with age illustrating the marked decrease in the peripheral response with chemical stimulation (methacholine) and by heating the legs in a water-bath at 43.5°C. (From Foster *et al.* (1976).)

explained by effector changes accompanying senile atrophy of the skin and by differences in the degree of sweat-gland training between young and old age groups in cross-sectional investigations.

REFERENCES

Allen, J. A., Armstrong, J. E., and Roddie, I. C. (1974). Sweat responses of a hyperhidrotic subject. *Br. J. Dermatol.* **90**, 277–81.

Aoki, T. (1962). Stimulation of human axillary apocrine sweat glands by cholinergic agents. *J. invest. Dermatol.* **38**, 41–4.

Benzinger, T. H. (1959). On physical heat regulation and the sense of temperature in man. *Proc. nat. Acad. Sci., Washington* **45**, 645–59.

Collins, K. J., Crockford, G. W., and Weiner, J. S. (1965). Sweat-gland training by drugs and thermal stress. *Arch. environ. Hlth* **11**, 407–22.

Collins, K. J. and Exton-Smith, A. N. (1981). Functional changes in autonomic nervous responses with ageing. *Age Ageing* **9**, 17–24.

Collins, K. J. and Weiner, J. S. (1961). Axon reflex sweating. *Clin. Sci.* **21**, 333–44.

Collins, K. J. and Weiner, J. S. (1962). Observations on arm-bag suppression of sweating and its relationship to thermal sweat-gland fatigue. *J. Physiol.* **161**, 538–56.

Coon, J. M. and Rothman, S. (1941). The sweat response to drugs with nicotine-like action. *J. Pharmacol. exp. Ther.* **23**, 1–11.

Craig, F. N. and Cummings, E. G. (1965). Speed of action of atropine on sweating. *J. appl. Physiol.* **20**, 311–15.

Dale, H. H. and Feldberg, W. (1934). The chemical transmission of secretory impulses to the sweat glands of the cat. *J. Physiol.* **82**, 121–8.

Ellis, H. (1979). Transaxillary sympathectomy in the treatment of hyperhidrosis of the upper limb. *Ann. Surg.* **45**, 546–51.

Foster, K. G., Ellis, F. P., Doré, C., Exton-Smith, A. N., and Weiner, J. S. (1976). Sweat responses in the aged. *Age Ageing* **5**, 91–101.

Foster, K. G. and Weiner, J. S. (1970). Effects of cholinergic and adrenergic blocking agents on the activity of the eccrine sweat glands. *J. Physiol.* **210**, 883–95.

Fox, R. H. and Hilton, S. M. (1958). Bradykinin formation in human skin as a factor in heat vasodilatation. *J. Physiol.* **142**, 219–32.

Hashimoto, K. (1978). The eccrine and apocrine glands and their function. In *The physiology and pathophysiology of the skin*, Vol. 5 (ed. A. Jarrett), pp. 1543–96. Academic Press, London.

Hillarp, N. A. (1959). The construction and functional organisation of the autonomic innervation apparatus. *Acta physiol. scand.* **Suppl 157**, 1–38.

Hökfelt, T., Johansson, O., Ljungdahl, A., Lundberg, J. M., and Schultzberg, M. (1980). Peptidergic neurones. *Nature* **284**, 515–21.

Hurley, H. J. and Shelley, W. B. (1960). *The human apocrine sweat gland in health and disease.* C. C. Thomas, Springfield, Illinois.

Kerslake, D. McK. (1972). *The stress of hot environments.* Cambridge University Press, Cambridge.

Kuno, Y. (1956). *Human perspiration.* C. C. Thomas, Springfield, Illinois.

Landis, S. C. and Keefe, D. (1983). Evidence for neurotransmitter plasticity *in vivo*: developmental changes in properties of cholinergic sympathetic neurones. *Develop. Biol.* **98**, 349–72.

Leithead, C. S. and Pallister, M. A. (1960). Observations on dehydration and sweating. *Lancet* **ii**, 114.

Lundberg, J. M., Hökfelt, T., Schultzberg, M., Uvnäs-Wallensten, K., Köhler, C., and Said, S. I. (1979). Occurrence of vasoactive intestinal polypeptide (VIP)-like immunoreactivity in certain cholinergic neurons of the cat: evidence from combined immunochemistry and acetylcholinesterase staining. *Neuroscience* **4**, 1539–59.

Prout, B. J. and Wardle, W. M. (1969). Sweating and peripheral blood flow in patients with phaeochromocytoma. *Clin. Sci.* **36**, 109–17.

Reas, H. W. and Trendelenburg, U. (1967). Changes in the sensitivity of the sweat glands of the cat after denervation. *J. Pharmacol. exp. Ther.* **156**, 126–36.

Robertshaw, D. (1974). Neural and humoral control of apocrine glands. *J. invest. Dermatol.* **63**, 160–7.

Sato, K. (1977). The physiology, pharmacology and biochemistry of the eccrine sweat gland. *Rev. Physiol. Biochem. Pharmacol.* **79**, 51–131.

Sato, K. (1980). Pharmacological responsiveness of the myoepithelium of the isolated human axillary apocrine sweat gland. *Br. J. Dermatol.* **103**, 235–43.

Sato, K. and Sato, F. (1979). Pharmacology and function of an isolated human apocrine gland *in vitro*. *Clin. Res.* **27**, 535A.

Seifert, G. (1967). Experimental sialadenosis by isoproterenol and other agents: histochemistry and electron microscopy. In *Secretory mechanisms of salivary glands* (ed. L. H. Schneyer and C. A. Schneyer), pp. 191–208. Academic Press, New York.

Shelley, W. B. and Hurley, H. J. (1953). The physiology of the human axillary apocrine sweat gland. *J. invest. Dermatol.* **20**, 285–95.

Shelley, W. B. and Hurley, H. J. (1975). Studies on topical antiperspirant control of axillary hyperhidrosis. *Acta dermatol., Stockholm* **55**, 241–60.

Uno, H. (1977). Sympathetic innervation of the sweat glands and piloerrector muscles of the macaque and human beings. *J. invest. Dermatol.* **69**, 112–20.

Uno, H. and Montagna, W. (1975). Catecholamine-containing nerve terminals of the eccrine sweat glands of macaques. *Cell Tissue Res.* **158**, 1–13.

Weiner, J. S. and Hellman, K. (1960). The sweat glands. *Biol. Rev.* **35**, 141–86.

Index